Neuropathology

Other books coming soon in this series:

Gastrointestinal and Liver Pathology

Dermatopathology

Breast Pathology

Bone and Soft Tissue Pathology

Genitourinary Pathology

Hematopathology

Gynecologic Pathology

Ear, Nose, and Throat/Endocrine Pathology

Fine Needle Aspiration Cytology

Pulmonary Pathology

Neuropathology

A Volume in the Series
Foundations in Diagnostic Pathology

Edited by

Richard A. Prayson, MD
Head, Section of Neuropathology
Department of Anatomic Pathology
The Cleveland Clinic Foundation
Cleveland Clinic Lerner College of Medicine
Case Western Reserve University
Cleveland, Ohio

Series Editor

John R. Goldblum, MD, FCAP, FASCP, FACG
Chairman, Department of Anatomic Pathology
The Cleveland Clinic Foundation
Cleveland Clinic Lerner College of Medicine
Case Western Reserve University
Cleveland, Ohio

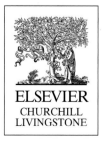

ELSEVIER
CHURCHILL
LIVINGSTONE

ELSEVIER
CHURCHILL
LIVINGSTONE

The Curtis Center
170 S Independence Mall W 300E
Philadelphia, Pennsylvania 19106

NEUROPATHOLOGY (A VOLUME IN THE
FOUNDATIONS IN DIAGNOSTIC PATHOLOGY
SERIES, Series Edited by John R. Goldblum)
Copyright © 2005, Elsevier Inc.

NOTICE

Pathology is an ever-changing field. Standard safety precautions must be followed, but as new research and clinical experience broaden our knowledge, changes in treatment and drug therapy may become necessary or appropriate. Readers are advised to check the most current product information provided by the manufacturer of each drug to be administered to verify the recommended dose, the method and duration of administration, and contraindications. It is the responsibility of the licensed prescriber, relying on experience and knowledge of the patient, to determine dosages and the best treatment for each individual patient. Neither the publisher nor the editor assumes any liability for any injury and/or damage to persons or property arising from this publication.

Library of Congress Cataloging-in-Publication Data

Neuropathology / editors, Richard A. Prayson, John R. Goldblum.
    p. ; cm.
    ISBN-13: 978–0–443–06658–0   ISBN-10: 0–443–06658–2
  1. Nervous system–Diseases. 2. Nervous system–Diseases–Diagnosis.
    [DNLM: 1. Nervous System Diseases–pathology. 2. Glioma–pathology. WL 140 N49375 2005]
I. Prayson, Richard A. II. Goldblum, John R.
    RC347.N47987 2005
    616.8′047–dc22   2004056215

ISBN-13: 978–0–443–06658–0
ISBN-10: 0–443–06658–2

Publisher: Natasha Andjelkovic
Developmental Editor: Heather Krehling
Publishing Services Manager: Tina Rebane
Project Manager: Jodi Kaye
Designer: Gene Harris

Printed in China

Last digit is the print number: 9   8   7   6   5   4   3   2

To Karen, Richard, Beth, Brigid, and Nicholas
for your tireless love, support, and encouragement.

Dimitri P. Agamanolis, MD
Professor of Pathology (Neuropathology)
Northeast Ohio Universities College of Medicine
Rootstown, Ohio
Director of Anatomical Pathology
Children's Hospital Medical Center of Akron
Akron, Ohio
Metabolic and Toxic Disorders

Daniel J. Brat, MD, PhD
Associate Professor
Department of Pathology and Laboratory Medicine
School of Medicine
Emory University
Atlanta, Georgia
Overview of Central Nervous System Anatomy and Histology

Elizabeth J. Cochran, MD
Associate Professor
Departments of Pathology and Neurological Sciences
Rush Medical College
Rush University Medical Center
Chicago, Illinois
Neurodegenerative Diseases

Mark L. Cohen, MD
Professor of Pathology
School of Medicine
Case Western Reserve University
Staff Pathologist
University Hospitals of Cleveland
Cleveland, Ohio
Skeletal Muscle and Peripheral Nerve Disorders

David Dolinak, MD
Assistant Professor
Department of Pathology
Southwestern Medical School
University of Texas
Deputy Chief Medical Examiner
Dallas County Medical Examiner Department
Dallas, Texas
Trauma

Rebecca D. Folkerth, MD
Associate Professor of Pathology
Harvard Medical School
Associate Pathologist
Brigham & Women's Hospital
Consultant Neuropathologist
Children's Hospital
Boston, Massachusetts
*Congenital Malformations, Perinatal Diseases,
and Phacomatoses*

Kymberly A. Gyure, MD
Assistant Professor and Director
Division of Neuropathology
School of Medicine
University of Maryland
Baltimore, Maryland
Infections

B. K. Kleinschmidt-DeMasters, MD
Professor of Pathology, Neurology, and Neurosurgery
Health Sciences Center
University of Colorado
Denver, Colorado
Dysmyelinating and Demyelinating Disorders

Arie Perry, MD
Associate Professor
Division of Neuropathology
School of Medicine
Washington University
St. Louis, Missouri
Glial and Glioneuronal Tumors

Richard A. Prayson, MD
Head, Section of Neuropathology
Department of Anatomic Pathology
The Cleveland Clinic Foundation
Cleveland Clinic Lerner College of Medicine
Case Western Reserve University
Cleveland, Ohio
Non-Glial Tumors

Jack H. Simon, MD, PhD
Professor of Radiology
Health Sciences Center
University of Colorado
Denver, Colorado
Dysmyelinating and Demyelinating Disorders

Anthony T. Yachnis, MD, MS
Associate Director of Anatomic Pathology
Chief, Neuropathology Section
Associate Professor
College of Medicine
University of Florida
Gainesville, Florida
Vascular Disease

Foreword

The study and practice of anatomic pathology is both exciting and overwhelming. Surgical pathology, with all of the subspecialties it encompasses, and cytopathology have become increasingly complex and sophisticated, and it is not possible for any individual to master the skills and knowledge required to perform all of these tasks at the highest level. Simply being able to make a correct diagnosis is challenging enough, but the standard of care has far surpassed merely providing a diagnosis. Pathologists are now asked to provide large amounts of ancillary information, both diagnostic and prognostic, often on small amounts of tissue, a task that can be daunting even to the most experienced pathologist.

Although large general surgical pathology textbooks are useful resources, by necessity they could not possibly cover many of the aspects that pathologists need to know and include in their reports. For this reason, the concept behind *Foundations in Diagnostic Pathology* was born. This series is designed to cover the major areas of surgical pathology and cytopathology, and each volume is focused on one major topic. The goal of every book in this series is to provide the essential information that any pathologist—whether general or subspecialized, in training or in practice—would find useful in the evaluation of virtually any type of specimen encountered.

My colleague, Dr. Richard Prayson, has edited an outstanding book on neuropathology that fulfills the goals and philosophy behind *Foundations in Diagnostic Pathology*. The book is an up-to-date text for understanding neoplastic and non-neoplastic conditions of the central and peripheral nervous systems and focuses on the practical aspects of specimen evaluation, culminating in an accurate diagnosis using morphologic, immunohistochemical, and molecular genetic techniques. Dr. Prayson, a renowned expert in the field, has assembled a premier group of neuropathologists to contribute to this edition. The book is organized into 11 chapters covering all of the major problems encountered in neuropathology, including vascular diseases, trauma, congenital malformations, demyelinating disorders, neurodegenerative diseases, infections, metabolic and toxic disorders, disorders of skeletal muscle and peripheral nerve, and glial and non-glial tumors. There is relative uniformity in the organization of these chapters, each of which includes practical information and photomicrographs that emphasize the essential points.

As a surgical pathologist and educator, I extend my heartfelt appreciation to Dr. Prayson and all of the authors who have contributed to this outstanding first edition of *Foundations in Diagnostic Pathology*. I am thoroughly impressed by the organization and practical nature of the information provided. As the first in a series of books that explore anatomic pathology subspecialties, including gastrointestinal, hepatobiliary, pulmonary, orthopedic, genitourinary, gynecologic, hematolymphoid and cytopathology, I could not have asked for a better book to serve as a model for the subsequent editions in this series. I sincerely hope you enjoy this first volume in the *Foundations in Diagnostic Pathology* series.

JOHN R. GOLDBLUM, M.D.

Preface

When I was first approached with the idea of editing this book, my first reaction was "not another neuropathology text. There are already several neuropathology books out there. How is this one going to be different?" Dr. Goldblum, as the editor for the *Foundations in Diagnostic Pathology* series, had a goal of creating something different from standard pathology books. In our case, he wanted us to envision a book that would present the broad spectrum of neuropathology in an updated, clear, templated, and highly illustrated fashion. The idea was not to present an exhaustive review of all neuropathology, nor did we want to merely sketch out the basics in an outline form. We wanted to give the reader an appreciation for the diversity of neuropathology while being aware of its complexity and the challenges it presents. The field of neuropathology is ever-expanding, and our collective powers of observation and inquiry add to what we know, enrich our understanding, and give us respect for what we do not yet know. We tried to touch on the highlights in this text, realizing that the full picture is always changing and is never really complete.

Being the first book in a series is a challenge. We had the task of taking a conceptualization and making it real, setting the tone for the volumes to follow. Our hope is that we have met the challenge and we look forward to the other volumes in the *Foundations in Diagnostic Pathology* series.

RICHARD A. PRAYSON, M.D.

Acknowledgments

This book was the result of the efforts of a number of individuals. First and foremost, to my coauthors, many thanks! The time, effort and expertise you invested and shared is much appreciated and makes this book what it is. Thanks to all those, from families to secretaries, who helped support the authors in their work. Special thanks to Denise Egleton for her help and to Heather Krehling who steered this project to completion.

RICHARD A. PRAYSON, M.D.

Contents

1 Overview of Central Nervous System Anatomy and Histology

Daniel J. Brat

The practice of neuropathology can be daunting. The spectrum of nervous system diseases is immense and spans all ages, ranging from congenital anomalies of the fetus to degenerative diseases of the elderly. Molecular mechanisms of neurologic disease continue to be unraveled, and such progress has given rise to new laboratory-based tests that not only improve our diagnostic capabilities but also require a continually updated knowledge bank. Furthermore, the recent neurosurgical and neuroradiologic techniques that have led to less invasive procedures often result in modest amounts of diagnostic tissue for the pathologist. Above all, the challenges of diagnostic neuropathology remain steep because the diseases affect the human central nervous system (CNS), a structure often called the most complex system in the universe. A sound comprehension of basic CNS organization is absolutely required to understand diseases that affect it. Of all the human organs, the brain is unrivaled in its intricacy, regional variation, and range of function (Table 1-1). Details regarding normal physiology of the brain that result in cognition, sensation, movement, and behavior remain incompletely understood. How, then, can we hope to understand and classify the entirety of pathologic conditions that affect the CNS?

Fortunately, the historical fascination of physicians and scientists with the human brain has generated a fundamental understanding of its normal anatomy, histology, and ultrastructure. Most often, but certainly not always, disease-related deficits correlate with structural alteration in the CNS. Recognition of abnormal conditions in the brain, whether by neuroimaging, gross inspection, or microscopy, rests on firm knowledge of the normal state, which can be learned and retained at a practical level. Current diagnostic neuropathology incorporates adjunctive laboratory-based studies to aid in diagnosis (Table 1-2). Nonetheless, microscopic examination of hematoxylin-eosin–stained tissue sections retains its central significance in neuropathology. This chapter introduces normal anatomy and histology of the human CNS at a depth necessary for routine diagnostic practice. Most of its content describes the normal adult brain, but certain aspects of age-related phenomena, artifacts, and developmental considerations that are routinely encountered in diagnostic neuropathology are also considered.

GROSS ANATOMY

The nervous system contains central and peripheral divisions. The CNS, the focus of the current chapter, is composed of the cerebrum, cerebellum, brain stem, spinal cord, and their meningeal coverings (see Chapter 11 for a discussion of peripheral nerves and skeletal muscle). The CNS is a complex three-dimensional structure that is normally viewed and described in two-dimensional representations. Most common for neuropathologic study is the coronal plane, a traditional view for brain cutting and gross examination. In today's clinical practice, firm knowledge of neuroanatomy in the sagittal and axial planes is also required because of the increasing role of multiplanar neuroimaging (computed tomography, magnetic resonance imaging, positron emission tomography) in clinical practice. Adding slightly to the complexity of neuropathology, human neuroanatomy introduces terminology from the veterinary world that is not commonly encountered in the study of other organ systems. Anterior, posterior, superior, and inferior retain their meanings in the CNS and are generally used in reference to a person in the standing position. Ventral is the anatomic side facing the floor when an individual is on all fours like a dog with eyes fixed on the horizon; dorsal is the side facing skyward. Rostral indicates a direction toward the superior pole of the vertically oriented CNS (toward the frontal lobe), whereas caudal implies the direction toward the inferior pole (i.e., the filum terminale of the spinal cord; literally, the "tail").

MENINGES

Initial inspection of the brain reveals its protective and functional coverings, the meninges (Fig. 1-1). Outermost is the dura mater ("hard mother"), which is tightly adherent to the inner aspect of the skull and vertebral column. It is composed of tough fibrous connective tissue (0.5 mm thick) that is glistening on its inner surface. The epidural and subdural spaces are defined

1

TABLE 1-1

Facts about the Brain

The average adult brain weight of a human is 1300-1400 g; an adult gorilla's brain weighs only 500 g.

The human CNS contains over 100 billion neurons.

Each neuron forms an average of 1000 synaptic connections (some up to 10^5), which results in 10^{14} neuronal connections per brain (100 trillion!).

Each synaptic vessel at the nerve terminal contains around 5000 neurotransmitter molecules.

Over 50 distinct types of neurons are present in the human brain; inhibitory neurons (most using GABA as a transmitter) account for 25%.

The length of myelinated tracts in the brain is 150,000-180,000 km—4 times the earth's circumference.

85,000 neurons are lost from the brain per day ($\approx$1 per second).

Glial cells are 10-50 times more numerous than neurons.

The brain expresses more genes than any other organ: >200,000 mRNA sequences.

Nerve impulses travel between 1 and 100 m/sec; an impulse starting in an anterior horn cell of the spinal cord travels to the big toe in 0.01 second.

Proteins and organelles are shuttled down nerve processes by axonal transport at a maximal rate of 400 mm/day; a protein produced in the anterior horn cell of the spinal cord reaches the big toe in 2 days.

Based on distinct layering patterns of the cerebral cortex, Korbian Brodmann subdivided the cerebral cortex into 47 cytoarchitectonic regions (this scheme is now believed to be overly simplified).

Cortical representation of sensory, motor, and higher cognitive function follows a general pattern in the human brain; however, cortical maps vary from person to person and can change in size and location with use or disuse.

The time to unconsciousness after complete cessation of blood flow to the brain is 8-10 seconds.

GABA, γ-aminobutyric acid.

by their locations outside and inside the dura, respectively. Embedded within the dura between its inner and outer layers are large dural sinuses, vascular channels that receive blood from bridging veins exiting the brain and represent the organ's main venous outflow. The superior sagittal sinus is the largest and runs the length of the cerebral hemispheres in the midsagittal plane. This vascular space—and to a lesser extent, the other large dural sinuses—contains numerous small inpouchings from the arachnoid space, the arachnoid villi (when larger, called arachnoid granulations). Arachnoid villi and granulations are lined only by endothelium and delicate connective tissue and function to resorb cerebrospinal fluid (CSF) from the subarachnoid space. Resorption occurs at a relatively brisk pace such that the half-life of CSF is only 3 hours. Four specific segments of dura deserve mention: the falx cerebri, the portion separating the two hemispheres in the midline, extends from the superior surface of the brain inferiorly to the corpus callosum; the falx cerebelli partially separates the cerebellar hemispheres in a similar manner; the tentorium cerebelli lies between the posterior fossa and the middle cranial fossa, thereby creating the infratentorial and supratentorial compartments; and the diaphragma sellae, which is the dural covering of the sella turcica overlying the pituitary gland.

The web-like meshwork underlying the dura that is loosely adherent to both the dura and the CNS surface is the arachnoid membrane ("spider-like"). Within the webs of arachnoid is the subarachnoid space, which normally contains only CSF, arteries and veins, and scattered native cellular elements. It can be completely removed from the underlying brain (sometimes a long, tedious process) to view the surface of the cortex more clearly. Despite its porous appearance the arachnoid membrane is relatively restrictive to fluid flow outside its domain; blood contained within this space is largely confined and does not freely exit. Finally, the pia mater ("soft mother") is a thin, delicate coating that rests directly on the surface of the CNS. It cannot be seen grossly, much less removed or inspected, and is best evaluated microscopically. The delicate trabeculae that form the arachnoid membranes fuse with the pia to form a singular unit, the pia-arachnoid or leptomeninges.

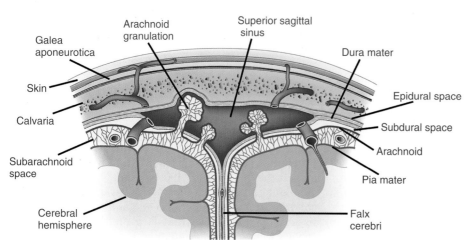

FIGURE 1-1

Anatomic relationships of the skull, meninges, and brain as demonstrated in a coronal view.

TABLE 1-2

Common Adjunctive Tests in Neuropathology

STAIN	HIGHLIGHTED STRUCTURE	STAIN	HIGHLIGHTED STRUCTURE
IMMUNOHISTOCHEMISTRY		**HISTOLOGIC STAINS**	
Aβ amyloid	Amyloid in senile plaques, blood vessels	Acid-fast stains	Mycobacteria
CAM5.2	Epithelial intermediate filaments	Bielschowsky	Silver stain for neurofibrillary pathology
CD3	T cells		
CD20	B cells	Bodian	Silver stain for neurofibrillary pathology
CD31	Endothelium		
CD45 (LCA)	Lymphocytes	Congo red	Amyloid
CD68	Macrophage lysosomes	Gram	Bacteria
Chromogranin	Neuronal vesicles	Hematoxylin-eosin	General histology
CMV	Cytomegalovirus	Iron	Iron
αβ-Crystallin	Glial inclusions	Luxol fast blue	Myelin
Cytokeratin (AE1/AE3)	Epithelial intermediate filaments	Methenamine silver	Fungus
Desmin	Muscle intermediate filament	Oil red O	Lipid stain (frozen tissue)
Epithelial membrane antigen (EMA)	Epithelial membranes	PAS/PAS-D	Glycogen/basement membrane
		Reticulin	Reticulin/basement membrane
Estrogen/progesterone receptor	Nuclear hormone receptors	Thioflavine S	Amyloid (fluorescence dye)
		Trichrome	Collagen and fibrin
GFAP	Glial intermediate filaments	von Kossa	Calcium
HMB-45	Melanocytic differentiation	**LABORATORY AND MOLECULAR STUDIES**	
Ham 56	Macrophages	Chemistry	Protein and glucose levels
HSV	Herpes simplex virus	Cytopathology	CSF examination
κ, λ Light chains	Immunoglobulin light chains	FISH or PCR/LOH	Chromosomal 1p and 19q
MIB-1	Nuclear marker of proliferation (Ki67)	FISH for oncogene amplification	c-MYC, EGFR
NeuN	Neuronal nuclei		
Neurofilament protein	Neuronal intermediate filament (axons)	Flow cytometry	Lymphoma, hematologic disorders
p53	Tumor suppressor protein accumulation	Hematology	Differential cell count
Polyomavirus	JC virus (progressive multifocal leukoencephalopathy)	Immunologic studies	Protein electrophoresis for oligoclonal bands; syphilis IgG
S-100	Melanocytic/neuroepithelial differentiation	Microbiology	Viral, mycobacterial, bacterial, and fungal culture; cryptococcal antigen
Smooth muscle actin	Smooth muscle		
Synaptophysin	Neuronal vesicle proteins	PCR detection of pathogens in CSF/brain	HSV, CMV, EBV, HIV, enterovirus, mycobacteria
α-Synuclein	Lewy bodies		
Tau	Neurofibrillary pathology, tangles		
Thyroid transcription factor-1 (TTF-1)	Nuclear factor in lung/thyroid differentiation		
Toxoplasmosis	Toxoplasmosis		
Ubiquitin	Glial and neuronal inclusions		

CSF, cerebrospinal fluid; EBV, Epstein-Barr virus; EGFR, epidermal growth factor receptor; FISH, fluorescence in situ hybridization; GFAP, glial fibrillary acidic protein; HIV, human immunodeficiency virus; HSV, herpes simplex virus; LCA, leukocyte common antigen; LOH, loss of heterozygosity; PAS, periodic acid–Schiff; PCR, polymerase chain reaction.

CEREBRUM

The structure most often referred to as "the brain" is the cerebrum, the portion of the CNS occupying the supratentorial compartment and consisting of large left and right cerebral hemispheres and the smaller midline diencephalon (Fig. 1-2). The outer view is dominated by numerous cerebral convolutions that add greatly to the human brain's cortical areas. In contrast, the diencephalon is largely hidden from external view because of its deep location. The outwardly projecting folds forming the cerebral hemispheric convolutions are gyri, whereas the infolded spaces between them are sulci (or fissures when large). Each hemisphere is divided by surface landmarks into frontal, parietal, temporal, and occipital lobes. The frontal and parietal lobes are separated by the central (rolandic) sulcus, the frontal and temporal lobes by the sylvian fissure, the temporal and parietal lobes by the continuation of the sylvian fissure posteriorly, and the parietal and occipital lobes by the parieto-occipital sulcus and calcarine fissures. At the intersection of the temporal, frontal, and parietal lobes, in the depth of the sylvian fissure, lies the insular cortex, which cannot be seen from the surface. The cortical gyri overlying the insula from each lobe are the opercula.

The gyri composing each lobe have specific designations largely based on anatomic location. Select gyri are better known for their functional significance. In the frontal lobe, the precentral gyrus, located anterior to the central sulcus, is the home of the primary motor cortex with its resident population of Betz cells (upper motor neurons). The cingulate gyrus, associated with limbic control of emotion and primal drives, is located on the mesial surface of the frontal, parietal, and occipital lobes, directly superior to the corpus callosum anteri-

orly. It follows a C-shaped path around into the temporal lobe, where it continues as the parahippocampal gyrus. Other frontal lobe gyri form premotor and prefrontal association regions, as well as the specialized language area of Broca. On the inferior surface are the orbitofrontal gyri, the most medial of which is the gyrus rectus. Lateral to the gyrus rectus is the olfactory sulcus, where the olfactory nerve (cranial nerve [CN] I) and olfactory bulb are found (Fig. 1-3). In the parietal lobe, the postcentral gyrus is the primary somatosensory cortex and has the same general body representation as the primary motor cortex: legs are represented on the mesial surface, the trunk and upper extremities on the superior lateral surface, and the face and oral cavity inferiorly on the lateral surface. Other parietal lobe gyri are sensory association cortices and those related to language comprehension. The main lateral subdivisions of the temporal lobe are simply referred to as the superior, middle, and inferior gyri, which together have functions in language, hearing, and vision. The medial surface of the temporal lobe is slightly more complex. It contains the parahippocampal gyrus, which is critical to both emotional and memory control and is often included as part of the functional limbic lobe. The anterior aspect of the parahippocampal gyrus contains the uncus, a small, medially projecting protrusion that has a slight horizontal notch on its surface because of contact with the tentorium cerebelli. The parahippocampal gyrus houses the amygdala anteriorly and the hippocampus more posteriorly. In the occipital lobe, the calcarine sulcus is the most prominent and functionally relevant: gyri on either side of this mesially located sulcus form the primary visual cortex. Other occipital lobe gyri are part of the visual association cortex.

As viewed from the inferior surface of the brain, dorsal to the brain stem and in the midline is the pineal

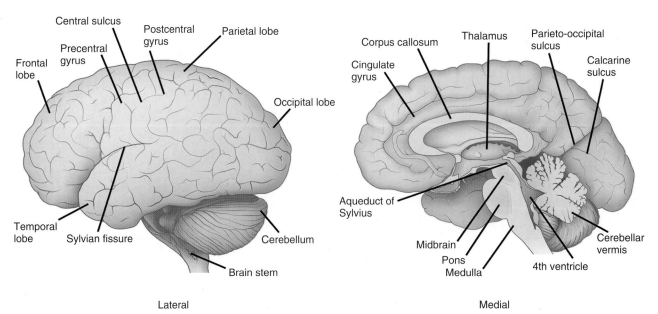

FIGURE 1-2

Lateral and medial views of the brain surface.

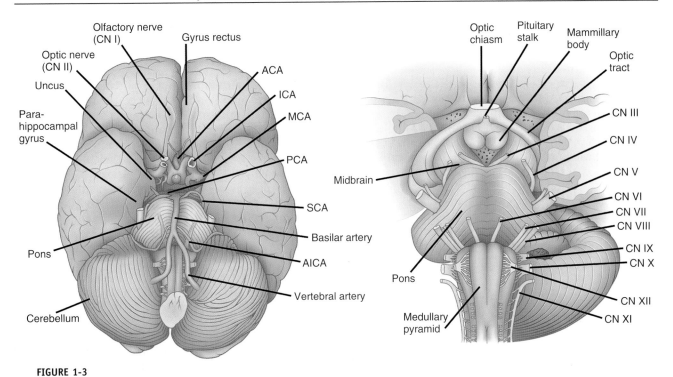

FIGURE 1-3

Inferior and ventral views of the brain surface. ACA, anterior cerebral artery; AICA, anterior inferior cerebellar artery; CN, cranial nerve; ICA, internal carotid artery; MCA, middle cerebral artery; PCA, posterior cerebral artery; SCA, superior cerebellar artery.

gland, a small (1 cm) piece of lobulated neural tissue. It sits immediately superior to the midbrain colliculi at the posterior aspect of the third ventricle. Ventral to the brain stem and riding the midline is the inferior aspect of the hypothalamus (see Fig. 1-3). This region includes the mammillary bodies, which are small hemispheric protrusions just anterior to the cerebral peduncles and the midline infundibular stalk. The latter is composed of inferiorly projecting processes from hypothalamic nuclei that traverse the suprasellar space, penetrate the diaphragma sellae, and extend into the sella turcica to form the posterior lobe of the pituitary gland (neurohypophysis). The anterior lobe of the pituitary (adenohypophysis) is larger than the posterior lobe, slightly red and lobulated, and together with the posterior lobe is contained within the sella underneath its dural covering. Optic tracts emerge from the thalamus, extend centrally and anteriorly, and merge to form the optic chiasm immediately anterior to the infundibular stalk. The optic chiasm separates into optic nerves (CN II) anteriorly, which course along the inferior frontal lobe a short distance before entering the orbital socket.

The inferior surface of the cerebrum gives the best view of the large arteries that supply blood to the brain (see Fig. 1-3). The two internal carotid arteries (ICAs) account for the anterior circulation, which supplies 85% of cerebral blood flow. The internal carotids give rise to the anterior cerebral arteries (ACAs), which course anteriorly between the frontal lobes and then loop back posteriorly along the corpus callosum, inferior to the cingulate gyrus, to supply the medial aspects of the frontal and parietal lobes. The left and right ACAs

are interconnected near their origins from the ICAs by the anterior communicating artery, which completes the anterior segment of the circle of Willis, an arterial network critical for collateral circulation. The middle cerebral artery (MCA) also comes from the ICA and travels first laterally and then posteriorly within the sylvian fissure to supply the lateral aspects of the cerebral hemispheres. Within its territory is a large portion of the primary sensory and motor cortex. Importantly, the MCA also gives rise to smaller, perforating branches, the lenticulostriate arteries, that supply the basal ganglia. The posterior circulation includes the two vertebral arteries, which merge at the level of the pons as the basilar artery. Along their route, the vertebral and basilar arteries give rise to penetrating arteries that supply the brain stem, as well as the superior, posterior inferior, and anterior inferior cerebellar arteries that supply the cerebellum. The basilar artery divides at the pons-midbrain junction to form two posterior cerebral arteries (PCAs). The PCAs supply most of the occipital lobes, the inferior aspects of the temporal lobes, including the hippocampus, and much of the thalamus and hypothalamus. Connecting the PCAs to the internal carotids and completing the circle of Willis are the posterior communicating arteries.

For classic anatomic study at brain cutting, the brain stem and cerebellum are removed from the cerebrum by slicing across the superior aspect of the midbrain in the axial plane. Such removal can be performed with the brain in its fresh state or after 7 to 10 days of fixation in 10% buffered formalin. The brain is more easily handled and cut after fixation, and its landmarks are better recognized. The cerebrum is traditionally cut in the coronal plane, beginning with a slice through the mammillary bodies and continuing anteriorly and posteriorly with 1.0- to 1.5-cm slices. Slices are placed with the anterior surface facing down so that the right side of the brain is on the examiner's right side (this technique is the opposite of neuroimaging studies, in which the brain's right side is on the examiner's left). Initial inspection reveals internal CNS structures that can be broadly subclassified as white matter, gray matter, or ventricular space (Fig. 1-4). Gray matter structures, including the cerebral and cerebellar cortices, deep nuclei of the cerebrum, cerebellum, and brain stem, and the internal components of the spinal cord, are all characterized microscopically by their high density of neuronal cell bodies and by their paucity of myelinated tracts. Together, these gray matter structures account

for 40% of the brain mass (but consume 94% of the oxygen). Grossly, gray matter is darker and tan-pink when compared with adjacent white matter. By contrast, white matter contains no neuronal cell bodies and is composed almost entirely of myelinated and unmyelinated axonal processes in transit to their connections. Its white color on gross inspection is due to the high lipid content present in myelinated tracts. By neuroimaging studies, the higher lipid content makes white matter relatively hyperintense on T1-weighted magnetic resonance images and hypointense on T2-weighted images (or fluid attenuated inversion recovery [FLAIR]), similar to fat. The higher relative content of water in gray matter makes it T1 hypointense and T2 (FLAIR) hyperintense (see Fig. 1-4).

The ventricular system is a macroscopic network of large interconnected channels within the CNS that

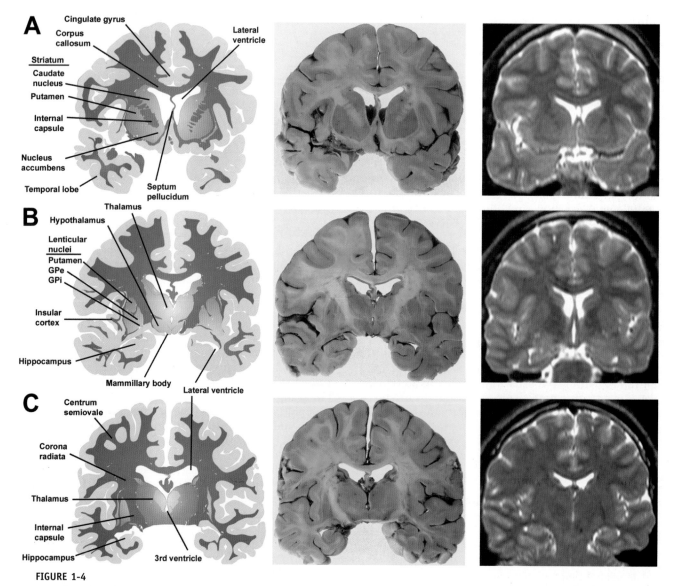

FIGURE 1-4

Coronal sections of the cerebrum at the level of the striatum (**A**), mammillary bodies (**B**), and thalamus (**C**). Labeled schematic representations (*left*), fixed postmortem brain slices (*middle*), and T2-weighted magnetic resonance images (*right*) are shown for each level. GPe, globus pallidus external; GPi, globus pallidus internal.

contains CSF and is continuous with the subarachnoid space. The entire CSF compartment contains 125 to 150 mL. Lateral ventricles are located within the cerebral hemispheres near the midline anteriorly and on each side; they form a C-shaped path from the frontal pole into the temporal lobe. An occipital horn extends posteriorly into the occipital lobe at the atrium (trigone), which represents the confluence of the temporal, parietal, and occipital components of the lateral ventricle. Anteriorly, the lateral ventricles are covered by the corpus callosum and separated from one another by the septum pellucidum, a single delicate translucent membrane that is occasionally split into two parallel membranes (cavum septum pellucidum, a normal variant). A foramen of Monro connects each lateral ventricle with the singular, midline third ventricle, located between the left and right lobes of the thalamus. In turn, the third ventricle is connected to the fourth ventricle by the aqueduct of Sylvius, a thin passageway that extends inferiorly from the posterior aspect of the third ventricle into the midbrain and empties into the superior aspect of the fourth ventricle. The latter is found between the cerebellum and brain stem and is bordered on its sides by the cerebellar peduncles. CSF maintains continuity with the subarachnoid space surrounding the brain stem through the fourth ventricle's lateral foramina of Luschka and its midline foramen of Magendie. Within the ventricles at specific locations are patches of choroid plexus, the tufts of specialized vascular networks covered by choroid epithelium that produce CSF. Choroid plexus carpets the portion of the lateral ventricular surface from the foramen of Monro to the tip of the temporal horn and expands to form a large aggregate (glomus) in the atrium. Choroid plexus also occupies the roofs of the third and fourth ventricles.

The cerebral cortex is the corrugated, outermost strip of brain parenchyma that covers the cerebrum; it ranges from 2 to 5 mm in thickness. The number and degree of cerebral infoldings (sulci and fissures) become more fully apparent on coronal sectioning, with some inward extensions measuring more than 2 inches. The subarachnoid space continues over the surface of the brain and deep into these infoldings. On gross examination, the cerebral cortex displays a fairly uniform thickness, texture, and color, with a sharp demarcation between it and the underlying white matter. Two grossly specialized regions deserve attention. First, in the primary visual cortex (Brodmann area 17) of the occipital lobe, the cortex contains a thin white line that runs parallel to the gray-white interface. This "line of Gennari" represents thickened myelinated tracts that are more prominent in the primary visual cortex than in other cortical regions and can be used reliably to identify the visual cortex. Second, in the inferior temporal lobe medially, specialized cortical regions are the amygdala and the hippocampal formation. The amygdala is an almond-shaped region of homogeneous gray matter near the anterior tip of the lateral ventricle's temporal horn that is medial and inferior to the lenticular nuclei and anterior to the hippocampus. The hippocampal formation is in the floor of the lateral ventricle's temporal horn and extends in an anterior-posterior direction

from the amygdala to the splenium of the corpus callosum. It is noted grossly as small wavy strips of gray and white matter anteriorly and as a curly structure of interlocking "C" shapes further posteriorly. The outward protrusion of the hippocampal formation is seen as the uncus on the surface of the anterior temporal lobe in the parahippocampal gyrus.

Underlying the cerebral cortex are large expanses of white matter formed largely by efferent, afferent, and cortical-cortical white matter tracts and their supporting structures. As neuronal processes travel from the cortex inward toward the internal capsule, they take the shape of a funnel. The most peripheral portion of white matter, near the gray-white junction and corresponding to the mouth of the funnel, is called the centrum semiovale. The more central region of white matter, corresponding to the narrowing portion of the funnel and located near the internal capsule, is called the corona radiata. The dominant white matter tract that connects the two hemispheres is the corpus callosum, which sits superior to the lateral ventricles and is subdivided in the anterior-posterior direction into the genu, body, and splenium. Other interhemispheric white matter connections are the anterior commissure, located inferior to the basal ganglia and superior to the basal forebrain, and the posterior commissure, located near the rostral midbrain.

The basal ganglia are the deep gray matter structures within the cerebrum and brain stem that are involved in the regulation of movement; they include the caudate nucleus, putamen, globus pallidus, subthalamic nucleus, and substantia nigra. In the cerebrum are the caudate nucleus, putamen, and globus pallidus. The caudate nucleus is located in the lateral wall of the lateral ventricle and follows it throughout its C-shaped course from the frontal pole into the temporal lobe. Although its head and body are readily noted grossly, the caudate tail in the temporal lobe is best identified microscopically across the lateral ventricle from the hippocampus. Lateral to the caudate and separated from it by the anterior limb of the internal capsule is the larger putamen. Together, the caudate, putamen, and internal capsule have a "striated" appearance and are called the striatum. At their anterior poles, the caudate and putamen form a continuum inferomedially with the nucleus accumbens, a functionally discrete nucleus with strong interconnections with limbic structures. Further posteriorly and medial to the insular cortex, the putamen is located peripherally to both the external and internal segments of the globus pallidus (GPe and GPi). This triad of nuclei—putamen, GPe, and GPi—takes the shape of a wedge and is referred to as the lenticular nucleus. The GPe is separated from the putamen by the lateral medullary lamina, whereas the medial medullary lamina separates the GPe and GPi. Peripheral to the putamen at the level of the insular cortex are the external capsule, the claustrum (a nucleus with largely undefined function), and the capsula extrema.

Located on the lateral aspects of the third ventricle are the constituents of the diencephalon, the thalamus and hypothalamus. The thalamus is a major throughput for nearly all cortical functions and contains numerous subdivisions of nuclei that extend from the foramen of Monro anteriorly to the brain stem posteriorly. Laterally and inferiorly, the posterior limb of the internal capsule separates the thalamus from the putamen and globus pallidus. Beneath the thalamus on the lateral and inferior aspects of the third ventricle is the hypothalamus, which has components that include bilateral mammillary bodies and the central, inferiorly projecting infundibular stalk. Finally, the pineal gland is located in the midline, posterior and inferior to the third ventricle and immediately superior to the midbrain colliculi. Also referred to as the "third eye" because of its embryologic relationship to the retina and as the "seat of the soul" because of its deep-seated location and mysterious function, the pineal is normally the size of a macadamia nut.

CEREBELLUM

The cerebellum is a fist-sized mass of neural tissue located in the posterior fossa, with functions that include muscle coordination and postural control (Fig. 1-5). It is connected to the more anteriorly positioned brain stem by the superior, middle, and inferior cerebellar peduncles. Slicing across the cerebellar peduncles bilaterally reveals the fourth ventricle between the dorsal pons and the ventral surface of the cerebellum. The cerebellar surface contains numerous deep and superficial fissures that create lobular subdivisions. The smallest lobules are folia—the fundamental structural units of the cerebellar cortex. Underlying the cortex in each folium are white matter tracts (medullary center) that extend from and to their cortical connections. Initial inspection reveals the dominant corpus cerebelli, which is formed by large left and right hemispheres, and a smaller midline lobe, the vermis ("worm"). The corpus cerebelli is separated from the smaller flocculo-nodular lobe by the posterolateral fissure. The two flocculi are located on the ventral surface inferior to the peduncles and are continuous in the midline with the nodulus, the vermian representation of the flocculo-nodular lobe. Opposite the flocculi are the tonsils of the cerebellar hemispheres; opposite the nodulus is the uvula. A major division of the corpus cerebelli is the primary fissure, which divides the anterior and posterior lobes of the cerebellar hemispheres and vermis.

The cerebellum is usually cut for examination in either the sagittal or axial plane. In sliced tissue sections, the white matter is seen beneath the highly convoluted surface folia. Embedded deep within the white matter and toward the midline are four nuclei that are difficult to distinguish from one another on gross inspection. Together they have a tortuous, ribbon-like appearance in the shape of a C, with the open mouth facing centrally and occupied by white matter. The largest and most peripherally located in each hemisphere is the dentate nucleus. More centrally placed, in order, are the emboliform and globose nuclei; the fastigial nucleus is a small nucleus located on either side of the midline in the vermis.

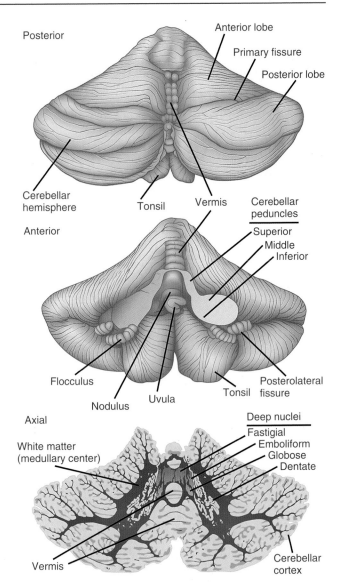

FIGURE 1-5

Posterior and anterior views of the cerebellar surface and an axial slice through the midportion of the cerebellum. The brain stem has been removed for the anterior view of the cerebellum. The ventral surface of the axial slice is pointed upward.

BRAIN STEM

From superior to inferior, the brain stem consists of the midbrain, pons, and medulla (Fig. 1-6; see also Fig. 1-3). Anterior in the midbrain are the cerebral peduncles, the main descending white matter tracts that run between the cerebral hemispheres, brain stem, and spinal cord. On the ventral surface, the oculomotor nerves (CN III) emerge from between the peduncles in the interpeduncular fossa. The trochlear nerve (CN IV) exits the midbrain on its dorsal surface immediately below the inferior colliculi. Gross inspection of axial slices of the midbrain reveals the pigmented substantia nigra immediately posterior to the large white matter tracts of the cerebral peduncles. This nucleus is normally brown-

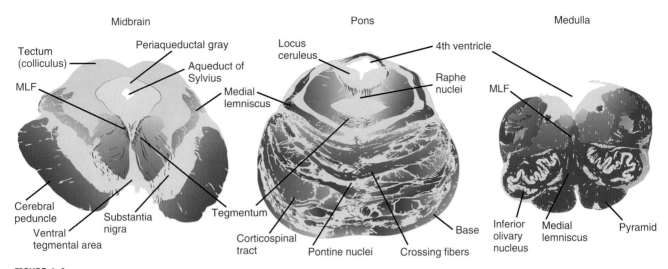

FIGURE 1-6

Axial slices through the midbrain, pons, and medulla. MLF, medial longitudinal fasciculus.

black in adulthood and composed of large dopaminergic neurons that project to the basal ganglia. Close to the midline in the most rostral aspect of the midbrain and posterior to the substantia nigra is the red nucleus, a distinctly round and demarcated gray matter structure. Surrounding the aqueduct of Sylvius in the dorsal aspect of the midbrain is the periaqueductal gray matter, a deep and primitive structure critical to pain perception and control. The superior and inferior colliculi are small hemisphere-shaped projections from the tectum that are seen on posterior views.

The pons has a larger circumference than the midbrain and medulla and bulges ventrally to give the impression of a "bridge" over the brain stem. From its ventral surface in the midline, near its inferior border, emerges the abducens nerves (CN VI). From the lateral aspect of the pons, the trigeminal nerve (CN V) exits superiorly and the facial (CN VII) and vestibulocochlear (CN VIII) nerves exit inferiorly in the region of the cerebellopontine angle. On cut section, the pons is dominated by its large base region anteriorly, which is characterized by a mixture of ascending, descending, and crossing white matter tracts and pontine nuclei that give the combined appearance of miniature tiger stripes in the axial plane. In the more posterior pontine tegmentum, within millimeters of the fourth ventricle, is the locus ceruleus, a small, darkly pigmented nucleus that houses large noradrenergic neurons. The cerebellar peduncles are large white matter tracts that solidly connect the posterolateral portion of the pons to the cerebellum, with the fourth ventricle enclosed between them.

The medulla tapers in circumference from its superior junction with the pons to its inferior border where it merges with the spinal cord. On the ventral surface in the midline is a deep groove, the anterior median fissure, that separates the medullary pyramids, a collection of descending white matter tracts. More lateral and dorsal

on each side are the olives, outward bulges of the inferior olivary nuclei. Between the pyramids and the olives is the hypoglossal nerve (CN XII). Arising from numerous thin filaments dorsal to the olive are, from superior to inferior, the glossopharyngeal (CN IX), vagus (CN X), and accessory (CN XI) nerves. On cut axial sections, the medulla is composed of the white matter tracts of the pyramids anteriorly; the more dorsolateral olivary nucleus, which is oval and consists of a peripheral convoluted ribbon of gray matter and central white matter; the tegmentum, which houses cranial and sensory nerve nuclei together with ascending and crossing white matter tracts; and the fourth ventricle, which is most dorsal.

SPINAL CORD

The spinal cord extends from its junction with the medulla superiorly to its tapering inferior tip, the conus medullaris (Fig. 1-7). The cord is divided into 31 segments based on its spinal roots and consists of 8 cervical, 12 thoracic, 5 lumbar, 5 sacral, and 1 coccygeal segment. Men have a slightly longer spinal cord (45 cm) than women do (43 cm). Along its length, the cord swells from its normal diameter in both the cervical and lumbar enlargements, where more neurons and fibers are present because of representation of the upper and lower extremities, respectively. The anterior surface of the cord is distinguished by its deep, single, midline anterior median fissure, which extends along its length and carries the anterior spinal artery. Posterior in the midline, the less distinct posterior median sulcus separates the left and right fasciculus gracilis, white matter tracts that bulge posteriorly. In the cervical region, the fasciculus gracilis is joined by the more lateral fasciculus

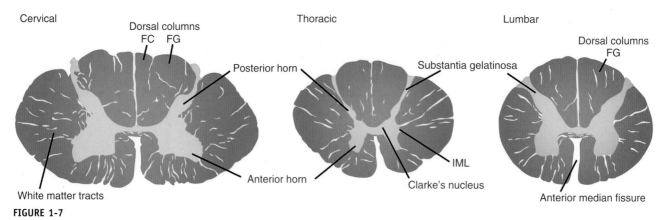

FIGURE 1-7

Cross sections of the cervical, thoracic, and lumbar spinal cord. FC, fasciculus cuneatus; FG, fasciculus gracilis; IML intermediolateral cell column.

cuneatus to form two distinct bulges on either side. Both anteriorly and posteriorly at each of its 31 segments, the spinal cord gives rise to numerous small anterior and posterior rootlets that fuse to form the anterior and posterior spinal roots. The anterior and posterior roots join together on exiting the spinal foramina to form functionally mixed spinal nerves. Because the dural sac is longer than the spinal cord, the more inferiorly located spinal roots course downward to their exit foramina. In the lumbar cistern, inferior to the spinal cord, the collection of roots is particularly dense and forms the cauda equina ("horse's tail"). In the middle of the cauda equina, the filum terminale—an extension of the spinal pia mater—extends from the inferior tip of the conus medullaris and attaches to the most inferior aspect of the dural sac.

On cross section, the spinal cord is separated into central neural tissue (gray matter) and peripheral white matter tracts throughout its length. The anterior horn is home to a collection of motor neurons, interneurons, and projection neurons, as well as the nerve terminals that end on them. The white matter represents the collection of ascending and descending axons that communicate among the spinal cord, peripheral nerves, and superior integrating networks of the cerebrum, cerebellum, and brain stem.

CELL TYPES

It may be somewhat surprising that an organ as complex as the brain would consist in large part of only two cell types, neurons and glia. Both are large families with many members having specific functions, yet the underlying structure and cell biology of each retain some central features. Most imposing for the pathologist are the large morphologic array, the geographic diversity, and the functional capacities of neurons that are disturbed by specific diseases. Recognizing normal and reactive states of glia can also be a challenge.

NEURONS

Neurons are the integrating and transmitting cells of the nervous system, and they communicate by chemical and electrical means. The spectrum of their morphology, connectivity, and function is enormous. As a rule, neurons have a cell body, branching processes called dendrites for integrating incoming signals, and a longer cell process—the axon—with a terminal synapse for conveying a signal over space. Cell body shape and size, as well as the number and arrangement of branching processes, vary considerably. For practicing pathologists, recognizing the major forms of neurons, many of which are described later, within their anatomic setting is requisite because individual populations show differential vulnerability and pathologic reaction in specific disease processes.

Pyramidal neurons are a morphologic prototype that are best known for their presence in the cerebral cortex and subfields CA1, CA2, and CA3 of the hippocampus (Fig. 1-8). In all cases, they have large, triangular cell bodies, a prominent apical dendrite extending toward the brain's surface, and numerous finer branching basal dendrites. Measuring approximately 10 to 50 µm in greatest dimension, their cell bodies contain abundant cytoplasm, variable hematoxiphilic Nissl substance (rough endoplasmic reticulum) near the entry zone to processes, and a large nucleus with open chromatin and a prominent nucleolus (a loose chromatin pattern and prominent nucleolus are typical of neurons and distinguish them from resting glia).

Cortical granular (stellate) neurons are the smaller counterparts to pyramidal neurons in the cortex, typically 15 µm or smaller. Being interneurons, they have numerous shorter processes that remain within the confines of the cortex.

Betz cells are the largest neurons of the cerebral cortex (70 to 100 µm) and are found in the primary motor cortex, where they dwarf their neighboring cortical pyramidal cells. Both the amount of cytoplasm and Nissl substance and the number of visible processes far

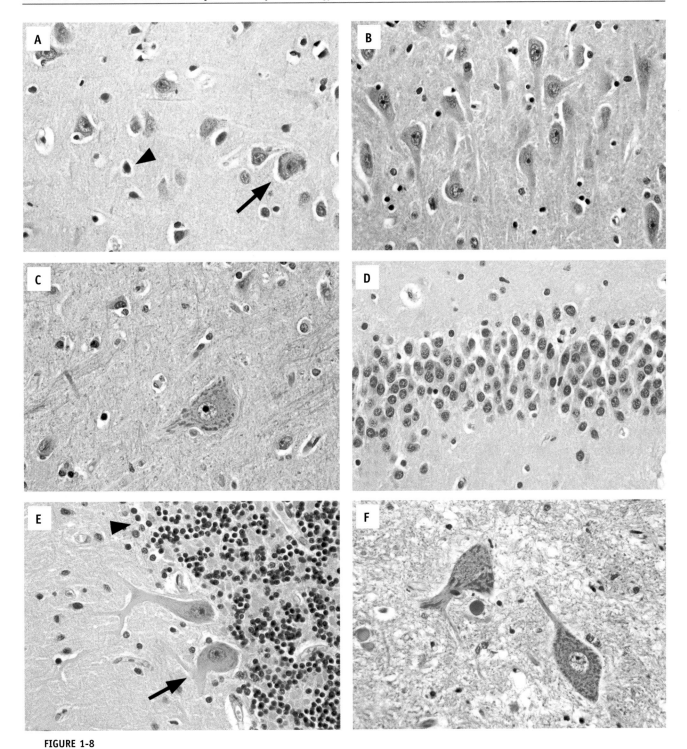

FIGURE 1-8

Neurons. **A**, Pyramidal neurons (*arrow*) and granular neurons (*arrowhead*) of the cerebral cortex. **B**, Pyramidal neurons of the hippocampus. **C**, Betz cells (upper motor neurons) of the motor cortex. **D**, Granular neurons of the dentate fascia of the hippocampal formation. **E**, Purkinje cells (*arrow*) and granular cells (*arrowhead*) of the cerebellar cortex. **F**, Anterior horn cells (lower motor neurons) of the spinal cord.

exceed that in normal pyramidal cells. Betz cells are upper motor neurons.

Small, tightly packed granular neurons form the stratum granulosum of the dentate gyrus in the medial temporal lobe and are intimately connected to the hippocampus proper. These neurons are nearly as small as cerebellar granular cells and have an extensive dendritic arbor that forms the adjacent molecular layer of the dentate gyrus.

Purkinje cells are large (50 to 80 μm), histologically distinctive neurons of the cerebellum with cell bodies that sit at the interface of the molecular and internal granular cell layers. Each neuron has a prominent pink cell body and an expansive dendritic tree with thick processes that extend into the molecular layer, as well as a large axon that travels centrally out of the cerebellar cortex.

The granular neurons of the cerebellar granular cell layer are tiny and densely packed, often displaying a linear arrangement or loose rosettes around delicate neuropil. Their sparse perinuclear cytoplasm gives the appearance of only nuclei on hematoxylin-eosin staining. This population can cause confusion on frozen section or cytologic preparations because they resemble "small round blue cell" lesions.

Anterior horn cells are large lower motor neurons (alpha motor neurons) that populate all levels of the spinal cord in the anterior horns and send long axonal processes via the anterior roots that eventually terminate on peripheral skeletal muscle end-plates.

The CNS contains a small number of highly specialized nuclei with neurons that produce specific bioaminergic neurotransmitters and project diffusely throughout the brain to affect global or regional tone. These nuclei include the substantia nigra, locus ceruleus, raphe nuclei, and nucleus basalis of Meynert (Fig. 1-9). The dopaminergic cells of the substantia nigra pars reticulata (and the ventral tegmental area) are large, heavily pigmented neurons with "neuromelanin" (not to be confused with the melanin of melanocytes), which accumulates in the cytoplasm as coarse brown granules and represents a combination of oxidized and polymerized dopamine within lysosomal granules. Similarly, the locus ceruleus, located near the fourth ventricle in the rostral pontine tegmentum, contains a population of large pigmented neurons that serve as a major source of norepinephrine in the brain. Neurons in the raphe nuclei, located along the midline of the brain stem, are similar in size and shape to the noradrenergic neurons of the locus ceruleus, but lack the pigmentation. These cells produce serotonin and have diffuse projections throughout the nervous system, but most heavily innervate the limbic and sensory regions. Within the basal forebrain, inferior to the anterior commissure in a region called the substantia innominata, is the nucleus basalis of Meynert, a collection of large cholinergic neurons that project throughout the cerebrum.

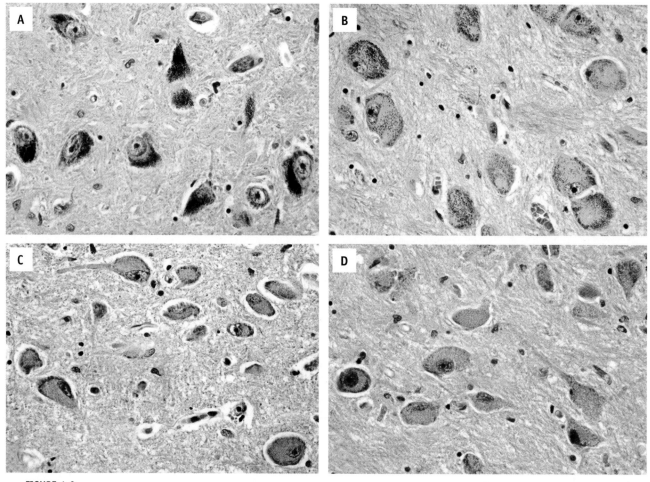

FIGURE 1-9

Diffusely projecting neurons producing specific bioaminergic neurotransmitters. **A,** Dopaminergic neurons of the substantia nigra are deeply pigmented because of the accumulation of neuromelanin. **B,** Neurons of the locus ceruleus are also pigmented and produce norepinephrine. **C,** Near the midline in the brain stem are serotonergic neurons of the raphe nuclei. **D,** Neurons of the nucleus basalis of Meynert produce acetylcholine.

GLIA

Glia account for approximately 90% of all CNS cells and have generally been regarded as "glue" because they provide structural and functional support for neuronal elements. It is now known that the role of glia is not so limited. Functions being elucidated include glia-neuronal signaling, extracellular buffering of electrolytes and metabolites, and turnover of neurotransmitters. Glia are divided into macroglia—astrocytes, oligodendrocytes, and ependyma—and microglia.

ASTROCYTES

Astrocytes are the multipolar, "star-like" glial cells of the CNS (Figs. 1-10 and 1-11). They are typically subdivided into protoplasmic and fibrillary families based on their location and morphology, although overlap between these divisions may outweigh their distinction. Protoplasmic astrocytes reside in the cortex, whereas fibrillary astrocytes populate the white matter. In addition to similar cell shapes and numerous processes, all astrocytes contain abundant cytoplasmic intermediate filaments largely composed of glial fibrillary acidic protein (GFAP). In the resting state, astrocyte nuclei are recognized on hematoxylin-eosin–stained sections, but the scant, delicate cytoplasm and processes are not readily seen because they blend with the surrounding neuropil. Nuclei are oblong and can be slightly angulated with a chromatin pattern that is lighter and looser than that of oligodendrocytes. The nucleoli that are typically seen in neuronal nuclei are not present in most resting astrocytes. Many astrocytes have processes that terminate as end-feet on blood vessel walls, where they contribute to the blood-brain barrier. Others have processes that extend end-feet to the pial surface of the

brain, thereby contributing to the glial limitans of the brain-CSF barrier. At these locations, astrocytes provide laminin, fibronectin, and proteoglycans for the limiting basement membrane.

Astrocytes are activated in response to a variety of pathologic conditions (see Fig. 1-11). The morphologic spectrum of reactive astrocytosis is critical to recognize because (1) it brings one's attention to pathologically affected tissue for further evaluation, (2) it serves as validation that a disease process is present in the CNS (i.e., rather than an artifact), and (3) reactive astrocytosis often causes a diagnostic dilemma as a result of its morphologic similarity to neoplastic conditions. Reactive astrocytosis involves both proliferation and hypertrophy of astrocytes, and its appearance varies with the chronicity and severity of the insult. The initial response is enlargement of the cell body, processes, nuclei, and nucleoli. In hematoxylin-eosin–stained sections, the presence of visible astrocytic cytoplasm and processes is almost always a pathologic finding. Immunohistochemistry for GFAP highlights the reactive nature of these astrocytes by demonstrating the extensive arborizing of their processes and the orientation of the reactive cells to the underlying injury. Reactive astrocytes of longer duration often take on a gemistocytic appearance, with large amounts of brightly eosinophilic cytoplasm in their cell bodies. Chronic reactive astrocytosis is more fibrillar in nature, with numerous long astrocytic processes forming a layer of dense gliosis adjacent to injury (often called piloid gliosis). Rosenthal fibers, which are large, flame-shaped or globular proteinaceous deposits, are often seen in this type of long-standing reactive astrocytosis.

Alzheimer type II astrocytes are a reactive form seen in states of elevated blood ammonia, usually related to renal or hepatic disease. They are present in highest concentration in the basal ganglia, where cells show nuclear

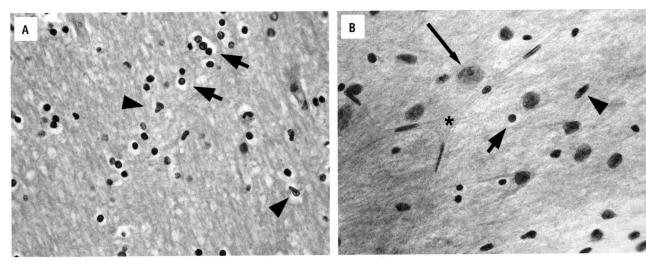

FIGURE 1-10

Normal glia. Normal white matter shows oligodendrocytes (*arrows*), which have round dark nuclei, often with a slight perinuclear halo, and astrocytes, which have oblong, irregularly shaped nuclei (*arrowheads*). **A,** Glial cytoplasm blends with the neuropil and typically cannot be noted in the resting state. **B,** A cytologic preparation of normal cortex demonstrates normal oligodendrocytes (*short arrow*), astrocytes (*arrowhead*), neuron (*long arrow*), and capillary (*asterisk*).

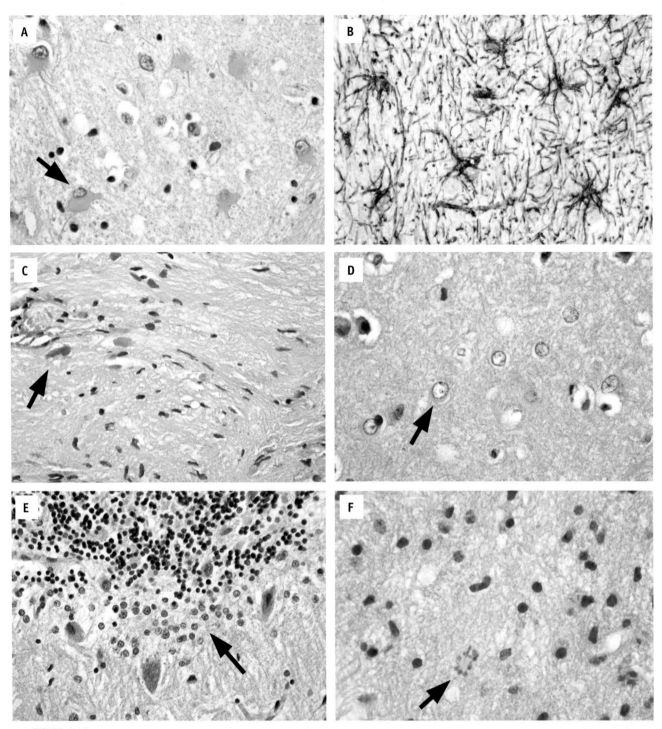

FIGURE 1-11

Reactive glia. **A**, Gemistocytic astrocytes (*arrow*) are one form of reactive change in which the astrocytic cytoplasm is distended and eosinophilic and its processes are readily identified. **B**, Immunohistochemistry for glial fibrillary acidic protein (GFAP) highlights reactive astrocytes and emphasizes their "star-like" quality. **C**, Piloid gliosis is a highly fibrillar form of reactive gliosis that is composed of dense, elongated astrocytic processes that are tightly packed together. Rosenthal fibers (*arrow*) can often be seen in piloid gliosis. **D**, Alzheimer type II astrocytes (*arrow*) have enlarged, clear nuclei and are seen in states of hyperammonemia. **E**, Bergmann's gliosis (*arrow*) occurs at the interface of the molecular and granular layers of the cerebellum, generally in response to Purkinje cell injury. **F**, Creutzfeldt cells (granular mitoses [*arrow*]) are reactive cells with fragmented nuclear material that can be mistaken for mitotic figures.

swelling, marked chromatin clearing, and micronucleoli. Cytoplasmic hypertrophy is not prominent in this form of astrocytosis.

The Bergmann glia consists of a layer of astrocytes located between the molecular and granular layers of the cerebellum. Cells are only one to two layers thick and can go unnoticed in resting states. In response to cerebellar injury, especially to individual Purkinje cell loss, the reactive proliferation of this cell layer is referred to as Bergmann's gliosis.

Creutzfeldt cells are another form of reactive astrocytes that have abundant cytoplasm and "granular mitoses," or the fragmenting of nuclear material that gives the impression of multiple micronuclei. They are seen in active inflammatory diseases (classic in demyelinating disease) and require recognition so that they are not mistaken for the mitoses of an infiltrating astrocytoma.

Markedly enlarged and atypical astrocytes can be seen in non-neoplastic conditions, including reactions to radiation (radiation atypia) and progressive multifocal leukoencephalopathy. In both conditions, nuclei can be wildly atypical with hyperchromatic nuclei that have irregular outlines. The context of additional microscopic changes and the clinical history are often required to avoid a misdiagnosis of neoplasm.

OLIGODENDROCYTES

Oligodendrocytes are the myelinating cells of the CNS and are therefore more numerous in white matter than in gray matter (see Fig. 1-10). With their cellular processes extending in all directions, oligodendrocytes provide internodes of myelination to multiple axonal processes in their environment. In hematoxylin–eosin–stained sections, only the nucleus of oligodendrocytes is usually visible because of the blending of cellular processes with the neuropil. A clear zone surrounding the nucleus—the so-called perinuclear halo—often highlights oligodendrocytes, as well as tumor derived from them (oligodendroglioma), and in either case is an artifact of fixation. Nuclei are generally round and regular but vary from small and darkly basophilic (accounting for the majority) to slightly larger with pale vesicular nuclei. Nucleoli are not usually visualized by standard light microscopy. In white matter, oligodendrocytes are disposed along the length of axonal processes, whereas in the cerebral cortex, they are scattered within the neuropil and concentrated immediately around neuronal cell bodies (satellite cells). In the latter location they may serve as a progenitor population.

EPENDYMA

The ependyma consists of cuboidal to columnar glial cells that form a single-layered covering of the ventricular system (Fig. 1-12). On its ventricular (apical) surface, the ependyma has microscopically visible cilia and microvilli, whereas the lateral surfaces are tethered to one another by desmosomes to form a functional CSF-brain barrier. Ependymal cytoplasm is pale to eosinophilic, and nuclei are oval and hyperchromatic. Within the supratentorial and infratentorial compartments, the ependyma is fairly homogeneous, with slight variation in cell height and degree of ciliation by anatomic location. In tissue sections along the lateral ventricles, especially posteriorly, it is fairly common to encounter either entrapped outpouchings of ependyma or small clusters forming canals. These findings do not represent hamartomas or malformations, only remnants of imperfect development that are clinically inconsequential. Within the spine, the central canal is lined by ependyma and serves as a conduit for CSF during childhood. In adulthood, the central canal is collapsed and

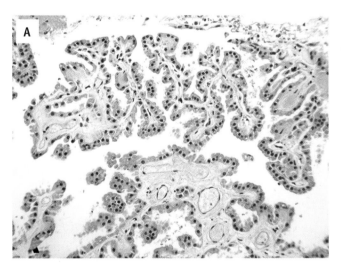
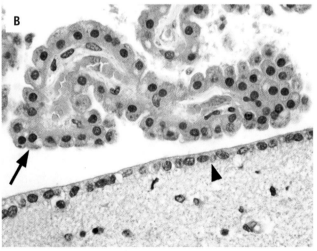

FIGURE 1-12

Choroid plexus and ependyma. **A**, The choroid plexus is a tufted aggregate of vascular channels lined by a single layer of choroid epithelium that contains large pink cells with a cobblestone shape (*arrow* in **B**). The ependyma is a single layer of cuboidal to columnar glial cells that line the ventricular system and form the brain-cerebrospinal fluid barrier (*arrowhead* in **B**). Cilia can usually be noted on the ventricular surface of the ependyma.

vestigial, with only a central collection of clustered ependyma remaining throughout the length of the spinal cord.

CHOROID PLEXUS

The choroid plexus is a functionally differentiated region of ependyma that extends into the ventricular space as frond-like tufts and functions to secrete the ultrafiltrate of CSF (see Fig. 1-12). On a daily basis, 400 to 500 mL is produced. Individual cells are found as a single layer on a fibrovascular core. When compared with the ependyma, the choroid plexus has larger cobblestone-shaped cell bodies and contains small, bland, basally located nuclei. Microvilli extend from the apical surface. Tight junctions and desmosomes are present between choroid plexus cells to ensure a viable blood-CSF barrier.

MICROGLIA

Microglia are small, elongated cells located throughout the CNS gray and white matter (Fig. 1-13). In the resting state, microglia are easily overlooked because of their small size and bland appearance, yet they account for nearly 20% of the glial population. In standard hematoxylin-eosin–stained sections, their nuclei are long, thin, and dark—leading to their designation as "rod cells"—but their cytoplasm is difficult to visualize. Special stains based on silver carbonate or lectins provide contrast to the small processes and delicate branches that extend from their tips. Microglia are not of neuroepithelial origin and are thought to derive from a monocyte/macrophage lineage incorporated into the CNS early in development. Once established, they serve as antigen-presenting cells for immune surveillance and participate in inflammatory responses, particularly against viral pathogens.

On activation, microglia proliferate and migrate to sites of damage, and in this state (microgliosis), cells are more readily identified. Activation also causes increased expression of proteins such as major histocompatibility complex class I and II molecules, which can be detected immunohistochemically. When microglia and astrocytes aggregate around a central focus of injury such as a virally infected neuron, they form a microglial nodule. Another population of monocyte/macrophage-derived cells resides in the perivascular compartment, between the outer basement membrane of the vessel and the glial limitans. In distinction to parenchymal microglia, these perivascular macrophages are in continuity with the circulating monocyte population. Both perivascular and circulating populations of monocytes are recruited into the CNS parenchyma in response to severe injury, where they differentiate as tissue macrophages to perform phagocytic and immunologic functions.

BLOOD VESSELS

Similar to other organs, the brain has a population of vascular and perivascular cells essential for its oxygen and nutrient supply. When compared with their extracranial counterparts, the large arteries that run within the subarachnoid space have thinner muscular walls and less adventitia and lack external elastic lamina (Fig. 1-14). As they penetrate into the brain parenchyma, larger arteries retain both a thin covering by the pia-arachnoid and a perivascular space, the Virchow-Robin space, that appears to represent a continuation of the subarachnoid space, although its function and content remain controversial. No such space exists once the vessels become small capillaries and the endothelium is intimately associated with the neuropil.

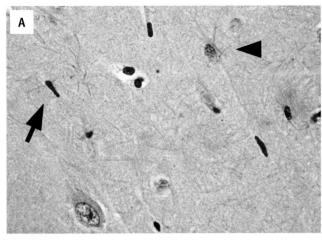
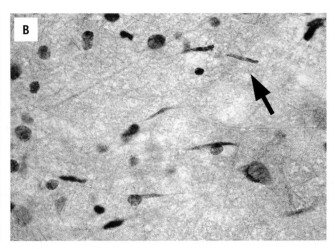

FIGURE 1-13

Microglia. **A,** Best seen in their activated state, microglia have thin, elongated, and hyperchromatic nuclei that stand out from the neuropil (*arrow*) and can be distinguished from reactive astrocytes (*arrowhead*). **B,** The rod-like quality of microglia is also appreciated on cytologic preparations (*arrow*).

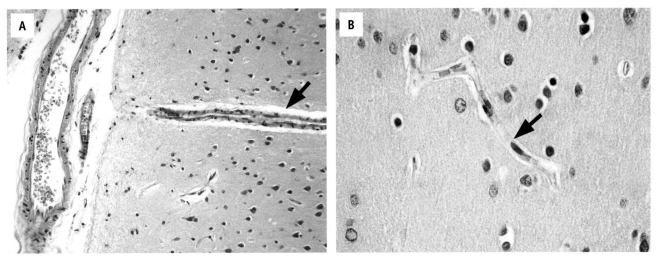

FIGURE 1-14

Blood vessels. **A**, Large arteries within the subarachnoid space (*left*) supply the brain by penetrating into the parenchyma, where they initially maintain a perivascular space (Virchow-Robin space) that separates the vessel from the neuropil (*arrow*). **B**, Smaller capillaries within the brain consist of a thin, delicate tube lined by a single layer of endothelial cells that appear to abut the brain parenchyma directly (*arrow*). The blood-brain barrier is due in large part to the specialized tight junctions between endothelial cells.

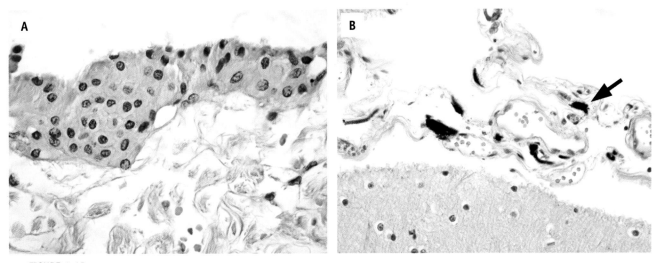

FIGURE 1-15

Meningothelial cells and melanocytes. **A**, Meningothelial cells are scattered within the arachnoid membranes and are most frequent within the uppermost layers as arachnoid cap cells. Meningothelial cells are spindled to polygonal in shape, have moderate amounts of eosinophilic cytoplasm and bland oval nuclei, and are usually found in small clusters. **B**, Melanocytes (*arrow*) are infrequent, flattened, highly pigmented cells of the pia and arachnoid membranes that are generally dispersed individually and are highest in density over the ventral portion of the brain stem.

Capillaries are created by individual endothelial cells forming delicate tubular structures with a width suitable only for the passage of individual circulating blood cells. The physiologically critical blood-brain barrier is formed predominantly by the specialized nature of CNS endothelial cell junctions and cannot be identified histologically. In particular, these endothelial cells lack fenestrations between them and are joined by specialized tight junctions that functionally preclude the free movement of substances between the vascular and CNS spaces. Astrocytic end-feet and basal lamina elements contribute to the integrity of this barrier.

MENINGOTHELIAL CELLS

Meningothelial cells are scattered within the arachnoid membranes throughout the neuraxis, but their concentration is higher at the tips of arachnoid granulations, where they are called arachnoid cap cells (Fig. 1-15). Meningothelial cells are epithelioid to slightly spindled and are typically seen in small clusters (10 to 20 cells), where they have a tendency to form whorls and psammoma bodies. Cells have moderate amounts of eosinophilic cytoplasm and oval nuclei with dispersed chromatin, often giving the appearance of central clearing.

MELANOCYTES

Melanocytes are normal, neural crest–derived constituents of the human leptomeninges that are intimately associated with the pia and subarachnoid membranes (see Fig. 1-15). They are widely scattered in most supratentorial regions and are noted histologically only after intense searching or fortuitous tissue sectioning. They are highest in density over the ventral surface of the superior portion of the spinal cord, brain stem, and base of the brain. Almost always seen as individual cells rather than clusters, leptomeningeal melanocytes are thin and elongated with slight branching and heavy pigmentation. The melanin pigment is made within cytoplasmic melanosomes and premelanosomes and is therefore similar to that in dermal melanocytes rather than the neuromelanin of the substantia nigra.

TISSUE ORGANIZATION

CEREBRAL CORTEX

The vast majority (>90%) of cerebral cortex in humans is neocortex, an evolutionarily late form of cortical development that is distinguished from paleocortex (mostly limbic and olfactory cortices) and archicortex (hippocampal structures), which are more primitive. Neocortex differs from primitive cortex in its anatomic location and architecture. All neocortical areas—also called isocortex—go through developmental periods in which their elements are laid down in six layers. Many regions retain this layered appearance throughout life. Paleocortex and archicortex do not share this developmental pattern or six-layered structuring in adulthood.

Cerebral cortex contains two dominant neuronal types, the granular (stellate) cell and the pyramidal cell (see "Neurons"). Pyramidal cells account for two thirds of the cerebral cortical neurons and are the primary output. They have prominent apical dendrites that extend toward the cortical surface and contain a network of dendritic spines for integrating synaptic input. Their axons extend long distances to terminate within the ipsilateral or contralateral cortex or travel to subcortical regions. Granular cells, in contrast, are smaller and are considered to be the primary interneurons of the neocortex. Other less common neurons are horizontal cells (of Cajal), common in the superficial cortex in development; fusiform cells, most frequent in the deepest cortical layers; and cells of Martinotti, present in lesser numbers in all cortical layers.

The practice of neuropathology requires a basic familiarity with neocortical structure because subtle abnormalities underlie diseases such as developmental migration disorders, cortical dysplasia, and epilepsy (Fig. 1-16). Moreover, this layered architecture is the substrate for the selective pathologic vulnerability that gives rise to laminar necrosis. The six layers of the cortex, from the surface to the white matter, are (I) the molecular layer, which has very few neurons in adulthood; (II) the outer granular cell layer; (III) the outer pyramidal cell layer; (IV) the inner granular cell layer; (V) the inner pyramidal cell layer; and (VI) the multiforme layer, which is populated primarily by fusiform neurons. These layers are more histologically apparent in some regions than others. Regions with primary output function, such as the primary motor cortex, have mostly pyramidal cells, whereas regions with primarily integrating or sensory function contain mainly granular cells. In either instance, dominance by a single cell type results in less apparent layering because of loss of architectural contrast. Regions with nearly equal complements of granular and pyramidal cells demonstrate the most apparent horizontal layering.

Afferents to the cortex arise in the ipsilateral and contralateral cortex and in subcortical structures, most notably the thalamus. Corticocortical afferents end mostly in layers II and III, whereas the majority of thalamic input terminates in layers I, IV, and VI. Among the efferents from the cortex, layer III gives rise to most corticocortical connections, layer V to corticostriate connections, and layer VI to most corticothalamic connections.

Myelin staining of the cortex reveals parallel horizontal bands of myelinated fibers that are not as readily apparent on hematoxylin-eosin–stained sections. The two most prominent bands are in layers IV and V and are referred to as the external and internal bands of Baillarger, respectively. The primary visual cortex (Brodmann area 17), located on either side of the calcarine fissure in the occipital lobe, is characterized by a greatly widened band of Baillarger in layer IV as a result of the large input of visual afferent fibers from the lateral geniculate nucleus (see Fig. 1-16). This enlarged zone divides layer IV into three distinct layers and can be seen grossly as the "line of Gennari."

WHITE MATTER

The white matter of the CNS is relatively uniform (Fig. 1-17). It is generally more deeply eosinophilic than the overlying cortex, and its matrix is coarser. Its architecture is dictated by the arrays of axonal processes that extend to and from gray matter structures. Individual axons themselves are difficult to appreciate on hematoxylin-eosin–stained sections of normal brain because they are thin and blend with the background neuropil (although they can be noted in disease states in which the neuropil is disrupted). Neurofilament immunohistochemistry or silver stains can highlight these struc-

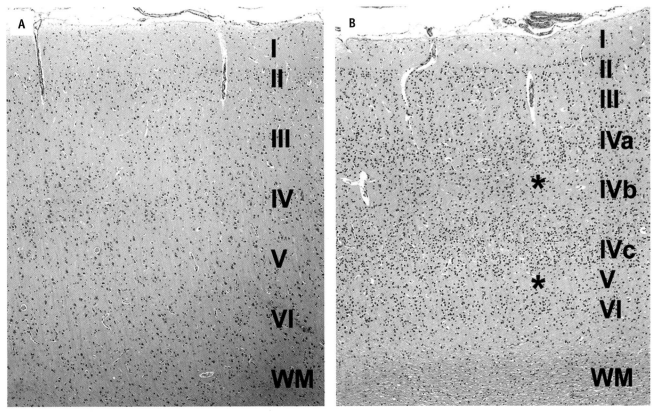

FIGURE 1-16

Cerebral cortex. **A**, The cerebral neocortex (isocortex) contains six layers, numbered sequentially from superficial to deep: I, molecular layer; II, external granular cell layer; III, external pyramidal cell layer; IV, internal granular cell layer; V, internal pyramidal cell layer; and VI, multi-forme layer. **B**, In the primary visual cortex of the occipital lobe, cortical layer IV is greatly expanded because of the high number of visual inputs and is divided into layers IVa, IVb, and IVc. Prominent bands of Baillarger are present in layers IV and V in the primary visual cortex (*asterisks*). The greatly expanded band of Baillarger in layer IV can be seen grossly as the line of Gennari. WM, white matter.

tures by enhancing contrast. Oligodendrocytes, fibrillary astrocytes, and microglia are all oriented along the length of axons with a fairly rigid periodicity. When viewed in the plane of white matter tracts, units of approximately 5 to 10 oligodendrocytes are disposed in linear, parallel arrays along axonal processes and interrupted by single interspersed fibrillary astrocytes. Microglia are also located at regular intervals, albeit with much less frequency than oligodendrocytes, and their cell bodies are oriented parallel to axons.

BASAL GANGLIA

The caudate, putamen, and nucleus accumbens are developmentally related and histologically similar (Fig. 1-18). They contain a variety of small and large neurons that have relatively uniform density. About 95% are small and medium-sized (10 to 18 μm) GABAergic spiny neurons that provide projections to the globus pallidus. These neurons have extensive dendritic trees packed with spines for connection with the large array of input fibers from the cerebral cortex, thalamus, and brain stem. Other populations consist of large cholinergic

neurons (approximately 2% of the neurons) and smaller cells containing neuropeptide Y, somatostatin, or nitric oxide synthetase. Interspersed among the neurons and neuropil of the striatum are small white matter bundles of the internal capsule that can only be seen microscopically. These "pencil fibers of Wilson" are specific for this region and serve as a guide to location when included in small biopsy specimens.

THALAMUS

The thalamus is the main integrator and relay of sensory information to the cortex and has more than 50 individual nuclei, each with its own specific function. Classic divisions are the anterior, medial, ventrolateral, and posterior groups of nuclei. Not included among these larger categories are the midline, intralaminar, and reticular nuclei. The histologic appearance of each of the lobes is relatively similar, with variations depending on specific functions (see Fig. 1-18). Thalamic neurons consist of two main types: large projection neurons with axons that exit the thalamus (75% of the neuronal population) and smaller, inhibitory (GABAergic) interneurons.

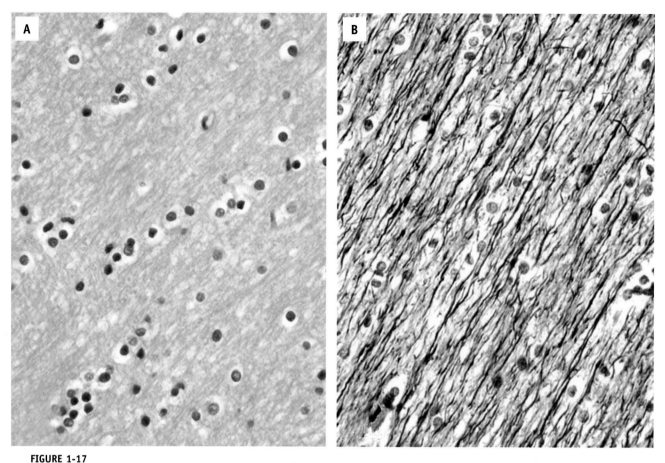

FIGURE 1-17
White matter. Sweeping linear arrays of axons are the backbone of the white matter but cannot be readily identified on hematoxylin-eosin staining. **A,** Oligodendrocytes, astrocytes, and microglia are dispersed along the length of axons with a fairly rigid periodicity. **B,** Axons in white matter are highlighted in black by silver staining.

Each large projection neuron extends its process to the cerebral cortex through the internal capsule.

HIPPOCAMPUS

The hippocampal formation consists of the hippocampus proper, subiculum, and dentate gyrus and is intimately associated with the entorhinal cortex (Fig. 1-19). The entorhinal cortex occupies most of the parahippocampal gyrus, is the largest source of input into the hippocampus, and contains a distinctive six-layered cortical architecture. Near its surface in layer II are numerous large, round neuronal clusters that can be seen as small protrusions on the brain's surface. Deeper are the remainder of its six layers, which contain pyramidal cells and a diverse array of smaller neurons. The subiculum sits at the base of the hippocampus and is a field populated largely by pyramidal neurons with an allocortical arrangement that transitions from the three-layered cortex of the hippocampal CA1 subdivision at one end to the six-layered entorhinal cortex at the other. The hippocampus is divided into CA1, CA2, and CA3 subfields,

each having distinct arrangements of pyramidal neurons and selective vulnerabilities to disease. CA3 emerges from the hilum of the dentate gyrus and contains the largest pyramidal neurons. The pyramidal neurons of CA2 form a narrow band that runs between CA1 and CA3. The transition to CA1 is characterized by a wider band of slightly smaller pyramidal neurons that are more spread out. CA1 (Sommer's sector) is generally much more sensitive to hypoxia, toxicants, seizures, and degenerative diseases than the other subfields are. The molecular layer of the hippocampal CA fields faces the dentate gyrus, whereas its white matter tracts form the alveus that runs within the space between the CA neurons and the lateral ventricle. The white matter tracts of the alveus converge to form the fimbria of the hippocampus, which continues as the fornix and travels in the septum pellucidum of the lateral ventricles to find its way to the hypothalamus and mammillary bodies.

The densely packed smaller granular cells arranged as a C-shaped structure in the dentate gyrus is the stratum granulosum. The hilar neurons that occupy the space within the C (these cells have alternatively been classified as the CA4 subdivision of the hippocampus) are a heterogeneous population of neurons that includes large pyramidal and smaller interneurons.

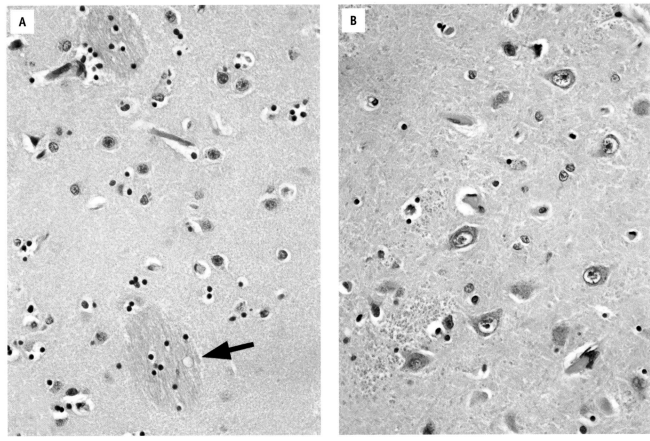

FIGURE 1-18

Basal ganglia and thalamus. **A**, The caudate, putamen, and globus pallidus contain a variety of small and large neurons interspersed in a rich neuropil. Pencil fibers of Wilson are small white matter bundles embedded within the gray matter neuropil that are unique to these deep nuclei of the cerebrum (*arrow*). **B**, The thalamus has large projection neurons, as well as a less frequent population of smaller, inhibitory interneurons.

FIGURE 1-19

Hippocampal formation. The hippocampus proper consists of the CA1, CA2, and CA3 sectors of pyramidal neurons. CA1 continues as the subiculum (SUB) at the base of the hippocampal formation. The dentate fascia (DF) contains a narrow, densely populated band of granular cells (stratum granulosum) that surround the hilum (H). The major white matter tract emerging from the hippocampus is the alveus (ALV), which is located between hippocampal pyramidal fields and the lateral ventricle (LV). Located across the lateral ventricle from the hippocampus are the tail of the caudate nucleus (CN) and the lateral geniculate nucleus (LGN).

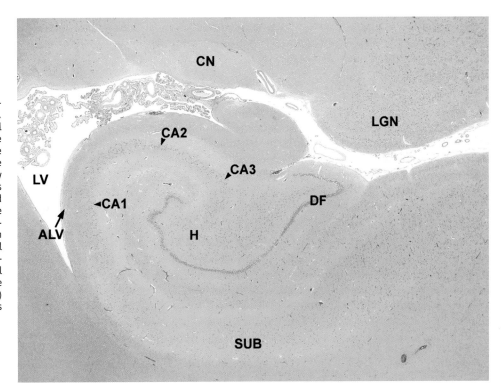

PINEAL GLAND

The pineal gland has a unique morphologic appearance that is unlike any other region in the CNS (Fig. 1-20). At low magnification, it has a lobulated arrangement with a prominent intralobular fibrovascular and glial stroma. The cellularity of a normal pineal gland is greater than that of most regions, which together with the unusual architecture can lead to misinterpretation as a neoplasm. The dominant lobular cell population, the pineocyte, is a medium-sized neuronal cell with round, regular "neuroendocrine" nuclei and delicate stippled chromatin. Pineocytes contain moderate amounts of pale pink cytoplasm with short processes and form pineocytic rosettes and linear arrays. At the periphery of nests and surrounding blood vessels is a higher density of fibrillarity. Interspersed among the nests and within the perivascular region are the less common pineal astrocytes.

PITUITARY GLAND

The pituitary gland is composed of anterior, intermediate, and posterior lobes (Fig. 1-21). The anterior and intermediate lobes (adenohypophysis) have a different embryogenesis, function, and microscopic appearance than the posterior lobe (neurohypophysis). The adenohypophysis is not of neuroectodermal origin, but rather is derived from stomodeal ectoderm that invaginates superiorly as Rathke's pouch and eventually finds its place within the sellar compartment. Notwithstanding their non-CNS origin, diseases of the sellar space often affect neurologic function.

The pituitary gland is connected to the more superior hypothalamus by the pituitary stalk, which is composed of the infundibulum, a superior extension of the neurohypophysis, and the pars tuberalis, an extension of the anterior gland. The stalk also carries a functionally vital vascular supply between the hypophyseal and hypothalamic compartments. Arterial supply to the pituitary is via the inferior and superior pituitary arteries, which branch from each internal carotid artery. These arteries give rise to a network of capillary loops within the gland (gomitoli), which in turn lead to a substantial network of venous sinuses that drain back to the hypothalamus and carry vital hormonal feedback. Thus, the vascular network of the pituitary is extensive and critical to endocrine function.

The anterior pituitary accounts for more than 75% of the sellar volume. It is composed of variably sized glandular arrangements interrupted by stromal and vascular septa. The majority of glands are filled with cellular elements and lack appreciable lumina. Only occasionally are follicles with central spaces noted, some containing mucinous or colloid material. The stroma surrounding individual glands can be highlighted by reticulin stains, a helpful adjunctive test for establishing a normal glandular arrangement and ruling out

adenoma. Individual cells of the anterior lobe are classified as acidophils (40%), basophils (10%), and chromophobes (50%) based on their hematoxylin-eosin staining. Hematoxylin-eosin–staining patterns are not specific for endocrine function or hormone production. Rather, glandular cells can be classified according to their immunohistochemical staining properties as lactotrophs (prolactin), thyrotrophs (thyroid-stimulating hormone), somatotrophs (growth hormone), corticotrophs (adrenocorticotropic hormone), or gonadotrophs (follicle-stimulating hormone or luteinizing hormone). Although gonadotrophs are diffusely spread throughout the gland with even density, other hormone-producing cells show regional variation. Corticotrophs and thyrotrophs are highest in density within the central portion of the gland, whereas lactotrophs and somatotrophs are highest in density laterally.

The thin intermediate lobe of the pituitary is derived from the posterior Rathke cleft. In humans, it is not well developed and contains only glandular and colloid-filled cystic remnants within a slightly fibrous stroma. Individual cells are cuboidal or columnar, some with apical cilia and others containing cytoplasmic mucin. When large or clinically symptomatic, these cystic spaces are termed Rathke's cleft cysts.

In contrast to the glandular anterior lobe, the posterior pituitary, or neurohypophysis, is an extension of the CNS and has a "neural" histology. It is composed of neuronal processes that extend from their cell bodies in the hypothalamus down the pituitary stalk (infundibulum) to occupy the posterior portion of the sella and terminate near blood vessels. Scattered in the neuropil are Herring bodies—subtle eosinophilic axonal dilations filled with lysosomes and neurosecretory granules containing vasopressin and oxytocin. The most prominent nucleated cells of the neurohypophysis are pituicytes—GFAP-expressing spindle or stellate glial cells that abut the basal lamina of blood vessels. Their cytoplasm engulfs the nerve terminals and regulates the release of hormones into the bloodstream. The overall histology of the neurohypophysis is complex, with a seemingly disorganized cell arrangement that includes sweeping axonal processes punctuated by more cellular perivascular regions. Confusion with neoplastic disease has occurred.

CEREBELLUM

Although the circuitry of the cerebellar cortex is exceedingly intricate, its histologic appearance is homogeneous and relatively simple throughout (Fig. 1-22). Outermost is the molecular layer, a rich neuropil network containing abundant axonal and dendritic processes, but only a few small neuronal cell bodies. The Purkinje cell layer is at the junction of the molecular layer and the deeper granular cell layer. Purkinje cells are large neurons with widely arborizing dendritic trees that extend into the molecular layer and serve as synaptic input for the parallel fibers of the granular

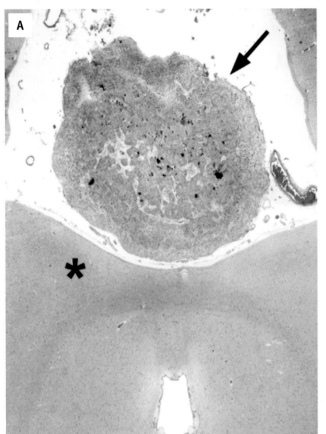

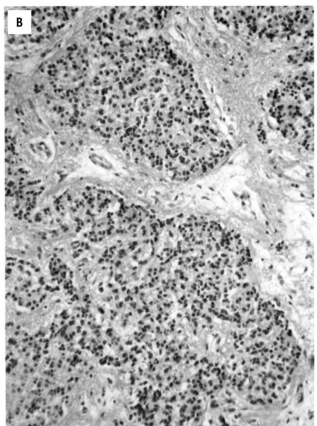

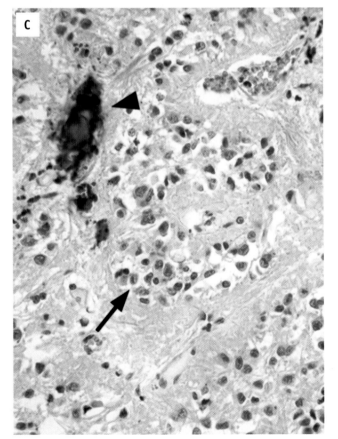

FIGURE 1-20

Pineal gland. **A**, The pineal gland (*arrow*) is located in the midline, posterior and superior to the midbrain tectum (*asterisk*). **B**, It consists of loose lobules of pineocytes arranged in rosettes and linear arrays and separated by glial and fibrovascular septa. **C**, Small clusters and rosettes of pineocytes (*arrow*) are seen adjacent to pineal calcification (*arrowhead*), which occurs normally with aging.

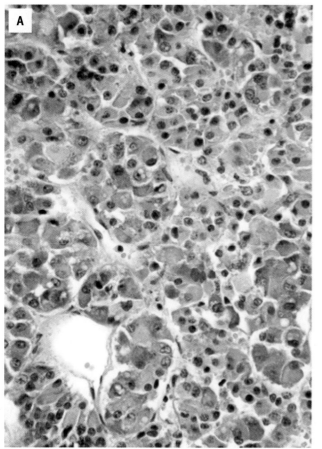

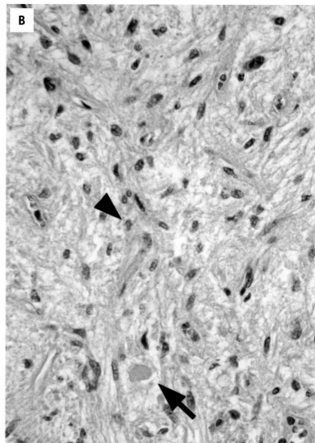

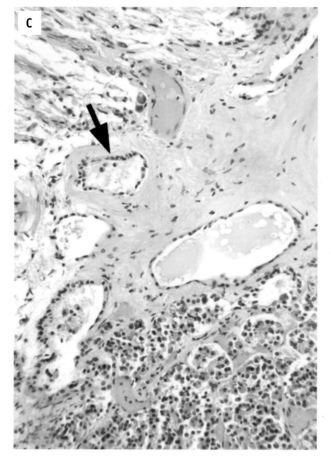

FIGURE 1-21

Pituitary gland. **A**, The anterior pituitary gland consists of tightly packed glandular arrangements of acidophils (pink), basophils (blue), and chromophobes (amphophilic) separated by a fine fibrovascular stroma. **B**, The posterior pituitary (neurohypophysis) is formed by the axonal projections of neurons located in the hypothalamus together with the primary glial cells, pituicytes, which are most commonly located in a perivascular distribution (*arrowhead*). Eosinophilic axonal dilations that store neurosecretory peptides (Herring bodies, *arrow*) can be seen distributed throughout the posterior gland. **C**, The intermediate lobe is small, often shows mild fibrosis, and contains cysts lined by flattened, Rathke-type epithelium (*arrow*).

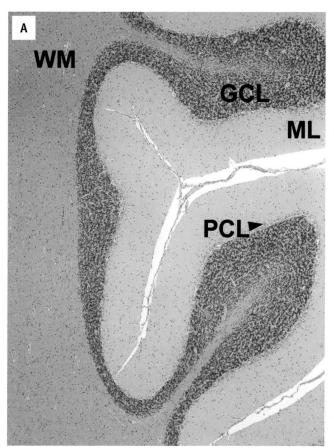
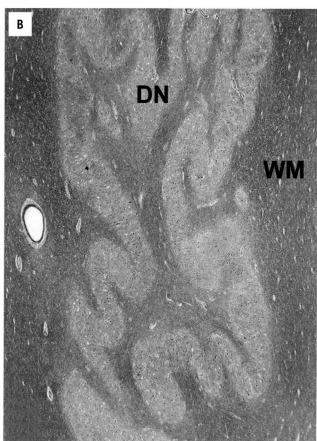

FIGURE 1-22

Cerebellum. **A**, From its outer surface, the cerebellar cortex contains a sparsely cellular molecular layer (ML), a Purkinje cell layer (PCL [*arrowhead*]), and a granular cell layer (GCL). Embedded in the deep white matter (WM) are the cerebellar nuclei. **B**, The largest, the dentate nucleus (DN), has a thin ribbon of gray matter surrounding a central hilum of exiting white matter tracts (Luxol fast blue/periodic acid–Schiff stain).

cells. Purkinje cell axons are the main output of the cerebellar cortex, and a majority have their termination on the neurons of the dentate nucleus. Granular cells of the cerebellum are the most common neuronal cell in the CNS and are present in high density central to Purkinje cells. Each granular cell sends an axon to the molecular layer, which then bifurcates to form the parallel fibers that synapse with numerous Purkinje cell dendritic trees.

The deep cerebellar nuclei are located on either side of the cerebellar midline in the midst of the white matter tracts of the medullary center that are entering and leaving the cerebellar cortex. These nuclei are seen as thin, undulating ribbons of gray matter containing large and small neurons. Within the gray matter ribbon is a central zone of white matter that projects out of the cerebellum. The largest and most lateral nucleus is the dentate nucleus, which has both developmental ties and morphologic similarity to the inferior olive of the medulla. It is the source of most efferents traveling out of the cerebellum via the superior peduncle. The other deep cerebellar nuclei, from lateral to medial, are the emboliform, globose, and fastigial nuclei.

BRAIN STEM

Throughout the brain stem, anatomic regions are broadly subdivided in the ventral-to-dorsal direction as base, tegmentum, and tectum (Fig. 1-23; see also Fig. 1-6). The base is located ventrally and consists mostly of long fiber tracts (cerebral peduncles, basis pontis, and medullary pyramids) that serve as the conduit function of the brain stem. The tegmentum lies dorsal to the base and ventral to the cerebral aqueduct or fourth ventricle. Among other structures, the tegmentum contains the reticular formation at all brain stem levels. This centrally located, relatively uniform gray matter lacks strict organization and boundaries, but it is critical to the control of basal body activity, including cardiovascular tone, respiration, and consciousness. The tectum is the area located dorsal to the brain stem ventricular compartments and serves as their roof. Together, the tectum and tegmentum house most of the integrative and cranial nerve nuclei components of the brain stem.

The locations of cranial nerve nuclei fall within the same general pattern throughout the brain stem. Nuclei

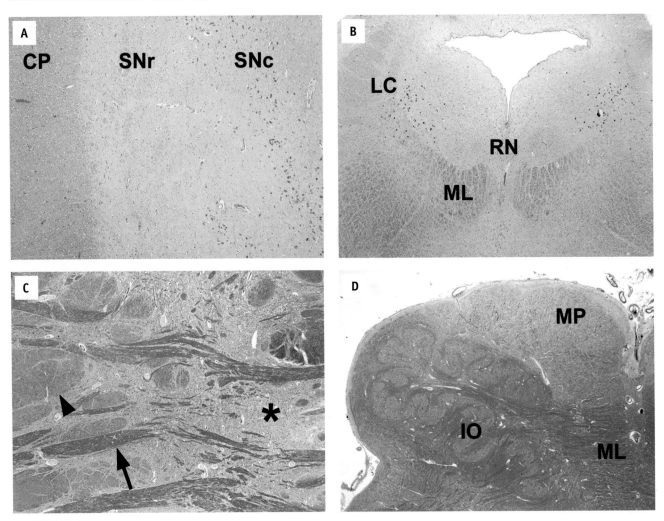

FIGURE 1-23

Brain stem. **A,** In the ventral aspect of the midbrain, the substantia nigra is composed of the reticulata (SNr), which resembles basal ganglia histologically, and the compacta (SNc), which contains a high density of large pigmented dopaminergic neurons. Ventral to the SNr is the cerebral peduncle (CP). **B,** The locus ceruleus (LC) is located in the pontine tegmentum, immediately ventral to the fourth ventricle, whereas the raphe nuclei (RN) are located at multiple brain stem levels near the midline. The medial lemniscus (ML) is located just off the midline at this level in the pons. **C,** The base of the pons contains numerous prominent pontine crossing fibers (*arrow*) that intertwine with the pontine nuclei (*asterisk*) and descending fibers, including the cortical spinal tracts (*arrowhead*, Luxol fast blue stain). **D,** The medulla contains the ventrally located medullary pyramids (MP), which house the descending corticospinal tracts. Lateral and dorsal to the MP is the inferior olivary nucleus (IO), which like the related dentate nucleus in the cerebellum, is made of a thin ribbon of undulating gray matter surrounding a white matter hilum (Luxol fast blue/periodic acid–Schiff stain). The medial lemniscus (ML) is located ventrally along the midline in the medulla.

are located in the dorsal tegmentum in the vicinity of the fourth ventricle. Motor nuclei are located medially, sensory nuclei are located laterally, and autonomic nuclei are found between them.

MIDBRAIN

At the most ventral aspect of the midbrain are the large cerebral peduncles, dense white matter bundles on either side composed predominantly of inferiorly projecting corticospinal and corticopontine fibers. Immediately dorsal is the substantia nigra (SN), a thin strip that extends laterally and dorsally from the midline (see Figs. 1-6 and 1-23). The SN is conventionally divided into two

compartments based on input, projections, and neuronal populations. The pars reticulata (SNr) is located ventrally, nearest the cerebral peduncle, and has histologic and functional similarity to the internal globus pallidus. The SNr contains mostly nonpigmented neurons. The pars compacta (SNc) is located more dorsally and contains a high density of large, heavily pigmented dopaminergic neurons that give rise to fibers that terminate mostly in the striatum (nigrostriatal pathway). In the midline between the right and left SN is the ventral tegmental area, which houses a functionally discreet population of pigmented dopaminergic neurons that project mostly to the cerebral cortex and limbic structures (mesocortical and mesolimbic pathways). The red nuclei are paired, round gray matter structures dorsal to the SN in the rostral midbrain. Around the ependymal-lined cerebral aqueduct is the periaqueductal gray matter, a collection of neurons involved in pain modulation. The midbrain tectum is almost entirely composed of inferior and superior colliculi, whereas the tegmentum contains predominantly white matter structures, including cerebellar projections, the medial longitudinal fasciculus, spinothalamic tracts, and the medial lemniscus.

PONS

The pons is dominated by its large base (basal pons or basis pontis) and by its large white matter connections to the cerebellum—the superior, middle, and inferior cerebellar peduncles. The basal pons consists of both transversely and longitudinally oriented white matter tracts (see Figs. 1-6 and 1-23). The majority of the longitudinal fibers are corticospinal tracts that continue as the medullary pyramids, but a smaller subset are corticopontine tracts that terminate on the interspersed pontine nuclei. The eye-catching transverse fibers represent white matter bundles arising from the pontine nuclei, crossing the midline, and entering the cerebellum via the middle cerebellar peduncle. Additional pontine white matter tracts are located more dorsally and include the spinothalamic tract, medial lemniscus, and medial longitudinal fasciculus. Near the fourth ventricle on each side of the pons is the locus ceruleus ("blue spot"), a small nucleus containing a high density of pigmented, noradrenergic neurons that project diffusely throughout the CNS. Near the midline throughout the brain stem but concentrated mostly in the dorsal pons are the midline raphe nuclei (midline "seam.") These nuclei contain large serotonergic neurons that project extensively throughout the brain.

MEDULLA

Anterior in the medulla are the paired medullary pyramids, which carry most of the fibers of the corticospinal tracts to their place of decussation at the medullary-spinal junction and then continue as the lateral corticospinal tracts in the spinal cord (see Figs. 1-6 and 1-23). Posterior to the pyramids in the midline is the medial lemniscus, a white matter tract projecting from the contralateral nucleus cuneatus and gracilis. More lateral in the rostral medulla are the dominant olivary nuclei, seen as bulges (olives) on the anterolateral medullary surface. Theses ovoid structures consist of a ribbon of convoluted gray matter with large pyramidal-type neurons surrounding a hilus of outwardly projecting white matter tracts that extend to the contralateral cerebellar peduncle. The olivary nucleus is developmentally and functionally related to the cerebellar dentate nucleus and bears resemblance to it histologically. Posteriorly, the fasciculus gracilis and cuneatus are continuations of the posterior columns and terminate in the nucleus gracilis and cuneatus, respectively. Fibers leaving these two nuclei for the medial lemniscus, combined with fibers leaving the inferior olive for the cerebellum, form the internal arcuate fibers that can be seen crossing through the reticular formation in the medulla. The medial longitudinal fasciculus is a white matter tract that rides the midline dorsally, whereas the spinothalamic tract maintains its anterolateral position in the brain stem, immediately dorsal to the olive in the medulla.

SPINAL CORD

The spinal cord has the same basic histologic organization throughout its length, with unique features superimposed at specific spinal levels (Fig. 1-24; see also Fig. 1-7). On cross section the cord contains central gray matter in the shape of an H and surrounding white matter tracts. The white matter tracts are functionally diverse and precisely organized in terms of sensory and motor function. Nonetheless, they are fairly uniform in histologic cross section and show mostly bundles of myelinated and unmyelinated fibers traveling in the superior-inferior direction with scattered oligodendrocytes and fibrillary astrocytes (see earlier). The anterior horns are the ventral extensions of the H-shaped gray matter. These structures contain the large anterior horn cells (lower motor neurons), as well as interspersed smaller gamma motor neurons, which innervate muscle spindles. The anterior horns are the largest and contain the most lower motor neurons at the cervical and lumbar enlargements because of their output to the arms and legs. The posterior horn contains large projection neurons and smaller interneurons. The substantia gelatinosa is a posteriorly located portion of the posterior horn that is distinguished by its lack of myelinated fibers, thus giving rise to its pale appearance. It continues dorsally into Lissauer's tract, another poorly myelinated region of white matter.

The gray matter region between the anterior and posterior horns contains cells of the autonomic nervous system. Located between levels T1 and L3 is the intermediolateral cell column, which extends off the central gray matter as a lateral horn. It contains the cell bodies of preganglionic sympathetic neurons, which project out through the ventral roots. The intermediate zone from S2 to S4 contains a mostly parasympathetic neuronal population. Finally, Clarke's nucleus is a medial extension of the intermediate gray matter found from spinal levels T1 to L2. It contains large neurons important for sensory processing with the cerebellum.

MENINGES

The dura mater has a histologic appearance unlike any other region of the nervous system (Fig. 1-25; see also Fig. 1-1). It consists of a thick, monotonous layer of dense fibrous connective tissue composed mostly of layered collagen with only scattered interspersed flattened

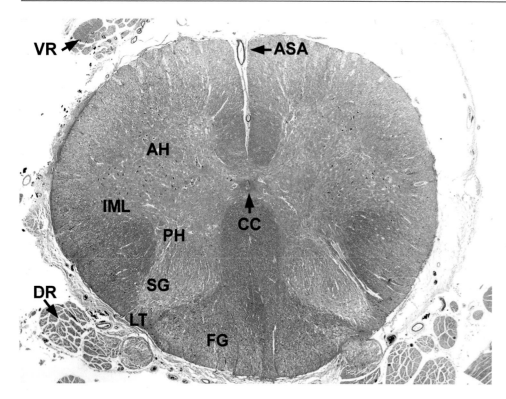

FIGURE 1-24

Spinal cord. A cross section of the thoracic spinal cord shows anterior horns (AH), posterior horns (PH), intermediolateral cell columns (IML), the ependymal-lined central canal (CC [*arrow*]), the substantia gelatinosa (SG), Lissauer's tract (LT), the fasciculus gracilis (FG) of the dorsal columns, the anterior spinal artery (ASA [*arrow*]), ventral roots (VR [*arrow*]), and dorsal roots (DR [*arrow*]).

fibroblasts. Because its appearance is so reliable, identification of it within a histologic section ensures the pathologist that the location of the surgically sampled lesion was peripheral and near the dural covering. The arachnoid membranes that traverse the space between the dura and underlying brain contain the arachnoid trabeculae, a delicate meshwork of thin connective tissue containing flattened fibroblast-like cells, scattered meningothelial cells, and rare melanocytes. The most superficial layer of cells forms a continuous lining that is tethered to the overlying dura and serves as a restrictive barrier to the flow of fluids between the subarachnoid and subdural spaces. The pial layer is found on the surface of the brain as a delicate fibrous coating that is slightly eosinophilic in comparison to the underlying cortex and contains only rare small flattened cells. It extends peripherally and fuses with the overlying arachnoid trabeculae to form a continuous pia-arachnoid network.

PERIPHERAL NERVE, SCHWANN CELLS, AND DORSAL ROOT GANGLIA

Within millimeters of their exit from the CNS, both cranial nerves and spinal nerve roots transition from a central to a peripheral nerve morphology and myelinating pattern (with the exception of CN VIII, which transitions at the internal auditory meatus). Schwann cells are the glial cells of the peripheral nervous system that provide an insulating coat of myelin around axons to improve conduction speed (Fig. 1-26). Together

with peripheral nerve fibroblasts and the collagen-rich network of endoneurium, perineurium, and epineurium, Schwann cells provide structural support to their underlying axonal processes (see Chapter 11 for a more detailed discussion of peripheral nerves). In contrast to oligodendrocytes, the myelin-rich cytoplasm of a single Schwann cell is flattened and concentrically laminated around a segment of a large axon at specific intervals between the nodes of Ranvier. Schwann cells also provide support to unmyelinated axons within peripheral nerves, but in this case numerous smaller axons are enveloped by individual Schwann cells and do not have laminated myelin sheaths. In standard hematoxylin-eosin–stained tissue sections, Schwann cells are the most numerous cell body within peripheral nerves and are seen in longitudinal section as elongated spindled cells containing cigar-shaped hyperchromatic nuclei. On cross section of nerve, their myelin-rich coating is seen as a clear donut-shaped ring around a central tiny eosinophilic axon. Stains for myelin (Luxol fast blue) dramatically improve the visibility of the myelin sheath.

Dorsal root ganglia are located near the spinal exit foramina, are invested within a dural sheath, and are the home of the cell bodies for the spinal afferent sensory neurons. Individual cell bodies are large, with abundant cytoplasm and Nissl substance, prominent vesicular nuclei, and large nucleoli. Peripheral extensions terminate in transducing sensory receptors that give rise to incoming signals. Large, long processes extend centrally via the dorsal roots into the spinal cord, with the largest myelinated tracts becoming the ascending posterior columns. Around the perimeter of each ganglion cell body are flattened satellite cells (specialized Schwann cells) that most likely serve a support role and

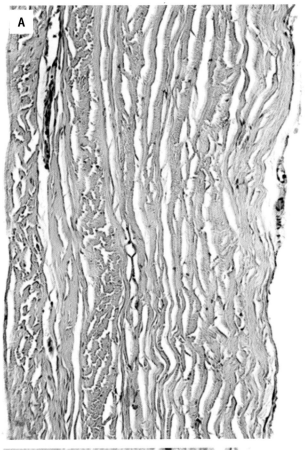

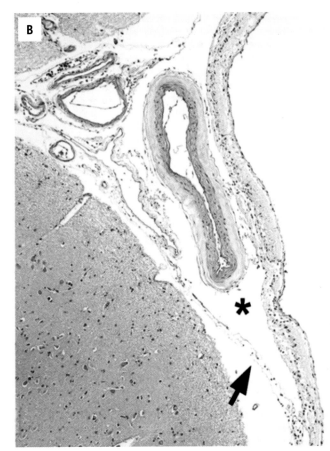

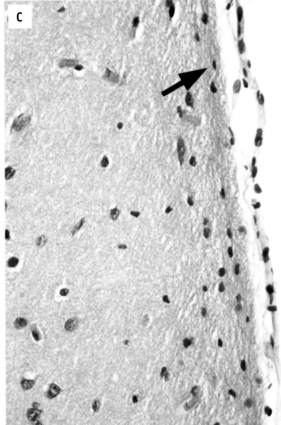

FIGURE 1-25

Meninges. **A**, The dura mater is a thick, dense, fibrous connective tissue covering for the brain with low cellularity. **B**, Arachnoid membranes are delicate fibrous bands (*arrow*) that traverse the subarachnoid space (*asterisk*), embed subarachnoid vessels, and have attachments to both the underlying pia and overlying dura. **C**, The pia mater (*arrow*) is a thin, fine coating on the surface of the brain that is brightly eosinophilic and merges with the arachnoid.

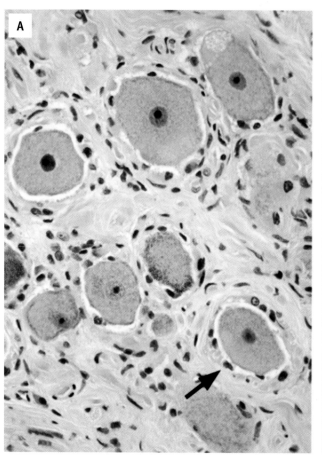

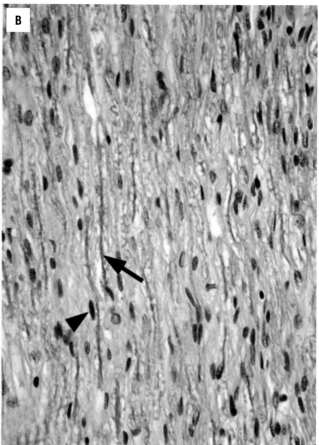

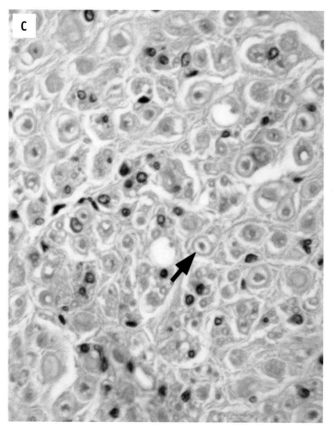

FIGURE 1-26

Dorsal root ganglia and peripheral nerve. **A**, Each large neuronal cell body (ganglion cell) of the dorsal root ganglion is surrounded by satellite cells, a specialized Schwann cell population (*arrow*). **B**, Peripheral nerve contains longitudinally oriented axons (*arrow*) that are only barely visible within their thicker, clear myelin sheath. Schwann cells have elongated nuclei with slightly bulbous ends and are oriented along the length of the axon to provide its myelination (*arrowhead*). **C**, On transverse section of peripheral nerve, a clear ring of bubbly myelin is seen surrounding a central zone occupied by the axon (*arrow*).

provide a committed stem cell source for repopulation of their more peripheral progeny.

FEATURES OF INFANCY AND CHILDHOOD

The size and surface complexity of the brain increase tremendously throughout the prenatal period. From midterm to full-term gestation, the brain increases from 60 to 400 g. The first major hemispheric subdivision, the sylvian fissure, does not develop until the 14th week, and the process continues at a rapid pace until the hemispheres are nearly completely gyrated by 32 weeks.

Tables in major textbooks of pediatric pathology categorize the brain by age as it relates to weight and surface convolutions.

The germinal matrix is a stem cell population that is adjacent to the lateral ventricles as a subependymal layer and gives rise to sequentially differentiated neuronal and glial precursors that migrate to their homes in the cerebrum (Fig. 1-27). The germinal matrix is prominent in early brain development and does not begin to thin out until the 26th week of gestation. The matrix persists as scattered cell islands and perivascular nests until term. After birth, most of the germinal matrix disappears except for a portion called the ganglionic eminence, which is located between the thalamus and caudate. It fragments and diminishes in size throughout the first year of life.

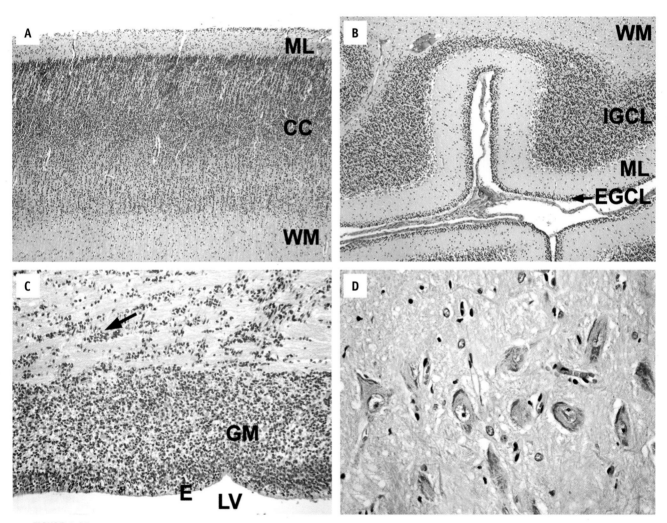

FIGURE 1-27

Features of development and infancy. **A,** The cerebral cortex undergoes gradual lamination during fetal development, with individual layers emerging in the fifth month of gestation. The cortex of a 30-week-gestation fetus shows a clearly formed molecular layer (ML), initial separation of the cerebrocortical layers (CC), and demarcation of the cortex from white matter (WM). **B,** The fetal and infant cerebellum contains an external granular cell layer (EGCL, *arrow*), a precursor cell population that migrates inward through the molecular layer (ML) to form the internal granular cell layer (IGCL) (cerebellum of a 6-week-old infant). **C,** The germinal matrix (GM) is a periventricular precursor cell population located directly adjacent to the ependyma (E) of the lateral ventricles (LV). Although heavily populated by neural precursors during fetal development, it diminishes and eventually disappears in the first year of postnatal life (germinal matrix of a 20-week-gestation fetus). Clusters of neuroblasts are noted migrating outward (*arrow*). **D,** The substantia nigra is not pigmented at birth and only slowly accumulates neuromelanin over the first 5 years of life (substantia nigra of a 3-year-old child).

The cerebral cortex is derived from neuroblasts that migrate outwardly along radial glia from the germinal matrix. The innermost neurons of the cortex are the first to arrive and are subsequently joined by neuroblasts migrating to progressively more superficial regions. By the fifth month, the cortex shows a superficial molecular layer and a deeper, densely cellular band. From the latter, a six-layered cortex gradually emerges starting in the sixth month. Cortical layering results from maturation of the cortical laminar neurons, selective cell death of neuronal populations, and expansion of the neuropil as a result of the growth of dendritic fields.

The process of axonal maturation and myelination within the CNS is not complete at birth. On gross examination of the fetal or infant brain, this lack of complete myelination results in a brain that is more gelatinous, does not fix as well, and has less demarcated borders between gray and white matter structures. Axon diameters and myelin sheaths continue to develop over the first 2 years of life. Many suggest that brain myelination continues into adolescence and may not be complete until adulthood.

Cerebellar cortical development occurs along two major pathways. Purkinje cells form early in embryonic life after migrating to their final location from the alar plate. Granular cells develop from the rhombic lip. They first form a precursor population as the external granular cell layer, which is located at the surface of the cerebellar folia, superficial to the molecular cell layer. External granular cells are actively dividing and give rise to inwardly migrating cells that form the internal granular cell layer—the granular cell population that persists in adulthood. Although the external granular cell layer begins to diminish at 2 to 3 months after birth, it does not totally disappear until 12 months.

The pigmented nuclei of the brain stem, the substantia nigra and locus ceruleus, do not contain visible neuromelanin at birth. Thus, gross examination of the brain stem should not reveal pigmented areas in the midbrain or pons. Pigmentation of these brain stem nuclei occurs gradually throughout the first 5 years of life as oxidized neuromelanin accumulates.

During the first 3 months of fetal life the spinal cord and dural sac are the same length. After this period, spinal cord growth slows in comparison, which results in a spinal cord that is shorter than its dural covering. By birth the cord ends at about L3, and at 2 months of life the cord ends at its mature level between L1 and L2. Consequently, most lumbar and sacral spinal roots travel inferiorly to exit their vertebral foramina and thus form the cauda equina inferior to the spinal cord.

NORMAL AGING AND COMMON ARTIFACTS

Some of the most confusing aspects of diagnostic neuropathology can involve distinguishing the histopathologic features of disease from those of the normal aging process (Table 1-3; Figs. 1-28 through 1-30). This problem is compounded by the fact that some findings are

---

TABLE 1-3
Nonpathologic Features of Normal Aging*

NEURONS

Neurofibrillary tangles

Granulovacuolar degeneration

Hirano bodies

Senile amyloid plaques

Ferrugination

Marinesco bodies

Lipofuscin accumulation

Pigment incontinence of substantia nigra

GLIA

Corpora amylacea adjacent to ependyma, brain surface, and
    vasculature

MENINGES

Fibrous thickening

Hyaline plaques

Arachnoid granulation collagenization (pacchionian bodies)

Meningothelial proliferation

Psammoma body formation

PITUITARY GLAND

Squamous cell metaplasia of pars tuberalis

Adenohypophyseal fibrosis

Glandular hyperplasia of pregnancy

OTHER

Perivascular mineralization, globus pallidus

Micronodular mineralization, globus pallidus and
    hippocampal molecular layer

Choroid plexus mineralization and cystic change

Pineal mineralization and cystic change

Hyaline sclerosis of vessels

Perivascular space enlargement

---

*See Figures 1-28 through 1-30.

---

present in both disease and normal aging, with only the clinical context and degree of change serving to distinguish them. For example, small amounts of neurofibrillary pathology, senile plaques, and other neurodegenerative changes can be part of the normal aging process. In the setting of clinical dementia, these pathologic findings in sufficient degree are used to establish the diagnosis of Alzheimer's disease.

Other causes of "diagnostic head-scratching" are the artifacts introduced into histologic sections as a result of tissue degeneration, tissue handling, inadequate fixation, and tangential sectioning (Table 1-4; Fig. 1-31). Only awareness of these common artifacts prevents their misinterpretation as disease.

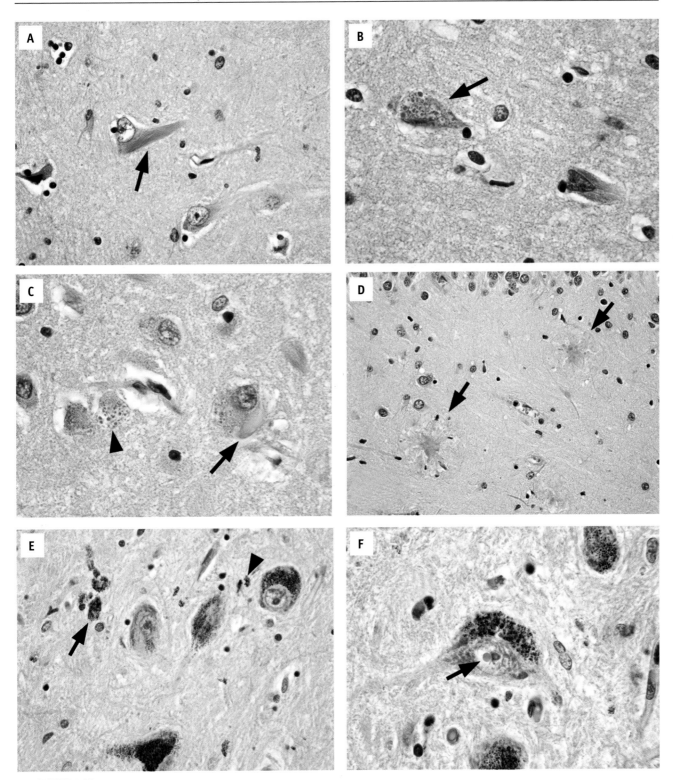

FIGURE 1-28

Findings of normal aging. **A**, Neurofibrillary tangles are slightly basophilic, crystalline inclusions that fill the neuronal cytoplasm, generally taking the shape of a flame (*arrow*). **B**, Granulovacuolar degeneration consists of small cytoplasmic vacuoles and basophilic granules and is noted most often in the hippocampal pyramidal cells of elderly individuals (*arrow*). **C**, In addition to granulovacuolar degeneration (*arrowhead*), these neurons will occasionally show Hirano bodies (*arrow*), eosinophilic, rod-shaped or ovoid cytoplasmic inclusions that often extend out of the cell into the neuropil. **D**, Amyloid plaques represent the extracellular accumulation of β-amyloid that is deposited in the normal aging process. Plaques can be diffuse, in which case they are difficult to identify without silver stains, or can contain amyloid cores, which stand out as central, brightly eosinophilic protein accumulations with hematoxylin-eosin staining (*arrows*). **E**, Pigment derived from cells in the substantia nigra and locus ceruleus is sometimes noted free in the neuropil (*arrowhead*) or engulfed within macrophage cytoplasm (*arrow*), findings called "pigment incontinence." **F**, The small eosinophilic intranuclear inclusions of the aging substantia nigra neurons are Marinesco bodies (*arrow*).

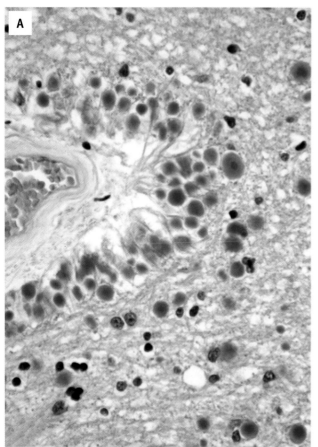

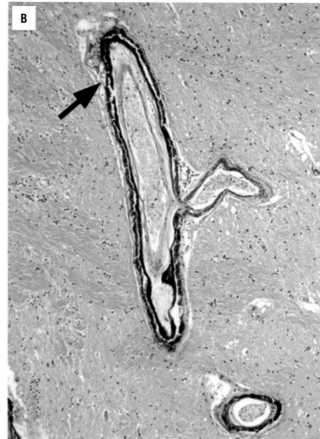

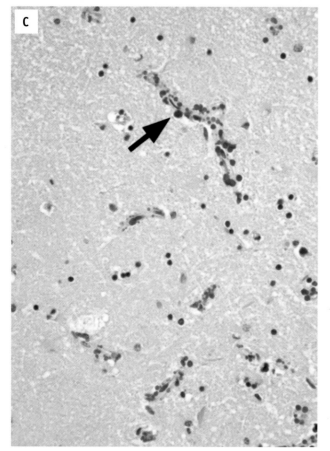

FIGURE 1-29

Findings of aging. **A**, Corpora amylacea are spherical basophilic polyglucosan bodies that accumulate as astrocytic inclusions during the aging process. Their highest density is around blood vessels, under the pial surface, and adjacent to the ventricles—locations where astrocytic foot processes are most common. **B**, These eye-catching laminated bodies are not always recognized as being intracellular and can accumulate to striking densities during aging. Perivascular mineralization of the large vessels of the globus pallidus is a normal aging process and can begin as early as childhood (*arrow*). **C**, Micronodular mineralization also occurs with increasing age and is seen most frequently in the hippocampus and the basal ganglia (*arrow*).

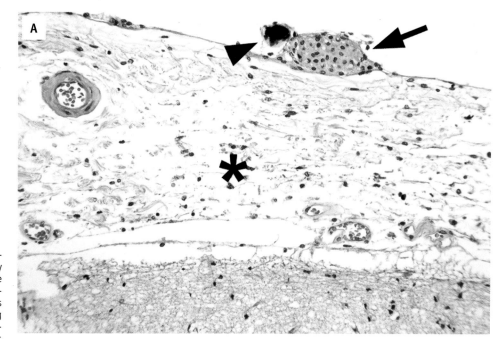

FIGURE 1-30

Aging of the meninges. **A**, The arachnoid membranes become slightly thickened and fibrous with age (*asterisk*). Both meningothelial clusters (*arrow*) and psammoma bodies (*arrowhead*) are seen with increasing frequency in the arachnoid membranes with age. **B**, Fibrous plaques (*arrow*) are a thick, densely hyalinized form of fibrosis that occurs in the most superficial layer of the arachnoid membranes (*asterisk*). They are noted most often over the median aspects of the superior frontal and parietal lobes and covering the spinal cord.

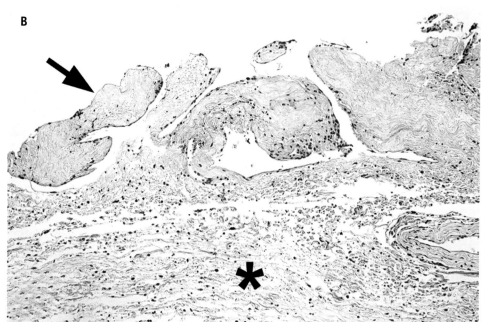

TABLE 1-4

Common Artifacts in Neuropathology*

Artifact	Mistaken for
"Bone dust" from skull removal/craniotomy*	Calcification
Neuronal shrinking from delayed fixation*	Neuronal ischemia
Pericellular halos from delayed fixation*	Neuronal ischemia/oligodendroglioma
Normal cortex in tangential section	Hypercellular brain/infiltrating neoplasm
"Swiss cheese brain" from prolonged postmortem/bacterial gases	Multiple cavitary lesions
Cerebellar granular cell conglutination from prolonged postmortem time*	Cerebellar degeneration
Tangential sectioning of the ventricular lining*	Hamartoma or ependymal rest

*See Figure 1-31.

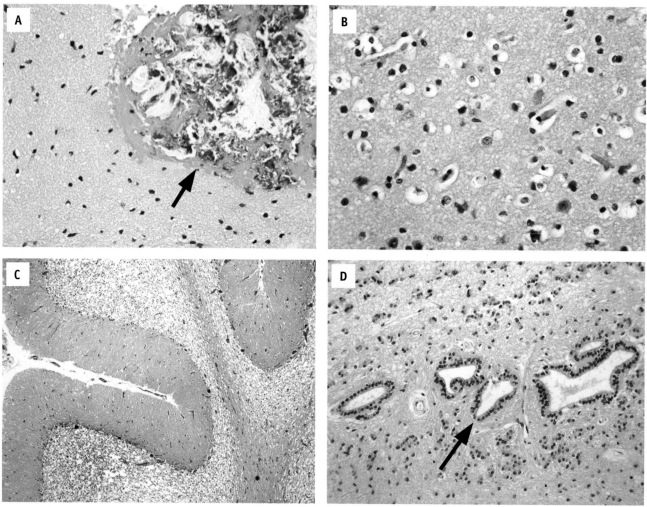

FIGURE 1-31

Common artifacts. **A**, "Bone dust" (*arrow*) from a craniotomy, bur hole, or skull removal can become embedded within brain parenchyma and be mistaken for calcification. **B**, Delayed or poor fixation can result in exaggerated perinuclear halos around oligodendrocytes, as well as neurons. **C**, Delayed fixation of the cerebellum results in nearly complete disappearance of the granular cell layer, known as granular cell conglutination. **D**, In the periventricular region, outpouchings of the ventricles can be seen as ependymal-lined spaces, which should not be confused with rests or hamartomas (*arrow*).

SUGGESTED READINGS

Friede RL: Developmental Neuropathology, 2nd ed. Berlin, Springer-Verlag, 1989.

Fuller GN, Burger PC: Central nervous system. In Sternberg SS (ed): Histology for Pathologists, 2nd ed. Philadelphia, Lippincott-Raven, 1997.

Graham DI, Lantos PL: Greenfield's Neuropathology, 7th ed. London, Arnold Publishers, 2002.

Kandel ER, Schwartz JH, Jessell TM: Principles of Neural Science, 4th ed. New York, McGraw-Hill, 2000.

Nelson JS, Mena H, Parisi JE, Schochet SS: Principles and Practice of Neuropathology, 2nd ed. New York, Oxford University Press, 2003.

Netter FH: The CIBA Collection of Medical Illustrations, vol 1, Nervous System, part 1, Anatomy and Physiology. West Caldwell, NJ, CIBA Pharmaceutical, 1991.

Nolte J: The Human Brain: An Introduction to Its Functional Anatomy, 5th ed. St Louis, CV Mosby, 2002.

2 Vascular Disease

Anthony T. Yachnis

Cerebrovascular disease ranks third behind heart disease and cancer as a cause of death in the United States and Europe. The terms "stroke," "brain attack," and "cerebrovascular accident" refer to an acute, nonepileptic alteration in neurologic status that lasts more than 24 hours and correlates with a sudden disruption in blood flow to a focal area of the brain. This can occur in two basic ways, both related to blood vessel pathology: (1) obstructed or stenotic blood vessels deprive the brain of oxygen and nutrients or (2) hemorrhage of diseased vessels may cause tissue destruction and oxygen deprivation.

This chapter begins with a review of brain pathology resulting from diffuse reductions in blood flow or oxygenation, followed by a survey of nervous system vascular diseases that are related to stroke.

CAUSES OF REDUCED BLOOD FLOW OR OXYGENATION

CEREBRAL HYPOXIA-ISCHEMIA

PATHOPHYSIOLOGIC AND REGIONAL CONSIDERATIONS

The brain receives about 15% of the total cardiac output and accounts for about 20% of the body's oxygen consumption. Neurons are absolutely dependent on a constant supply of oxygen for proper function. Any systemic or central nervous system (CNS) process that reduces the oxygen supply to some or all of the brain will interfere with the function of this vital organ and, when severe enough, can cause the death of brain cells (the most vulnerable being neurons). Anoxia refers to the absence of oxygen, whereas hypoxia describes a reduced concentration of oxygen. The term "hypoxia" tends to be more widely used because it encompasses a range of reduced oxygen concentrations that may be encountered clinically. Ischemia is defined as absence of blood flow, whereas oligemia connotes reduced flow.

Hypoxia-ischemia may affect the brain in a diffuse (or global) fashion as with cardiac arrest, shock, or severe hypotension. In contrast, focal hypoxia-ischemia results from a loss or marked reduction of blood flow to circumscribed areas of the brain. The latter occurs with

---

CEREBRAL HYPOXIA-ISCHEMIA: LOCATION AND PATHOPHYSIOLOGY—FACT SHEET

Regional Distribution of Lesions
- ▶ Diffuse (global): for example, cardiac arrest, shock, severe hypotension
- ▶ Focal: for example, cerebral infarction in a vascular territory

Types of Cerebral Hypoxia
- ▶ Stagnant hypoxia: decreased blood flow
  - ▶ Ischemic hypoxia (no flow)
  - ▶ Oligemic hypoxia (reduced flow)
- ▶ Hypoxic hypoxia: reduced blood oxygen content (cardiopulmonary disease)
- ▶ Anemic hypoxia: reduced oxygen-carrying capacity (CO poisoning)
- ▶ Histotoxic hypoxia: inability of tissues to use oxygen (cyanide poisoning)
- ▶ Hypoglycemic hypoxia: decreased ability to metabolize oxygen under conditions of reduced blood glucose

Selective Vulnerability of Neural Cell Types to Hypoxic-Ischemic Injury
- ▶ Neurons > oligodendrocytes > astrocytes > endothelial cells (most vulnerable) (least vulnerable)
- ▶ Most sensitive neuronal populations
  - ▶ Hippocampal pyramidal cells of Sommer's sector (area CA1)
  - ▶ Purkinje cells (cerebellar cortex)
  - ▶ Neurons of cortical layers III, V, and VI

---

thromboembolic occlusion of cerebral blood vessels (i.e., cerebral infarction in a vascular territory). Clinical characteristics of cerebral hypoxia-ischemia vary widely depending on the severity and duration of hypoxia, the size of the lesion, whether brain involvement is diffuse or focal, and the availability of collateral circulation.

A practical classification of the pathophysiologic types of cerebral hypoxia is as follows. Stagnant hypoxia includes conditions in which there is no flow ("ischemic hypoxia") or significantly reduced flow ("oligemic hypoxia"). "Hypoxic hypoxia" refers to the reduced blood oxygen content that may result from pulmonary disease or conditions that lead to reduced oxygen-carrying capacity of the blood ("anemic hypoxia"). Cyanide poisoning, which prevents cells from using oxygen to produce adenosine triphosphate, is an example of "histotoxic hypoxia." "Hypoglycemic hypoxia" refers to a reduced ability of the brain to use oxygen in conditions of low blood glucose.

Perhaps the most common clinical scenario associated with diffuse or global cerebral hypoxia occurs in survivors of acute cardiopulmonary arrest who have acute hypotension or hypoperfusion (a combination of stagnant and hypoxic anoxia). Consequently, the term "hypoxia-ischemia" or "hypoxic-ischemic encephalopathy" is used to reflect reduced blood oxygen content as well as reduced blood flow. Other important causes include drug overdose, birth injury, shock, and carbon monoxide (CO) poisoning.

PATHOLOGIC FEATURES

In the acute stage of diffuse (global) hypoxia-ischemia, the brain will appear congested and dusky (Fig. 2-1). There is diffuse cerebral swelling with gyral widening and sulcal narrowing as a result of the cytotoxic effect of oxygen deprivation on neurons, which lose the ability to regulate ions, accumulate water, and swell ("cytotoxic edema"). The border zones or "end-artery" regions of supply between the anterior, middle, and posterior cerebral arteries in the cerebrum and those of the vertebrobasilar regions of supply in the brain stem and cerebellum are preferentially affected. The patchy areas of softening and discoloration that occur in such border zones are referred to as "watershed infarcts" (Fig. 2-2).

Brain cells differ in their susceptibility to hypoxia. Neurons are most sensitive, followed by oligodendrocytes, astrocytes, and endothelial cells. In addition, subtypes of neurons display a striking selective vulnerability to hypoxia. The most sensitive neurons in adults are the pyramidal cells in area CA1 of the hippocampus ("Sommer's sector") (Fig. 2-3) and the Purkinje cells of the cerebellum. In relatively mild hypoxic injury, only

---

CEREBRAL HYPOXIA-ISCHEMIA, DIFFUSE— PATHOLOGIC FEATURES

Gross Findings

▶ Diffuse brain swelling with widened gyri and narrow sulci
▶ "Watershed" infarction in end-artery regions of the vascular supply
▶ Necrosis of vulnerable regions: CA1 (Sommer's sector), Purkinje cells
▶ Laminar necrosis of the cerebral cortex
▶ "Respirator brain"

Microscopic Findings

▶ Acute changes (12 to 24 hours after significant hypoxia-ischemia): acute neuronal cell change, eosinophilic (ischemic) cell change
▶ Subacute changes (2 days to 2 weeks): appearance of macrophages, capillary proliferation, astrocytes
▶ Chronic changes (months to years): removal of necrotic tissue by macrophages with resulting cavitation (liquefaction necrosis)

---

these two areas of the brain may be affected. With more severe insults, however, laminar necrosis of layers III, V, and VI of the cerebral cortex will occur.

If a patient dies within 12 hours of severe hypoxia, no apparent changes are observed by routine light microscopy. The alterations associated with acute hypoxia-ischemia will first become apparent 12 to 24 hours after significant hypoxia and, at low magnification, consist of pallor and vacuolation of the neuropil. High-magnification study will reveal neuronal shrinkage with cytoplasmic hypereosinophilia and nuclear

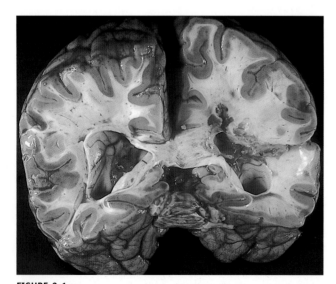

FIGURE 2-1
Diffuse hypoxia-ischemia: diffuse dusky and congested appearance of the cerebral cortex in a patient dying of cardiopulmonary arrest.

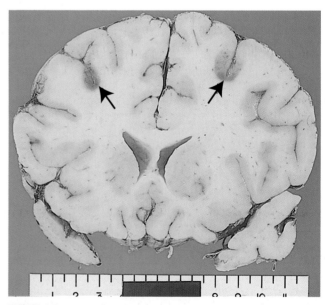

FIGURE 2-2
Border zone (watershed) infarcts: bilateral foci of congestion and softening at the border zones between the anterior and middle cerebral artery regions of supply.

pyknosis (Figs. 2-4 and 2-5). This neuronal reaction has been referred to as ischemic cell change, acute neuronal cell change, eosinophilic cell change, or simply "red dead" neurons. The latter indicates that irreversible damage has occurred. Eosinophilic neurons may persist for several days after an acute hypoxic-ischemic event.

In the days to weeks after severe hypoxia (defined as the subacute period), macrophages enter the lesion to engulf necrotic tissue. Capillaries proliferate and hypertrophic (reactive) astrocytes become prominent in residual brain tissue. Removal of necrotic debris by macrophages ultimately results in cavitation of cortical layers II to VI with sparing of the subpial layer and per-

sistence of thread-like capillaries. Macrophages may persist in the resulting cavity for years after the original event. The formation of a cavity in the region of severe hypoxia-ischemia is referred to as "complete liquefaction necrosis," whereas necrosis of the most vulnerable population of cells (the neurons) with sparing of astrocytes and other cellular elements of the neuropil is called "incomplete necrosis."

Prolonged severe hypoperfusion results in widespread cerebral cortical necrosis. However, other organ systems may continue to function with the support of mechanical ventilation. Under such conditions the brain will undergo autolysis at body temperature ("intravitum" autolysis). The dusky necrotic appearance of the entire cerebrum has been referred to as "respirator brain." Such patients may survive for prolonged periods in a persistent vegetative state and display the clinical characteristics of brain death, including absent reflexes, absent respiratory drive, and an isoelectric electroencephalogram. The brain exhibits extensive cavitary necrosis of the cerebral cortex and deep nuclear structures with compensatory ventricular dilatation because of the loss of brain substance ("ex vacuo hydrocephalus") (Fig. 2-6).

CO poisoning represents a toxic insult that results in decreased oxygen-carrying capacity of the blood (anemic hypoxia). The affinity with which CO binds to hemoglobin is about 100-fold more than oxygen, thus making the latter less available to tissues. If death occurs acutely, the high concentration of carboxyhemoglobin produces a bright red color to the tissues. Edema may also be seen for several days after the insult as a manifestation of diffuse hypoxia. In patients who die in the subacute or chronic state, CO poisoning produces a

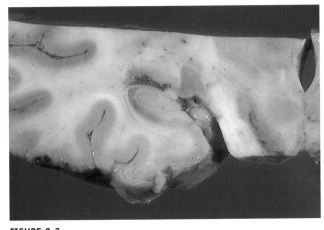

FIGURE 2-3

Acute hippocampal necrosis: dusky discoloration and softening in the region of Sommer's sector (area CA1) of the hippocampus. (Courtesy of Dr. Richard A. Prayson.)

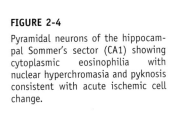

FIGURE 2-4

Pyramidal neurons of the hippocampal Sommer's sector (CA1) showing cytoplasmic eosinophilia with nuclear hyperchromasia and pyknosis consistent with acute ischemic cell change.

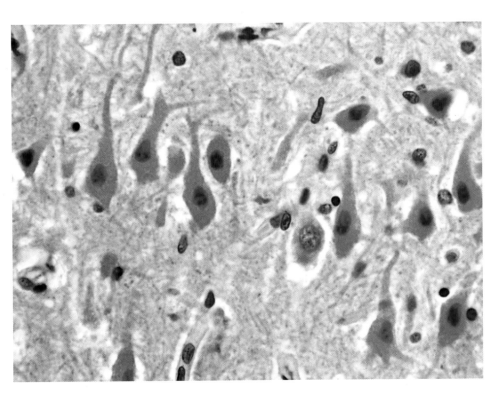

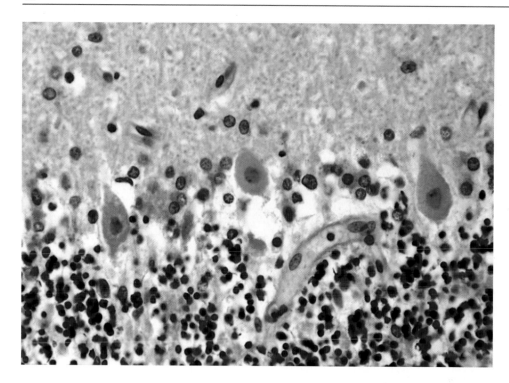

FIGURE 2-5
Cerebellar Purkinje cells with acute ischemic (eosinophilic) cell change.

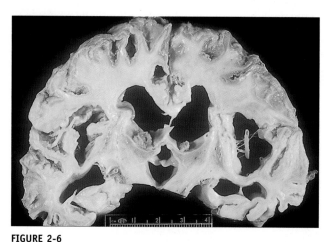

FIGURE 2-6
Widespread cerebral necrosis with cavitation of gray matter structures and "ex vacuo" hydrocephalus in a patient who survived 2 years after an episode of severe diffuse hypoxia. (Courtesy of Dr. Elizabeth Rushing.)

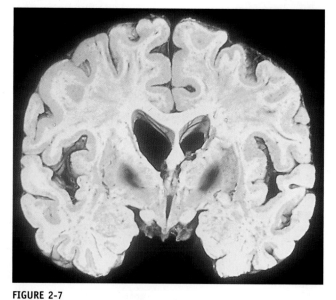

FIGURE 2-7
Bilateral necrosis of the globus pallidus in a case of carbon monoxide poisoning. (Courtesy of Dr. Richard A. Prayson.)

characteristic pattern of bilateral cystic necrosis of the globus pallidus (Fig. 2-7). Multifocal, patchy white matter demyelination and destruction may also occur ("Grinker's myelinopathy").

CEREBRAL INFARCTION

CLINICAL FEATURES

A cerebral infarct is defined as a circumscribed focus or area of brain tissue that dies as a result of localized hypoxia-ischemia caused by cessation of blood flow. The onset of an infarct is sudden, and the spectrum of acute neurologic signs and symptoms depends on the amount of brain compromised, the location of the lesion, the duration of reduced flow, the status of the collateral circulation, and the intrinsic vulnerability of brain cells. In contrast to arterial border zone infarcts caused by diffuse brain ischemia, infarcts resulting from embolization or intrinsic cerebrovascular disease occur in circumscribed vascular territories within the distributions of major cerebral arteries.

CEREBRAL INFARCTION—FACT SHEET

Definition

▶ A circumscribed focus or area of brain tissue that was rendered nonviable as a result of localized hypoxia-ischemia from cessation of blood flow

Incidence and Location

▶ Accounts for 70% of all strokes
▶ Incidence: 70 per 100,000 persons between the ages of 45 and 55 years; 2 per 100 persons 85 years or older
▶ Location: well-defined vascular territories of the major cerebral blood vessels

Gender and Risk Factors

▶ Male > Female (highly dependent on risk factors)
▶ Risk factors: diabetes, hypertension, smoking, family history, hyperlipidemia, obesity

Clinical Features

▶ Highly variable depending on
  ▶ Amount of brain compromised
  ▶ Location of the lesion
  ▶ Duration of reduced flow
  ▶ Status of collateral circulation
  ▶ Intrinsic vulnerability of brain cells

Prognosis and Treatment

▶ Significant reduction in mortality with early diagnosis and thrombolytic therapy
▶ Aspirin and antiplatelet agents reduce risk in susceptible individuals
▶ Control risk factors: blood pressure control in hypertensive patients, reduction of blood lipids, cessation of smoking, regulation of blood glucose in diabetics

In the United States, cerebral infarction is 10 times more common than spontaneous brain hemorrhage. The incidence increases with age, being about 70 per 100,000 between the ages of 45 and 55 and about 2 per 100 in those older than 85 years. Brain infarction accounts for almost 70% of strokes and is more common in men than in women. However, the gender distribution is highly dependent on other risk factors (see later). Almost any neurologic syndrome may be produced, including unilateral hemiplegia, focal aphasia, coma, hemispheric cerebellar ataxia, and visual changes, to name a few.

The main causes of cerebral infarction are atherosclerosis of large vessels or embolic occlusion of distal vessels, or both. Thus, the risk factors for cerebral infarction are the same as those for atherosclerotic cardiovascular disease and include diabetes, hypertension, smoking, family history, hyperlipidemia, and truncal obesity. Chronic hypertension aggravates the atherosclerotic changes in both extracranial and intracranial blood vessels and leads to a more distal arterial distribution of atheromatous changes.

Most infarcts are believed to result from disruption and embolization of platelet thrombi or friable plaque material, or both, with subsequent obstruction of intracranial arteries. Thrombosis may occur in extracranial atherosclerotic blood vessels such as the bifurcation of the carotid artery or within the heart. Occasionally, emboli may arise from calcified, marantic, or infected heart valves. Transient ischemic attacks cause reversible neurologic deficits lasting less than 24 hours and are believed to result from embolization of microscopic plaque material in patients with significant carotid artery disease. Symptoms of a major stroke last more than 24 hours, and the degree of reversibility and the magnitude of residual deficit depend on the location and extent of the lesion.

RADIOGRAPHIC FEATURES

Patients with neurologic signs and symptoms of a stroke are typically evaluated by computed tomography (CT) to determine the extent of the lesion and the amount of mass effect and to exclude the possibility of some other pathology. About 60% of scans are normal during the first few hours after a cerebral infarct. Within 6 to 8 hours of the ictus, the infarcted area becomes hypodense, consistent with focal brain swelling as a result of cytotoxic edema. Enhancement after contrast administration is observed within a week of the event and may persist as long as 2 months. Magnetic resonance imaging (MRI) is performed if there is a discrepancy between the CT findings and the clinical picture or if aggressive thrombolytic therapy is being considered.

PATHOLOGIC FEATURES

Gross changes are not detectable if the patient dies within 6 to 8 hours after an infarct. The first indication of

CEREBRAL INFARCTION—PATHOLOGIC FEATURES

Gross Findings

▶ Acute cerebral infarct: focal swelling and congestion in a well-defined vascular territory
▶ Subacute: circumscribed regions of congestion, softening, and early cavitation with separation of cortex from the underlying white matter
▶ Chronic (remote) infarct: complete cavitation with sparing of the subpial layer of cortex

Microscopic Findings

▶ Acute changes (12 to 24 hours after significant hypoxia-ischemia): tissue pallor with acute neuronal necrosis—eosinophilic (ischemic) cell change
▶ Subacute changes (2 days to 2 weeks): appearance of macrophages, capillary proliferation, and early astrocytic reaction at the lesion edge
▶ Chronic changes (months to years): removal of necrotic tissue by macrophages with resulting cavitation (liquefaction necrosis); residual reactive astrocytes form a gliotic scar at the infarct edges

abnormality is subtle blurring of the gray-white junction and swelling of affected tissues. Within 1 or 2 days of infarction there is congestion with dusky discoloration of the gray matter and slight softening of the tissues. At this time, gross examination reveals a well-circumscribed area of swelling and hyperemia in the gray matter of a well-defined vascular territory (Fig. 2-8). Large acute infarcts may be associated with a significant mass effect and herniation. A combination of focal infarcts in a specific vascular territory and border zone lesions may be present. If little or no reperfusion occurs in an area of ischemia, the infarct is called "bland." However, if reperfusion occurs, as is the case for most embolic infarcts, the area of ischemia will appear hemorrhagic.

With organization of the lesion, macrophages enter the tissue to remove necrotic material. Such removal results in softening and disruption of the tissues and a circumscribed pattern of laminar necrosis in which the cortex appears detached from the underlying white matter (Fig. 2-9). The subpial region of the cortex usually remains intact. With further elimination of necrotic tissue, the cerebral surface becomes depressed and cavitated (Fig. 2-10).

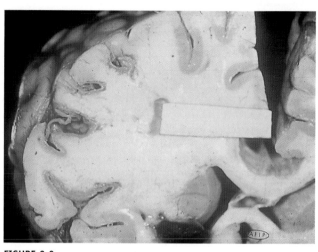

FIGURE 2-9

Organizing cerebral infarct in the middle cerebral artery distribution showing early cavitation and separation of the cortex from the underlying white matter. (Courtesy of Dr. Elizabeth Rushing.)

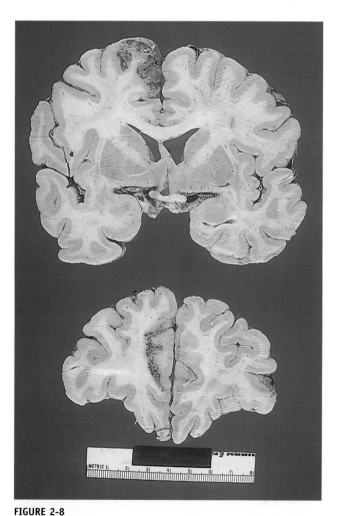

FIGURE 2-8

Recent cerebral infarct manifested as a well-circumscribed focus of hyperemia and softening in the anterior cerebral artery distribution.

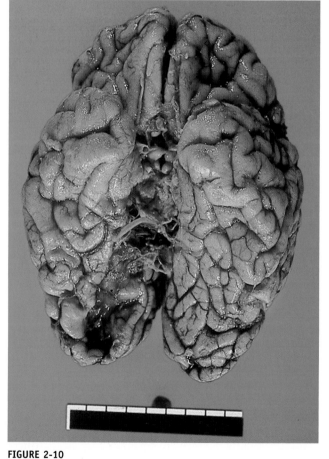

FIGURE 2-10

Cavitated (remote) cerebral infarct in a posterior cerebral artery distribution.

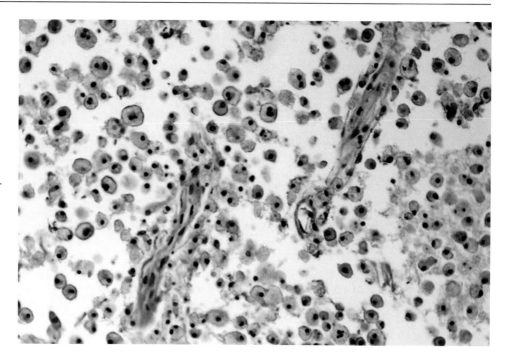

FIGURE 2-11

Organizing cerebral infarct containing foamy macrophages.

The histopathologic changes that occur with acute, subacute, and organized cerebral infarcts are similar to those described earlier for diffuse (global) hypoxia-ischemia. In the acute stage (1 to 4 days), there is pallor of the neuropil with ischemic (eosinophilic) neuronal cell change. During the subacute or organizing stage (5 to 30 days), microglia become transformed to foamy macrophages, which begin to remove necrotic material (Fig. 2-11). Capillary proliferation occurs during the first 2 weeks after infarction. Astrocytic hyperplasia and hypertrophy become apparent at the edges of the lesion a week to 10 days after the insult (Fig. 2-12). In the chronic phase (weeks to years), scattered macrophages, some containing hemosiderin, are found within organized areas of cavitation. Thin strands of residual blood vessels often traverse such areas, and reactive astrocytes are scattered at the lesion edge.

The venous side of the circulation may also undergo thrombosis and cause significant cerebral ischemia. A particularly striking example is thrombosis of the superior sagittal sinus (Fig. 2-13), which can occur with some infections and various hypercoagulation states,

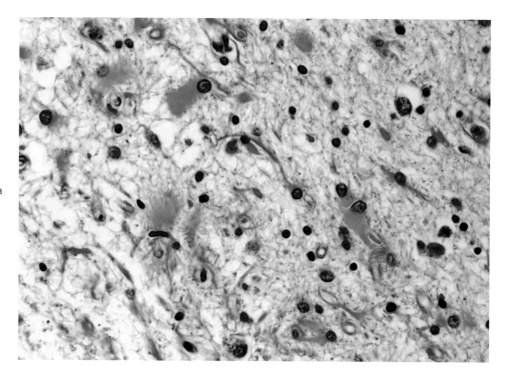

FIGURE 2-12

Reactive astrocytes at the edge of a remote infarct.

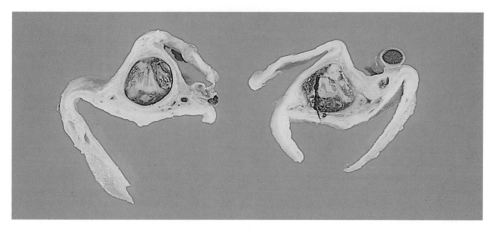

FIGURE 2-13
Superior sagittal sinus thrombosis: cross sections of the superior sagittal sinus containing an organizing thrombus.

including systemic malignancies. Here, venous outflow from superficial veins of the superior median aspect of the cerebral hemispheres is obstructed, thereby resulting in marked congestion and hemorrhagic infarction in this region.

DIFFERENTIAL DIAGNOSIS

A hemorrhagic infarct may be difficult to distinguish from a primary brain hemorrhage. Occasionally, a glioma that diffusely infiltrates the cerebral cortex and subcortical white matter may give the radiographic appearance of an acute organizing infarction.

PROGNOSIS AND THERAPY

Early diagnosis and immediate thrombolytic therapy have led to a significant reduction in mortality from acute cerebral infarction. In addition, treatment with aspirin and other antiplatelet agents plays a significant role in preventive therapy. Treatment of diabetes and hypertension, lowering of cholesterol, cessation of smoking, and other measures to control risk factors for stroke are important preventive measures.

VASCULAR DEMENTIA (INCLUDING BINSWANGER'S DISEASE)

CLINICAL FEATURES

Patients in whom multiple subcortical infarcts develop, especially in the deep nuclei and white matter, may be susceptible to the development of a chronic progressive dementing illness. A number of terms have been use to describe this phenomenon, including "subcortical atherosclerotic encephalopathy," "multi-infarct dementia," "vascular dementia," and "small vessel disease." This pattern of infarction includes atherothrombotic/embolic,

coagulopathic, hypertensive, and vasculitic causes. Various sporadic or familial arteriopathies, including cerebral autosomal dominant arteriopathy with subcortical infarcts and leukoencephalopathy (CADASIL) and cerebral amyloid angiopathy (CAA), are also associated with dementia. The brains of demented patients with vascular pathology may also show changes consistent with neurodegenerative disorders such as Alzheimer's disease. Because of the multiple possible causes and

---

VASCULAR DEMENTIA (INCLUDING BINSWANGER'S DISEASE)—FACT SHEET

Definition
▶ A heterogeneous group of chronic progressive dementing diseases characterized by multiple subcortical ischemic lesions. Binswanger's disease is a clinicopathologic subtype of subcortical vascular dementia

Incidence and Location
▶ Incidence of Binswanger's disease: 2.5 to 3.8 per 1000
▶ Incidence as high as 6 to 12 per 1000 in patients older than 70 years
▶ Multifocal ischemic lesions of the deep nuclei and white matter

Gender and Age Distribution
▶ Most common in the sixth and seventh decades of life
▶ Affects men and women equally

Clinical Features
▶ Stepwise deterioration in memory, mood, and cognition
▶ Psychiatric symptoms such as affective disorders early in the disease course
▶ Focal motor signs with occurrence of multiple infarcts
▶ Strong association with systemic hypertension

Radiologic Features
▶ Nodular or confluent areas of white matter hyperintensity ("leukoaraiosis")

Prognosis and Treatment
▶ Control of hypertension and atherosclerosis risk factors

overlap with neurodegenerative diseases, the concept of "subcortical vascular dementia" is still evolving.

Binswanger's disease can be thought of as a clinico-pathologic subtype of subcortical vascular dementia. It is a form of vascular dementia that typically begins in the sixth and seventh decades and affects men and women equally. Although the exact incidence is uncertain, a large Canadian study estimated the incidence of vascular dementia to be 2.5 to 3.8 per 1000. The incidence increases with age, rising to 6 to 12 per 1000 in patients older than 70 years. Clinically, patients experience a stepwise deterioration in memory, mood, and cognition. Psychiatric symptoms and signs such as affective disorders may occur early in the course of the disease. Focal motor signs and partial resolution of symptoms coincide with the occurrence of multiple infarcts. Although not all patients with Binswanger's disease have high blood pressure, there is an association with systemic hypertension and systemic atherosclerotic vascular disease.

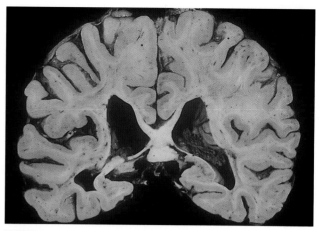

FIGURE 2-14

Binswanger's disease: coronal section at the level of the splenium of the corpus callosum showing bilateral ventricular dilatation as a result of extensive white matter vascular disease. (Courtesy of Dr. Elizabeth Rushing.)

RADIOLOGIC FINDINGS

The descriptive term "leukoaraiosis" refers to the imaging finding of nodular or confluent areas of hyperintensity in the periventricular white matter. This appearance is nonspecific for a particular cause but is characteristic of Binswanger's disease. Other conditions that may produce similar radiographic findings include demyelinating diseases, leukodystrophies, postradiation effects, encephalitis secondary to acquired immunodeficiency syndrome (AIDS), and normal-pressure hydrocephalus.

PATHOLOGIC FINDINGS

Patients with multi-infarct dementia characteristically have numerous lesions of the white matter and deep nuclear structures, but occasionally the cortex may also be involved, and examples of dementia associated with a single large infarct have been reported. The brain shows diffuse ventriculomegaly with hydrocephalus ex vacuo because of the marked reduction in white matter volume (Fig. 2-14). Multifocal lacunar infarcts are encountered in about 90% of cases. Classic histopathologic descriptions of Binswanger's disease have referred specifically to extensive atherosclerotic microvascular changes ("hyaline arteriolosclerosis"; see later) that involve the periventricular and deep white matter. Nonspecific ischemic changes in the white matter and hypertensive vascular pathology are common (see "Hypertensive Cerebrovascular Disease" later).

PROGNOSIS AND TREATMENT

No definitive treatment is available for this progressive dementia. Control of hypertension and modification of

atherosclerosis risk factors are important preventive measures.

CAUSES OF CEREBRAL HEMORRHAGE

This section focuses on the major causes of acute cerebral hemorrhage that relate to abnormalities of blood vessels. Such causes include hypertensive cerebrovascular disease, aneurysms, vascular malformations, and CAA. Hemorrhage caused by trauma, tumor, or systemic coagulopathies is not discussed.

VASCULAR DEMENTIA (INCLUDING BINSWANGER'S DISEASE)—PATHOLOGIC FEATURES

Gross Findings

► Cerebral atrophy and ex vacuo hydrocephalus from reduced volume of white matter
► Multifocal lacunar infarcts of periventricular white matter or deep nuclei, or both, in 90% of cases

Microscopic Findings

► Extensive atherosclerotic or hypertensive microvascular changes, or both:
  ► Hyaline arteriolosclerosis
  ► Lipohyalinosis

Differential Diagnosis

► The radiographic differential diagnosis includes demyelinating disease, leukodystrophies, postradiation effects, AIDS encephalitis, and normal-pressure hydrocephalus
► Pathology confirmed by characteristic gross and microvascular changes

HYPERTENSIVE CEREBROVASCULAR DISEASE

CLINICAL FEATURES

Spontaneous intracranial hemorrhage affects about 37,000 patients in the United States and is believed to account for 10% to 20% of all strokes. Hypertension is the most important underlying cause of acute nontraumatic intracerebral hemorrhage (ICH). More than 50% of spontaneous acute cerebral hemorrhages occur in hypertensive individuals. The incidence of ICH is around 9 per 100,000, and 70% to 90% of patients with ICH have high blood pressure. Cerebral hemorrhage accounts for 15% of deaths in patients with chronic hypertension. Spontaneous ICH reaches a peak incidence around 60 years of age and is 5% to 20% higher in men.

HYPERTENSIVE CEREBROVASCULAR DISEASE—FACT SHEET

Definition
▶ Cerebrovascular disease associated with acute or chronic hypertension
▶ May result in
  ▶ Spontaneous intracranial hemorrhage
  ▶ Lacunar infarcts

Incidence and Location
▶ Believed to account for 10% to 20% of all strokes
▶ Annual incidence of about 9 per 100,000 persons
▶ Affects about 18,000 to 20,000 individuals in the United States
▶ Location of spontaneous intracranial hemorrhage:
  ▶ Deep cerebral nuclei (putamen, thalamus): 60%
  ▶ Cerebrum (lobar): 20%
  ▶ Cerebellum: 13%
  ▶ Pons: 7%
▶ Location of lacunar infarcts:
  ▶ Basal ganglia in the distribution of the lenticulostriate branches of the middle cerebral arteries
  ▶ Periventricular and deep cerebral white matter

Gender and Age Distribution
▶ 5% to 20% increased incidence in men
▶ Peak incidence at 60 years of age

Clinical Features
▶ Rapid demise with massive intracranial hemorrhage
▶ Internal capsule, basal ganglia stroke syndromes
▶ Hypertensive encephalopathy

Radiologic Features
▶ Highly variable depending on the location of hemorrhage or infarction, or both

Prognosis and Treatment
▶ Depends on extent of the lesion
▶ Preventive measures include antihypertensive therapy

Acute hypertensive hemorrhage typically occurs in the distribution of the lenticulostriate branches of the middle cerebral artery and in the pontine perforators of the basilar artery. Accordingly, hypertensive hemorrhage arises in the deep cerebral nuclei (60%; putamen, thalamus), cerebrum (lobar, 20%), cerebellum (13%), and pons (7%). The clinical picture of hypertensive brain disease varies widely from massive, acute ICH resulting in rapid death to a chronic, slowly progressive dementing illness. Between these two extremes lies a syndrome of "hypertensive encephalopathy" caused by an acute increase in systemic pressure. Involvement of the deep nuclei may produce hemiparesis, hemisensory deficits and a visual field defect (putamen) or gaze abnormalities, and vomiting (thalamus). Headache, vomiting, and truncal or limb ataxia may occur with cerebellar hemorrhage, and coma with quadriparesis may signal a pontine hemorrhage. Patients usually have a clinical history of systemic hypertension and may have cardiac and renal manifestations of this disease.

Hypertensive encephalopathy is an acute neurologic syndrome characterized by diffuse cerebral dysfunction, severe headache, confusion, and vomiting precipitated by a sudden and severe increase in systemic blood pressure. It can occur in patients with kidney disease, eclampsia, disseminated vasculitis, or catecholamine-secreting tumors such as pheochromocytoma or after discontinuation of antihypertensive therapy (i.e., "rebound effect"). Untreated, the syndrome may progress to coma or fatal hemorrhage.

PATHOLOGIC FEATURES

Two types of gross lesions associated with hypertension include acute cerebral hemorrhage and lacunar infarcts. Massive hemorrhages involving the deep nuclei are manifested as circumscribed areas of acutely clotted blood that cause tissue disruption, a significant mass effect, and herniation (Fig. 2-15). Blood may dissect medially into the ventricles but only rarely dissects outward through the cortex and into the subarachnoid space. In nonfatal cases, the region of hemorrhage undergoes cavitation and will demonstrate yellow-brown hemosiderin staining. Pontine and cerebellar hemorrhages are associated with significant brain stem compression (Fig. 2-16).

Lacunar infarcts are classically located in the deep cerebral nuclei, especially in the putamen (Fig. 2-17). They may also be found in the periventricular white matter. In some cases, lacunes represent small areas of ischemic infarction (Fig. 2-18) that organize by liquefaction necrosis and cavitation. Frequently, "lacunes" are actually widened perivascular spaces of the lenticulostriate arteries (Fig. 2-19). Careful autopsy studies of the brains of hypertensive individuals have demonstrated that the perivascular spaces were widened because of increased tortuosity of parenchymal arteries.

Hypertension is associated with a number of histologic abnormalities in cerebral blood vessels. Because

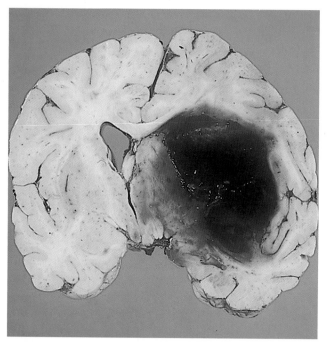

FIGURE 2-15

Acute hypertensive hemorrhage arising in the region of the basal ganglia. There is a striking mass effect, herniation, and focal extension to the lateral ventricle.

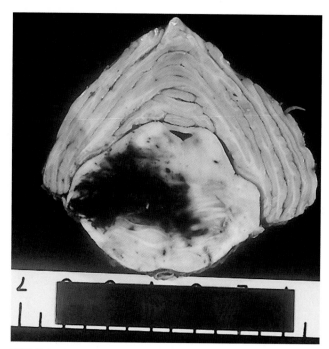

FIGURE 2-16

Acute hypertensive hemorrhage of the pons, which resulted in acute brain stem swelling and death of the patient.

HYPERTENSIVE CEREBROVASCULAR DISEASE— PATHOLOGIC FEATURES

Gross Findings

▶ Acute, extensive cerebral hemorrhage of the deep nuclei, cerebellum, or pons
▶ Lacunar infarcts of the basal ganglia or periventricular white matter, or both

Microscopic Findings

▶ Acute hemorrhage with acute blood clot and disruption and dissection through CNS tissue, sometimes with intraventricular or subarachnoid extension
▶ Lacunar lesions may represent foci of ischemic infarction or widened perivascular spaces as a result of increased tortuosity of affected arteries
▶ Blood vessel changes may include
　▶ Hyaline arteriolosclerosis
　▶ Lipohyalinosis
　▶ Charcot-Bouchard aneurysms (rarely observed in routine practice)

Pathologic Differential Diagnosis

▶ Lobar hemorrhage in patients with cerebral amyloid angiopathy or coagulopathies may mimic hypertensive hemorrhage

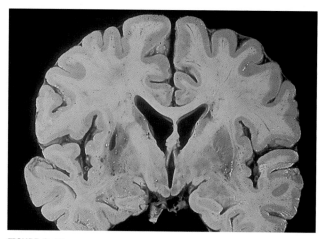

FIGURE 2-17

Lacunar infarcts of the left putamen and right caudate nuclei in a patient with chronic hypertension. (Courtesy of Dr. Elizabeth Rushing.)

---

of the strong association of diabetes and hypertension with accelerated atherosclerosis, atheromatous changes extend more distally and involve smaller superficial and parenchymal arteries, as well as large vessels at the base. Hyaline arteriolosclerosis consists of concentric thick-ening of small arteries and arterioles and is one of the more common cerebrovascular changes associated with hypertension (see Fig. 2-19). To some extent, this change may be seen with aging and may occur with concentric mineralization of the media of small arteries in the globus pallidus (Fig. 2-20).

Lipohyalinosis (fibrinoid necrosis) affects vessels between 40 and 300 mm in diameter and is associated with lacunar lesions. Based on experimental studies, it is believed that chronic hypertension promotes the accumulation of serum proteins (including fibrin) in the

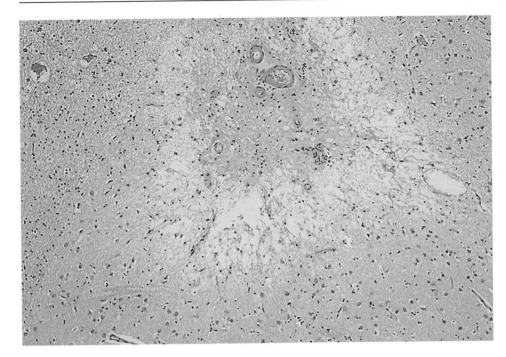

FIGURE 2-18
Low-power photomicrograph showing a circumscribed area of organizing lacunar infarction.

basement membranes of cerebral arterioles. Continued protein deposition results in microvascular fibrinoid necrosis. Healing of such a lesion includes the transient appearance of foamy or lipid-laden macrophages and eventually progresses to fibrosis and hyalinization (Fig. 2-21). With acute hypertension, "onion-skinning" of the vessel wall occurs.

The traditional view that local weakening of damaged blood vessels in hypertensive patients leads to focal microscopic aneurysmal dilatations at branch points ("Charcot-Bouchard aneurysms") has recently been questioned. Such aneurysms are only rarely identified in routine autopsy material (Fig. 2-22). The known tortuosity of blood vessels in patients with chronic

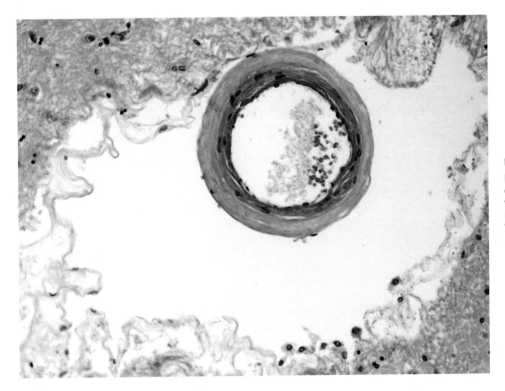

FIGURE 2-19
Low-power photomicrograph showing concentric arteriolosclerosis and widening of the perivascular space (as a result of increased vascular tortuosity) in chronic hypertension.

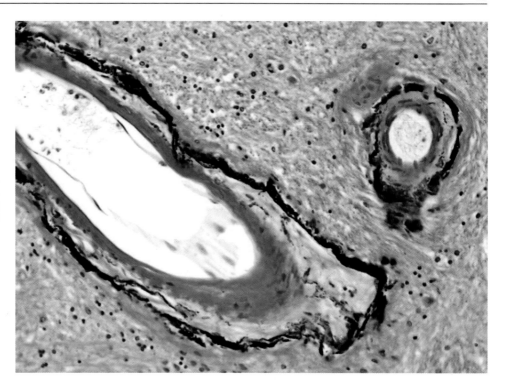

FIGURE 2-20

Concentric calcification of the lenticulostriate arteries in the globus pallidus. This nonspecific change may be encountered in patients with chronic hypertension.

hypertension could be mistaken for an aneurysmal dilatation in histologic sections. It is possible that Charcot-Bouchard aneurysms develop rapidly, possibly just before a fatal hemorrhage, and are obliterated thereafter. The cause of massive deep nuclear hemorrhages associated with hypertension is most likely multifactorial, with vascular hyalinization and fibrinoid changes causing decreased wall compliance and increased fragility.

PROGNOSIS AND TREATMENT

The prognosis is variable and related to disease manifestations. Medical control of hypertension and atherosclerosis risk factors is the mainstay of preventive therapy.

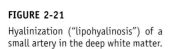

FIGURE 2-21

Hyalinization ("lipohyalinosis") of a small artery in the deep white matter.

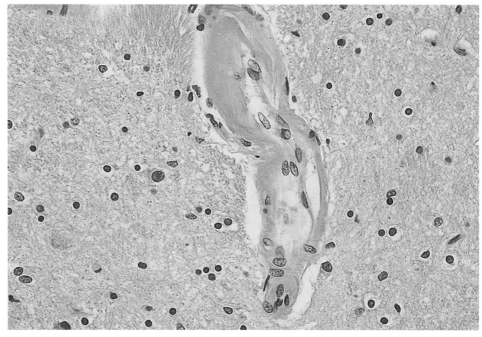

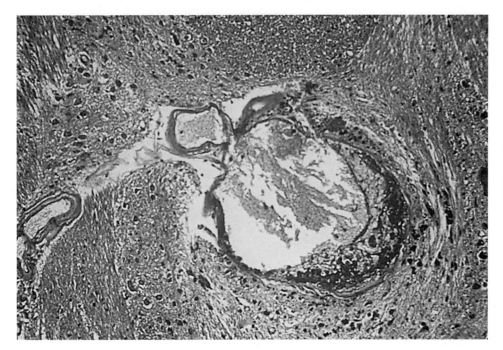

FIGURE 2-22

Charcot-Bouchard aneurysm in a patient with chronic hypertension (trichrome stain). (Courtesy of Dr. Elizabeth Rushing.)

CEREBRAL ANEURYSMS

An aneurysm is defined as an abnormally dilated segment of a blood vessel. Included in this group of CNS vascular diseases are saccular (congenital), fusiform (atherosclerotic), infectious, and traumatic types. We will focus on saccular aneurysms since they are the most frequent cause of clinically significant subarachnoid hemorrhage.

SACCULAR ("BERRY") ANEURYSMS

CLINICAL FEATURES

A saccular (berry) aneurysm is by far the most common type of cerebral aneurysm. Approximately 3% to 5% of the population is believed to have some type of cerebral aneurysm, and they are about twice as common in women. About 25% of all cerebrovascular deaths are due to ruptured aneurysms, with an annual incidence of about 7 to 10 per 100,000 and a peak incidence in the sixth decade.

Although a congenital cause is widely accepted, such aneurysms are rare in infancy and childhood and most common in adults older than 30 years. Multiple aneurysms have been identified in 20% to 30% of autopsied individuals with berry aneurysms. Risk factors for the development of saccular aneurysms and spontaneous subarachnoid hemorrhage include chronic hypertension, cigarette smoking, female sex, and African American race. Although the pathogenesis is not well understood, genetic factors are suggested by an increased occurrence in first-degree relatives (especially siblings) and well-known associations of berry aneurysms with autosomal dominant polycystic kidney disease, Ehlers-Danlos syndrome type IV, neurofibromatosis type I, and Marfan's syndrome. About 6% to 9% of arteriovenous malformations (AVMs) may occur together with one or more saccular aneurysms. The latter also arise in the setting of extracranial vascular diseases such as fibromuscular dysplasia and coarctation of the aorta.

Typically occurring at branch points in large arteries of the circle of Willis, turbulent flow may contribute to aneurysmal dilatation. The most common locations include branch points between (1) the anterior cerebral and anterior communicating arteries (40%), (2) the M1 and M2 divisions of the middle cerebral artery within the sylvian fissure (34%), and (3) the internal carotid and posterior communicating arteries (20%). Saccular aneurysms arising at the site of the bifurcation of the basilar artery into the posterior cerebral arteries account for about 4% of cases.

Most saccular aneurysms remain asymptomatic until rupture. However, about 50% of patients experience mild symptoms related to an initial small bleed ("sentinel hemorrhage") days to months before a large subarachnoid hemorrhage. The latter is heralded by an acute, severe headache and sometimes loss of consciousness. Stiff neck, nausea/vomiting, muscle weakness, decreased sensation, lethargy, seizures, speech impairment, and impulsivity may also occur. Blood in the subarachnoid space can stimulate vasospasm of the basal arteries, a feared complication of aneurysm rupture that can result in significant cerebral ischemia, infarction, and brain swelling. Occasionally, aneurysms may cause symptoms by compression of adjacent structures. For example, a posterior communicating artery aneurysm may cause ipsilateral third nerve compression. Symptoms of parenchymal or ventricular hemorrhage may also be observed.

SACCULAR (BERRY") ANEURYSMS—FACT SHEET

Definition

▶ Abnormal sac-like dilatations of cerebral arteries believed to be congenital in origin

Incidence and Location

▶ Ruptured aneurysms account for 25% of cerebrovascular deaths
▶ The annual incidence of rupture is 7 to 10 per 100,000 persons
▶ The annual risk of rupture is 0.05% to 2%, depending on size
▶ Multiple aneurysms occur in 20% to 30% of patients with cerebral aneurysms
▶ Saccular aneurysms are found in 6% to 9% of patients with arteriovenous malformations
▶ Arise at *branch points* of major arteries of the circle of Willis:
  ▶ Anterior cerebral–anterior communicating arteries: 40%
  ▶ M1-M2 divisions of the middle cerebral artery: 34%
  ▶ Internal carotid–posterior communicating arteries: 20%
  ▶ Basilar artery–posterior cerebral arteries: 4%
  ▶ Other branch points: 2%

Gender and Age Distribution

▶ Female preponderance (female-to-male about 2:1)
▶ Most common in adults older than 30 years, with a peak incidence in the sixth decade
▶ Rare in childhood

Clinical Features

▶ Most aneurysms remain asymptomatic until rupture
▶ Mild symptoms are occasionally related to an initial small bleed ("sentinel hemorrhage")
▶ Acute aneurysm rupture results in severe headache with or without loss of consciousness
▶ Other symptoms may include stiff neck, nausea/vomiting, muscle weakness, decreased sensation, lethargy, seizures, speech impairment, and impulsivity

Radiographic Features

▶ Cerebral angiography is the most sensitive and specific method for localization

Prognosis and Treatment

▶ About 25% of patients die within 24 hours of acute aneurysm rupture
▶ About 25% die within 3 months of rupture
▶ Emergency therapy includes stabilization of cardiorespiratory function and prevention of further bleeding
▶ Aneurysms larger than 10 mm in diameter carry a 50% annual risk of hemorrhage
▶ Patients with aneurysms 6 mm or larger are considered candidates for neurosurgical "clipping" to prevent further bleeding
▶ Endovascular embolization is sometimes an option

RADIOGRAPHIC FEATURES

CT or MRI may be used to determine the extent of subarachnoid hemorrhage and the presence of parenchymal or ventricular extension of the bleeding. However, the most sensitive and specific method of identifying a saccular aneurysm is cerebral angiography.

PATHOLOGIC FEATURES

Variable amounts of basal subarachnoid hemorrhage are found in patients dying acutely (Fig. 2-23). Identification of a ruptured aneurysm is greatly facilitated by removal of blood in the fresh state under a gentle stream of water. A berry aneurysm consists of a thin-walled sac-like structure that is attached to an arterial branch point via a narrow neck. The sac may be spherical, oval, or lobulated, and multiple aneurysms may be present (Fig. 2-24A and B). The rupture site is usually apparent at the apex of the sac, and there may be evidence of previous surgical clipping. If the bleeding point of the ruptured aneurysm is oriented toward the cerebral surface, hemorrhage under arterial pressure dissects into the brain parenchyma and may extend into the ventricular system (Fig. 2-25). Most saccular aneurysms are between 0.1 and 2.5 cm in diameter. Those measuring more than 2.5 cm are called "giant aneurysms."

Microscopically, the aneurysm sac may contain thrombotic material, and fibrocalcific atheromatous plaque material may be found in the wall. The junction between an adjacent normal artery and the aneurysm neck will show loss of elastin fibers and smooth muscle, with the neck ultimately being composed of hyalinized, collagenous tissue (Fig. 2-26).

Basal subarachnoid hemorrhage causes vasospasm of major branches of the circle of Willis. The pathogenesis

---

SACCULAR ("BERRY") ANEURYSMS—PATHOLOGIC FEATURES

Gross Findings

▶ Thin-walled sac attached to an arterial branch point via a narrow neck
▶ The sac may be spherical, oval, or lobulated, and the rupture site may be apparent
▶ Aneurysm rupture is associated with extensive basal subarachnoid hemorrhage
▶ Cerebral infarction is due to arterial spasm caused by subarachnoid blood
▶ Dissection of blood through CNS parenchyma occurs if the rupture site is oriented toward the brain
▶ Hemorrhage may extend into the ventricles
▶ With prolonged survival, organizing basal subarachnoid hemorrhage may obstruct flow of cerebrospinal fluid and cause hydrocephalus

Microscopic Findings

▶ The aneurysm sac typically has a fibrocollagenous wall and may contain thrombotic or fibrocalcific material
▶ The junction between the aneurysm neck and an adjacent artery shows loss of elastin fibers and smooth muscle

Pathologic Differential Diagnosis

▶ Other forms of cerebral aneurysm, including fusiform and infective, are described further in the text
▶ Aneurysms may mimic tumors radiographically when embedded in brain parenchyma or when they involve the parasellar region

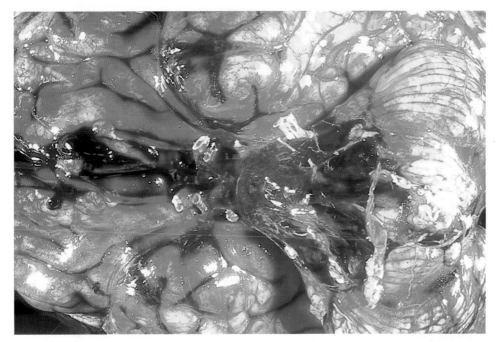

FIGURE 2-23

Saccular (berry) aneurysm: extensive acute basal subarachnoid hemorrhage that resulted from a ruptured saccular aneurysm. (Courtesy of Mr. Joseph DiRienzi.)

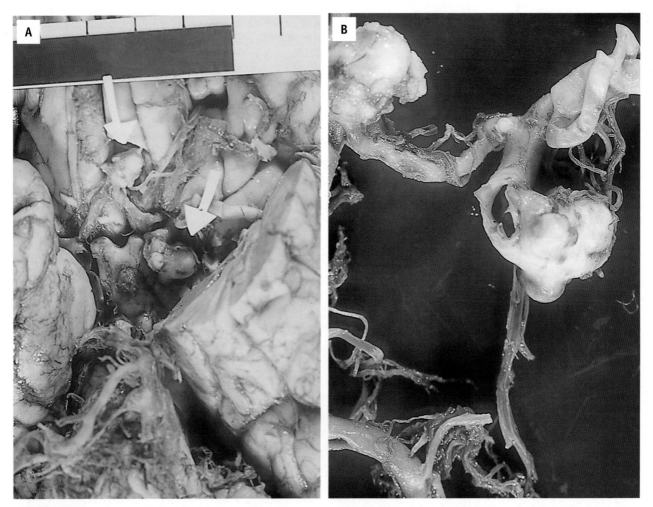

FIGURE 2-24

Saccular (berry) aneurysm. **A**, Gross specimen showing the base of the brain and the locations of two saccular aneurysms. The one toward the top of the figure (*arrow*) involves the anterior communicating artery, and a second arose from the branch point of the internal carotid artery and the middle cerebral artery (*arrow*). **B**, Gross dissection of the circle of Willis showing the same two saccular aneurysms as in **A**. Note the lobular appearance of the aneurysms.

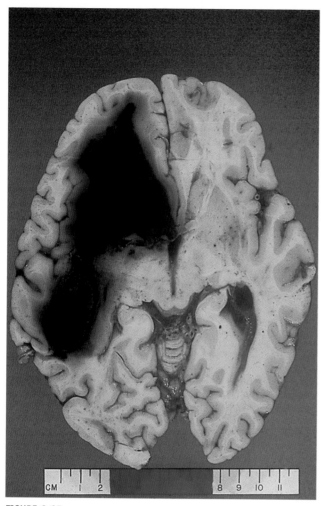

FIGURE 2-25

Extensive acute parenchymal and ventricular hemorrhage caused by rupture of a saccular aneurysm. The rupture site was oriented toward the brain and dissected into the lateral ventricle.

of vasospasm involves a number of mediators, including endothelin-1. With prolonged survival, organizing subarachnoid hemorrhage features accumulations of hemosiderin and reactive (fibrotic) meningeal changes.

PROGNOSIS AND THERAPY

About 25% of patients die within the first 24 hours after aneurysm rupture, with another 25% dying within 3 months. Of the survivors, about half have some sort of permanent neurologic deficit. Emergency therapeutic measures include stabilization of cardiorespiratory function and prevention of further bleeding. Once the aneurysm has been located by angiography, depending on its size and the extent of bleeding, endovascular embolization may be attempted, but adequate occlusion occurs in only 50% to 70% of cases. More definitive therapy consists of placing a surgical clip at the aneurysm neck, which controls bleeding and eliminates the risk of rebleeding. The prognosis relates to the patient's clinical status on admission.

The annual risk of aneurysm rupture is 0.05% to 2%, depending on the size and type of lesion. Aneurysms larger than 10 mm in diameter have a 50% yearly risk of hemorrhage. Patients discovered to have aneurysms 6 to 7 mm or larger are considered to be candidates for neurosurgical clipping.

FUSIFORM ANEURYSMS

Cerebral fusiform aneurysms are rare. In contrast to saccular aneurysms, they are believed to be atherosclerotic in nature, are more likely to cause significant brain compression and mass effect, do not usually produce subarachnoid hemorrhage, and most often involve the

FIGURE 2-26

Low-power histologic section of a saccular aneurysm. The sac is located toward the left of the figure, the neck is on the right (elastin stain). (Courtesy of Dr. Elizabeth Rushing.)

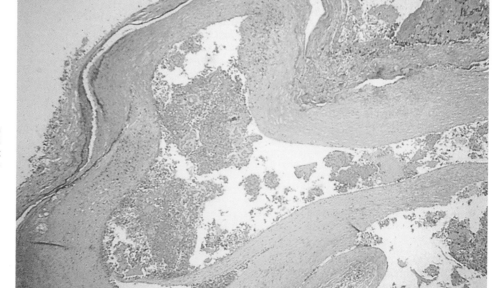

vertebrobasilar system. Symptoms relate to brain stem and cranial nerve compression and ischemia as a result of atherothrombotic occlusion. Grossly, there is diffuse dilatation of the basilar artery and, occasionally, extension to involve the vertebral vessels. Atheromatous plaque with associated thrombosis, varying degrees of calcification, and nonspecific inflammatory changes are observed. Despite surgical intervention the mortality rate is high.

INFECTIVE ANEURYSMS

Vascular invasion by infectious organisms and the associated inflammatory reaction can lead to focal dilatations of cerebral blood vessels and symptomatic hemorrhage. Also referred to as "mycotic" aneurysms, such lesions may be caused by bacteria as well as fungi. They account for 5% to 6% of all intracranial aneurysms and may rupture and result in subarachnoid hemorrhage or multiple hemorrhagic infarcts with disseminated disease. Vasoinvasive fungi such as *Aspergillus* species directly invade the vessel wall and cause thrombosis and hemorrhage. The clinical course can be rapidly progressive with high mortality (90% for fungal and 30% for bacterial aneurysms).

VASCULAR MALFORMATIONS

Vascular malformations are traditionally classified into four groups: AVMs, cavernous angiomas, capillary telangiectasia, and venous angiomas. The basis for classification takes into account the caliber and configuration of the component blood vessels, the relationship of abnormal vessels to brain parenchyma, and the presence or absence of arteriovenous shunting. A variety of cerebrovascular malformations that do not fit neatly into the following four subtypes may also be encountered.

ARTERIOVENOUS MALFORMATIONS

CLINICAL FEATURES

AVMs are the most clinically important brain vascular malformations. They account for 1.5% to 4% of all brain masses, with a peak incidence in adults between 20 and 40 years of age. In one large study, the mean age at diagnosis was 31.2 years. Most AVMs are supratentorial and occur within the distributions of the major cerebral arteries (middle cerebral artery > anterior > posterior). Less common sites may include the corpus callosum, choroid plexus, or the optic nerve (the latter associated with Wyburn-Mason syndrome). Multiple AVMs may be present in 4% of individuals with an AVM.

About 50% of patients present with a cerebral hemorrhage, and this finding is typical of younger individuals. Some patients experience a subtle onset of headache or focal neurologic deficits. Progressive symptoms may

---

ARTERIOVENOUS MALFORMATIONS—FACT SHEET

Definition

► Tangled mass of abnormal arterial and venous channels without intervening capillaries typically separated by gliotic brain parenchyma

Incidence and Location

► Account for 1.5% to 4% of all brain masses
► The annual incidence of symptomatic AVMs is 1.1 per 100,000 persons
► About 0.14% of the U.S. population is believed to be affected
► Most AVMs are located in the distributions of the major cerebral vessels: middle cerebral artery > anterior cerebral artery > posterior cerebral artery
► Uncommon locations: corpus callosum, choroid plexus
► Optic nerve involvement in Wyburn-Mason syndrome

Gender and Age Distribution

► Males and females affected equally
► Peak incidence in adults between 20 and 40 years of age
► The mean age at diagnosis is about 30 years

Clinical Features

► 50% of patients present with acute hemorrhage (typical of younger individuals)
► There may be a subtle onset of headaches and focal deficits
► Symptoms may occasionally be progressive because of AVM growth

Radiographic Features

► Cerebral angiography reveals a high-flow vascular lesion with arteriovenous shunting

Prognosis and Treatment

► The yearly risk of acute hemorrhage is 2% to 4%
► The risk of hemorrhage is higher in patients younger than 45 years
► Two thirds of patients with AVM have significant hemorrhage
► Immediate mortality with hemorrhage occurs in 10%
► Therapies include surgical resection, endovascular embolization, and radiosurgery

---

be encountered as the AVM grows slowly. This progressive enlargement probably involves the development of collateral arteries and veins. Large AVMs produce ischemia of surrounding brain tissue because of the "steal" phenomenon. Seizures may occur in 25% of patients with supratentorial AVMs, especially older individuals. About 6% to 9% of AVMs occur with saccular (berry) aneurysms, and aneurysms may occur at the branch points of feeding arteries.

RADIOGRAPHIC FEATURES

MRI and cerebral angiography are the diagnostic methods of choice. MRI usually shows abnormal collections of large blood vessels, whereas angiography will clearly demonstrate the high-flow character of these arteriovenous shunts.

PATHOLOGIC FEATURES

Grossly, the surface of the brain in the region of an AVM contains dilated, thick-walled veins, which represent draining vessels of the lesion. On cut section, AVMs consist of a tangled mass of blood vessels of varying diameter and wall thickness (Fig. 2-27). There may be evidence of remote or recent hemorrhage, or both. Superficial AVMs tend to have a broad base near the cortical surface where they drain into surface veins, whereas deeper lesions drain into the deep venous system.

Microscopically, the variability in size and configuration of the abnormal blood vessels is usually quite striking (Fig. 2-28). In addition, a characteristic feature is the presence of gliotic CNS tissue between the abnormal blood vessels (Fig. 2-29). Arterial elements may have variable amounts of smooth muscle proliferation, collagen deposition, and reduplication of the internal elastic lamina (Fig. 2-30), whereas large "arterialized" veins are thick walled and collagenized. Thrombosis with varying stages of recanalization and sometimes calcification may be present. If embolization was performed before surgery, there will be evidence of endovascular material, which may incite a foreign body giant cell reaction (Fig. 2-31).

AVMs represent a congenital failure of vascular differentiation that results in arteriovenous shunting without an intervening capillary network. Although the pathogenesis is poorly understood, abnormal cerebral arteriovenous shunts developed in mice lacking the gene for activin receptor–like kinase-1 (a member of the transforming growth factor-β family).

ARTERIOVENOUS MALFORMATIONS—PATHOLOGIC FEATURES

Gross Findings
▶ An AVM is a tangled mass of thick-walled blood vessels of varying caliber
▶ More superficially located AVMs are associated with dilated draining veins on the cerebral surface
▶ Deep AVMs drain into the deep venous system
▶ There may be evidence of remote or recent hemorrhage

Microscopic Findings
▶ Thick-walled arteries with variable smooth muscle proliferation, collagen deposition, and reduplication of the internal elastic membrane
▶ Thick-walled "arterialized" veins
▶ Abnormal blood vessels may show thrombosis, recanalization, or evidence of previous embolization
▶ Gliotic CNS tissue between abnormal blood vessels

Genetics and Pathogenesis
▶ Poorly understood
▶ Arteriovenous shunts develop in mice lacking an activin receptor–like kinase

Pathologic Differential Diagnosis
▶ Highly vascular neoplasms
▶ Other vascular malformations

DIFFERENTIAL DIAGNOSIS

Highly vascular neoplasms may mimic an AVM. However, the high flows demonstrated by angiography are usually well in excess of those encountered in tumors. Other types of vascular malformations may enter the differential diagnosis.

FIGURE 2-27

Arteriovenous malformation: gross appearance of a large arteriovenous malformation arising in the region of the sylvian fissure and extending toward the lateral ventricle.

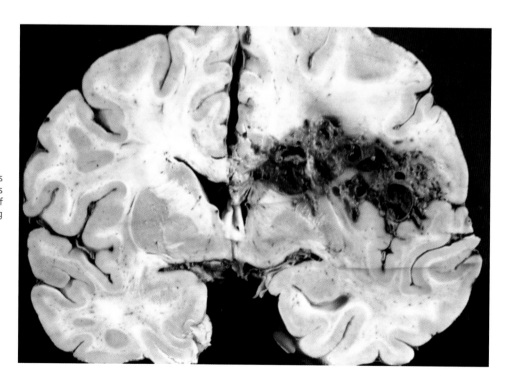

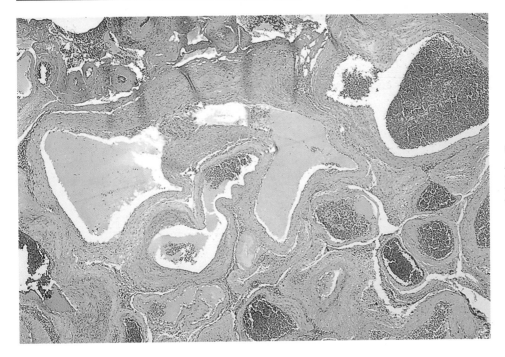

FIGURE 2-28

Arteriovenous malformation: low-power photomicrograph showing thick-walled arterial and venous vessels.

PROGNOSIS AND THERAPY

Two thirds of patients with AVMs suffer clinically significant hemorrhage with an immediate mortality rate of 10%. The yearly risk of an acute bleeding episode is between 2% and 4%. This risk is higher in younger individuals (<45 years of age), and treatment options include surgical resection, endovascular embolization, or radiosurgery. Sometimes a combination of these options is used. In general, more superficially located AVMs in noneloquent locations carry a better prognosis than do deep lesions or those that involve the brain stem.

OTHER TYPES OF ARTERIOVENOUS MALFORMATIONS

The so-called vein of Galen aneurysm is really a congenital AVM that has extensive "feeder arteries" arising from the posterior and occasionally the middle cerebral

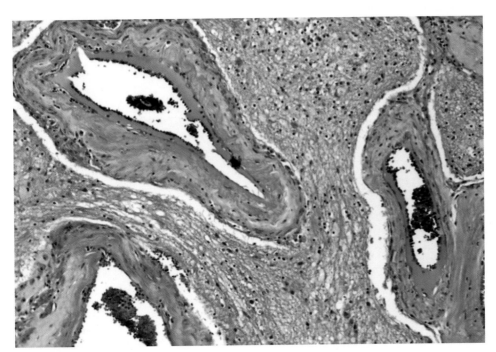

FIGURE 2-29

Arteriovenous malformation: high-power view showing three profiles of thickened blood vessels that are separated by gliotic brain tissue.

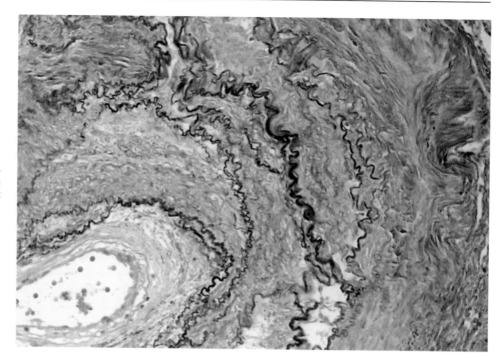

FIGURE 2-30

Arteriovenous malformation: high-power photomicrograph showing dispersal of the internal elastic membrane (elastin stain).

arteries; these feeder arteries drain into an enlarged residual vein ("of Galen") of the deep venous system (Fig. 2-32). Infants born with this condition usually have cardiomegaly and congestive heart failure as a result of the excessive degree of arteriovenous shunting. The prognosis is poor and depends somewhat on the complexity and extent of the lesion and the associated "steal" effect of the arteriovenous shunt. The latter usually results in cerebral ischemia and infarction. One treatment approach involves embolization of the vascu-

lar malformation with surgical coils to induce thrombosis and curtail shunting.

Spinal cord AVMs consist of enlarged, thick-walled blood vessels located on the posterior aspect of the spinal cord ("long dorsal" type). Thrombosis of the abnormal vessels may result in a stepwise, progressive myelopathy that correlates with multifocal spinal cord infarctions (Foix-Alajouanine syndrome). Dural arteriovenous fistulas may also result in significant spinal cord pathology.

FIGURE 2-31

Arteriovenous malformation: high-power photomicrograph showing intravascular embolization material (black particles) in a patient who had undergone endovascular treatment before surgery.

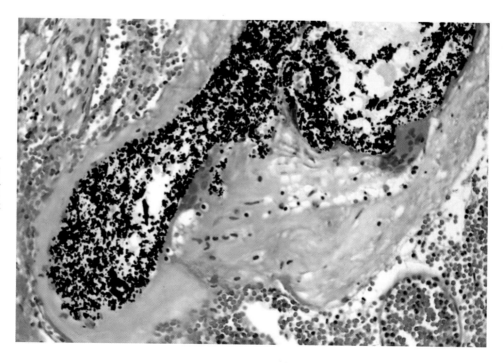

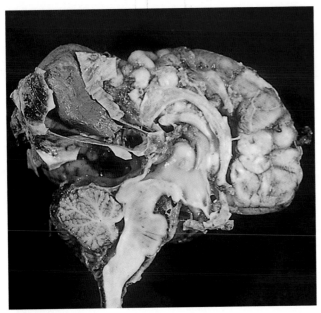

FIGURE 2-32

Vein of Galen aneurysm: midsagittal gross section showing a vein of Galen aneurysm that has been opened to reveal a large thrombus. There were extensive ischemic changes of the cerebral hemispheres as a result of the "steal" effect of the arteriovenous shunt.

CAVERNOUS ANGIOMA

CLINICAL FEATURES

Cavernous angiomas (also called cavernous malformations, cavernous hemangiomas, and cavernomas) arise most commonly in young adults, with a slight male preponderance. A third of patients present with focal epilepsy. The annual risk of an acute hemorrhage is about 1%. Surgery is performed to control seizures and reduce the risk of hemorrhage. Cavernous angiomas may occur anywhere in the nervous system and leptomeninges but most typically cause seizures when the cerebral cortex is involved.

Although the cause is not known, some familial forms of cavernous angioma are associated with mutations of the *CCM1* gene on chromosome 7q11-21. This gene encodes KRIT1, which interacts with proteins of the RAS family of guanine triphosphatases (GTPases). *CCM1* mutations may result in altered regulation of angiogenic factors such as β_1-integrin via abnormal KRIT1 interaction with the integrin-binding protein ICAP-1. Other possible genetic disease–related loci have been identified on chromosomes 7p15-p13 (*CCM2*) and 3q25.2-27 (*CCM3*).

RADIOGRAPHIC FEATURES

On T2-weighted MRI, the lesion consists of a compact focus of increased vascularity with variable density that is surrounded by a "ring" of hypodensity (Fig. 2-33).

The latter corresponds to hemosiderin deposition in the adjacent brain tissue ("ferruginous penumbra"). This radiographic appearance is virtually pathognomonic for cavernous angioma.

PATHOLOGIC FEATURES

In contrast to AVMs, cavernous angiomas have no direct arterial contribution. They consist of a compact mass of dilated, thin-walled, variably hyalinized vascular channels with little intervening brain tissue (Fig. 2-34). There is no muscular hypertrophy or elastic lamina, but vessels may be calcified or thrombosed. The surrounding brain tissue is gliotic and shows evidence of remote hemorrhage with scattered hemosiderin-laden macrophages. Cavernous angiomas may occur together with venous angiomas or capillary telangiectases. Occasionally, patients with cerebral cavernous angiomas may have similar vascular lesions in other organs such as the kidney, liver, lung, or skin.

DIFFERENTIAL DIAGNOSIS

The distinctive MRI appearance of cavernous angiomas usually leaves little doubt regarding the diagnosis. However, a focal remote cerebral hemorrhage or hemorrhagic

---

CAVERNOUS ANGIOMA—FACT SHEET

Definition
► An abnormal compact collection of thin-walled vascular channels without intervening brain parenchyma and peripheral hemosiderin

Incidence and Location
► Annual incidence estimated at 0.4% to 0.5%
► May occur anywhere in the brain but typically involves the cerebral cortex
► Supratentorial: 80%; infratentorial: 20%

Gender and Age Distribution
► Slight male preponderance
► Young adults are most commonly affected
► One fourth of patients are children

Clinical Features
► One third of patients present with focal epilepsy

Radiographic Features
► Compact focus of increased vascularity with variable central density and peripheral hypodensity as a result of hemosiderin accumulation
► MRI findings are sensitive and specific

Prognosis and Treatment
► The annual risk of acute hemorrhage is about 1%
► The prognosis is excellent for surgically resectable, symptomatic lesions

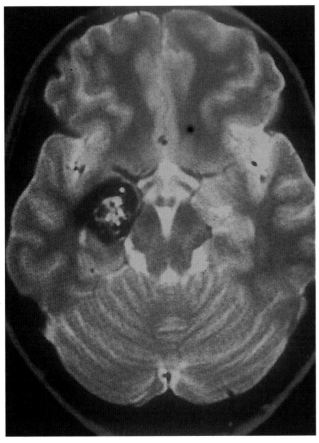

FIGURE 2-33

Cavernous angioma: T2-weighted magnetic resonance image showing classic central irregular enhancement corresponding to vascular flow voids and peripheral hypodensity consistent with hemosiderin deposition.

<table>
<tr><td colspan="1">

CAVERNOUS ANGIOMA—PATHOLOGIC FEATURES

Gross Findings

▶ Circumscribed hemorrhagic-appearing lesion

Microscopic Findings

▶ Compact mass of dilated, thin-walled blood vessels with no intervening brain tissue
▶ Vessels may be calcified or thrombosed
▶ The surrounding brain is gliotic and contains hemosiderin

Genetics and Pathogenesis

▶ Familial cavernous angiomas are associated with *CCM1* gene mutations (chromosome 7q11-21)
▶ The encoded protein is KRIT1, which interacts with the RAS family of GTPases
▶ Other possible genetic loci: *CCM2* (7p15-p13) and *CCM3* (3q25.2-27)

Pathologic Differential Diagnosis

▶ Hemorrhagic tumor
▶ Organizing cerebral hemorrhage
</td></tr>
</table>

tumor with perilesional hemosiderin might be possible mimics that can be distinguished histologically.

PROGNOSIS AND THERAPY

The prognosis is usually excellent after surgical resection. Cavernous malformations are not typically embolized, and the role of radiosurgery for such lesions is uncertain.

FIGURE 2-34

Cavernous angioma: low-magnification view showing a cluster of dilated, thin-walled blood vessels without intervening brain tissue.

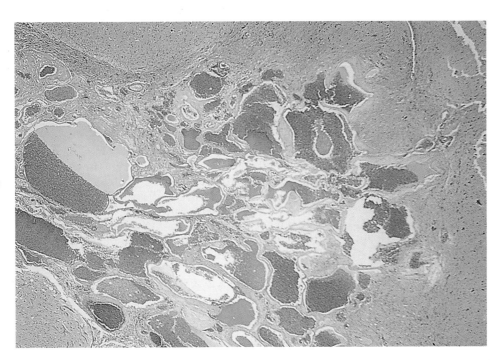

CAPILLARY TELANGIECTASES

These vascular malformations are typically incidental findings of little clinical significance and only rarely become symptomatic. They are believed to account for 16% to 20% of all brain vascular malformations, with an estimated prevalence of about 0.4%.

Capillary telangiectases are most commonly found in the ventromedial pons or subcortical white matter and grossly resemble a focal petechial hemorrhage. Microscopically, they consist of dilated capillaries separated by normal brain tissue. Hemorrhage from such lesions is rare.

VENOUS ANGIOMAS

This term refers to dilated veins of the superficial or subcortical cerebral vasculature, which are usually asymptomatic. Venous angiomas are similar to varicose veins elsewhere in the body and may be associated with other vascular malformations in the same patient. Surgical pathologists do not usually encounter venous angiomas because removal of these functional blood vessels would result in rather extensive hemorrhagic infarction of the underlying brain.

CEREBRAL AMYLOID ANGIOPATHY (FORMERLY CALLED "CONGOPHILIC ANGIOPATHY")

CLINICAL FEATURES

CAA predisposes patients to large lobar hemorrhages, which account for 12% to 15% of all cerebral hemorrhages in the elderly. This disease should be considered in any older, nonhypertensive adult with spontaneous ICH. In contrast to the deep cerebral hemorrhages of chronic hypertension, hemorrhages associated with amyloid angiopathy are more peripheral and involve the cerebral cortex and adjacent structures. Clinical symptoms reflect the anatomic extent and location of the hemorrhage. Lobar hemorrhage can occur acutely as a massive acute stroke, most often involving the frontal or frontoparietal regions, or as recurrent hemorrhagic infarctions that take place over a period of years. Large hemorrhages of the right parietal lobe may result in a classic contralateral neglect syndrome in which patients fail to recognize the left side of their body as their own.

Although more than 20 proteins or protein products can form amyloid fibrils in humans, at the present time, about a half a dozen are associated with CAA. The most common form of amyloid associated with sporadic and some familial forms of CAA is the Aβ-amyloid peptide (Aβ), which is a cleavage product of the β-amyloid precursor protein encoded on chromosome 21. In this regard, it should be noted that the Aβ that accumulates in CAA is the same type of amyloid found in neuritic (senile) plaques of Alzheimer's disease. Rare inherited

---

CEREBRAL AMYLOID ANGIOPATHY—FACT SHEET

Definition
► A disorder characterized by deposition of β-amyloid protein in the walls of cortical and leptomeningeal arteries, which predisposes patients to spontaneous lobar hemorrhage

Incidence and Location
► The incidence is about 20 per 100,000 in patients older than 60 years
► Accounts for 12% to 15% of all cerebral hemorrhages in the elderly
► Hemorrhages typically affect the cerebral cortex and subcortical white matter
► Underlying cause of large "lobar" hemorrhages

Gender and Age Distribution
► Men and women equally affected
► Most common in patients older than 60 years

Clinical Features
► Symptoms reflect the anatomic extent of hemorrhage and range from massive lobar "stroke" to progressive dementia
► Parietal lobe involvement may result in contralateral "neglect" syndrome
► Commonly found in demented individuals with Alzheimer-like neurofibrillary pathology

Prognosis and Treatment
► Acute lobar hemorrhage may result in death as a result of mass effect and herniation
► Smaller hemorrhages are treated symptomatically
► No definitive therapy at present

---

forms of CAA result from amyloid composed of cystatin C, transthyretin, gelsolin, and prion protein.

CAA often occurs together with the neurofibrillary pathology of Alzheimer's disease, and the clinical symptomatology may reflect the additive effects of the vascular and neurodegenerative diseases. Rarely, CAA may occur together with CNS vasculitis.

PATHOLOGIC FEATURES

Amyloid is a pathologic protein in which abnormal folding produces an extensive β-pleated sheet secondary structure. In this conformation, protein polymers form highly insoluble fibrils 8 to 10 nm in diameter. Amyloid deposition occurs in the walls of arteries and arterioles of the cerebral cortex and meninges. On routine hematoxylin-eosin staining, affected vessels show mural thickening and effacement by acellular, homogeneous eosinophilic material (Fig. 2-35). Capillaries and veins are less often involved, and blood vessels of the deep white matter are typically spared. Arterial and arteriolar amyloid accumulation initially appears in the basement membrane around smooth muscle cells at the peripheral aspect of the media and adventitia. There is progressive destruction of smooth muscle cells but, generally, sparing of the endothelium until late stages of the disease. Affected vessels become rigid and fragile and often assume a rounded or "double-barrel contour" (Fig. 2-36). Some vessels ultimately undergo fibrinoid necrosis and rupture with hemorrhage. Vascular amyloid accumulation is also likely to alter the function of cerebral autoregulation.

ANCILLARY STUDIES

Amyloid deposition can be confirmed by the characteristic "apple-green" birefringence under polarized illumination with Congo red staining. This characteristic led to the designation "congophilic angiopathy." Green fluorescence is seen with thioflavin S stain. Since most sporadic and some familial CAAs are due to abnormal accumulations of Aβ-amyloid, detection of this peptide by immunohistochemistry has greatly facilitated the histopathologic diagnosis. Immunostaining for Aβ-amyloid will often reveal neuritic (senile) plaques in the cortex of individuals with CAA (Fig. 2-37).

DIFFERENTIAL DIAGNOSIS

The hemorrhages associated with CAA may be accompanied by ischemic lesions that mimic CNS vasculitis, and there is evidence that CAA may coexist with vasculitis. Occasionally, white matter lesions may occur in a distribution suggesting a Binswanger-like leukoencephalopathy. The relatively noninflammatory character of CAA

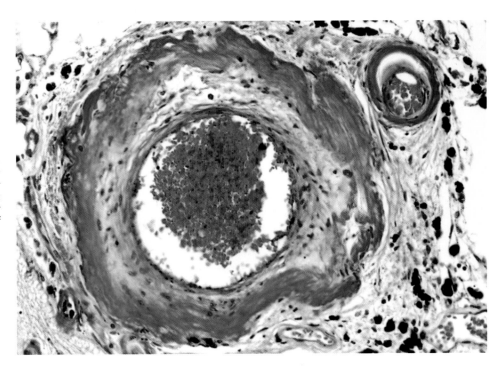

FIGURE 2-35

Cerebral amyloid angiopathy: irregularly thickened leptomeningeal artery with effacement of normal vascular structure by amorphous eosinophilic material. Note the perivascular hemosiderin deposition suggestive of previous hemorrhage.

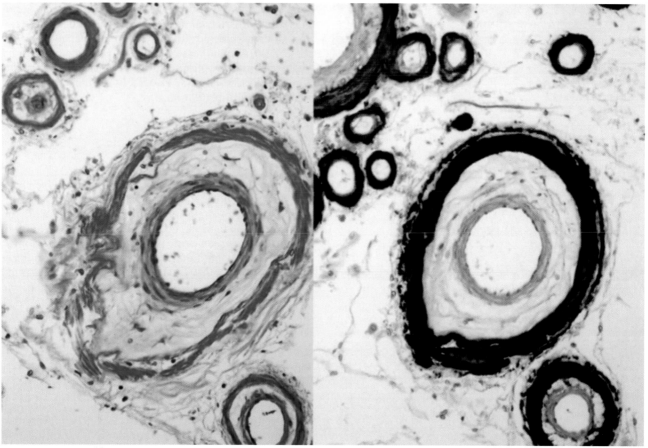

FIGURE 2-36

Cerebral amyloid angiopathy: composite photomicrograph with a hematoxylin-eosin–stained section on the left and a parallel Aβ-amyloid–immunostained section on the right. Note the "double-barrel" appearance of the vessel caused by separation of the endothelium from the heavily affected muscularis.

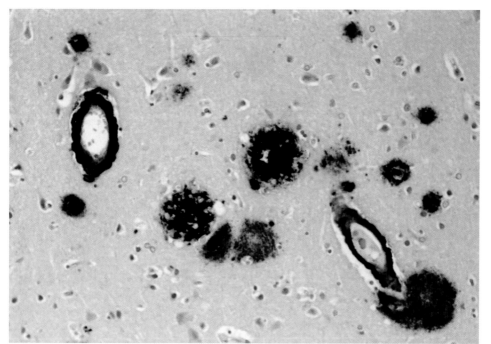

FIGURE 2-37

Cerebral amyloid angiopathy: immunohistochemical stain for Aβ-amyloid peptide showing positive staining of two small cortical arteries and several neuritic (senile) plaques. Cerebral amyloid angiopathy often occurs together with the neuritic plaques and neurofibrillary tangles associated with Alzheimer's disease.

and detection of Aβ-amyloid peptide by immunohisto-chemistry confirms the diagnosis in most cases.

PROGNOSIS AND THERAPY

Acute parenchymal brain hemorrhage may cause death because of mass effect and herniation. Excessive bleeding of amyloid-laden blood vessels may complicate surgery for removal of acutely clotted blood. Management of smaller hemorrhages is mainly symptomatic because no specific therapies are available at present.

VASCULITIS

Inflammation of the blood vessel wall may occur as a primary systemic disorder such as giant cell arteritis and polyarteritis nodosa or may be localized to cerebral blood vessels or to those of peripheral nerves. Alternatively, inflammatory changes of nervous system blood vessels may represent secondary involvement by collagen vascular disease, infection, tumor, and substance abuse. Primary vasculitides may preferentially affect large (elastic), medium (muscular), or small (<0.5 mm in diameter) arteries.

GIANT CELL (TEMPORAL) ARTERITIS

Giant cell arteritis is the most common primary vasculitis that affects the nervous system. It occurs almost exclusively in adults older than 50 years and has a peak incidence between 75 and 85 years of age. Women are affected twice as often as men. The incidence is 15 to 25 per 100,000. Extracranial branches of the aorta are typically involved, especially the external and internal carotid arteries (large and medium-sized arteries). Inflammatory changes in these vessels lead to vascular compromise and local end-organ ischemia, which result in the classic symptoms of blindness, headache, scalp tenderness, and jaw claudication. Involvement of the vertebral arteries is associated with vertigo, dizziness, transient ischemic attacks, and stroke. Malaise, fever, night sweats, anorexia, and weight loss are nonspecific manifestations of this systemic inflammatory disorder. Levels of acute phase proteins such as C-reactive protein are elevated along with the sedimentation rate. About 30% to 40% of patients with giant cell arteritis also have polymyalgia rheumatica.

A definitive diagnosis can be made by temporal artery biopsy (Fig. 2-38). Giant cell arteritis is a panarteritis with transmural infiltration by mononuclear cells, including lymphocytes and monocyte/macrophages (Fig. 2-39). Granulomas composed of T cells and multinucleated giant cells form in close proximity to a fragmented internal elastic lamina. The disease appears to represent a disorder of cell-mediated immunity, with CD4$^+$ T lymphocytes playing a key pathogenetic role in

---

GIANT CELL (TEMPORAL) ARTERITIS—FACT SHEET

Definition
► The most common primary systemic vasculitis that affects the nervous system

Incidence and Location
► The incidence is 15 to 25 per 100,000 population
► Extracranial branches of the aorta are affected, especially the external and internal carotid arteries

Gender and Age Distribution
► Female preponderance (female-to-male about 2:1)
► Occurs exclusively in adults older than 50 years
► Peak incidence between 75 and 85 years of age

Clinical Features
► Blindness, headache, scalp tenderness, jaw claudication
► Involvement of the vertebral arteries associated with vertigo, dizziness, transient ischemic attacks, or stroke
► Nonspecific systemic symptoms include malaise, fever, night sweats, anorexia, and weight loss
► Elevation of the sedimentation rate and C-reactive protein
► 30% to 40% of patients will also have polymyalgia rheumatica

Prognosis and Treatment
► Good response to steroids

GIANT CELL (TEMPORAL) ARTERITIS—PATHOLOGIC FEATURES

Gross Findings
► Multiple nodular swellings of the affected artery

Microscopic Findings
► Panarteritis with transmural mononuclear cell infiltrates
► Granulomas with multinucleated giant cells
► Fragmentation and phagocytosis of the internal elastic lamina
► Intimal proliferation and reduced luminal diameter

Pathogenesis
► Disorder of cell-mediated immunity with CD4$^+$ T lymphocytes playing a key pathogenetic role

Pathologic Differential Diagnosis
► The diagnosis is straightforward in the appropriate clinicopathologic setting
► Granulomatous endarteritis may occur with tuberculous, fungal, and treponemal infections

---

the activation of monocyte/macrophages and the formation of multinucleated giant cells. The granulomatous reaction results in marked intimal proliferation with reduced luminal diameter and resultant ischemic phenomena. The disease responds well to corticosteroids, and aspirin has some benefit.

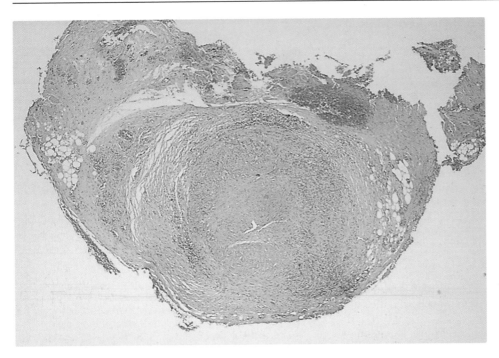

FIGURE 2-38

Giant cell (temporal) arteritis: low-magnification cross-sectional view of a temporal artery biopsy specimen showing marked mural thickening by an inflammatory process.

Takayasu's disease is a rare vasculitis that affects the aorta and its major branches and is considered to be the "classic" large vessel vasculitis. It typically affects young women in the second or third decades of life (female-to-male ratio about 9:1). A systemic phase of the disease marked by nonspecific constitutional symptoms is followed by an occlusive phase characterized by ischemic symptoms. The pathologic features are similar to those of giant cell arteritis. Therapy includes corticosteroids and immunosuppressive agents. The disease is self-limited in some cases, and the 10-year survival rate is about 90%.

PRIMARY ANGIITIS OF THE CENTRAL NERVOUS SYSTEM

Although quite rare, primary angiitis of the CNS is the most common vasculitis that by definition exclusively involves CNS blood vessels. Patients can present with headaches, stroke-like episodes, or multifocal myelopathies with spinal cord involvement. Males are predominantly affected, and there is a wide age range with a peak incidence of diagnosis during the fifth to sixth decades of life. Although the prognosis was considered to be poor, modern immunosuppressive therapy is effective in some cases.

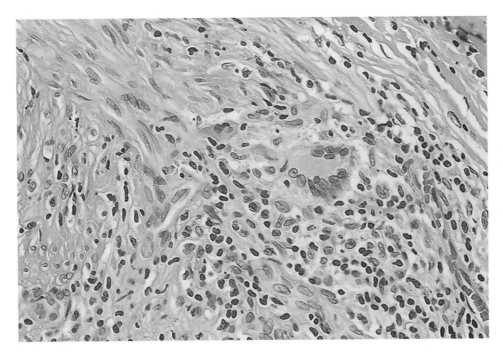

FIGURE 2-39

Giant cell (temporal) arteritis: high-magnification view showing a mononuclear infiltrate composed of mature T lymphocytes and a multinucleated giant cell.

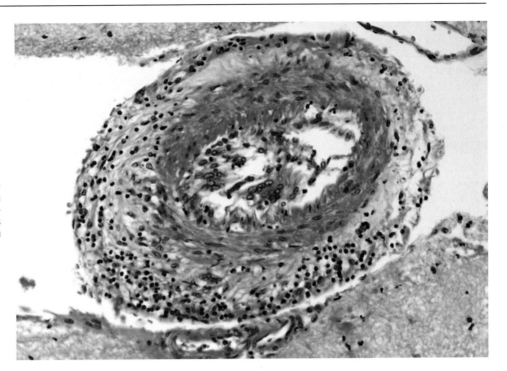

FIGURE 2-40

Primary angiitis of the central nervous system: low-power view of a leptomeningeal artery showing mononuclear inflammatory cell infiltrates and early intimal proliferation with a giant cell reaction.

Medium-sized and small blood vessels of the leptomeninges and superficial cortex show focal segmental granulomatous changes. A transmural infiltrate of mature lymphocytes is typically present, and multinucleated giant cells are often seen within a significantly thickened intima (Figs. 2-40 and 2-41). Ischemic microinfarcts result from vascular stenosis and obstruction.

Sarcoidosis, infectious granulomatous meningitis, and intravascular lymphoma are in the differential diagnosis. The diagnostic workup includes imaging studies and cerebral angiography. However, a definitive diagnosis can be made only by histologic study of biopsy or autopsy material. Special stains for acid-fast bacilli and fungi should be performed to help exclude an infectious cause. Intravascular lymphoma is recognized by the intravascular location and immunohistochemical phenotype (CD20 positive, B cells) of the atypical lymphoid cells.

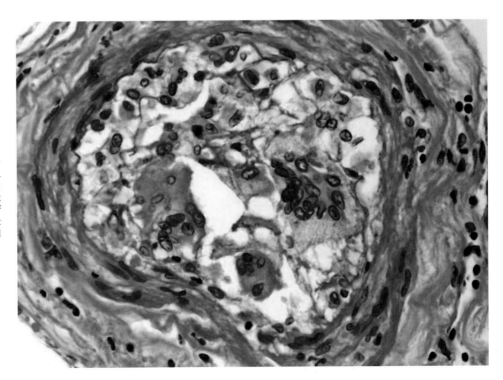

FIGURE 2-41

Primary angiitis of the CNS: high-power view of a small parenchymal artery showing intimal proliferation with several multinucleated giant cells. Stenosis and obstruction of such a vessel lead to microscopic ischemic lesions of the brain and spinal cord.

PRIMARY CENTRAL NERVOUS SYSTEM ANGIITIS—FACT SHEET

Definition

▶ An inflammatory disorder that primarily affects small and sometimes medium-sized arteries of the central nervous system

Incidence and Location

▶ Very rare
▶ May affect the brain and spinal cord

Gender and Age Distribution

▶ Males more commonly affected
▶ Usually affects adults most often in the fifth and sixth decades

Clinical Features

▶ Nonspecific: headaches, stroke-like episodes, multifocal myelopathy

Prognosis and Treatment

▶ Considered to be poor; some cases respond to immunosuppressive therapy

PRIMARY CENTRAL NERVOUS SYSTEM ANGIITIS—PATHOLOGIC FEATURES

Gross Findings

▶ Nonspecific multifocal ischemic lesion

Microscopic Findings

▶ Transmural lymphocytic infiltration of small to medium-sized arteries
▶ Intimal granulomatous proliferation
▶ Multifocal ischemic infarctions

Genetics and Pathogenesis

▶ Unknown, probably multifactorial

Pathologic Differential Diagnosis

▶ Sarcoidosis, infectious granulomatous meningitis, intravascular lymphoma

POLYARTERITIS NODOSA

This immune complex vasculitis can involve any organ system except the lung and spleen. The CNS may be affected in 20% to 40% of cases, whereas peripheral nerve damage occurs in more than 50% of cases. About 30% of patients in the United States are positive for serum hepatitis B antigen. Peripheral nerve involvement may result in the syndrome of mononeuritis multiplex. Vasculitic changes consist of focal, segmental inflammation with an infiltrate of polymorphonuclear neutrophils and fibrinoid necrosis (Figs. 2-42 and 2-43). Thrombotic occlusion leads to ischemic damage in the affected nerve.

CADASIL (CEREBRAL AUTOSOMAL DOMINANT ARTERIOPATHY WITH SUBCORTICAL INFARCTS AND LEUKOENCEPHALOPATHY)

CLINICAL FEATURES

This hereditary cerebrovascular disease occurs worldwide and may affect many ethnic groups, but the largest

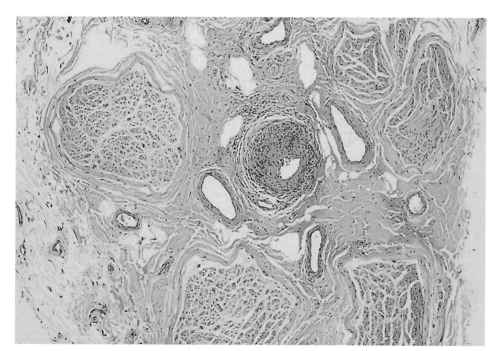

FIGURE 2-42

Polyarteritis nodosa: low-magnification view of a peripheral nerve showing active vasculitis of a small epineurial artery (center of image).

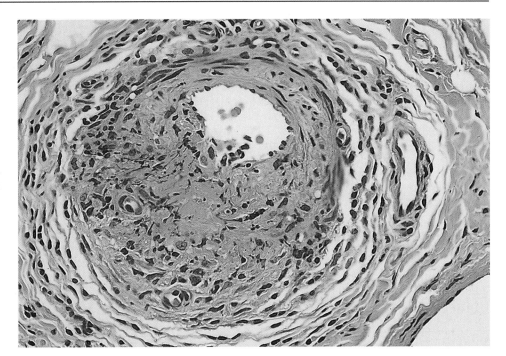

FIGURE 2-43

Polyarteritis nodosa: high-power view of a vessel from Figure 2-42 showing neutrophilic inflammation with fibrinoid necrosis.

CADASIL (CEREBRAL AUTOSOMAL DOMINANT ARTERIOPATHY WITH SUBCORTICAL INFARCTS AND LEUKOENCEPHALOPATHY)—FACT SHEET

Definition

▶ Familial arteriopathy associated with *Notch 3* gene mutations and characterized by deposition of abnormal granular osmiophilic material in blood vessels walls

Incidence and Location

▶ Exact incidence uncertain; the prevalence is about 4 per 100,000
▶ Ischemic lesions of white matter and deep cerebral nuclei

Gender and Age Distribution

▶ Both sexes affected roughly equally
▶ The mean age of onset is 45 years
▶ Cognitive decline between the ages of 40 and 70 years

Clinical Features

▶ Migraine with aura may be the initial symptom and appears most commonly in the third decade
▶ Ischemic attacks peak between 40 and 50 years of age
▶ Dementia occurs in 80% of CADASIL patients older than 65 years
▶ Depression and mood disturbance in 20% of patients
▶ Seizures as a late finding in less than 10% of patients

Radiographic Features

▶ T2-hyperintense lesions of white matter and deep nuclei

Prognosis and Treatment

▶ The clinical course is usually progressive
▶ Life expectancy is 15 to 25 years after the onset of symptoms
▶ Acetazolamide is used for severe migraine headaches

---

and most thoroughly studied families are from Europe. Although the exact prevalence of the disease is not known, it is estimated that about 500 families are affected worldwide with an estimated prevalence of 4 per 100,000. Both sexes are affected equally. The four major symptoms of CADASIL are migraine with aura, ischemic attacks (transient or strokes), psychiatric findings, and dementia. Migraine headaches may begin in late childhood but most commonly arise in the third decade. The first ischemic attacks occur with a peak between 40 and 50 years of age. Dementia may develop without identified stroke-like episodes in 10% to 15% of patients. Cognitive decline becomes apparent between the ages of 40 and 70 years, with about 80% of CADASIL patients older than 65 years being demented. Depression is the most common psychiatric symptom, and mood disturbances occur in more than 20% of patients. Seizures develop in less than 10% of affected individuals, usually at late stages of the disease. The life expectancy is 15 to 25 years after the onset of symptoms.

CADASIL is caused by point mutations or small deletions in the *Notch 3* gene on chromosome 19p13. The encoded protein is a transmembrane receptor that plays a critical role in regulating cell differentiation during development. In adults, Notch 3 protein is expressed almost exclusively in vascular smooth muscle cells and may promote cell survival. On binding to its ligand, Notch 3 is cleaved at two sites, and the released and intracellular fragment may enter the nucleus and regulate transcription. The mechanism by which *Notch 3* mutations lead to the vascular pathology of CADASIL is not yet known.

RADIOGRAPHIC FEATURES

Hyperintense lesions of the subcortical and deep white matter may be seen on T2-weighted MRI. Periventricular lesions reminiscent of those seen in multiple sclerosis are also typical of CADASIL. Lacunar infarcts of the basal ganglia may likewise be seen. T2-hyperintense areas of the white matter, especially the anterior temporal lobes and periventricular regions, may be identified in asymptomatic individuals with the *Notch 3* mutation.

PATHOLOGIC FEATURES

Lacunar infarcts of the white matter and deep cerebral nuclei may be seen grossly in CADASIL (Fig. 2-44). Hydrocephalus ex vacuo may occur as a result of multi-

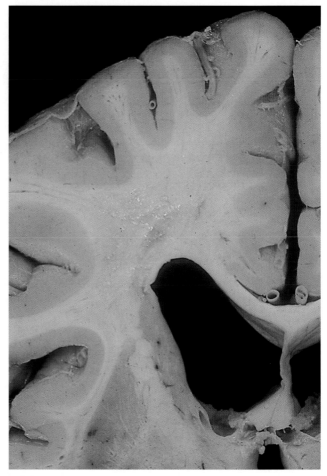

FIGURE 2-44

CADASIL: gross brain section showing focal softening (infarction) in the periventricular white matter. (Courtesy of Dr. Elizabeth Rushing.)

CADASIL (CEREBRAL AUTOSOMAL DOMINANT ARTERIOPATHY WITH SUBCORTICAL INFARCTS AND LEUKOENCEPHALOPATHY)—PATHOLOGIC FEATURES

Gross Findings
▶ Lacunar infarcts of white matter and deep nuclei with ex vacuo hydrocephalus
▶ Usually little or no hemorrhage

Microscopic Findings
▶ Parenchymal arteries are thickened and contain granular periodic acid–Schiff–positive material
▶ Multiple foci of ischemic necrosis

Ultrastructural Features
▶ Focal accumulations of granular osmiophilic material (GOM) between vascular smooth muscle cells or within the thickened basal lamina are virtually pathognomonic

Genetics and Pathogenesis
▶ Point mutations or small deletions on the *Notch 3* gene (chromosome 19p13)
▶ Notch 3 protein is expressed in vascular smooth muscle cells and may promote survival

Immunohistochemical Features
▶ Granular vascular material is reactive for Notch 3 protein

Pathologic Differential Diagnosis
▶ The distribution of ischemic lesions is somewhat similar to multi-infarct dementias (Binswanger's disease)
▶ Mitochondrial disorders such as MELAS (mitochondrial encephalopathy, lactic acidosis, and stroke-like episodes) may present a similar distribution of lesions
▶ Skin biopsy with ultrastructural demonstration of GOM in deep dermal arteries has facilitated the diagnosis

---

ple infarcts. The cerebral cortex is typically uninvolved, usually with little or no evidence of hemorrhage.

Microscopically, affected parenchymal and leptomeningeal arteries are thickened (Fig. 2-45) and contain granular, periodic acid–Schiff–positive material, which replaces smooth muscle cells of the media (Fig. 2-46). This granularity corresponds to the pathognomonic accumulation of granular osmiophilic material (GOM) by electron microscopy (see later). Accumulation of collagen and laminin contributes to the arterial wall thickening. Multiple areas of infarction in various stages of organization are typically present. Although CADASIL is primarily a neurologic disease, involvement of systemic arteries has allowed for a definitive diagnosis of CADASIL by skin biopsy. Characteristic GOM is well demonstrated in dermal arterioles.

ANCILLARY STUDIES

The granular material in the walls of affected blood vessels is immunoreactive for Notch 3 protein. Degen-

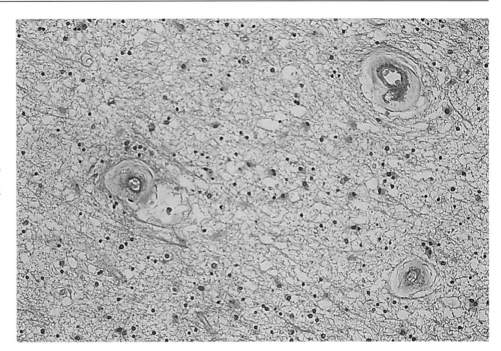

FIGURE 2-45

CADASIL: low-magnification view showing two thick-walled blood vessels in the white matter. (Courtesy of Dr. Elizabeth Rushing.)

eration of smooth muscle cells may be demonstrated by smooth muscle actin immunostain. The pathognomonic feature of CADASIL, revealed by electron microscopy, is the presence of GOM between degenerating vascular smooth muscle cells or within the thickened basal lamina (Fig. 2-47). GOM varies in size from 0.2 to 0.8 μm and is composed of nonfilamentous 10- to 15-nm granules (Fig. 2-48). Although the molecular components of GOM are not known, Notch 3 is probably one constituent.

DIFFERENTIAL DIAGNOSIS

The presence of GOM in dermal arterioles is virtually pathognomonic in the appropriate clinical setting. Multiple subcortical white matter and deep nuclear infarcts may have a thromboembolic or hypertensive cause. However, in neither condition would GOM be identified. The vascular hyalinization typical of hypertension corresponds to collagenous fibrosis and is not granular

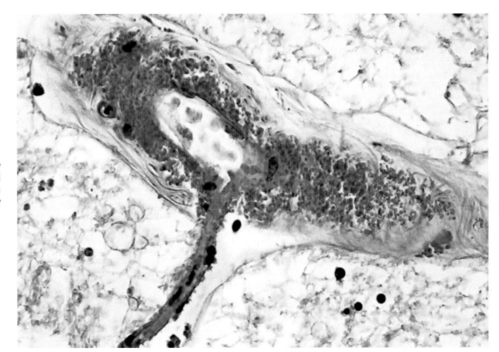

FIGURE 2-46

CADASIL: high-magnification view of a periodic acid–Schiff–stained section showing granular material in the wall of a small artery. (Courtesy of Dr. B.K. Kleinschmidt-DeMasters.)

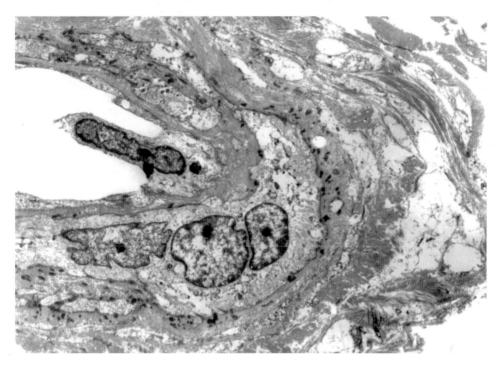

FIGURE 2-47

CADASIL: low-magnification electron micrograph showing dot-like granular osmiophilic material (GOM) in the wall of a dermal arteriole. This neurologic disease can be diagnosed by skin biopsy.

in nature. CADASIL differs from CAA by virtue of its relative lack of hemorrhage and deep (rather than superficial) location of the lesions. Immunohistochemical stains for Aβ-amyloid peptide would confirm CAA. Mitochondrial disorders such as MELAS should be considered in the differential diagnosis. A rare familial disorder associated with migraine and stroke-like episodes (familial hemiplegic migraine) is characterized by a mutation in the *CACNLA4* gene.

PROGNOSIS AND THERAPY

CADASIL is a slowly progressive disorder, and death typically occurs within 15 to 25 years of the initial strokes. Anticoagulants have been used to prevent thrombotic complications, but with minimal change in the ultimate outcome. Acetazolamide has been used to treat acute severe migraine headaches.

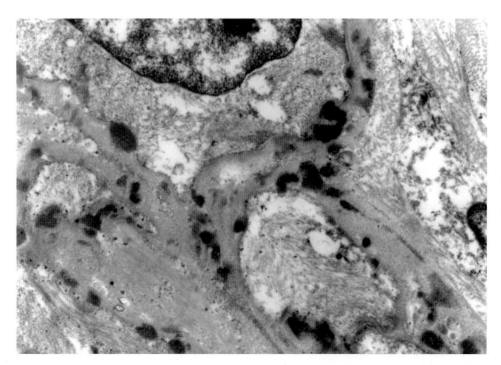

FIGURE 2-48

CADASIL: high-magnification electron micrograph showing deposits of granular osmiophilic material (GOM), which are diagnostic of CADASIL.

MOYAMOYA SYNDROME

This disease is defined by the angiographic finding of abnormal collateral vessels at the base of the brain. The syndrome was first described in Japan, where the term "moyamoya" was used to describe the angiographic findings as "something hazy" like a puff of smoke. Moyamoya syndrome has now been identified in all major ethnic groups. Included under this term are cases of so-called primary moyamoya syndrome and other disorders that may manifest the characteristic radiographic findings. The latter may include neurofibromatosis type 1, tuberous sclerosis, sickle cell anemia, Alpert's syndrome, Marfan's syndrome, Fanconi's anemia, and Schimke's immuno-osseous dysplasia.

Clinically, patients present in the first decade of life with cerebral ischemia or hemorrhage. About 50% of patients are children younger than 15 years, with a second peak of incidence during the fourth decade. A syndrome of alternating hemiparesis results from cerebral ischemia. The prognosis is related to the extent of vascular involvement and is poor if the anterior and posterior branches of the circle of Willis are affected.

The vascular pathology is characterized by stenosis or occlusion of distal branches of the internal carotid arteries, combined with an abundance of dilated, thin-walled collateral branches of the posterior circle of Willis. Arterial stenosis is due to fibrointimal proliferation complicated by platelet-fibrin thrombi.

SUGGESTED READINGS

Hypoxia-Ischemia

Garcia JH, Mena H: Injuries to the brain and spinal cord associated with ischemia. In Nelson J, Mena H, Parisi JE, Schochet SS (eds): Principles and Practice of Neuropathology, 2nd ed. New York, Oxford University Press, 2003, pp 112-121.

Kalimo H, Kaste M, Haltia M: Vascular diseases. In Graham DI, Lantos PL (eds): Greenfield's Neuropathology, 7th ed. London, Arnold, 2002, pp 281-355.

Marti-Vilalta JL, Arboix A, Garcia JH: Brain infarcts in the arterial border zones: Clinicopathologic correlations. J Stroke Cerebrovasc Dis 1994;4:114-120.

Petito CK: Cerebrovascular disease. In Nelson J, Mena H, Parisi JE, Schochet SS (eds): Principles and Practice of Neuropathology, 2nd ed. New York, Oxford University Press, 2003, pp 122-139.

Vinters HV: Cerebrovascular disease—practical issues in surgical and autopsy pathology. Curr Top Pathol 2001;95:51-99.

Cerebral Infarction

Barnett HJM, Yatsu FM, Mohr JP, Stein BM: Stroke: Pathophysiology, Diagnosis, and Management, 3rd ed. New York, Churchill Livingstone, 1998.

Ellison D, Love S, Chimelli L, et al: Neuropathology: A Reference Text of CNS Pathology, 2nd ed. Edinburgh, CV Mosby, 2004.

Ginsberg MD: Adventures in the pathophysiology of brain ischemia: Penumbra, gene expression, neuroprotection. Stroke 2003;34:214-223.

Kalimo H, Kaste M, Haltia M: Vascular diseases. In Graham DI, Lantos PL (eds): Greenfield's Neuropathology, 7th ed. London, Arnold, 2002, pp 281-355.

Vascular Dementia and Binswanger's Disease

Mirra SS, Hyman BT: Ageing and dementia. In Graham DI, Lantos PL (eds): Greenfield's Neuropathology, 7th ed. London, Arnold, 2002, pp 195-271.

Okeda R, Murayama S, Sawabe M, Kuroiwa T: Pathology of the cerebral artery in Binswanger's disease in the aged: Observation by serial sections and morphometry of the cerebral arteries. Neuropathology 2004;24:21-29.

Pantoni L, Garcia JH: The significance of white matter abnormalities 100 years after Binswanger's report: A review. Stroke 1995;26:1293-1301.

Pantoni L, Garcia JH: Pathogenesis of leukoraiosis. A review. Stroke 1997;28:652-659.

Roman GC, Erkinjuntti T, Wallin A, et al: Subcortical ischaemic vascular dementia. Lancet Neurol 2002;1:426-436.

Hypertensive/Atherosclerotic Angiopathy

Ellison D, Love S, Chimelli L, Harding BN, et al: Neuropathology: A Reference Text of CNS Pathology, 2nd ed. Edinburgh, CV Mosby, 2004.

Lammie GA: Hypertensive cerebral small vessel disease and stroke. Brain Pathol 2002;12:358-370.

Manolio TA, Olson J, Longstreth WT: Hypertension and cognitive function: Pathophysiologic effects of hypertension on the brain. Curr Hypertens Rep 2003;5:255-261.

Spangler KM, Challa VR, Moody DM: Arteriolar tortuosity of the white matter in aging and hypertension. A microradiographic study. J Neuropathol Exp Neurol 1994;53:22-26.

Aneurysms

Barnes B, Cawley CM, Barrow DL: Intracerebral hemorrhage secondary to vascular lesions. Neurosurg Clin N Am 2002;13:289-297.

Janjua N, Mayer SA: Cerebral vasospasm after subarachnoid hemorrhage. Curr Opin Crit Care 2003;9:113-119.

Maurice-Williams RS, Lafuente J: Intracranial aneurysm surgery and its future. J R Soc Med 2003;96:540-543.

Mitchell P, Gholkar A, Vindlacheruvu RR, Mendelow AD: Unruptured intracranial aneurysms: Benign curiosity or ticking bomb? Lancet Neurol 2004;3:85-92.

Rhoton AL Jr: Aneurysms. Neurosurgery. 2002;51(4 Suppl):S121-S158.

Vascular Malformations

Al-Shahi R, Bhattacharya JJ, Currie DG, et al: Prospective, population-based detection of intracranial vascular malformations in adults: The Scottish Intracranial Vascular Malformation Study (SIVMS). Stroke 2003;34:1163-1169.

Fleetwood IG, Steinberg GK: Arteriovenous malformations. Lancet 2002;359:863-873.

Kondziolka D, Lunsford LD, Kestle JR: The natural history of cerebral cavernous malformations. J Neurosurg 1995;83:820.

Maruyama K, Kondziolka D, Niranjan A, et al: Stereotactic radiosurgery for brainstem arteriovenous malformations: Factors affecting outcome. J Neurosurg 2004;100:407-413.

Zawistowski JS, Serebriiskii IG, Lee MF, et al: KRIT1 association with the integrin binding protein ICAP-1: A new direction in the elucidation of cerebral cavernous malformations (CCM1) pathogenesis. Hum Mol Genet 2002;11:389-396.

Cerebral Amyloid Angiopathy

Ghiso J, Frangione B: Cerebral amyloidosis, amyloid angiopathy, and their relationship to stroke and dementia. J Alzheimers Dis 2001;3:65-73.

Rensink AA, de Waal RM, Kremer B, Verbeek MM: Pathogenesis of cerebral amyloid angiopathy. Brain Res Brain Res Rev 2003;43:207-223.

Revesz T, Ghiso J, Lashley T, et al: Cerebral amyloid angiopathies: A pathologic, biochemical, and genetic view. J Neuropathol Exp Neurol 2003;62:885-898.

Van Nostrand WE, Melchor JP, Romanov G, et al: Pathogenic effects of cerebral amyloid angiopathy mutations in the amyloid beta-protein precursor. Ann N Y Acad Sci 2002;977:258-265.

Weller RO, Nicoll JA: Cerebral amyloid angiopathy: Pathogenesis and effects on the aging and Alzheimer brain. Neurol Res 2003;25:611-616.

Vasculitis

Calabrese LH: Vasculitis of the central nervous system. Rheum Dis Clin North Am 1995;21:1059-1076.

Carolei A, Sacco S: Central nervous system vasculitis. Neurol Sci 2003;24:S8-S10.

Chu CT, Gray L, Goldstein LB, Hulette CM: Diagnosis of intracranial vasculitis: A multidisciplinary approach. J Neuropathol Exp Neurol 1998;57:30-40.

Jennette JC, Falk RJ: Small-vessel vasculitis. N Engl J Med 1997;337:1512-1522.

Kelley RE: CNS vasculitis. Front Biosci 2004;9:946-955.

Lie JT: Primary (granulomatous) angiitis of the central nervous system: A clinicopathologic analysis of 15 new cases and a review of the literature. Hum Pathol 1992;23:164-171.

Nadeau SE: Neurologic manifestations of vasculitis and connective tissue disease. In Joynt RJ, Griggs RC (eds): Baker's Clinical Neurology on CD-ROM. Philadelphia, Lippincott Williams & Wilkins, 2000.

Weyland CM, Goronzy JJ: Medium and large vessel vasculitis. N Engl J Med 2003;349:160-169.

CADASIL

Chabriat H, Vahedi K, Iba-Zizen M, et al: Clinical spectrum of CADASIL: A study of 7 families. Lancet 1995;346:934-939.

Dichgans M: CADASIL: A monogenic condition causing stroke and subcortical vascular dementia. Cerebrovasc Dis 2002;13(Suppl 2):37-41.

Joutel A, Dodick DD, Parisi JE, et al: De novo mutation in the Notch 3 gene causing CADASIL. Ann Neurol 2000;47:388-391.

Joutel A, Favrole P, Labauge P, et al: Skin biopsy immunostaining with a Notch3 monoclonal antibody for CADASIL diagnosis. Lancet 2001;358:2049-2051.

Kalimo H, Ruchoux M-M, Viitanen M, Kalaria RN: CADASIL: A common form of hereditary arteriopathy causing brain infarcts and dementia. Brain Pathol 2002;12:371-384.

Ruchoux M-M, Maurage C-A: CADASIL: Cerebral autosomal dominant arteriopathy with subcortical infarcts and leukoencephalopathy. J Neuropathol Exp Neurol 1997;56:947-964.

Moyamoya Syndrome

Fukui M, Kono S, Sueishi K, Ikezaki K: Moyamoya disease. Neuropathology 2000;20(Suppl):S61-S64.

Gosalakkal JA: Moyamoya disease: A review. Neurol India 2002;50:6-10.

Yonekawa Y, Kahn N: Moyamoya disease. Adv Neurol 2003;92:113-118.

3 Trauma

David Dolinak

Traumatic head injury is a major cause of morbidity and mortality in the United States. Every year there are an estimated 500,000 victims of closed head injury, with an annual estimated mortality of more than 100,000. Motor vehicle accidents are the most common cause of closed head injury and involve young adults and teenagers in particular. Falls are also common and often involve intoxicated and elderly individuals. Head injury can be divided into two main categories—closed head injury and penetrating/perforating head injury, which primarily involves gunshot wounds. In this chapter, for ease of discussion and understanding, head injuries are presented in an "outward-in" format, with illustration and discussion of injuries to the scalp and skull fractures, followed by discussion of various types of bleeding between the skull and the brain (epidural hemorrhage, subdural hemorrhage, and subarachnoid hemorrhage), and then discussion of focal and diffuse injuries to the brain parenchyma (cerebral contusions and diffuse traumatic brain injury, respectively). Discussion of head injuries in child abuse is covered in a separate section, followed by the various sequelae of traumatic head injury, including brain swelling with herniation, cerebral infarcts, hypoxic-ischemic encephalopathy, post-traumatic seizure disorder, and post-traumatic meningitis.

during a complete autopsy, and investigative information to determine whether the injuries were inflicted or accidental. If inflicted, one may see a patterned abrasion on the skin or tool marks on the skull that may give a clue regarding the type of implement used in the assault. More often, however, one may only be able to say that the injury is consistent with a certain implement.

SCALP INJURY—FACT SHEET

Definitions
► Abrasion: a scrape of the skin; a surface injury
► Contusion: a bruise of the skin and underlying tissues
► Laceration: a blunt force injury causing a tear in the skin and underlying tissues; may be associated with extensive blood loss
► Avulsion: large tear of tissue, often creating a "tissue flap"; may be associated with extensive blood loss

Etiology
► Blunt force injury/impact

SCALP INJURY

A scalp injury occurs at the point of contact between the head and another force. If the impact is severe enough, injury to the scalp results and has a varying appearance based on the type of impacting force and the magnitude of the impact. Blunt force injuries to the scalp may result in abrasions, contusions, and lacerations.

Penetrating injuries such as gunshot wounds and impaling objects leave a circular to ovoid defect in the skin, whereas stab wounds and incised wounds usually appear slit-like or cut-like. It is often advantageous to shave hair from around a scalp wound to better observe the details of the wound and better document the findings photographically.

Examining a scalp wound is only one bit of information gleaned at autopsy. One often needs more information such as the pattern of skull fractures, the extent and nature of the brain injury, other findings detected

---

SCALP INJURY—GROSS PATHOLOGIC FEATURES

Abrasion
► Reddened "scrape-like" appearance of skin (Fig. 3-1A)
► May have a pattern (such as the outline of a rope in a hanging victim)
► Rolled skin at the edge of the abrasion may give an indication about the direction of the force

Contusion
► Red-purple, sometimes swollen bruise
► It is not reliable to predict the age of a contusion based on its color
► Microscopic examination may give an approximate indication regarding its age

Laceration
► A tear in skin and subcutaneous tissue, frequently with abrasion along the edges of the wound (Fig. 3-1A)
► Often with tissue bridging (Fig. 3-1B)

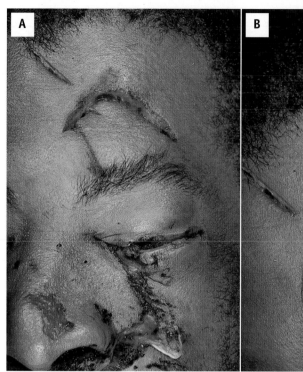
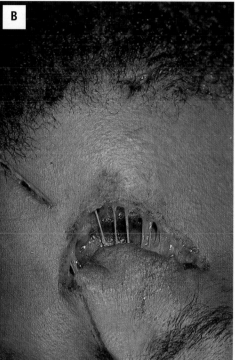

FIGURE 3-1

A, Note the laceration over the left eyebrow in this motor vehicle crash victim. There is also a laceration below his left eye and an abrasion on his nose. **B**, With the ends of the laceration separated, note the tissue bridging between the two sides of the laceration. Tissue bridges usually consist of blood vessels, nerves, and strands of connective tissue that remain intact; the tissues around them are torn as they are compressed underneath the impacting surface. Sharp force injuries such as incised wounds and stab wounds do not have tissue bridging.

SKULL FRACTURE

A skull fracture reflects the fact that the head sustained an impact significant enough to fracture bone. A fracture by itself does not necessarily mean that a person sustained a particularly severe injury. A person with a skull fracture may be seemingly unaffected and able to ambulate and converse without any difficulty and without any sequelae. On the contrary, it is not unusual for a person to sustain a traumatic head injury severe enough to be fatal without sustaining a skull fracture. Although skull fractures all represent the same finding—a crack or separation in the bone—their significance lies in their location, pattern, size, and how the injury was sustained.

SKULL FRACTURE—FACT SHEET

Definition and Etiology

▶ Fracture: A traumatic crack or separation of bones at a site of impact; the character of the fracture may give an indication regarding the nature of the impacting force

▶ Linear fracture: Most skull fractures are linear or curvilinear and involve the calvaria; often seen in individuals who fall and hit their head on a flat surface or in individuals struck by an object; most commonly seen after impact of the head with a flat and blunt surface such that the forces are spread over a large surface area

▶ Depressed fracture: A more focal (compact) impacting force such as with a hammer tends to fracture the bone directly under the area that it impacts and presses the broken pieces of bone downward, into brain tissue; this type of fracture is referred to as a depressed skull fracture; if many widely displaced pieces of fractured bone are present, it is referred to as a comminuted fracture

▶ Basilar fracture: Fractures at the base of the skull are generally associated with great force and many times are associated with unconsciousness. Among the most common are roughly transverse or oblique fractures from one side of the skull to the other, usually adjacent to the petrous ridges; if this fracture is severe enough and the bones are separated and displaced, the front and back of the base of the skull can be separated and brought back together, as though on a hinge—hence the common designation "hinge" fracture; hinge fractures are generally seen in victims of motor vehicle accidents and reflect the great forces sustained during vehicular crashes (see Fig. 3-2C)

▶ Ring fracture: A ring fracture occurs at the base of the skull and encircles or nearly encircles the foramen magnum; reflect severe forces causing either the head to be pressed downward onto the vertebral column or the vertebral column being thrust upward into the base of the skull (as is sometimes seen in individuals descending from heights onto the ground) (see Fig. 3-2C)

Clinical Features

▶ Varies from virtually asymptomatic to immediately fatal, depending on the location and severity of the fracture and the nature of the incident

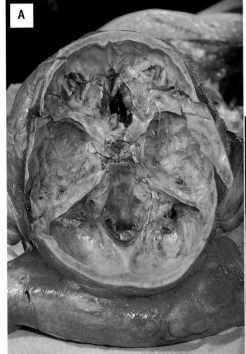

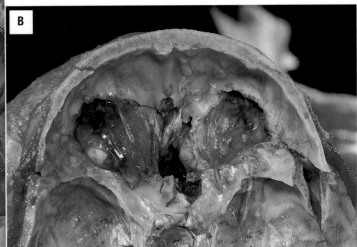

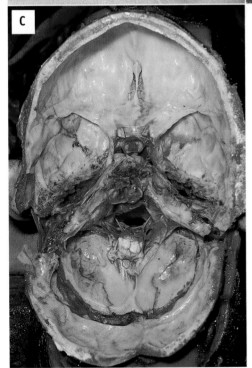

FIGURE 3-2

A and **B**, Note the fractures in the base of the skull involving the anterior cranial fossa in this victim of a gunshot wound. With the bones of the orbital plates removed, note the hemorrhage in the periorbital tissues (**B**). The bones of the orbital plates are particularly thin (in some cases almost paper thin) and are easily fractured. When fractures occur, it is not uncommon to see bleeding in the underlying orbital soft tissues. The blood may leak out into the subcutaneous tissues around the eyes and produce periorbital ecchymoses that may resemble "black eyes." However, one must be reminded that in this scenario, the bleeding has originated from an internal injury extending outward, not from direct trauma to the eyes. The orbital plates may also be fractured by extension from other fractures at the base of the skull. In addition, they may be fractured by sudden increases in intracranial pressure, as can occur with a pressure wave caused by a bullet as it traverses the head. They may also be of a "contrecoup" nature and occur in someone who has fallen and struck the back of the head on the ground. In this situation, the thin orbital plate bones are probably fractured by the frontal lobes of the brain as they "rebound" and impact the front of the inside of the skull after the initial impact to the back of the head on striking the ground. Alternatively, they may originate from the direct transmission of forces through the head at the time of impact. **C**, In this motor vehicle crash victim, note the gaping hinge fracture extending transversely across the base of the skull just anterior to the petrous ridges. There is also a displaced circular fracture extending through the occipital bones. In essence, the fracture in the occipital bones and the hinge fracture together create a wide "ring" fracture encircling the foramen magnum.

SKULL FRACTURE—GROSS PATHOLOGIC FEATURES

- ► Linear: may have branching fractures
- ► Basilar: general term for fractures involving the base of the skull
- ► Hinge: gaping fracture across the base of the skull, often along the petrous ridges
- ► Ring: circular fracture around the foramen magnum
- ► Depressed: focal area of fractured bone pushed inward; often seen after severe force or focal impacts with hard, compact objects
- ► Comminuted: "crush" injury from severe force

EPIDURAL HEMORRHAGE

An epidural hemorrhage is a collection of blood between the inner table of the skull (externally) and the dura (internally). If the collection of blood is space occupying, the hemorrhage is referred to as a hematoma. Epidural hemorrhages are usually located at the sides of the head, but they may occur at any location and usually underlie a skull fracture. The reason that they are preferentially located at the sides of the head is twofold. First, the temporal and sphenoid bones

---

EPIDURAL HEMORRHAGE—FACT SHEET

Definition
- ► Hemorrhage or hematoma (if space occupying) located between the inner table of the skull and the dura (Fig. 3-3)
- ► 90% to 95% associated with skull fracture

Clinical Features
- ► The victim may have a lucid interval
- ► May take time (many minutes to hours) to tear the adherent dura from the inner table of the skull as the hematoma expands
- ► Often with eventual headache, obtundation, and a comatose state if the epidural hematoma expands and remains untreated
- ► Frequently considered a neurosurgical emergency necessitating evacuation

Etiology
- ► Usually arise from a torn middle meningeal artery
- ► Rarely arise from a dural sinus tear or a tear in a middle meningeal vein
- ► Posterior fossa epidural hematomas usually arise from tears in a dural sinus

Imaging
- ► On computed tomography (CT), appears as a biconvex, or lens-shaped, hyperintensity (collection of blood) lying along the inner aspect of the skull

---

EPIDURAL HEMORRHAGE—PATHOLOGIC FEATURES

Gross
- ► If acute, typically a maroon clot of gelatinous blood not adherent to the dura or skull
- ► If chronic, may appear rust colored or brown and adherent to the dura
- ► If chronic, may have autolyzed blood replaced to a variable extent by fibrous tissue

Microscopic
- ► Acutely, red blood cells
- ► After several days, macrophages, hemosiderin, and endothelial cells
- ► After a week or so, fibroblasts, venules, membrane formation (see Fig. 3-3E)

---

at the sides of the head are relatively thin and more susceptible to fracture. Second, the course of the middle meningeal artery is along vascular grooves located along the inner aspect of the temporal and sphenoid bones. When these bones are fractured, the middle meningeal artery may be torn.

The prognosis/treatment is good if the epidural hematoma is evacuated before it enlarges enough to cause herniation symptoms. Generally speaking, epidural hematomas are regarded as neurosurgical emergencies and are evacuated on discovery rather than waiting and observing whether the hematoma will expand significantly or not.

SUBDURAL HEMORRHAGE

A subdural hemorrhage is a collection of blood between the dura (externally) and the meninges (internally). If the collection of blood is space occupying, the hemorrhage is referred to as a hematoma. Subdural hemorrhages are usually located over the vertices and lateral aspects of the cerebral hemispheres, but they may also occur in the interhemispheric fissure and over the base of the skull. In contrast to epidural hematomas, subdural hematomas are not usually well circumscribed and do not have distinct borders (Fig. 3-4A-D).

Individuals with head trauma and resultant subdural blood can have a range of clinical features, depending on the mechanism of injury. In the case of a severe head injury that is rapidly fatal (within minutes), the subdural hemorrhage may be only a thin film of blood. In individuals surviving a head injury for longer periods (many minutes to hours), the bleeding blood vessel or vessels may have enough time to hemorrhage significantly and form a large hematoma. In this scenario, the person is likely to progress through a series of symptoms ranging from headache to decreased responsiveness and finally to a comatose state and death if untreated.

The prognosis of a subdural hematoma depends on the severity of the head injury and how soon treatment is initiated. A small collection of subdural blood (a thin film of blood) may be seen in a rapidly fatal head injury, with death attributed to a severe diffuse traumatic brain injury. In this situation, the subdural blood is a marker of the generalized severe traumatic brain injury, which may have resulted in apnea or disruption of cardiovascular regulation, or both. The person may have died before the subdural hematoma had sufficient time to enlarge. Alternatively, a small amount of subdural blood may be seen in a person sustaining a much milder and survivable traumatic head injury, and surgical evacuation may not be necessary.

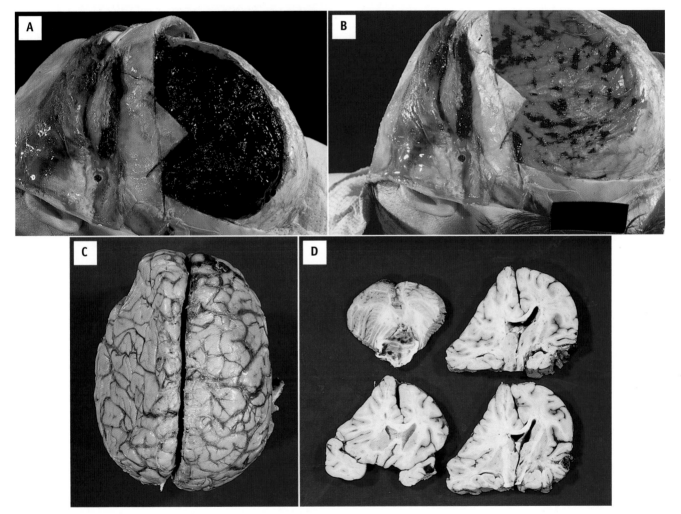

FIGURE 3-3

A, This man was struck on the head by a large, heavy object. Note the large maroon clotted epidural hematoma overlying most of the left cerebral hemisphere. The hematoma rests on top of the dura, which remains attached and is covering the brain. The hematoma measured 230 mL in volume. As is typical, an epidural hematoma has a well-circumscribed border because the hematoma must tear the dura away from the inner table of the skull as it enlarges. **B**, With the epidural hematoma removed, note the resultant concave, crater-like depression on the left side of the brain, evidence of the massive compressive effects that the epidural hematoma had on the brain. **C**, After fixation in formalin, the compression of the left cerebral hemisphere is obvious. **D**, On coronal sections, note the compressive effects that the epidural hematoma had on the left cerebral hemisphere. There is a massive left-to-right shift of the midline structures, left cingulate gyrus herniation, and left parahippocampal gyrus herniation. Note how the edge of the compressed left cerebral hemisphere is very flat. This flatness occurs because the epidural hematoma is pressing on the dura, which then presses on the surface of the brain. The dura transmits the forces evenly over the surface of the brain and produces a very flat cerebral surface. This appearance should be compared with the coronal sections of the brain from a subdural hematoma, in which case the brain surface is compressed, yet maintains its surface gyral undulations.   *Continued*

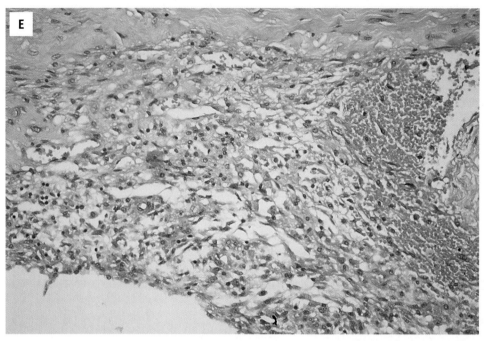

FIGURE 3-3, cont'd

E, In a different case, note the organizational changes on microscopic examination that have taken place in this 10-day-old epidural hematoma. There is a proliferation of fibroblasts and capillary formation. Note that if the hematoma persists for days to weeks, it will begin to organize. Its blood becomes autolyzed and is eventually resorbed and replaced by membranes of fibrous tissue that will eventually form a flat fibrous membrane firmly adherent to the outer surface of the dura. This process takes weeks to months. Microscopically, during the course of organization, macrophages appear and engulf red blood cells within a few days or so. Hemosiderin is identifiable with an iron stain. Along with this process, endothelial cells appear and form capillaries and then venules, and fibroblasts proliferate and eventually form a tough fibrous membrane adherent to the dura.

SUBDURAL HEMORRHAGE—FACT SHEET

Definition

▶ Hemorrhage or hematoma (if space occupying) located between the dura (externally) and the meninges (internally) (Fig. 3-4A-D)

▶ May or may not be associated with a skull fracture

Clinical Features

▶ If the person is conscious, headache is often a complaint, followed by progressive obtundation and a comatose state if the subdural hematoma expands and remains untreated

Etiology

▶ Usually caused by tears in cortical bridging veins

▶ May also arise from tears in cortical surface veins or cortical arteries, or tears in a dural sinus

Imaging

▶ On CT, an acute subdural hematoma typically appears as a hyperdense crescentic collection of blood that curves along the inner table of the skull. An organizing (subacute or chronic) subdural hematoma appears as a hyperdensity within an isodense collection

Prognosis

▶ If the subdural hematoma is large enough and detected early enough, surgical evacuation is usually recommended to decrease the mass effect and control further hemorrhage and brain swelling

▶ A larger subdural hematoma usually reflects a longer postinjury survival interval and possibly an increased number of torn and bleeding blood vessels

▶ The hematoma may be particularly large in those with a coagulopathy

---

FIGURE 3-4

A, In this motor vehicle accident victim, note the large maroon clotted subdural hematoma lying underneath the dura on the right side of the head. **B**, With the dura reflected, note the large subdural hematoma covering the right cerebral hemisphere. **C**, After formalin fixation and reflection of the dura, the subdural hematoma is seen to extend from the front to the back of the brain. **D**, The mass effect of this subdural hematoma is evident when the brain is viewed from its inferior aspect. Note the shift of the midline structures, including the midbrain to the right side of the image (away from the subdural hematoma). There is also a large parahippocampal gyrus herniation (also referred to as uncal herniation) on the side of the brain. **E**, This subdural hematoma has had a chance to organize for 2 months. Note how it has become variably brown and tan/yellow and is now adherent to the dura. As a subdural hematoma organizes, it becomes rusty brown and adherent to the overlying dura. As the organization proceeds, inner (meninges side) and outer (dura side) membranes of fibrous tissue are formed. Eventually, in many cases the bloody fluid is resorbed, with nothing left but a layer of organizing fibrous tissue attached to the inner lining of the dura. In some cases there may be a persistent accumulation of watery fluid in the area, a condition termed "subdural hygroma," that may need to be surgically drained. **F**, Microscopically, this organizing subdural hematoma consists largely of fibroblasts, capillaries, and hemosiderophages. Usually within a few days or so, early macrophages migrate into the area and engulf blood (the hemosiderin is readily identified on iron stain). Soon thereafter, the macrophages become more prominent, and endothelial cells form capillaries and eventually venules as fibroblasts proliferate and the blood continues to be resorbed. Finally, a membrane of fibrous tissue is firmly attached to the dura after having replaced the original liquid blood.

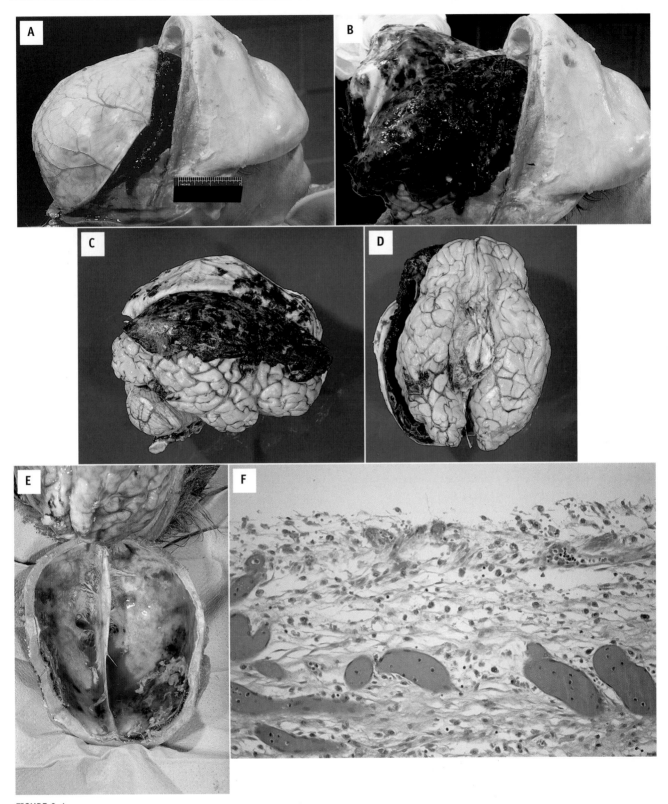

FIGURE 3-4
For legend see opposite page

SUBDURAL HEMORRHAGE—PATHOLOGIC FEATURES

Gross

▶ If acute, maroon clot of gelatinous, nonadherent blood
▶ If chronic, variably liquid/watery tan/rusty fluid with adherent fibrous membranes (see Fig. 3-4E)

Microscopic

▶ If acute, red blood cells
▶ If days old, macrophages, endothelial cells, capillaries, hemosiderin (see Fig. 3-4F)
▶ If weeks old, membranes of fibrous tissue, venules (see Fig. 3-4F)

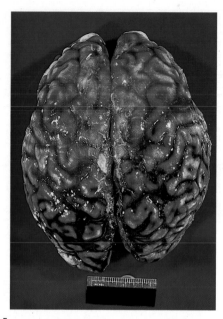

FIGURE 3-5

Note how the subarachnoid hemorrhage has imparted a red appearance to the brain.

SUBARACHNOID HEMORRHAGE

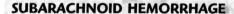

A subarachnoid hemorrhage is blood located between the meninges (externally) and the surface of the brain (internally) (Fig. 3-5). Subarachnoid blood may be due either to natural disease such as a ruptured cerebral artery berry aneurysm, to trauma, or to a combination of natural disease and trauma.

SUBARACHNOID HEMORRHAGE—PATHOLOGIC FEATURES

▶ Imparts a red color to the brain
▶ Identify the source (often cortical contusion).
▶ A small ruptured berry aneurysm may be difficult, if not impossible to identify

SUBARACHNOID HEMORRHAGE—FACT SHEET

Definition

▶ Subarachnoid blood is located between the meninges (externally) and the surface of the brain (internally)

Clinical Features

▶ Often accompanied by headache

Etiology

▶ Most commonly arises from cerebral contusions
▶ May be caused by a ruptured berry aneurysm or other natural disease process

Imaging

▶ On imaging, CT has high sensitivity and specificity for subarachnoid blood, with sensitivity approaching 95%. However, occasional false positives occur because imaging may falsely suggest subarachnoid blood in cases of cerebral anoxia and cerebral edema and in cases in which a contrast study has previously been performed
▶ If blood has pooled in the posterior cranial fossa, consider a torn vertebral artery (may be evaluated by postmortem angiography) or a torn basilar artery

Prognosis

▶ Depends on the cause and extent of injury
▶ May cause cerebral artery vasospasm and result in ischemic brain injury

CEREBRAL CONTUSION

A cerebral contusion is a bruise of the brain and is most commonly located on the surface of the brain, but it may be present as a deep (intracerebral) hematoma. Contusions may form hematomas ("contusion hematomas") that can enlarge over time. Contusions may occur at the site of impact or opposite the site of impact. The most common situation involving the latter scenario occurs when a person falls backward and strikes the back of their head on the ground. Although the impact is to the back of the head, contusions in this instance are often seen at the front of the brain, namely, the frontal poles, temporal poles, and orbital gyri (Fig. 3-6A,B). It is theorized that these contusions are formed by "rebounding" of the brain against the inner table of the front of the skull, bruising it, thereby, after the initial impact at the back of the head. Contusions are also likely to be formed in the frontal and temporal lobes of the brain because of the relatively rough, irregular, undulating, and sometimes relatively sharp bony surfaces of the orbital plates and middle cranial fossa. These contusions that are located opposite the site of impact are called "contrecoup" contusions. This theory may also explain the occasional occurrence of fractures of the thin orbital plates in such a scenario (contrecoup fractures).

DIFFUSE TRAUMATIC BRAIN INJURY

The term diffuse traumatic brain injury refers to a pattern of injury throughout the brain caused by

---

CEREBRAL CONTUSION—FACT SHEET

Definition

▶ A contusion is a bruise of the brain with disruption of tissue and hemorrhage (see Fig. 3-6A-D)

Etiology

▶ A fracture contusion underlies a skull fracture and is the most common type of contusion
▶ A "coup" contusion occurs at the site of impact (but without an associated skull fracture)
▶ A "contrecoup" contusion occurs opposite the site of impact
▶ May form a contusion hematoma; this injury is more common in those who have a coagulopathy (natural or therapeutic)
▶ Deeply situated contusions (in deep nuclei or deep white matter) usually associated with severe traumatic brain injury (see Fig. 3-6E)

Prognosis

▶ Varies, depending on the extent and location of contusions, the amount of associated brain injury, and the degree of any associated multisystem trauma
▶ A contusion may not be present on initial CT scan of the head and may be identified only on repeated scanning at later times and dates as the contusion evolves and enlarges
▶ A contusion may cause no mass effect initially, only to enlarge over the course of a few days after the injury, as edema develops and blood vessels necrose
▶ Cerebral contusions are not necessarily associated with clinical deterioration
▶ There may be pericontusional cerebral edema that may further compromise the blood supply to the area and cause additional ischemia and swelling
▶ May lead to a seizure disorder or debilities of cognition and/or motor function

Imaging

▶ Contusions may not be evident on initial CT, but become apparent on repeat studies. Pericontusional cerebral edema may develop. Contusions appear as parenchymal blood

---

DIFFUSE TRAUMATIC BRAIN INJURY—FACT SHEET

Definition

▶ Diffuse pattern of axonal injury throughout the brain

Clinical Features

▶ Immediate decreased level of consciousness or loss of consciousness, depending on the severity of the injury
▶ May lead to cognitive or physical debilities, or both, or may result in a persistent vegetative state

Etiology

▶ Head injury causing traumatic shifting of brain regions relative to each other, with stretching and damage of brain tissue
▶ Commonly seen in motor vehicle accidents
▶ Often occurs in association with ischemic brain injury

Imaging

▶ On imaging, may see scattered areas of blood, particularly in regions of white matter tracts; there may be intraventricular blood, effacement of the sulci or diffuse cerebral swelling, and loss of the differentiating features between gray and white matter

---

CEREBRAL CONTUSION—PATHOLOGIC FEATURES

Gross

▶ Focal bloody disruptions of brain tissue, usually on the surface of the cortex (see Fig. 3-6A, inferior right temporal lobe and anterior frontal lobes)
▶ Usually involve the crest of gyri and spare the sulci, but they may also involve the sulci (see Fig. 3-6C)
▶ Remote contusions appear as shrunken, partially cavitated, dark tan–discolored regions, often with tissue loss (see Fig. 3-6F and G)

Microscopic

▶ Acute contusions are characterized by bloody disruptions of the surface brain tissue with perivascular hemorrhage (see Fig. 3-6D)
▶ Remote contusions are characterized by gliosis, hemosiderophages, and eventual tissue loss (see Fig. 3-6H and I)
▶ When analyzing a remote contusion in the cortical ribbon, note how the contusion preferentially involves the superficial layers of cortex—this finding is in contrast to a remote infarct, which usually spares the most superficial layer of cortex (Fig. 3-6H)

DIFFUSE TRAUMATIC BRAIN INJURY—PATHOLOGIC FEATURES

Gross

▶ May have hemorrhages of the corpus callosum and superior cerebellar peduncle region (Fig. 3-7A and B)
▶ May have hemorrhages of the deep nuclei (see Fig. 3-6E)
▶ May have gliding contusions in the parasagittal white matter (see Fig. 3-6E)
▶ May have small hemorrhages scattered throughout the cerebral hemispheric white matter and brain stem (see Fig. 3-7C and D)

Microscopic

▶ Widespread dystrophic axons
▶ Dystrophic axons are visible on routine hematoxylin-eosin–stained sections after approximately 1 day's survival time (see Fig. 3-7E and F)
▶ Dystrophic axons can be visible with β-amyloid precursor protein immunohistochemistry (BAPP) after approximately 2 hours' survival time (see Fig. 3-7G-I)
▶ Injured axons undergo physiologic changes over time, becoming gradually more swollen and varicose before disconnecting
▶ Must distinguish diffuse traumatic axonal injury from vascular axonal injury or other causes of axonal injury (see Fig. 3-7J and K)

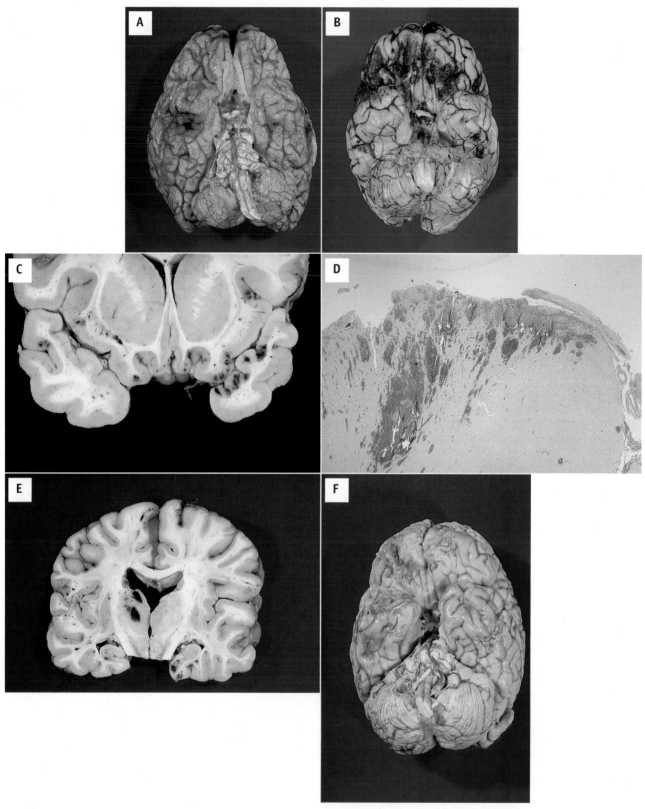

FIGURE 3-6

A, In this older person who fell and hit the back of his head on the ground, note the small bloody red acute contusions of the anterior frontal lobes and the right temporal lobe. The contusions are in a classic contrecoup distribution—on the side of the brain opposite the site of impact. Also note the subarachnoid hemorrhage, which invariably occurs with cortical contusions. **B**, In this fixed brain, note the bloody contusions of the orbital gyri. It is not unusual for the olfactory nerves to also be contused and result in an impaired sense of smell. **C**, On coronal sections, contusions often appear grossly as linear bloody streaks extending perpendicularly though the cortical ribbon. **D**, Microscopically, the contusions generally appear as perivascular hemorrhages that streak perpendicularly through the cortical ribbon. If the contusion is extensive, its fine details may not be evident, and instead, it may appear simply as a large hemorrhage. **E**, Deep cerebral contusions are also known as "intermediary coup" contusions and "basal ganglia" contusions and represent a great amount of force imparted onto the brain, often seen in high-speed motor vehicle accidents. In this case, note the two contusions in the left thalamus. Also note the curvilinear contusion in the left parasagittal white matter. This injury is often referred to as a "gliding" contusion and is likewise frequently seen in high-speed motor vehicle accidents. **F**, In this fixed brain, note the remote contusions of the orbital gyri and the right temporal lobe. Remote contusions that are months to years old appear as shrunken, disrupted, tan/brown-discolored lesions that often have fibrous adhesions to the overlying meninges or to the dura.

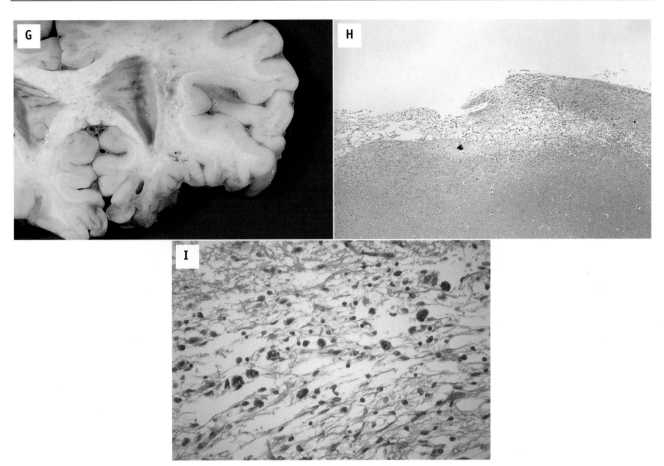

FIGURE 3-6, cont'd

G, On coronal section, a remote contusion appears as a disruption of the cortical ribbon and sometimes the underlying white matter, often with tissue loss. The adjacent tissues are soft and tan/brown discolored. **H**, Microscopically, note that this remote contusion characteristically involves the crest of the gyrus. Notice how in a remote contusion, the most superficial layers of cortex are disrupted. This finding is in contrast to a remote infarct, in which the most superficial layer or layers of cortex are usually spared because of their ability to glean nutrients and oxygen from the circulating cerebrospinal fluid. **I**, The affected tissues are disrupted, with the remaining tissue partially vacuolated, gliotic, and with hemosiderophages.

traumatic disruption of its nerve cells, identified as axonal disruptions. This pattern of injury is seen most commonly with motor vehicle accidents or any other mechanism of injury in which a large amount of force is imparted to the head and causes stretching/twisting of the brain tissue within the confines of the skull. It may also be seen with assaults or other mechanisms of great force. There may be other evidence of severe head injury, such as skull fractures, subdural blood, subarachnoid blood, and cortical contusions, but such additional injuries are not necessary for the diagnosis.

GUNSHOT WOUNDS

Gunshot wounds of the head are not uncommon and usually have a devastating outcome. Proper evaluation of a gunshot wound of the head begins with good scene investigation and, if possible, knowledge of what type and caliber of weapon was used. Careful collection of

evidence may include hand wipings (to be examined for gunshot residue) and collection of scalp hair from around the entrance wound (to be examined for gunpowder). Careful examination of the entrance and exit wounds and a radiograph of the head will provide additional important information before the internal examination is performed.

The available weapons and ammunition are seemingly endless, but generally consist of handguns, low- and high-power rifles, and shotguns. Handguns are most common and are of varying caliber ranging from .22 to .40 and larger. When a gun is fired, not only the bullet comes out of the end of the muzzle but also heated gas and unburned, burning, and burned gunpowder and soot. The presence or absence of these other substances on the victim's body or clothing may be helpful in determining the range of fire. The range of fire refers to the distance from the end of the muzzle to the body surface when the gun was fired.

The gunshot entrance wound is typically a circular to ovoid defect in the skin surrounded by a rim of

Text continued on p. 88

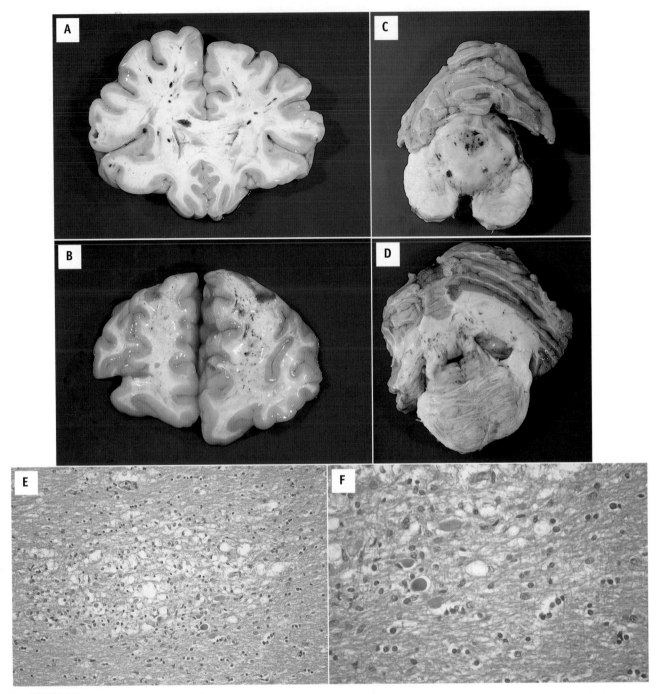

FIGURE 3-7

A, Note the hemorrhage in the corpus callosum in this victim of a car accident who survived for 15 hours. In severe closed head injury, many times there is both microscopic and macroscopic evidence of brain injury. Hemorrhages in the corpus callosum, deep nuclei, and brain stem in the region of the superior cerebellar peduncle are characteristic of severe primary traumatic brain injury. Also note the small hemorrhages scattered throughout the cerebral hemispheric white matter. Such scattered hemispheric white matter hemorrhages have been referred to as diffuse vascular injury. Diffuse vascular injury may be seen in patients with severe brain injuries and short survival time. The hemorrhages are scattered throughout the cerebral hemispheric white matter, but they are characteristically most pronounced in the anterior frontal lobes (**B**). **C**, Note the small hemorrhages scattered around the cerebral aqueduct in the midbrain of this bicyclist hit by a car. Hemorrhages in this location are typical of primary traumatic injury and are generally reflective of diffuse axonal injury. These hemorrhages are in contrast to streaky hemorrhages in the midline of the midbrain, which are often due to increased intracranial pressure (secondary brain stem hemorrhages or "Duret" hemorrhages). **D**, In the brain stem at the level of the pons in the same bicyclist, note the small hemorrhages in the superior cerebellar peduncles and around the cerebral aqueduct. Hemorrhages in these locations most commonly reflect primary traumatic brain injury. **E**, Microscopically, diffuse traumatic axonal injury is characterized by swollen, disconnected, traumatically injured axons found throughout the brain. They are most easily seen in the long white matter tracts such as the corpus callosum, internal capsules, and cerebral and cerebellar peduncles. One may also see scattered tiny areas of parenchymal disruption, referred to as microtears or microglial scars. Note the small remote tear in the tissue in the corpus callosum of this motor vehicle accident victim who survived for 6 weeks. **F**, At higher power, note the scattered pink swollen axons (dystrophic axons) and the gliosis. In months to years, the dystrophic axons will either become resorbed or become mineralized. It usually takes approximately 18 to 24 hours' survival time for dystrophic axons to become visible on routine hematoxylin–eosin–stained sections. With the help of β-amyloid precursor protein (BAPP) immunostaining, the dystrophic axons can become visible as early as 2 hours after injury. With immunostaining it is also easier to appreciate the pattern of axonal staining.

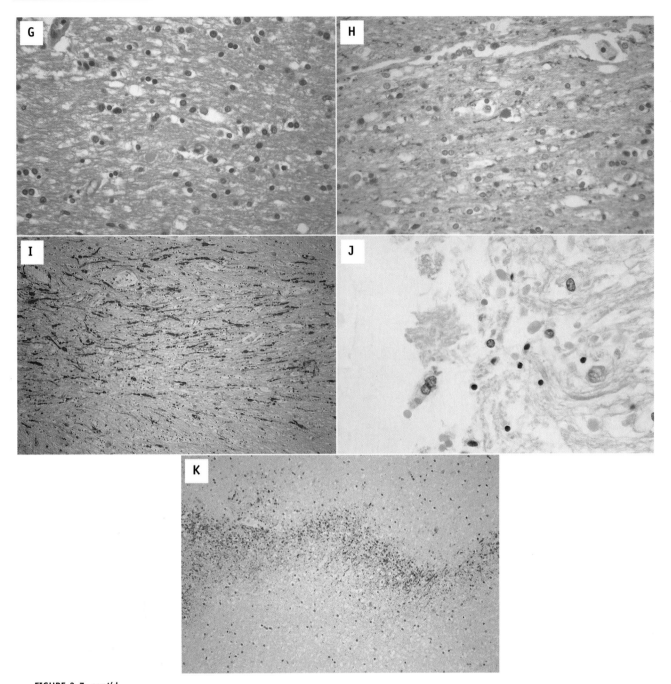

FIGURE 3-7, cont'd

G, In this motor vehicle accident victim, note the swollen axons in the central region of the image on a routinely stained section. **H**, In the same section as in **G** stained with BAPP, note not only the swollen bulb-like axons but also an extensive number of axons that are swollen to a lesser degree. Injured axons swell, become varicose, and eventually separate at varying rates. The BAPP immunostain helps identify injured axons at various stages of their injury evolution. Such observation is not possible with routine hematoxylin-eosin staining. **I**, After the injury, in most cases the axons are not "sheared" immediately, but rather sustain a disruption of their cytoarchitecture (their microtubules and neurofilaments). Axonal transport is slowed or stopped, and the axon begins to take on a varicose appearance and eventually "balloons" with accumulating intracellular substances. Eventually, the axon may separate at the site of injury and achieve a transected appearance. In this motor vehicle accident victim, note the classic pattern of traumatic axonal injury highlighted with BAPP immunostain. The axonal injury is diffuse and widespread. **J**, Axons can be injured for reasons other than trauma. Axonal injury may be caused by ischemia and hypoglycemia, among other things. Note the numerous dystrophic axons in this section of corpus callosum. There was no trauma in this case. The section was taken from a region of infarct. **K**, The pattern of axonal BAPP immunostaining can help differentiate traumatic from ischemic axonal injury. In this section of corpus callosum, note the curvilinear border of axonal staining in an early infarct. The prominent axonal staining will map out the border of ischemic/infarcted tissue. Contrast this appearance to the diffuse axonal staining characteristic of traumatic injury (**I**). The pattern of axonal injury has been given different names based on its origin. In this example, the term "vascular axonal injury" reflects the ischemic nature of the axonal injury. Diffuse traumatic axonal injury reflects traumatically injured axons throughout the brain. One must be reminded that BAPP immunostaining is not specific for trauma and will stain axons injured for virtually any reason.

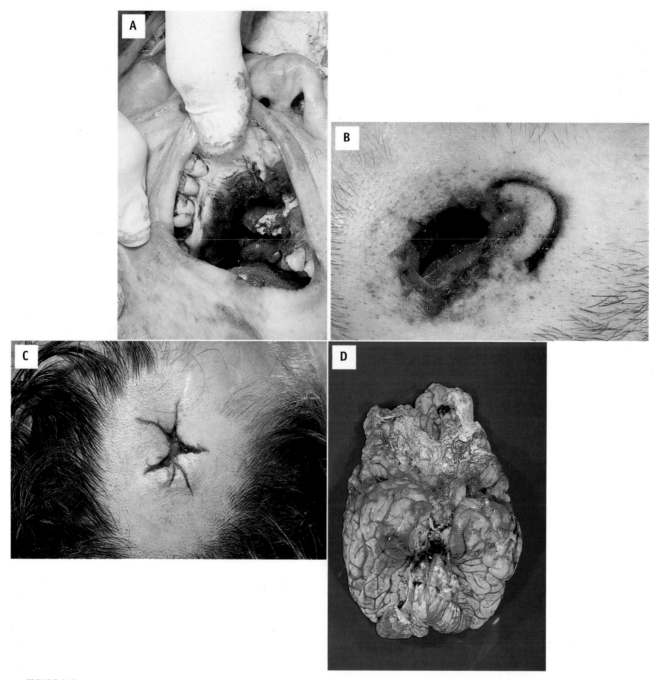

FIGURE 3-8

A, Note the black soot deposited on the roof of the mouth in this contact intraoral gunshot wound. **B**, In this contact gunshot wound of the right temple, note the muzzle imprint, characterized by a curvilinear abrasion at the right side of the wound. Also note the marginal abrasion surrounding the wound, which is typical of an entrance wound, and the faint black soot deposited along the edges of the wound. **C**, In this exit wound, note the tear-like appearance of the tissue defect created as the bullet exits the body. Entrance wounds usually leave a circular to ovoid defect in the tissue, whereas exit wounds generally leave a slit-like tear in the tissue that can usually be easily reapproximated to leave no central defect. **D**, A gunshot injury to the brain is generally characterized as a tract of bloody disrupted brain tissue. Note the brain tissue disruption and subarachnoid hemorrhage in the frontal lobes of the brain in this person who sustained a gunshot wound of the head.

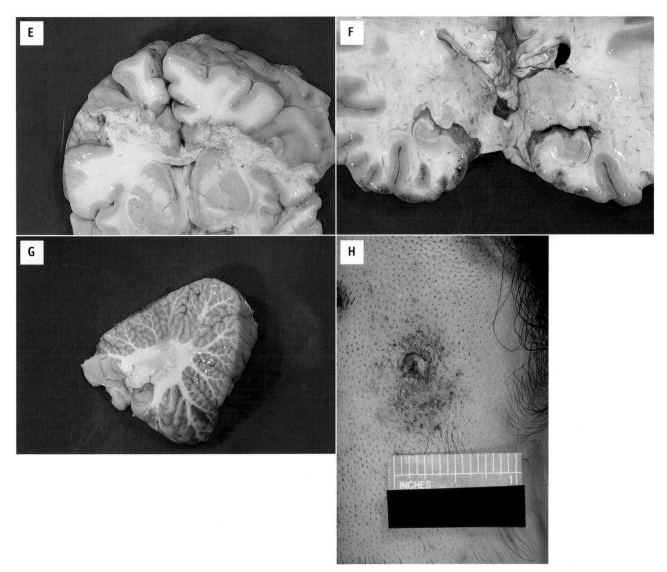

FIGURE 3-8, cont'd

E, On coronal sections, in a different case, note the tract of bloody, disrupted brain tissue along the path of the bullet through the frontal lobes. When examining a brain that has a gunshot wound, it is often advantageous to make a slice in the brain connecting the entrance and exit wounds, whatever the plane, to more accurately describe the path of the bullet through various brain structures. **G**, The bullet destroys brain tissue along its path through the brain. However, brain damage is also produced by the pressure wave created by the bullet as it imparts its energy to the tissue. The pressure wave extends outward in all directions from the bullet's path through the brain and creates a "temporary cavity" in the brain tissue that is present for a split second. This pressure wave can cause extensive damage, particularly if the bullet has high velocity. The pressure wave can create herniation contusions of brain tissue far away from the path of the bullet. In this case of a gunshot wound through the brain, note the herniation contusions of the parahippocampal gyri bilaterally (**F**) and the herniation contusion of the cerebellar tonsils (**G**). These contusions are due to the pressure wave causing rapid and forceful displacement of brain tissue against the tentorium and the edge of the foramen magnum, respectively. **H**, Note the small red disruptions of the skin around this gunshot wound to the head. This pattern is referred to as stippling and is usually seen in medium-range gunshot wounds in which the end of the muzzle is a few inches to a few feet from the surface of the skin when the bullet is fired. The stippling is caused by tiny pieces of burned, burning, and unburned gunpowder that impact the skin and injure it. In distant-type gunshot wounds there is no muzzle imprint, no soot, and no stippling. All that is present is the entrance wound in the skin, which is usually circular to ovoid.

abraded skin. The edges of the wound cannot be reapproximated. The underlying bony defect, if in the calvaria, typically demonstrates inward beveling as the bullet pushes bony fragments into the brain. When the bullet exits the calvaria, it usually creates a defect with external beveling as it pushes bony fragments out into the scalp tissue. The exit wound in the skin is caused by tearing of the skin as the bullet exits the body. In an exit wound, there is usually no marginal abrasion, and the edges of the exit wound can generally be easily reapproximated. The bullet creates a path of bloody disrupted brain tissue as it courses through the brain. The bullet also creates an expanding pressure wave around it that displaces brain tissue and can lead to herniation contusions located far away from the actual path of the bullet (Fig. 3-8F and G).

GUNSHOT WOUNDS—FACT SHEET

Definition
► Penetrating (into, but not through, the head) or perforating (through the head) missile injury caused by a bullet
► The amount of tissue injury depends largely on the velocity of the bullet and to a lesser extent on the size of the bullet

Clinical Features
► Often unconscious/comatose, particularly if the bullet track is perforating, high velocity, through the basal ganglia, or through the posterior cranial fossa/brain stem

Imaging
► Skull fracture, tracks of bone, missile fragments, or intact projectiles
► May have cerebral contusions at the entrance and exit sites

GUNSHOT WOUNDS—GROSS PATHOLOGIC FEATURES

► Entrance wounds are usually round/ovoid defects with marginal abrasion (see Fig. 3-8B)
► Exit wounds are usually tears in the skin (see Fig. 3-8C)
► Internal/external beveling of the calvaria may help differentiate an entrance from an exit wound
► Contact wound (soot in the depth of the wound, muzzle imprint, tears in the skin): end of the muzzle directly on the skin (see Fig. 3-8A and B)
► Close-range wound (soot/searing on the skin around the wound): end of the muzzle usually within a few inches of the skin
► Medium-range wound (stippling around the wound): end of the muzzle a few inches to a few feet from the skin (see Fig. 3-8H)
► Distant-range wound (no gunpowder residue or other defects on the skin—but may be on overlying clothing)
► Temporary cavitation may cause herniation contusions
► Brain injury consists of a tract of bloody, disrupted brain tissue (see Fig. 3-8D and E)

The prognosis depends on the caliber and muzzle velocity of the weapon and the location of the injury. Gunshot wounds to the infratentorial region are particularly poorly tolerated, as are wounds to the deep nuclei. Small-caliber, low-velocity wounds of the anterior frontal lobes or tangential wounds of the brain may be better tolerated.

CHILD ABUSE

Although many of the head injuries sustained by an infant or young child during an assault are similar to those seen in an adult, child abuse is discussed in its own section because of the subtle differences in anatomy of infants or young children and adults, the unique types of trauma that may be inflicted on a small body, and the different reaction to injury in the young and still-developing brain. Because an infant or young child is often unconscious after a head injury or is too young to talk, circumstances regarding the injury are often gleaned from parents or caretakers who may not be forthright or honest to protect themselves from accusations of wrongdoing and possible punishment. In addition, because these injuries are often sustained in the home, there is rarely an independent witness. It is important to be able to differentiate accidental from inflicted injury. Such differentiation is usually accomplished only after careful and complete analysis of all information available regarding the case, including good and proper investigation, interviews of all potential witnesses, and a complete autopsy, and then interpreting the injuries in the context of the complete case and considering whether the injuries are consistent with the scenario provided. Accidental fatal head injuries in the home that occur during normal daily activities are rare, and one must carefully consider inflicted injury, often despite the parents' or caretakers' stories or recollection of events.

Inflicted fatal head injuries in infants and young children can take many forms and range from severely comminuted skull fractures with brain lacerations and a large amount of subdural blood to those with no evidence of an impact site, no skull fractures, and only a smear of subdural blood. Characteristic markers of severe inflicted head injury include subdural blood and retinal or optic nerve hemorrhage, or both. These conditions are not diagnostic of severe inflicted head injury but are commonly seen in this setting. Skull fractures are indicative of an impact and may be seen in both accidental and inflicted head injury.

The mechanism of head injury varies, but impact injury is usually involved. Even in cases reported to be "shaken baby syndrome," the majority of victims at autopsy have been found to have skull fractures or scalp contusions, or both. Pure shaking is probably a rare event inasmuch as most of these cases have evidence of head impact injury. Moreover, all the autopsy findings identified in reportedly shaken babies can be seen with severe impact injury alone. There are no pathologic findings diagnostic of shaking. Regardless of the mechanism of injury, the head injuries sustained during an assault that prove to be fatal should be well documented photographically and descriptively.

The head injury leading to death in these cases is often attributed to diffuse traumatic brain injury, and the cause of this injury is frequently believed to be diffuse axonal injury; however, injured axons are often not easily demonstrated and often requires the use of β-amyloid precursor protein (BAPP) immunohistochemistry. Even then, one may not be able to document axonal injury because the death may have occurred too quickly or the brain may have swelled so quickly that the blood supply to the brain was limited or stopped before the necessary reactive changes could take place. Select studies have shown that injured axons are more readily demonstrable in axonal tracts in the medulla. This finding may reflect the fact that during an assault the brain stem is physically damaged, which may lead to apnea or other types of dysfunctional breathing or cardiac dysfunction with hypotension, or both. Because victims of child abuse with severe head injury are often apneic or hypoxic when first seen by medical personnel, one must consider the possibility that at least some component of the brain injury is secondary to hypoxic-ischemic damage arising as a result of trauma-induced apnea. Indeed, the brain in these victims is frequently swollen, intracranial pressure is high, and there is often evidence of ischemia or infarction on microscopic examination. Often, traumatic and ischemic injury coexist in the brains of these victims, but all the changes still stem from the initial traumatic injury.

Cases of severe accidental head injury that prove to be fatal most commonly involve infants and young children injured in high-speed motor vehicle accidents,

---

CHILD ABUSE—PATHOLOGIC FEATURES

Gross

▶ Scalp contusions (Fig. 3-9A and B)
▶ Subdural blood common (often only a small amount) (see Fig. 3-9C)
▶ Perioptic nerve hemorrhage and retinal hemorrhage common (see Fig. 3-9D-F). Note the normal appearance of retinas in D.
▶ Skull fractures may or may not be present (see Fig. 3-9G)
▶ Often have hypoxic-ischemic brain injury
▶ The extent of internal injury often does not correlate with the extent of external injury

---

pedestrians run over by motor vehicles, or those who have fallen from great heights (such as a second- or third-floor balcony). Occasionally, an accidental crush injury is caused by a heavy object such as a precariously positioned television falling on a playing child. These types of accidental head injuries usually involve severe skull fractures, often through the base of the skull. Accidental head injuries that occur during normal daily activities are rarely very significant or fatal. Activities such as falling off a couch or chair should not normally prove to be fatal, and such stated scenarios should prompt further investigation to rule out inflicted head injury.

SEQUELAE OF TRAUMATIC BRAIN INJURY

The direct effect of traumatic head injury may be fatal or may lead to varying degrees of physical and/or mental debilities. Immediately after a head injury, brain swelling may lead to increased intracranial pressure and various types of brain herniation. After the acute injury, having survived the initial effects of the head injury, one may still die or suffer varying amounts of additional injury or illness from delayed complications that arise from the head injury. Such complications may include post-traumatic seizure disorder, post-traumatic meningitis, and various complications related to being comatose or in a persistent vegetative state.

Severe head injury may lead to the development of a persistent vegetative state. The most common injury leading to such a state is diffuse traumatic axonal injury. In persistent vegetative state, the person maintains regular sleep/wake cycles but is not aware of the environment and requires total care. In this bedridden state, patients are susceptible to complications such as bronchopneumonia, mucous plugs in their airways, deep venous thrombosis, and pulmonary artery thromboemboli. Additionally, decubitus ulcers, malnutrition, or other wasting conditions may develop. If somebody dies of delayed complications of remote head injury, it is important to attribute the underlying cause and manner of death to the head injury and how it was sustained.

CHILD ABUSE—FACT SHEET

Definition

▶ Abusive head injury is inflicted injury

Clinical Features

▶ With severe head injury, there is often initial loss of consciousness and the victim may present with apnea or hypotension/bradycardia, or both
▶ The history of the incident is often wrong or incomplete
▶ Clinically, infants and young children with a head injury severe enough to prove to be fatal will not have a lucid interval and will be observed, at the very least, to be acting "not right"; a possible exception to this statement is an expanding epidural hematoma, which is rare in this situation

Prognosis

▶ Victims of inflicted head injury usually have a worse outcome than those with accidental head injury
▶ May lead to varying degrees or combinations of cognitive and motor dysfunction and blindness or other sensory deficits

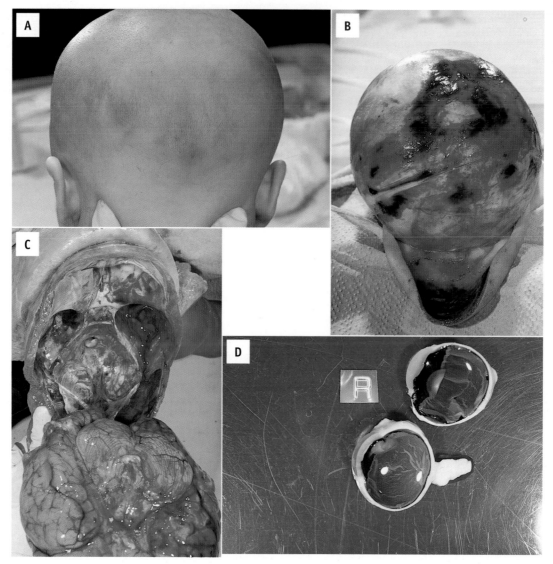

FIGURE 3-9

A, Note the contusions of the scalp at the back of the head. Contusions at the back of the head are not uncommon, particularly if the child's head was slammed or otherwise impacted backward onto a surface. **B**, Note the large amount of subscalp blood in this case. Sometimes, the surface of the scalp can show no contusion or abrasion or only mild contusion, whereas the undersurface of the scalp shows severe contusion. Even if no scalp impact site can be identified, it does not mean that a significant head impact did not occur. Such may be the case for a number of reasons. The skin and subcutaneous tissues of infants and young children are elastic and may not bruise easily. The head may have been impacted against a soft surface or a surface with "give" such as a couch cushion, which would diffuse the force over a greater surface area and lessen the chance of forming a distinct contusion. This possibility underscores the importance of autopsy in sudden and unexplained death in infants and young children because the extent of injury is not reliably determined by external examination of the body. **C**, The subdural blood is often just a film of blood and may be located over the vertices of the cerebral hemispheres or the base of the skull, or both. The subdural blood is generally regarded as a marker of the rotational effects of the brain within the skull sustained during severe head injury, with tearing of bridging veins. Sometimes, however, the accumulation of subdural blood is sufficient to form a hematoma, which may be surgically evacuated. **D**, Normally, when eyes are sectioned, there will be no hemorrhages of the retina or the optic nerves.

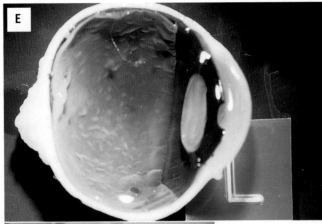

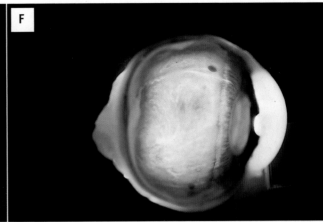

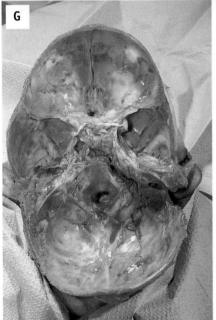

FIGURE 3-9, cont'd

E, Note the small, scattered retinal hemorrhages in this 2-year-old chid with severe traumatic head injury. **F**, The retinal hemorrhages can be highlighted by illuminating the eye from behind. Although retinal hemorrhages often occur with abusive head injury in infants and young children, they may also be seen in other conditions, and may be seen up to a few weeks after birth, in those with a coagulopathy, and in those with sepsis, and they may rarely occur after severe accidental head injury, such as high-speed motor vehicle accidents. Retinal hemorrhages are not specific for abusive head injury. **G**, Skull fractures may or may not be present in cases of severe inflicted head injury. In cases of fatal accidental head injury, such as those sustained in high-speed motor vehicle accidents or falls from great heights, the skull fractures are usually severe and often involve the base of the skull and may form a hinge fracture, as seen in this case. Note the hinge fracture extending transversely across the base of the skull, along the petrous ridges.

SEQUELAE OF TRAUMATIC BRAIN INJURY—FACT SHEET

► Meningitis may arise following traumatic head injury
  ► More common when there is a skull fracture or a tear in the dura
► Seizures may arise in post-traumatic head injury
  ► Occur in up to 10% of those with traumatic brain injury
  ► Usually occur soon after the injury (within 1 to 2 weeks) and are associated with hypoxia, hemorrhage, and physical disruption of tissues
  ► May be late in onset (weeks, months, and even years after the injury) because of scarring in brain tissue with imperfect reorganization of the electrical circuitry
  ► May require treatment with anticonvulsants
  ► Rarely, may be fatal (sudden unexpected death in epilepsy or "SUDEP")
  ► More common in those with penetrating head injury, intracerebral hemorrhage, cortical contusion, and depressed skull fracture

SEQUELAE OF TRAUMATIC BRAIN INJURY—PATHOLOGIC FEATURES

Gross

► Remote contusions
► Secondary brain stem hemorrhages (Fig. 3-10A)
► Diffuse white matter degenerative changes (see Fig. 3-10B)
► Types of herniations (see Fig. 3-10C):
  ► Subfalcial (cingulate gyrus) herniation: herniation of the cingulate gyrus under the falx cerebri
  ► Transtentorial (uncal or parahippocampal gyrus) herniation: herniation of the uncus or parahippocampal gyrus over the edge of the tentorium (see Fig. 3-10C)
  ► Tonsillar herniation: herniation of the cerebellar tonsils into the foramen magnum

---

Microscopic

► Diffuse gliosis of white matter (see Fig. 3-10E)

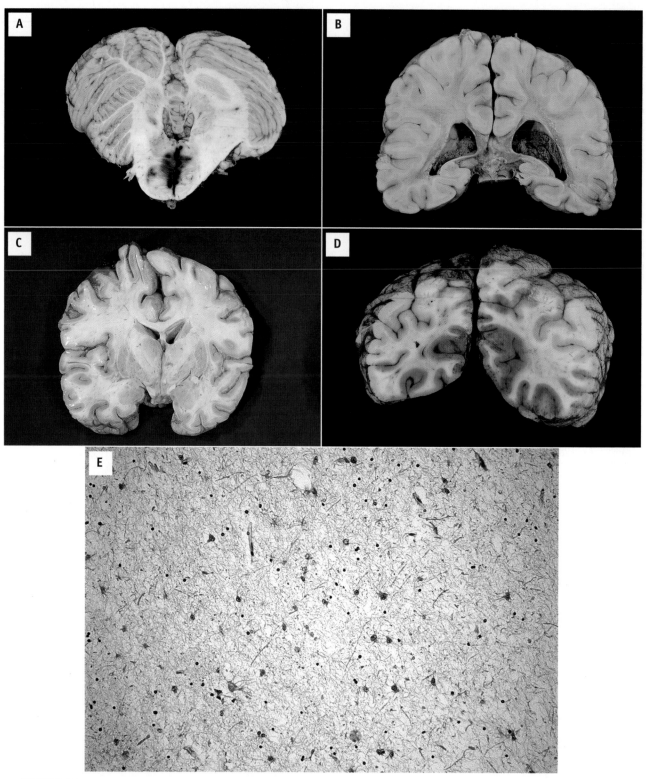

FIGURE 3-10

A, Note the hemorrhage in the central region of the pons in this brain stem. This is a typical location of a secondary brain stem hemorrhage resulting from increased intracranial pressure. **B**, Note the gray, waxy discoloration of the hemispheric white matter and the relative preservation of the overlying cortical ribbon in this person who survived for many years in a persistent vegetative state following diffuse traumatic brain injury sustained in a motor vehicle accident. This white matter damage is reflective of remote diffuse traumatic axonal injury. **C**, Note the shift of the midline structures to the right in this swollen brain from a person with a left subdural hematoma. There is also compression of the left lateral ventricle, a left-to-right subfalcial (cingulate gyrus) herniation, and a left-to-right transtentorial (parahippocampal gyrus or "uncal") herniation. As a result of the traumatic brain injury as well as ischemic brain injury, the brain swells, often to the point of creating high intracranial pressure that impairs cerebral perfusion and creates further cerebral ischemia. This may result in cerebellar tonsillar herniation as the brain tissue is forced down through the foramen magnum. Hypoxic-ischemic brain injury is frequently associated with traumatic brain injury, often because the head-injured person is unconscious, cannot protect the airway, and may also be hypotensive, bradycardic, apneic, or bradypneic before resuscitation is attempted. **D**, Note the dusky brown discoloration of the cortical ribbon in the distribution of the posterior cerebral arteries as a result of infarction in this coronal section of the parieto-occipital region. This finding is not uncommon in a swollen brain and is caused by the herniated parahippocampal gyri compressing the posterior cerebral arteries against the edge of the tentorium. **E**, On microscopic examination of the white matter, note the small number of cells and the widely scattered reactive astrocytes.

Bronchopneumonia may seem like a natural cause of death, but when it is related to debility from a gunshot wound to the head inflicted by another person months or years ago, the death is still considered a homicide.

The brain is encased within a hard, bony, unyielding skull. As a subdural hematoma (or any other mass lesion) expands or the brain swells for any other reason, intracranial pressure can increase quickly. The first response is for cerebrospinal fluid to be displaced out of the intracranial region as the cerebral ventricles are compressed. Cerebrospinal fluid is also resorbed. Subsequently, the gyri flatten. If intracranial pressure continues to increase, brain tissue herniates over the dural flaps from a region of high pressure to a region of lower pressure. The most common herniations are herniation of the cingulate gyrus underneath the falx cerebrum (subfalcial herniation), herniation of the parahippocampal gyrus over the edge of the tentorium (transtentorial or "uncal" herniation), and herniation of the cerebellar tonsils into the foramen magnum (cerebellar tonsillar herniation). Eventually, as intracranial pressure increases enough or mean arterial pressure falls, or both, cerebral ischemia may result. Complications of head trauma are varied but often readily recognized.

SUGGESTED READINGS

Scalp Injury

DiMaio VJM, Dana SE: Handbook of Forensic Pathology. Georgetown, TX, Landes Bioscience, 1998.
Knight B: Forensic Pathology. London, Oxford University Press, 1996.

Skull Fracture

Ezzat W, Ang LC, Nyssen J: Pontomedullary rent: A specific type of primary brainstem traumatic injury. Am J Forensic Med Pathol 1995;16:336-339.
Gurdijian ES, Webster JE, Lissner HR: The mechanism of skull fracture. Radiology 1950;54:313-338.
Harvey FH, Jones AM: "Typical" basal skull fracture of both petrous bones: An unreliable indicator of head impact site. J Forensic Sci 1980;25:280-286.
Hirsch CS, Kaufman B: Contrecoup skull fractures. J Neurosurg 1975;42:530-534.
McElhaney JH, Hopper RH, Nightingale RW, Myers BS: Mechanisms of basilar skull fracture. J Neurotrauma 1995;12:669-678.
Voigt GE, Skold G: Ring fractures of the base of the skull. J Trauma 1974;14:494-505.

Epidural Hemorrhage

Cruz J: Neurologic and Neurosurgical Emergencies. Philadelphia, Saunders, 1998.
Hirsch CS, Adelson L: Ethanol in sequestered hematomas. Am J Clin Med 1973;59:429-433.
Paterniti S, Falcone MF, Fiore P, et al: Is the size of an epidural hematoma related to outcome? Acta Neurochir 1998;140:953-955.
Pearl GS: Traumatic neuropathology. Clin Lab Med 1998;18:39-64.
Rivas JJ, Lobato RD, Sarabia R: Extradural hematoma: Analysis of factors influencing the courses of 161 patients. Neurosurgery 1988;23:44-51.
Wijdicks EFM: Neurologic Catastrophes in the Emergency Department. Boston, Butterworth Heinemann, 2000, pp 231-252.

Subdural Hemorrhage

Avis SP: Nontraumatic acute subdural hematoma—a case report and review of the literature. Am J Forensic Med Pathol 1993;14:130-134.
Buchsbaum RM, Adelson L, Sunshine I: A comparison of postmortem ethanol levels obtained from blood and subdural specimens. Forensic Sci Int 1989;41:237-243.
Gennarelli TA, Thibault LE: Biomechanics of acute subdural hematoma. J Trauma 1982;22:680-686.
Kleiven S: Influence of impact direction on the human head in prediction of subdural hematoma. J Neurotrauma 2003;20:365-379.
Maxeiner H: Detection of ruptured cerebral bridging veins at autopsy. Forensic Sci Int 1997;89:103-110.
Maxeiner H, Wolff M: Pure subdural hematomas: A postmortem analysis of their form and bleeding points. Neurosurgery 2002;50:503-509.
O'Brien PK, Norris JW, Tator CH: Acute subdural hematomas of arterial origin. J Neurosurg 1974;41:435-439.
Seravadei F: Prognostic factors in severely head injured adult patients with acute subdural hematomas. Acta Neurochir 1997;139:279-285.

Subarachnoid Hemorrhage

Al-Yamany M, Deck J, Bernstein M: Pseudo-subarachnoid hemorrhage: A rare neuroimaging pitfall. Can J Neurol Sci 1999;25:57-59.
Contostavlos DL: Massive subarachnoid hemorrhage due to laceration of the vertebral artery associated with fracture of the transverse process of the atlas. J Forensic Sci 1970;16:40-56.
Mant AK: Traumatic subarachnoid hemorrhage following blows to the neck. J Forensic Sci Soc 1972;12:567-572.
Nanda A, Vannemreddy PS, Polin RS, Willis BK: Intracranial aneurysms and cocaine abuse: Analysis of prognostic indicators. Neurosurgery 2000;46:1063-1069.
Opeskin K, Burke MP: Vertebral artery trauma. Am J Forensic Med Pathol 1998;19:206-217.
Vanezis P: Techniques used in the evaluation of vertebral artery trauma at post-mortem. Forensic Sci Int 1979;13:159-165.

Cerebral Contusion

Adams JH, Doyle D, Graham DI, et al: Gliding contusions in nonmissile head injury in humans. Arch Pathol Lab Med 1986;110:485-488.
Adams JH, Doyle D, Graham DI, et al: Deep intracerebral (basal ganglia) hematomas in fatal non-missile head injury in man. J Neurol Neurosurg Psychiatry 1986;49:1039-1043.
Courville CB, Blomquist OA: Traumatic intracerebral hemorrhage (with particular reference to its pathogenesis and its relation to "delayed traumatic apoplexy.") Arch Surg 1940;41:1-28.
Dawson SL, Hirsch CS, Lucas FV, Sebek BA: The contrecoup phenomenon—reappraisal of a classic problem. Hum Pathol 1980;2:155-166.
Gudeman SK, Kishore PRS, Miller JD, et al: The genesis and significance of delayed traumatic intracerebral hematoma. Neurosurgery 1979;5:309-312.
Gurdjian ES: Cerebral contusions: Re-evaluation of the mechanism of their development. J Trauma 1976;16:35-51.
Lindenberg R, Freytag E: The mechanism of cerebral contusions. AMA Arch Pathol 1960;69:440-469.
Oertel M, Kelly DF, McArthur D, et al: Progressive hemorrhage after head trauma: Predictors and consequences of the evolving injury. J Neurosurg 2002;96:109-116.

Diffuse Traumatic Brain Injury

Adams JH, Doyle D, Ford I, et al: Diffuse axonal injury in head injury: Definition, diagnosis, and grading. Histopathology 1989;15:49-59.
Adams JH, Doyle D, Graham DI, et al: Deep intracerebral (basal ganglia) hematomas in fatal non-missile head injury in man. J Neurol Neurosurg Psychiatry 1986;49:1039-1043.

Dolinak D, Smith C, Graham DI: Global hypoxia per se is an unusual cause of axonal injury. Acta Neuropathol 2000;100:553-560.

Geddes JF: What's new in the diagnosis of head injury? J Clin Pathol 1997;50:271-274.

Geddes JF, Vowles GH, Beer TW, Ellison DW: The diagnosis of diffuse axonal injury: Implications for forensic practice. Neuropathol Appl Neurobiol 1997;23:339-347.

Geddes JF, Whitwell HL, Graham DI: Traumatic axonal injury: Practical issues for diagnosis in medicolegal cases. Neuropathol Appl Neurobiol 2000;26:105-116.

Maxwell WL, Povlishock JT, Graham DI: A mechanistic analysis of nondisruptive axonal injury: A review. J Neurotrauma 1997;14:419-439.

Niess C, Grauel U, Toennes SW, Bratzke H: Incidence of axonal injury in human brain tissue. Acta Neuropathol 2002;104:79-84.

Povlishock JT: Traumatically induced axonal injury: Pathogenesis and pathobiological implications. Brain Pathol 1992;2:1-12.

Schreiber MA, Aoki N, Scott BG, Beck JR: Determinants of mortality in patients with severe blunt head injury. Arch Surg 2002;137:285-290.

Vitaz TW, Jenks J, Raque GH, Shields CB: Outcome following moderate traumatic brain injury. Surg Neurol 2003;60:285-291.

Gunshot Wounds

Adelson L: A microscopic study of dermal gunshot wounds. Am J Clin Pathol 1961;35:393-402.

Davis JH: Forensic pathology in firearms cases. J Int Wound Ballistics Assoc Wound Ballistics Rev 1998;3(4):5-15.

DiMaio VJM: Gunshot Wounds—Practical Aspects of Firearms, Ballistics, and Forensic Techniques, 2nd ed. Boca Raton, FL, CRC Press, 1999.

Karger B: Penetrating gunshots to the head and lack of immediate incapacitation 1. Wound ballistics and mechanisms of incapacitation. Int J Legal Med 1995;108:53-61.

Karger B: Penetrating gunshots to the head and lack of immediate incapacitation 2. Review of case reports. Int J Legal Med 1995;108:117-126.

Nathoo N, Chite SH, Edwards PJ, et al: Civilian infratentorial gunshot injuries: Outcome analysis of 26 patients. Surg Neurol 2002;58:225-233.

Oehmichen M, Meissner C, Konig HG: Brain injury after gunshot wounding: Morphometric analysis of cell destruction caused by temporary cavitation. J Neurotrauma 2000;17:155-162.

Surgical management of penetrating brain injury. J Trauma 2001;51:S16-S25.

Child Abuse

Alexander R, Sato Y, Smith W, Bennett T: Incidence of impact trauma with cranial injuries ascribed to shaking. Am J Dis Child 1990;144:724-726.

Atkinson JLD, Anderson RE, Murray MH: The early critical phase of severe head injury: Importance of apnea and dysfunctional respiration. J Trauma 1998;45:941-945.

Case ME, Graham MA, Hardy TC, et al: Position paper on fatal abusive head injuries in infants and young children. Am J Forensic Med Pathol 2001;22:112-122.

DiMaio VJ, DiMaio D: Forensic Pathology, 2nd ed. Boca Raton, FL, CRC Press, 2001, pp 358-362.

Duhaime AC, Eppley M, Margulies S, et al: Crush injuries to the head in children. Neurosurgery 1995;37:401-407.

Duhaime AC, Gennarelli TA, Thibault LE, et al: The shaken baby syndrome. J Neurosurg 1987;66:409-415.

Emerson MV, Pieramici DJ, Stoessel KM, et al: Incidence and rate of disappearance of retinal hemorrhages in newborns. Ophthalmology 2001;108:36-39.

Geddes JF, Hackshaw AK, Vowles GH, et al: Neuropathology of inflicted head injury in children 1. Patterns of brain damage. Brain 2001;124:1290-1298.

Geddes JF, Hackshaw AK, Vowles GH, et al: Neuropathology of inflicted head injury in children 2. Microscopic brain injury in infants. Brain 2001;124:1299-1306.

Gilles EE, Nelson MD: Cerebral complications of nonaccidental head injury in childhood. Pediatr Neurol 1998;19:119-128.

Gilliland MG, Luckenbach MW, Chenier TC: Systemic and ocular findings in 169 prospectively studied child deaths: Retinal hemorrhages usually mean child abuse. Forensic Sci Int 1993;69:117-132.

Hadley MN, Sonntag VKH, Rekate HL, Murphy A: The infant whiplash-shake injury syndrome: A clinical and pathological study. Neurosurgery 1989;24:536-540.

Harwood-Nash DC, Hendrick EB, Hudson AR: The significance of skull fractures in children. Radiology 1971;101:151-155.

Hymel KP, Abshire TC, Luckey DW, Jenny C: Coagulopathy in pediatric abusive head trauma. Pediatrics 1997;99:371-375.

Lindenberg R, Freytag E: Morphology of brain lesions from blunt trauma in early infancy. Arch Pathol 1969;87:298-305.

Maxeiner H: Demonstration and interpretation of bridging vein ruptures. In cases of infantile subdural bleedings. J Forensic Sci 2001;46:85-93.

Reichard RR, White CL, Hladik CL, Dolinak D: Beta-amyloid precursor protein staining in nonhomicidal pediatric medicolegal autopsies. J Neuropathol Exp Neurobiol 2003;62:237-247.

Reichard RR, White CL, Hladik CL, Dolinak D: Beta-amyloid precursor protein staining of nonaccidental central nervous system injury in pediatric autopsies. J Neurotrauma 2003;20:347-355.

Rustamzadeh E, Truwit CL, Lam CH: Radiology of nonaccidental trauma. Neurosurg Clin N Am 2002;13:183-199.

Tarantino CA, Dowd D, Murdock TC: Short vertical falls in infants. Pediatr Emerg Care 1999;15:5-8.

Willman KY, Bank DE, Senac M, Chadwick DL: Restricting the time of injury in fatal inflicted head injuries. Child Abuse Neglect 1997;21:929-940.

Sequelae of Traumatic Brain Injury

Abe M, Udono H, Tabuchi K, et al: Analysis of ischemic brain damage in cases of acute subdural hematomas. Surg Neurol 2003;59:464-472.

Adams J, Jennett B, McLellan DR, et al: The neuropathology of the vegetative state after head injury. J Clin Pathol 1999;52:804-806.

Atkinson JLD: The neglected prehospital phase of head injury: Apnea and catecholamine surge. Mayo Clin Proc 2000;75:37-47.

Friede RL, Roessmann U: The pathogenesis of secondary midbrain hemorrhages. Neurology 1966;16:1210-1216.

Graham DI, Ford I, Adams JH, et al: Ischemic brain damage is still common in fatal non-missile head injury. J Neurol Neurosurg Psychiatry 1989;52:346-350.

Hirsch CS, Martin DL: Unexpected death in young epileptics. Neurology 1971;21:682-689.

Jennett, WB, Lewin W: Traumatic epilepsy after closed head injuries. J Neurol Neurosurg Psychiatry 1960;23:295-301.

Kimmelberg HK: Current concepts of brain edema. J Neurosurg 1995;83:1051-1059.

Lindenberg R: Compression of brain arteries as pathogenetic factor for tissue necroses and their areas of predilection. J Neuropathol Exp Neurol 1955;14:223-243.

Liu Z, Mikati M, Holmes GL: Mesial temporal sclerosis: Pathogenesis and significance. Pediatr Neurol 1995;12:5-16.

Marmarou A, Fatouros PP, Barzo P, et al: Contribution of edema and cerebral blood volume to traumatic brain swelling in head-injured patients. J Neurosurg 2000;93:183-193.

Matschke J, Tsokos M: Post-traumatic meningitis: Histomorphological findings, postmortem microbiology, and forensic implications. Forensic Sci Int 2001;115:199-205.

Pohlmann-Eden B, Bruckmeir J: Predictors and dynamics of posttraumatic epilepsy. Acta Neurol Scand 1997;95:257-262.

General Reference

Dolinak D, Matshes E: Medicolegal Neuropathology. Boca Raton, FL, CRC Press, 2002.

4

Congenital Malformations, Perinatal Diseases, and Phacomatoses

Rebecca D. Folkerth

The range of disorders affecting the developing nervous system is as broad as that seen in the adult, yet includes primary malformations as well. In addition, the capacity of the immature brain to respond to environmental insults differs in some important respects from that of adults. This chapter discusses brain malformations in groups according to their known etiopathogenesis or, when such is not known or only partially elucidated, according to shared morphologic or clinical features. Acquired perinatal diseases are also considered, as is hippocampal sclerosis (a lesion with probable origin in childhood) and heritable syndromes characterized by developmental anomalies and tumor diatheses involving the central nervous system (CNS).

MICROCEPHALY/MACROCEPHALY

CLINICAL FEATURES

The terms microcephaly and macrocephaly (or megalocephaly) are merely descriptive rather than diagnostic. They are be briefly explained in this section, with the understanding that they each may reflect a wide spectrum of underlying brain diseases, which are further discussed in the following sections. *Microcephaly* refers to a head circumference 2 or more standard deviations (SD) below the mean for age and sex. Consideration must be made for intrauterine growth retardation, low birth weight, and body length. Head circumference is influenced by head shape, normal development of which is dependent on a normal sequence of closure of the fontanelles and cranial sutures (beyond the scope of this chapter). *Micrencephaly* (Fig. 4-1) refers to a brain weight 2 SD below the normal for age and is thought to be a reflection of decreased neuronal proliferation. In general, a small cranium and small brain occur in parallel and are discussed under the term microcephaly.

Microcephaly can reflect an insult to the brain during intrauterine life, in which case head circumference is small at birth, or it can develop postnatally, with a normal head circumference at birth followed by failure of normal head growth thereafter. Processes interfering with normal neuronal growth and proliferation, known

as primary microcephaly, include Down syndrome and other trisomies (see the section on trisomies later), malformations, and inherited factors, which may be either autosomal recessive or dominant. Secondary (destructive) microcephaly results from environmental factors such as prenatal exposure to radiation, intrauterine infections (TORCH [toxoplasmosis, rubella, cytomegalovirus, herpesvirus], human immunodeficiency virus, syphilis), maternal alcohol abuse, and maternal anticonvulsant therapy. Postnatal deceleration in head growth may be a sign of metabolic, nutritional, or neurodegenerative disorders, although some metabolic diseases may result in enlargement of the brain (see later). Clinically, as a rule, microcephalic patients tend to be mentally retarded, but they may also exhibit symptoms, such as seizures or hydrocephalus, related to the underlying cause of the small brain.

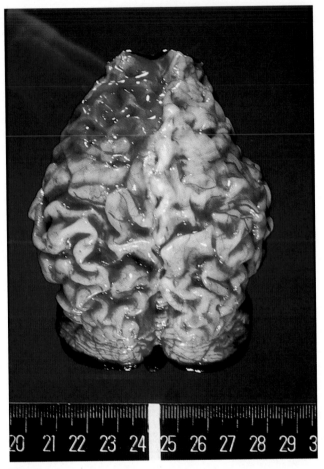

FIGURE 4-1

Micrencephaly: dorsal view of a micrencephalic brain from a 7-year-old girl with microcephaly and developmental delay from birth. Note the widened sulci and narrow gyri indicative of atrophy, as well as poor brain growth.

Macrocephaly is a term indicating an enlarged head, greater than 2.5 SD above the mean for age and sex. Enlargement of the head can reflect an enlarged brain (megalencephaly, or brain weight >2.5 SD above the mean for age and sex) or expanded CSF spaces, either in the ventricles (hydrocephalus) or as extracerebral fluid collections (e.g., subdural hygromas, arachnoid cysts). Primary megalencephaly (Fig. 4-2) can be sporadic, autosomal dominant, autosomal recessive, or part of a recognized syndrome or disease. It may be found in a subject with a normal body habitus, as well as in the setting of achondroplasia, with a large head circumference noted at birth. Males are affected twice as frequently as females. Secondary megalencephaly (not caused by hydrocephalus) develops postnatally and may be due to neuronal storage, as in the gangliosidoses and mucopolysaccharidoses; to degenerative and metabolic disorders such as Alexander's, Canavan's, and Schilder's diseases; to lead encephalopathy; and to some heritable syndromes ("phakomatoses"; see the later section "Familial Malformation/Tumor Syndromes"). Rarely, megalencephaly may be unilateral (hemimegalencephaly), with hemihypertrophy of the body. Clinically, mental retardation, seizures, spasticity, and failure to thrive may be seen in any of the aforementioned underlying conditions.

The most frequent reason for postnatal acceleration in head circumference giving rise to macrocephaly, however, is hydrocephalus. Causes of hydrocephalus are numerous and include primary (congenital) aqueductal atresia (see the section "Posterior Fossa Malformations" later), secondary obstruction of the aqueduct or outflow points at the foramina of Luschka and Magendie (e.g., perinatal intraventricular hemorrhage causing hemosiderosis and scarring; see the section "Disruptions of Developing Gray and White Matter"), TORCH infections causing scarring and calcification of the ependymal lining of the ventricles, and congenital or rapidly growing infantile brain neoplasms. Of course, these conditions may also result in an enlarged head at the time of birth and cause difficulties with normal delivery.

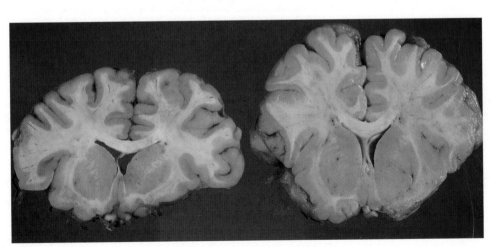

FIGURE 4-2

Megalencephaly: coronal sections of a proportionally enlarged brain (*right*) next to a normal-sized control (*left*) at the level of the corpus striatum. (Courtesy of Dr. C. Pierson, Boston.)

RADIOLOGIC FEATURES

On neuroimaging, the features of microcephaly and macrocephaly reflect the underlying cause and are discussed in more detail later in the corresponding sections or elsewhere in this text.

PATHOLOGIC FEATURES

A micrencephalic brain is 2 SD less than the age- and gender-related norm at birth. It may have a normal gyral pattern, evidence of atrophy (see Fig. 4-1), or another pattern specific to the underlying abnormality (e.g., holoprosencephaly, lissencephaly; see the corresponding sections later). Microscopic findings are appropriate to the underlying cause. Generalized megalencephaly (see Fig. 4-2) refers to increased brain weight (brain weight at birth >2.5 SD above the age- and gender-related norm), as well as diffuse broadening of the cerebral gyri with increased white and gray matter volume; the ventricles are normal in size. The brain is usually microscopically normal, although some reports have suggested increased cell density, increased volume, or both.

DIFFERENTIAL DIAGNOSIS, PROGNOSIS, AND THERAPY

The differential diagnosis is broad for either microcephaly or macrocephaly. Detailed macroscopic examination of the gyral patterns, gray and white matter volume, patency of the aqueduct, and ventricular size, for example, allows preliminary determination of the underlying condition, especially in light of other systemic (i.e., syndromic) pathologic findings, chromosomal studies, or family history. Microscopic evaluation of cortical cytoarchitecture, of neurons for storage or degenerative processes, and of the ventricular lining and leptomeninges for hemosiderin, for instance, helps identify the type of process, many of which are discussed in subsequent sections. Seizures may require anticonvulsant therapy. Shunting of the ventricular system to either the peritoneum or venous circulation treats hydrocephalus. Otherwise, the prognosis and treatment depend on the underlying cause of the abnormal head and brain size.

NEURAL TUBE CLOSURE DEFECTS

In this section, malformations resulting from defective formation of the neural tube are discussed, including *anencephaly*, *encephalocele*, *myelocele*, *meningocele*, and the *Chiari II malformation*.

CLINICAL FEATURES

Neural tube defects (NTDs) are among the most common malformations and account for 0.001% to 1% of all human malformations, depending on the population studied. Although several environmental factors have been associated with abnormalities in neural tube closure, including maternal diabetes, hyperthermia, and anticonvulsant therapy with valproic acid and carbamazepine, elimination of some of these minor risk factors is inadequate to account for the observed decrease in incidence in recent years. Currently, treatment of expectant mothers with vitamin supplementation, particularly folate, is thought to underlie the reduced risk of delivering a second child with an NTD. Preliminary data indicate that folate supplementation may reduce the risk in first pregnancies as well. The mechanisms underlying the protective effect of maternal vitamin supplementation are not understood. Genetic factors may also contribute to the risk for NTDs inasmuch as chromosome aberrations (trisomy 13 and 18) and monoallelic disorders (deletions of 22q11) are occasionally associated with these defects; an X-linked form of spina bifida has been suggested. Most data, however, support a multifactorial cause.

Prenatal detection relies on screening by serum and amniotic chemistry and prenatal ultrasound. Elevated maternal serum or amniotic fluid α-fetoprotein and increased amniotic fluid acetylcholinesterase are found in almost all cases with "open" NTDs (i.e., those lacking a covering of skin over the exposed meninges or central neuroglial tissue). Even though α-fetoprotein levels are highly sensitive for open NTDs, they are not specific; if combined with acetylcholinesterase determination, however, the specificity is improved. Fetal ultrasonography as early as 14 to 16 weeks' gestation can detect the defects themselves, if large, as well as associated changes (see the next section). High-level fetal ultrasonography, fetal magnetic resonance imaging (MRI), and amniocentesis may be required for confirmation. Polyhydramnios is a common, although inconsistent, finding in pregnancies with NTDs.

MICROCEPHALY/MACROCEPHALY—PATHOLOGIC FEATURES

Gross Findings
▶ May have normal gyration, polymicrogyria, or lissencephaly/pachygyria, depending on the underlying cause, or may have a relatively normal gyral pattern
▶ The cerebellum may or may not be affected as well, depending on the cause of the small or enlarged brain

Microscopic, Ultrastructural, and Immunohistochemical Features and Genetics
▶ Depend on the underlying cause

NEURAL TUBE CLOSURE DEFECTS—FACT SHEET

Definition

▶ Failure of closure of some portion of the neural tube: rostral and complete (anencephaly); rostral and partial, with displacement of brain tissue through the defect (encephalocele); and spinal, with herniation of the meninges, meningocele, or central neural tissue (myelocele or myelomeningocele) associated with secondary crowding of the posterior fossa contents (Chiari II malformation)

▶ Caused by incomplete neurulation (fusion of the neural folds) at any point in the neuraxis at the end of the first 4 weeks of embryonic life

▶ May be "closed" or "open" (i.e., with or without a covering of skin, subcutis, and bone)

Incidence/Prevalence

▶ Incidence of anencephaly, 0.1 to 0.7 per 1000 live births; that of spinal dysraphism, somewhat less

▶ Together, anencephaly and spinal dysraphism account for 0.001% to 1% of human malformations, depending on the population studied

▶ Risk increased if an affected sibling

▶ M/F ratio of 1:3 to 1:7

Clinical Features

▶ Associated with maternal diabetes, hyperthermia, anticonvulsant therapy

▶ Prenatal detection by elevated maternal serum α-fetoprotein and amniotic fluid acetylcholinesterase, prenatal ultrasound, MRI

▶ Anencephaly is fatal, whereas encephaloceles cause seizures, mental retardation, blindness, or other signs and symptoms, depending on the site of the cranial defect and the extent of displacement of brain tissue

▶ Spinal defects in which cord tissue is present show paresis below the level of the lesion and Chiari II malformation in >90% of cases

▶ A Chiari II malformation consists of hindbrain crowding from a small posterior fossa (secondary to loss of expansion by CSF, which has leaked through the spinal defect in utero) leading to displacement of cerebellar vermis tissue into the foramen magnum and distortion of the brain stem with hydrocephalus

▶ Risk is reduced by periconceptional folate supplementation

Radiologic Features

▶ On prenatal ultrasound, bony cranial and spinal defects are visible as hypoechoic regions; the "lemon sign" (symmetric bifrontal narrowing) may be a clue to Chiari II malformation if a spinal defect is not well visualized

▶ Encephaloceles show displaced brain tissue and variable amount of CSF; brain adjacent to the defect may be abnormal by ultrasound or fetal MRI

▶ By prenatal ultrasound or fetal MRI: anencephaly associated with a flattened, sloping skull base and protuberant eyes

▶ Postnatal MRI of Chiari II malformation demonstrates hydrocephalus, beaking of the tectum, a Z-shaped or kinked medulla, and displaced cerebellar vermis below the level of the foramen magnum, as well as local spinal abnormalities (hydromyelia, diplomyelia) at the site of the myelomeningocele

Prognosis and Treatment

▶ No treatment of anencephaly because it is uniformly fatal

▶ Encephaloceles may be surgically removed for cosmesis and control of seizures

▶ Open myelomeningoceles may require surgical closure for prevention of infection and preservation of function; affected children usually require a wheelchair unless the lesion is at the low lumbar levels

▶ The hydrocephalus of Chiari II malformation requires shunting

NTDs can arise at any point along the neuraxis, although some sites are preferred. In general, they are either cranial (*anencephaly* [Fig. 4-3], *encephalocele* [Fig. 4-4], or *cranial meningocele*) or caudal (*myelocele* or *spinal meningocele* [Fig. 4-5]), with the occasional case involving the entire length of the neuraxis (*craniospinal rachischisi*s [Fig. 4-6]). Spinal NTDs can be occult (*spina bifida occulta*), defined as a defect in the dorsal bony elements of the vertebral column not involving the cord or meninges. Spina bifida occulta may be found only incidentally on radiographic studies, or it may be suspected on finding a tuft of hair, cutaneous angioma, or subcutaneous lipoma in the midline of the back overlying the occult bony defect. Occasionally, a sinus tract may communicate between the skin and underlying thecal sac. For all NTDs, the clinical deficits naturally relate to the level of involvement.

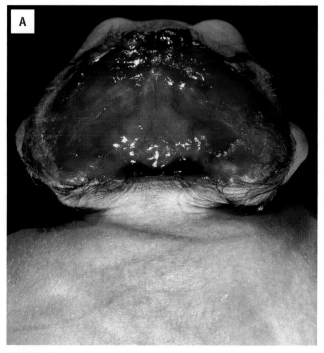

FIGURE 4-3

Anencephaly. **A,** Dorsal view of the cranium showing complete absence of the cranial vault, congested membranous tissue (area cerebrovasculosa) covering the cranial base, and prominence of the eyes.

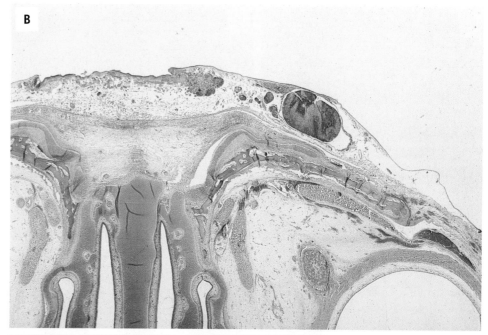

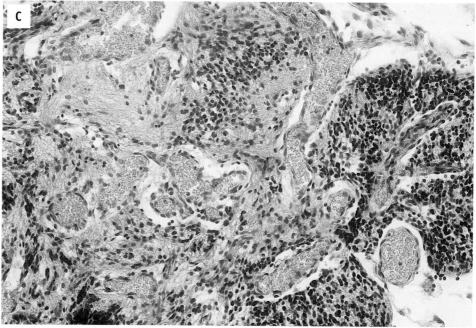

FIGURE 4-3, cont'd

B, Microscopic section through cranial base, including the paranasal sinuses and orbit (*right lower corner*), illustrating an overlying area cerebrovasculosa containing vessels and disorganized central neuroglial tissue, seen at higher power in **C**.

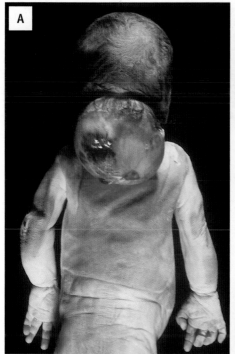

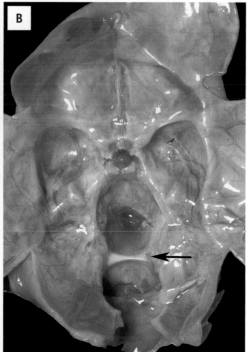

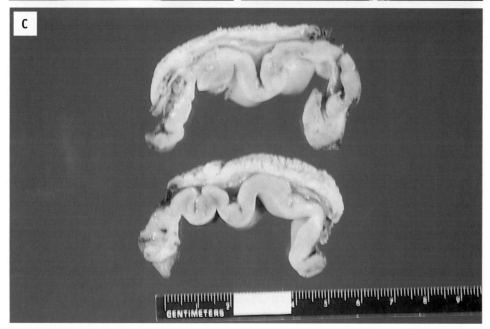

FIGURE 4-4

Encephalocele. **A**, Term stillborn infant with a massive posterior (occipital) encephalocele and focal ulceration of the overlying skin. **B**, View of the base of the skull at autopsy after removal of the brain and encephalocele; note the large defect (*arrow*) at the margins of the lambdoid sutures, through which the encephalocele protruded. **C**, Surgical specimen from a surviving infant with encephalocele: cross section revealing the underlying cerebral gray and white matter (occipital lobe tissue) within the encephalocele sac.

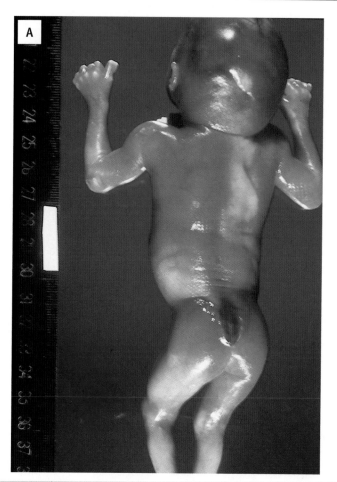

FIGURE 4-5

Lumbosacral myelomeningocele. **A**, Dorsal view of a 20-week-gestation fetus with an open spinal defect in the lumbosacral region and enlargement of the head (as a result of hydrocephalus) (Chiari II malformation). **B**, Microscopic section of the edge of the spinal defect showing the transition between the epidermis (on the *right*) and disorganized central neuroglial tissue and congested vessels (area medullovasculosa) on the *left*.   *Continued*

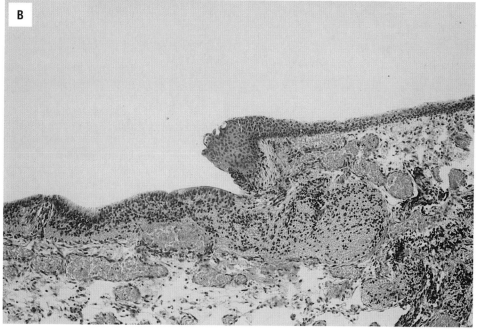

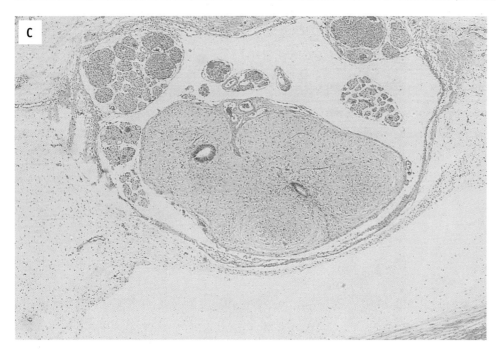

FIGURE 4-5, cont'd

C, Rostral to the open defect, the spinal cord is partially duplicated (diastematomyelia); note the two central canals.

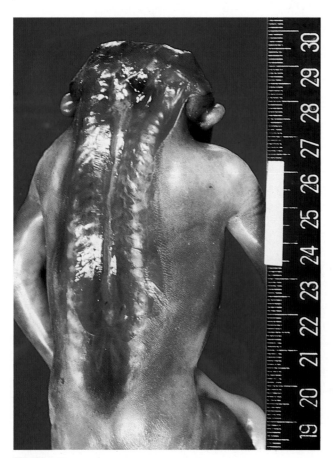

FIGURE 4-6

Complete cerebrospinal rachischisis: dorsal aspect of the spine and cranium demonstrating complete failure of neural tube closure in this spontaneously aborted 24-week-gestation fetus.

Anencephalic infants have only rudimentary brain stem reflexes that are incompatible with life. Seizures resembling infantile spasms have been observed in infants surviving a few hours. Encephaloceles arising from incomplete closure of the most anterior aspect of the neural tube consist of protrusion of the frontal lobes into the paranasal sinuses or even the nasal cavity and may be asymptomatic until adult life, when an intranasal mass, pharyngeal obstruction, or recurrent meningitis develops. Hypertelorism, a median cleft lip, or hypothalamic dysfunction can be seen with this type of anterior encephalocele, the incidence of which is much higher in Southeast Asia than elsewhere, for obscure reasons. Encephaloceles involving defects in the occipital bone may include the cerebellum or calcarine cortex (or both), thereby leading to visual defects, and may rarely include the brain stem, a life-threatening occurrence. The presence of cortex within or adjacent to the displaced brain tissue may cause seizures. Spinal dysraphisms generally lead to paralysis below the level of the lesion, as well as bladder and bowel dysfunction. Defects at or above L2 are usually accompanied by skeletal deformities, including kyphosis and scoliosis, dislocated hips, and clubfeet. Moreover, open spinal NTDs are nearly always associated with hindbrain crowding leading to displacement of the cerebellar vermis into the foramen magnum and hydrocephalus, a combination known as the Chiari II (or Arnold-Chiari) malformation (Fig. 4-7). Clinically, infants with the Chiari II malformation have dysfunction of the lower cranial nerves, facial paralysis, and downbeat nystagmus related to compression of the displaced cerebellar and brain stem tissue. Pure spinal meningoceles (i.e., not involving spinal neural tissue) may be asymptomatic.

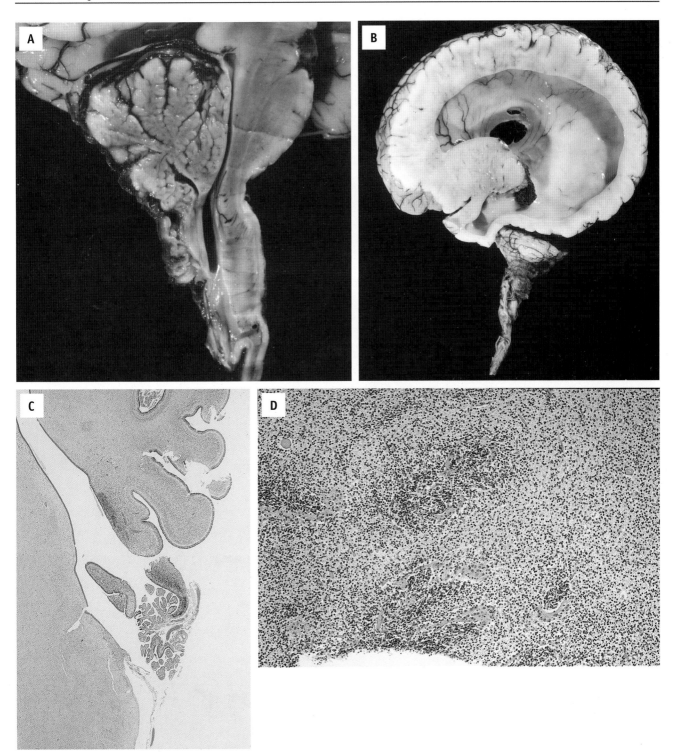

FIGURE 4-7

Chiari II malformation. **A**, Midsagittal aspect of the cerebellum and upper cervical spinal cord showing displacement of cerebellar tissue into the spinal canal and partially covering the dorsal surface of the cord. **B**, Right lateral view of dilated ventricles in the same case. (Courtesy of Dr. U. De Girolami, from the collection of the late Dr. E. P. Richardson, Jr., Boston.) **C**, Microscopic section of displaced vermian tissue and choroid plexus closely apposed to the underlying cervicomedullary region. **D**, Disorganization of the displaced cerebellar cortex.

RADIOLOGIC FEATURES

Anencephalic fetuses are easily recognized on prenatal ultrasound or fetal MRI by absence of the cranial vault, prominence of the orbits and eyes, and a flattened, downwardly sloping appearance of the skull base (Fig. 4-8). Likewise, encephaloceles in the parietal or occipital regions may be readily detected by either method (Fig. 4-9). Nasal or ethmoidal (anterior) encephaloceles may be difficult to identify by prenatal ultrasound or even by computed tomography (CT) in the neonatal period because the anterior skull base is primarily cartilaginous. MRI using 2- to 3-mm sections and T1- and T2-weighted images may be useful.

Spinal defects may be identified by prenatal ultrasound as focal loss of normal echogenicity of the posterior vertebral elements; a meningocele is a hypoechoic mass of variable size and may or may not have denser material corresponding to dysraphic neural tissue. Fetal MRI easily demonstrates the spinal mass (Fig. 4-10). Associated changes such as the "lemon sign" (symmetric bifrontal narrowing of the skull), as well as a small posterior fossa and herniation of cerebellar tissue into the foramen magnum and cervical canal, can be clues to the Chiari II malformation (see Fig. 4-10), even if the spinal myelomeningocele is not well seen.

The cranial bones in infants with spinal NTDs and Chiari II malformation may show multifocal thinning resulting in radiographic lucencies known as lückenschädel, especially in the presence of hydrocephalus, that are detectable on prenatal and postnatal imaging. The hindbrain manifestations of Chiari II malformation are visible by CT or MRI in the midsagittal plane as an abnormally small posterior fossa resulting in a narrow fourth ventricle, flattening of the colliculi dorsally and the basis pontis ventrally, and kinking of the dorsal aspect of the medulla. The vermis may be small, with much of it displaced inferiorly across the foramen magnum (see Fig. 4-10).

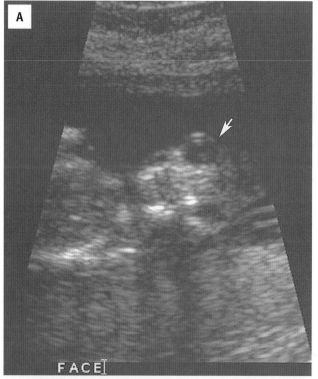

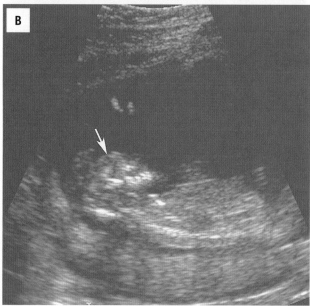

FIGURE 4-8

Anencephaly. **A** and **B**, Coronal and sagittal prenatal ultrasound images from the late second trimester showing prominent orbits (*arrow*) and absence of the cranial vault. (Courtesy of Dr. D. Levine, Boston.)

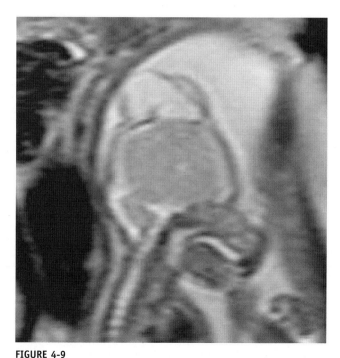

FIGURE 4-9

Encephalocele: fetal MRI of a protruding occipital encephalocele. (Courtesy of Dr. D. Levine, Boston.)

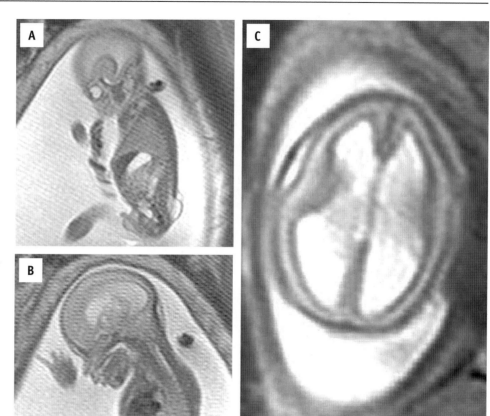

FIGURE 4-10

Chiari II malformation. **A**, Fetal brain and spine MRI, sagittal view, revealing a lumbosacral myelomeningocele. **B**, Fetal brain MRI, sagittal view, showing a small posterior fossa with hindbrain crowding and hydrocephalus. **C**, Fetal brain MRI, axial view, demonstrating ventricular expansion and anteroposterior elongation of the head. (Courtesy of Dr. D. Levine, Boston.)

On plain radiographs, spinal NTDs show absence of the dorsal spinous processes with lateral splaying of the transverse processes, findings lending an "unzipped" appearance to the spine.

PATHOLOGIC FEATURES

NTDs are believed to represent failure of the neural folds to come together to form the neural tube, as opposed to the splaying open of a previously closed neural tube. Closure of the neural folds is a very early event in embryogenesis; it begins on day 20 and ends by approximately day 28 postfertilization. Experimental data indicate that neural tube closure occurs at multiple sites and in a coordinated pattern rather than as a continuous "zipping up" from one end. Each site may be under the control of different genes and could be susceptible to different environmental factors. The sites of closure correlate well with locations of craniospinal closure defects.

Complete absence of the brain and overlying skull is known as *anencephaly* (see Fig. 4-3). Some cases may have relative sparing of supratentorial or more commonly the infratentorial structures. The anterior pituitary, eyes, and brain stem are nearly always spared and lie beneath a highly vascular, disorganized film of tissue called the area cerebrovasculosa (see Fig. 4-3). It is thought that this substance remains after degeneration of the brain tissue at the "open" edges of the defect because of direct contact between the neural epithelium and amniotic fluid. As mentioned earlier, *craniorachischisis* refers to anencephaly with a contiguous spinal defect, which can extend from the cervical spine region all the way down the spinal column (see Fig. 4-6).

Encephaloceles (containing brain and meningeal tissue) (see Fig. 4-4) and *cranial meningoceles* (harboring only meninges and often filled with CSF, similar to a cyst) differ from anencephaly in having an epidermal covering over the cranial defects (i.e., they are "closed"). Both entities are associated with a defect in the skull, usually at the midline sutures or fontanelles (see Fig. 4-4). Occasionally, no clear bony defect or contiguity with the underlying brain can be identified. Polymicrogyric cortex may be present at the edges of the displaced brain tissue and may generate seizure activity. The size of the encephalocele can vary from an inconspicuous bump to a mass larger than the infant's head. Some syndromes are associated with encephaloceles at typical locations, such as occipital encephaloceles in the Meckel-Gruber and Walker-Warburg syndromes and anterior encephaloceles in Roberts' syndrome. Parietal encephaloceles occur only rarely.

Spinal NTDs can involve the meninges alone (*meningocele*) or the meninges and underlying spinal cord (*myelomeningocele*) (see Fig. 4-5). Most NTDs

NEURAL TUBE CLOSURE DEFECTS—PATHOLOGIC FEATURES

Gross Findings

▶ Anencephaly: absence of the cranium and most of the brain tissue, with replacement by area cerebrovasculosa; the eyes are protuberant

▶ Encephaloceles: vary in size from small skin-covered bumps to large masses overlying the cranial sutures/fontanelles or in the sinonasal region

▶ Spinal defects: may be skin-covered (occult) defects in vertebral body closure or open plaque-like areas in which neural tissue and nerve roots are visible (placode), with replacement by area medullovasculosa

▶ Chiari II malformation: midline cerebellar tissue displaced into the foramen magnum dorsally, small posterior fossa and cerebellar hemispheres, flattened or kinked brain stem, variable expansion of the ventricular system

Microscopic Features

▶ Area cerebrovasculosa (in anencephaly) or medullovasculosa (in spinal NTDs) is made up of ectatic, thin-walled vessels in loose connective tissue, often containing disorganized central neuroglial tissue

▶ Spinal NTDs may contain peripheral nerve bundles

▶ With encephaloceles, the brain, often disorganized, and the overlying meninges are in contact with dermal tissue

▶ The cerebellum, especially the vermis, may be disorganized in Chiari II malformation

Genetics

▶ Not well defined, although deletions of 22q11 are associated with some spinal dysraphisms

Differential Diagnosis

▶ For anencephaly, amniotic band sequence with disruption of the normally closed cranial vault

▶ Aplasia cutis (localized defect in the dermal and subcutaneous tissue of the scalp)

occur in the lumbar region, followed by the lumbosacral region, but they can also be located at the cervical or thoracic level. Those arising in the lumbosacral region are often associated with other defects in the surrounding mesoderm, including vascular telangiectases, as well as other abnormalities of the spinal cord, such as *hydromyelia* (cystic dilation of the central canal) and *syringomyelia* (a glial-lined cavity within the parenchyma of the spinal cord). These lesions may extend rostrally to involve the brain stem (syringobulbia). It is should be noted that these conditions are not specific to NTDs and can be found after trauma or in association with spinal tumors. Iniencephaly refers to failure of closure of the posterior vertebral arches of the rostral cervical vertebrae and is usually associated with abnormalities of the brain stem and the medulla. *Diplomyelia* refers to duplication of the spinal cord segments (Fig. 4-11), occasionally in association with myelomeningocele; midline pegs of vertebral bone and connective tissue may result in partial duplications or splitting of the cord (diastematomyelia) (see Fig. 4-5).

The *Chiari II* (or *Arnold-Chiari*) *malformation* consists of the association of a spinal NTD with a small posterior fossa, hindbrain crowding, and secondary abnormalities of the brain stem and cerebellum. The cerebellar vermis is displaced caudally into the spinal canal through an enlarged foramen magnum and often has disorganized cortical Purkinje and granule cells (see Fig. 4-7). Also noted are lengthening of the cerebellar peduncles, a "Z-shaped" deviation or flattening of the medulla oblongata, and a beaked tectum, as well as cerebellar hypoplasia (see Fig. 4-7). Forking of the aqueduct, aqueductal stenosis, aqueductal atresia, or any combination of these findings may be present. This complex association is further characterized by hydrocephalus,

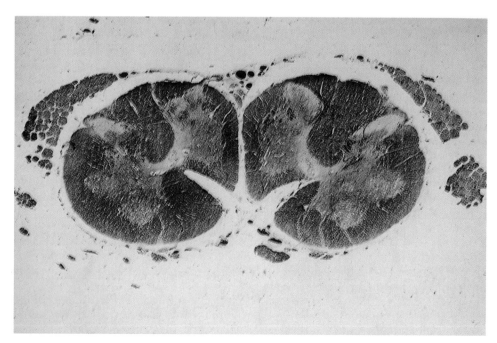

FIGURE 4-11

Diplomyelia. Rarely, neural tube closure abnormalities may be manifested by nearly complete duplication of the spinal cord. (Courtesy of Dr. U. De Girolami, Boston.)

sometimes with a microgyric pattern of the cerebral convolutions and subependymal heterotopia. The presumed cause of this constellation of findings is leakage of CSF from the open defect causing failure of expansion of the basal cisterns, chronic "herniation" of caudal hindbrain structures into the foramen magnum interfering with their normal bulk growth and causing hindbrain crowding, compression of the fourth ventricle and aqueduct, and chronic expansion of the upper ventricular system.

DIFFERENTIAL DIAGNOSIS

The diagnosis of an NTD is usually straightforward, except in rare cases of small encephaloceles, dural sinus tracts, or aplasia cutis congenita, in which bony skull defects can occur without the protrusion of meningeal or central neuroglial tissue. Caudal lipomas, teratomas, and dermoid cysts, although often markers of an underlying spinal dysraphism, can occur in isolation.

The amniotic band sequence can disrupt normally developed structures rostrally and result in loss of cranial tissue and brain resembling anencephaly. Such amniotic band disruptions can be distinguished from true NTDs by the asymmetry of involvement and by the presence of facial clefts or extremity amputations (Fig. 4-12).

PROGNOSIS AND THERAPY

Anencephalic fetuses have a high incidence of intrauterine demise and, if liveborn, die within a few hours, even with intensive care. These short-term survivals have created controversy over the use of anencephalic infants as organ donors.

If a dysraphic disorder has been diagnosed prenatally and the pregnancy continued, an atraumatic delivery may be planned to improve the neurologic outcome in children with myelomeningoceles. Large encephaloceles may also be managed in this way, although the clinical context in which they occur (i.e., associations and syndromes) also influences the decision making. Overall, surgical excision (see Fig. 4-4) is recommended to prevent breakdown of skin over the lesion (particularly in occipital encephaloceles) and secondary infection, including meningitis, in the affected infant. The prognosis is significantly better with anterior (sinonasal) encephaloceles, which may be asymptomatic.

Spinal dysraphism is best treated by surgical closure as soon after birth as feasible, again to prevent infection and limit the extent of disability, because cognitive function in survivors of spinal NTDs has been shown to be negatively affected by meningitis or ventriculitis. In general, lesions above the L3 level make ambulation impossible, whereas lesions below S1 usually allow for unaided ambulation. With lesions between S1 and L3,

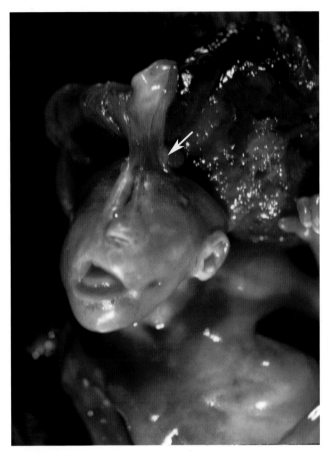

FIGURE 4-12

Amniotic band sequence. Although resembling anencephaly, this second-trimester fetus acquired this facial and cranial disruption from a constricting band of amnion (*arrow*) and does not have a true neural tube defect.

assisted walking is possible. Concurrent or eventual shunting of coexisting hydrocephalus is often required. Surgical decompression of the accompanying cerebellar displacement in the Chiari II malformation may become necessary when prominent cerebellar or brain stem signs persist despite adequate treatment of the hydrocephalus. Because of the risk of serious recurrent upper and lower urinary tract infections as a result of the paralysis, aggressive urologic management plays an important role in the care of affected children. A bowel care program is necessary as well. Late sequelae of myelomeningoceles include scoliosis and traction on the cord from tethering at the level of the defect, the latter occurring either as a "primary" abnormality or as a consequence of previous surgery and scarring. In either case, surgical release of the tethered cord is recommended to prevent exacerbation of deficits, which can sometimes be precipitous and irreversible. Unusual, but significant, postsurgical complications include spinal cord infarction, compression of the cord by arachnoid cysts arising in the scar, and inclusion cysts originating from trapped skin appendages.

HOLOPROSENCEPHALY SEQUENCE

CLINICAL FEATURES

The holoprosencephaly sequence refers to a spectrum of malformations resulting from failure of normal induction and patterning of the prosencephalon by the mesodermal floor plate in the fifth to sixth gestational weeks. Because of the interrelated development of the forebrain and underlying mesodermal structures, patients frequently exhibit specific craniofacial anomalies, including midline facial clefts, cyclopia (Fig. 4-13), and nasal

---

HOLOPROSENCEPHALY SEQUENCE—FACT SHEET

Definition

▶ Failure of normal forebrain induction/patterning resulting in a spectrum of abnormalities (from least to most severe): arrhinencephaly (absence of the olfactory bulbs and tracts), lobar holoprosencephaly, semilobar holoprosencephaly, alobar holoprosencephaly (complete failure of separation of two cerebral hemispheres with fusion of the midline diencephalic structures)
▶ Usually associated with midline facial defects ranging from a single midline incisor or hypotelorism, to a midline cleft lip and palate, to cyclopia with a proboscis (nasal anlage)

Incidence/Prevalence

▶ 0.48 to 0.88 per 10,000 live births and 1 in 200 spontaneous abortions
▶ Associated with trisomies 13 and 18 (see the later section on trisomies)
▶ Familial occurrence, inherited as autosomal dominant
▶ Gender distribution is apparently equal

Clinical Features

▶ Associated with maternal diabetes, alcoholism, Smith-Lemli-Opitz syndrome (defect in cholesterol biosynthesis)
▶ Most severe forms detectable on prenatal ultrasound or MRI
▶ Opisthotonos, spasticity, seizures, mental delay

Radiologic Features

▶ Crescent-shaped holoventricle (absence of the septum pellucidum and corpus callosum) and fusion of the thalami and basal ganglia in the semilobar and alobar forms on transfontanelle ultrasound or MRI
▶ Absence of the rostrum of the corpus callosum with a dorsal interhemispheric cyst in the lobar and semilobar forms
▶ Abnormal nasal bones in arrhinencephaly on ultrasound, CT, or MRI

Prognosis and Treatment

▶ High incidence of fetal wastage in the most severe forms (i.e., alobar holoprosencephaly with cyclopia)
▶ Profound mental retardation, apneic spells, and hypothalamic dysfunction in severe forms; lesser degrees of cognitive delay and seizures in the limited forms

---

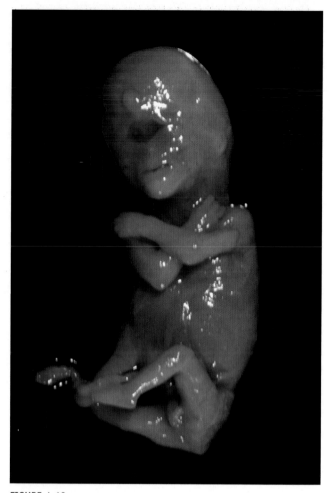

FIGURE 4-13

Cyclopia: 11-week-gestation fetus with a single orbit and proboscis.

---

anomalies, in addition to the brain "holosphere" or undivided prosencephalic vesicle (Fig. 4-14). The pathogenesis of this disorder has been elucidated in numerous recent experimental studies of neural tube patterning and by the identification of mutations in several genes. The malformation runs in families, although the degree of involvement among affected individuals can vary widely within the same family. The incidence is approximately 0.48 to 0.88 per 10,000 liveborn children with normal chromosomes. There is a high rate of fetal wastage, however, with the incidence of holoprosencephaly in intrauterine demise estimated at 40 per 10,000.

Several environmental/maternal factors, including maternal diabetes and maternal ethanol consumption, have been associated with the holoprosencephaly sequence. Experimental ethanol exposure in mice and macaques can produce craniofacial and CNS anomalies resembling holoprosencephaly. An outbreak of cyclopia in lambs in the early 1960s led to the identification of a holoprosencephaly-inducing teratogen in the forage plant *Veratrum californicum*, on which the pregnant ewes were feeding. The plants were found to contain the

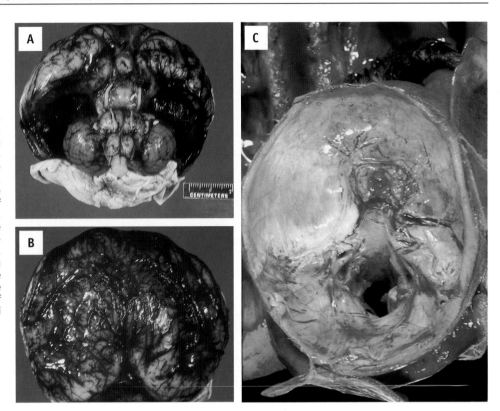

FIGURE 4-14

Alobar holoprosencephaly. **A**, Anterior aspect of the brain from a term infant showing absence of the olfactory bulbs and tracts (arrhinencephaly) and midline fusion of the cerebral hemispheres, optic nerves, and cerebral peduncles; note the relatively normal development of the pons, medulla, and cerebellum. **B**, Dorsal view of the holosphere (fused hemispheres with slight separation between the occipital poles). **C**, View of the skull base with the brain removed to illustrate the absence of separation between the anterior and middle fossa and lack of the cribriform plate and crista galli in the anterior midline.

alkaloid cyclopamine, which can result in similar anomalies in rodents, chickens, and rabbits. This alkaloid interferes with molecular signaling along the sonic hedgehog (SHH) pathway (see later). Similarly, the administration of cholesterol biosynthesis inhibitors to pregnant rats results in skeletal and craniofacial anomalies, pituitary agenesis, and holoprosencephaly in the pups. Thus, cholesterol biosynthetic pathways and SHH signaling appear to be important in the pathogenesis of the holoprosencephaly sequence.

In the human cases not resulting from maternal diabetes or fetal alcohol exposure, many may have a genetic cause recognizable in conjunction with other systemic anomalies. For example, the Smith-Lemli-Opitz syndrome, which is due to a defect in cholesterol biosynthesis at the level of 3β-hydroxysteroid-Δ⁷-reductase, has a link to the SHH signaling pathway; these patients have severe hypocholesterolemia, and cholesterol is required for normal SHH signaling, a process critical for normal forebrain patterning (see later).

The most common nonrandom chromosomal abnormality in patients with holoprosencephaly is trisomy 13, which is reported in 24% to 45% of affected liveborn infants. In addition to trisomy 13, several other chromosomal anomalies, including trisomy 18, trisomy 13-15, trisomy 13-15 mosaicism, ring chromosome 13 or 18, and deletion of chromosome 13 or 18, have been identified in patients with holoprosencephaly.

Numerous chromosomal regions on several chromosomes contain genes that may play a role in the pathogenesis of holoprosencephaly. Seven different loci have been identified and are designated *HPE1* (21q22.3),

HPE2 (2p21, causing mutation in the *SIX3* gene), *HPE3* (7q36, site of *SHH*), *HPE4* (18p), *HPE5* (*ZIC2* on chromosome 13), *HPE6* (2q), and *HPE7* (*PTCH* mutation). In particular, mutations in the *SHH* gene have been found in some patients with autosomal dominant holoprosencephaly, as well as in one sporadic case.

The pathogenesis of the holoprosencephaly sequence has been shown to be related to failure of induction of the ectoderm overlying the ventral neural tube by the notochord. The notochord secretes the signaling molecule SHH, which mediates ventral patterning of the midbrain and the forebrain. SHH appears to be necessary and sufficient for forebrain development in zebra fish and mice. SHH also appears to directly participate in craniofacial and eye development. To become functional, the SHH molecule must undergo autoproteolytic cleavage mediated by its C-terminal domain, which requires attachment of a cholesterol tag. As mentioned previously, blockers of cholesterol biosynthesis cause cyclopia and, in some cases, holoprosencephaly in experimental animals, as can disruptions in genes involved in cholesterol transport. Finally, holoprosencephaly may occasionally be seen in the Smith-Lemli-Opitz syndrome in humans, a metabolic defect in cholesterol biosynthesis characterized by severe hypocholesterolemia. Failure of dorsal induction and patterning of the prosencephalon, which is mediated in part through bone morphogenetic proteins, also appears to result in holoprosencephalic phenotypes in experimental animals.

Clinically, opisthotonos and spasticity may be prominent, as may seizures and mental delay. Milder forms of the holoprosencephaly sequence may be associated with normal neurologic and cognitive function.

RADIOLOGIC FEATURES

In *alobar holoprosencephaly*, prenatal and transfontanelle sonograms and fetal MRI may demonstrate absence of the falx cerebri and interhemispheric fissure, as well as a crescent-shaped holoventricle and fused diencephalon (Fig. 4-15). By ultrasound, *semilobar holoprosencephaly* may show disordered cerebral cortical gyration and thalamic midline fusion, with or without a dorsal cyst. In semilobar holoprosencephaly, the posterior portion (splenium) of the corpus callosum forms normally, whereas the anterior (body and genu) is absent, best seen on sagittal T1-weighted MRI; this pattern is opposite the situation in partial callosal agenesis (see the section "Midline/Commissural Defects" later). The septum pellucidum is absent on MRI in both the alobar and semilobar forms. *Arrhinencephaly* is detectable on MRI as absence of the olfactory sulcus and tracts; CT may demonstrate absence or hypoplasia of the nasal bones.

PATHOLOGIC FEATURES

The neuropathologic features of holoprosencephaly range from isolated absence of the olfactory bulbs and tracts (*arrhinencephaly*), to *lobar holoprosencephaly* (in which the cerebral lobes can be identified) (Fig. 4-16), to a single telencephalic ventricle with absence of the

---

HOLOPROSENCEPHALY SEQUENCE—PATHOLOGIC FEATURES

Gross Findings

▶ Absence of the olfactory bulbs and tracts and straight sulci of the orbitofrontal cortex in arrhinencephaly, as well as in the more severe forms

▶ Fusion of the inferior frontal cortex and occasionally the basal ganglia across the midline in lobar holoprosencephaly

▶ Absence of the anterior interhemispheric fissure with continuity of the cerebral convolutions across the midline and thalamic or more extensive diencephalic fusion in semilobar holoprosencephaly

▶ Complete absence of the interhemispheric fissure, septum pellucidum, and corpus callosum (holosphere) with fusion of the diencephalon and absence of the third ventricle; occasional fusion of the optic nerves (in cyclopia)

▶ Abnormal fan-like array of blood vessels over the anterior aspect of the holosphere (rete mirabile) in the most severe forms

Microscopic Features

▶ The inferomedial aspect of the lip of the holosphere may contain hippocampal structures and entorhinal cortex

▶ Some cases have abnormalities in cerebral neocortical cytoarchitecture, as well as pia/subarachnoid glioneuronal heterotopia

▶ Fused diencephalic structures have disorganized neuronal cytoarchitecture

▶ The brain stem and cerebellum are usually spared

Genetics

▶ Most common are trisomy 13 (24% to 45% of affected liveborn infants) and trisomy 18 (see the section on trisomies)

▶ Numerous chromosomal regions may contain genes important in holoprosencephaly, including *HPE1* (21q22.3), *HPE2* (2p21, which causes mutation in the *SIX3* gene), *HPE3* (7q36, site of SHH), *HPE4* (18p), *HPE5* (*ZIC2* on chromosome 13), *HPE6* (2q), and *HPE7* (*PTCH* mutation)

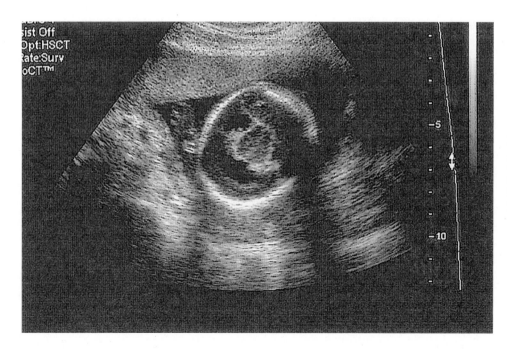

FIGURE 4-15

Alobar holoprosencephaly: second-trimester fetal MRI, axial view, showing paired diencephalic structures but no interhemispheric fissure or lobes. (Courtesy of Dr. D. Levine, Boston.)

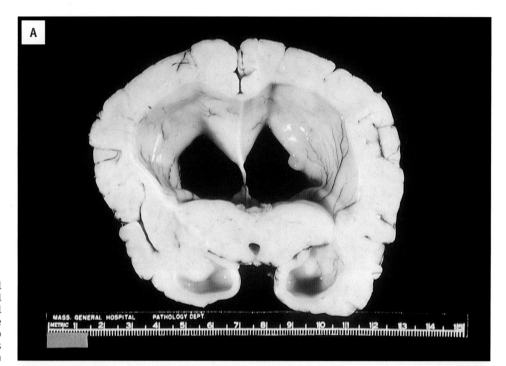

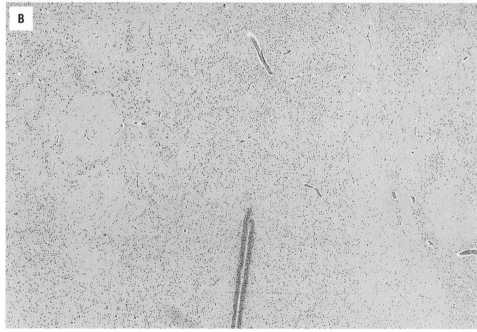

FIGURE 4-16

Lobar holoprosencephaly. **A,** Coronal section with fusion of the dorsal aspect of the thalamus and a small third ventricle. There is complete separation of the hemispheres into recognizable lobes, and the corpus callosum is present, although thinned; the ventricles are expanded. (Courtesy of Dr. U. De Girolami, from the collection of the late Dr. E. P. Richardson, Jr., Boston.) **B,** Histologic section through the dorsally fused and disorganized thalamus and narrow third ventricle.

interhemispheric fissure and continuity of the cerebral convolutions across the midline (*alobar holoprosencephaly*) (see Fig. 4-14). An intermediate-severity form showing partial midline division by an interhemispheric fissure is known as *semilobar holoprosencephaly* (Fig. 4-17). In general, the craniofacial abnormalities associated with each category are stereotypic and, with some exceptions, "predict" the underlying brain malformation. For example, the mildest craniofacial abnormality, such as a single midline maxillary incisor, might be associated with arrhinencephaly, whereas at the other end of the spectrum, the most severe craniofacial anomalies,

such as cyclopia lying below a proboscis (nasal anlagen) (see Fig. 4-13), would accompany complete alobar holoprosencephaly. In the semilobar forms, the facial abnormalities may include cebocephaly (elongated nose with a single nostril) and hypotelorism (Fig. 4-18). This spectrum of associations constitutes the holoprosencephaly sequence or syndrome.

In all forms of holoprosencephaly, the brain is small (micrencephaly); in the alobar and semilobar forms, brain weight averages less than 100 g at full term (normal, 380 to 410 g). The olfactory bulbs and tracts, as well as the straight sulci, are absent in virtually all

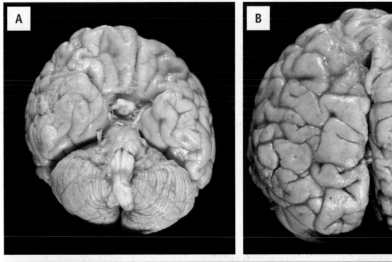

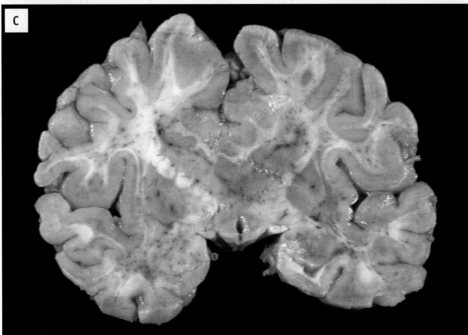

FIGURE 4-17

Semilobar holoprosencephaly. **A**, Ventral aspect of the brain illustrating absence of the olfactory bulbs and tracts. **B**, Dorsal view showing continuity of the cerebral gyri across the midline in the frontal lobes, but normal separation of the parieto-occipital lobes. **C**, Coronal section of the cerebral hemispheres at the level of the basal ganglia demonstrating absence of the corpus callosum, continuity of gray matter in the dorsal midline, and partial midline fusion of the medial portion of the thalamus and caudate nuclei.

cases (arrhinencephaly) (see Figs. 4-15 and 4-16). The optic nerves may be hypoplastic, or fused in the case of cyclopia, whereas the remaining cranial nerves are usually normally formed. The middle and anterior cerebral arteries may be disorganized and form a fan-like cluster of vessels (*rete mirabile*) extending over the ventral forebrain and orbitofrontal regions. A single anterior cerebral artery may course over the rostral midline of the cerebral hemispheres.

In *alobar holoprosencephaly*, the interhemispheric fissure separating the two cerebral hemispheres is absent, as are the sylvian fissures. There is generally no delineation of the lobes of the cerebral hemisphere (see Fig. 4-14). In infants and older individuals, the gyri are usually distinct; however, their patterns are abnormal. The most inferior medial gyri frequently contain displaced cells of the hippocampus and entorhinal cortex

coursing along the lateral aspect of a cyst-like membrane over the dorsal-posterior aspect of the brain. Viewed posteriorly, the cerebrum is shaped like a horseshoe, with the rim contiguous with the cyst-like membrane representing the roof of the single midline ventricle (see Fig. 4-14). The basal ganglia and thalamus lie beneath the membrane and vary from distinct paired structures to poorly defined masses that are fused along the midline (see Fig. 4-16). Rarely, the basal ganglia cannot be identified. The corpus callosum and anterior commissure are generally absent; however, rudimentary crossing fiber bundles may occasionally be seen. The brain stem and cerebellum are relatively normal, except for hypoplastic or absent corticospinal tracts.

Semilobar holoprosencephaly represents a lesser degree of the same CNS malformation. Usually, a partial interhemispheric fissure separates the parieto-occipital

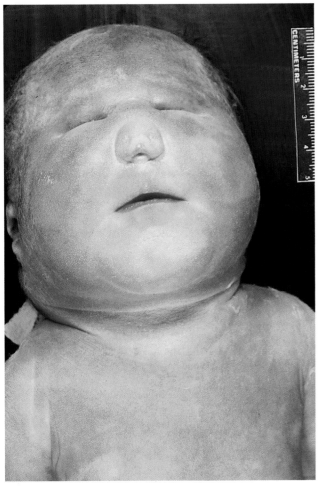

FIGURE 4-18

Holoprosencephaly: facies of an infant with alobar holoprosencephaly (see Fig. 4-15) consisting of hypotelorism (close-set eyes), a narrow palpebral fissure, and a single nostril.

Microscopically, the cytoarchitecture of the cerebral cortex may be normal, although displaced from its usual location. Some cases, however, may have significant disorganization of the cerebral cortex, possibly representing abnormal cell migration, secondary injury to the cerebral cortex, or an abnormality in connections into and out of the cerebral cortex. Pial glioneuronal heterotopia may form a "crust" over the surface of the brain, seen more commonly in late gestation and postnatally (see the section "Neuronal Migration Defects" later).

The hippocampus is microscopically identifiable, although it is often displaced and may show incomplete or abnormal development. The histopathology of the basal ganglia and thalamus varies with the severity of the hemispheric malformation. In alobar holoprosencephaly (see Fig. 4-18), the basal ganglia may be microscopically unidentifiable or recognized only as a fused midline mass with disorganized cytoarchitecture (see Fig. 4-16). In less severe forms of holoprosencephaly, the basal ganglia are present, although the head of the caudate may be fused and the septal region indistinct. The septum pellucidum is generally absent in all forms. Microscopically, the cerebellum may have focal cortical disorganization or heterotopia, or both, especially in the setting of trisomy 13 and other cytogenetic anomalies. Abnormalities of the brain stem are limited to hypoplastic or absent corticobulbar and corticospinal tracts or fused colliculi or peduncles at the midbrain level (see Fig. 4-14).

DIFFERENTIAL DIAGNOSIS

The gross appearance of alobar holoprosencephaly is sufficiently distinctive that little can be confused with it. In contrast, isolated arrhinencephaly may be overlooked, especially in very immature brains in which the olfactory bulbs and tracts are soft and easily avulsed from the brain at the time of removal. Arrhinencephaly is confirmed by evaluating the anterior fossa and demonstrating absence of the cribriform plate (see Fig. 4-14). In lobar holoprosencephaly, the midline fusion of the thalamus or basal ganglia may be subtle and also overlooked on coronal section of the brain.

PROGNOSIS AND THERAPY

Surviving liveborn infants with the most severe variants (alobar holoprosencephaly) generally have profound mental retardation and often suffer from seizures, which may be difficult to treat. They may have apneic spells and hypothalamic dysfunction with diabetes insipidus, poikilothermy, and inappropriate secretion of antidiuretic hormone. Their life span can be reduced. Patients with intermediate forms of holoprosencephaly and pure arrhinencephaly may have a normal life span and very limited clinical deficits, such as cognitive delay and seizures.

lobes, whereas the cerebral cortex crosses the midline in continuity over the frontal lobes (see Fig. 4-17). Variable degrees of midline fusion of diencephalic structures may be demonstrable. Occasionally, the separated parieto-occipital lobes may have an intervening dorsal midline cyst.

The *lobar form* of holoprosencephaly is characterized by an interhemispheric fissure that divides virtually the entire brain with the exception of the most rostral and ventral regions of the frontal lobes. Beneath the apparent interhemispheric fissure, however, cerebral cortex may still cross the midline (see Fig. 4-17). There may be a segment of well-developed corpus callosum posteriorly where the cerebral hemispheres are truly separated. The lobes of the cerebral hemispheres may be recognizable and have the semblance of a normal gyral pattern. Cross sections of the brain continue to show abnormal communication between the lateral ventricles with fusion of the basal ganglia rostrally. The thalami may have an enlarged massa intermedia.

NEURONAL MIGRATION DEFECTS

Cerebral cortical developmental anomalies are extremely diverse and include the *lissencephalies, pachygyria, polymicrogyria, cortical dysplasia,* and *neuronal heterotopia.* Recent experimental work on the lissencephalies has shed a great deal of light on the sequences of normal as well as abnormal cerebral cortical development.

CLINICAL FEATURES

As a group, the exact incidence of cortical neuronal migrational abnormalities is unknown. They have a variety of inheritance patterns or may be sporadic. A number of environmental risk factors have been associated with the development of neuronal migrational disorders, including maternal exposure to ethanol, retinoic acid, heavy metals, and x-irradiation. Viral infections and bilateral carotid ischemia in utero before the third trimester have also been associated with migrational disturbances, although strictly speaking, such processes are generally considered to represent disruptions (discussed further in the later section "Disruptions of Developing Gray and White Matter").

Although many disorders of cerebral cortical development are referred to as cortical migrational anomalies, an actual defect in cell migration has been demonstrated in only a few genetic conditions, so other factors such as cellular proliferation, cell death, post-migrational intracortical growth and development, axonogenesis, and dendritogenesis may in fact cause the phenotype. Nevertheless, in this section the term cortical neuronal migration anomaly is used to collectively designate conditions in which the cortical gray matter is maldeveloped, including *lissencephaly/pachygyria, polymicrogyria, cortical dysplasia,* and *neuronal heterotopia.* Lissencephalies are divided into type I and type II, both characterized by markedly widened gyri (pachygyria), which in the most severe widespread form gives an overall smooth appearance to the surface of the cerebrum (Fig. 4-19). Polymicrogyria refers to numerous, small disorganized convolutions not corresponding to

---

NEURONAL MIGRATION DEFECTS—FACT SHEET

Definition
- ▶ Lissencephaly is a smooth-surfaced brain, without cortical gyri; it may be partial or complete. Type I is smoother, whereas type II has a fine "cobblestone" appearance
- ▶ Pachygyria is abnormally broad gyri, usually occurring with areas of lissencephaly or polymicrogyria
- ▶ Polymicrogyria is numerous, narrow convolutions in a complex pattern

---

- ▶ Focal cortical dysplasia of the Taylor type is a localized area of thickened cortical width (pachygyria) and disturbed neuronal cytoarchitecture
- ▶ Neuronal heterotopia are collections of neurons in abnormal places (i.e., along the pial surface, in white matter, or beneath the ependyma)

Incidence/Prevalence and Gender Distribution
- ▶ The exact incidence is not known
- ▶ Some subtypes (e.g., Walker-Warburg syndrome) have a high incidence of intrauterine demise and neonatal lethality
- ▶ For X-linked lissencephaly, affected patients are female (the defect is lethal in males)

Clinical Features
- ▶ Associated with genetic factors; with maternal exposure to alcohol, retinoic acid, heavy metal, and x-irradiation; and with intrauterine infection and bilateral carotid ischemia
- ▶ Lissencephaly:
  - ▶ Manifested as neonatal hypotonia with later spasticity, seizures, and mental retardation
  - ▶ Miller-Dieker (type I) syndrome has characteristic facies (upturned nose, bitemporal hollowing, small chin, long upper lip, and low-set ears)
  - ▶ X-linked lissencephaly (also type I) is lethal in males, whereas females demonstrate subcortical band heterotopia ("double cortex")
  - ▶ Type II includes Walker-Warburg syndrome, the Finnish muscle-eye-brain disease of Santavuori, and Fukuyama's muscular dystrophy, all of which are associated with eye abnormalities, including coloboma, retinal dysplasia, or cataracts
- ▶ Pachygyria is seen as a component of many different types of cortical malformation, including Zellweger's syndrome (peroxisome deficiency), and is not specific
- ▶ Polymicrogyria is associated with areas of destruction (porencephaly) or ischemia (i.e., bilateral middle cerebral artery ischemia or perisylvian polymicrogyria) (see the later section "Disruptions of Developing Gray Matter")
- ▶ Focal cortical dysplasia is manifested as seizures, usually in early childhood

Radiologic Features
- ▶ In type I lissencephaly, a smooth cortical surface is visible on prenatal ultrasound in the third trimester and on CT or MRI
- ▶ In type II lissencephaly, irregularity of cortical gray matter corresponds to a "cobblestone" appearance; hydrocephalus is also seen
- ▶ Gyral widening (pachygyria, focal cortical dysplasia) or narrowing and complexity (polymicrogyria) are detectable on CT and MRI
- ▶ Periventricular nodular or subcortical band heterotopia are visible as gray matter signals in the white matter

Prognosis and Treatment
- ▶ Seizures may be severe and life-threatening in all neuronal migration disorders
- ▶ Only focal cortical dysplasia is amenable to surgical therapy for seizure control
- ▶ Zellweger's syndrome also has an accumulation of plasmalogens and very long chain fatty acids as a result of abnormal peroxisome function, with hepatorenal failure and death ensuing within 1 to 2 years
- ▶ Eye involvement in type II lissencephaly can be source of morbidity
- ▶ Muscular weakness in Fukuyama's muscular dystrophy can result in death in infancy

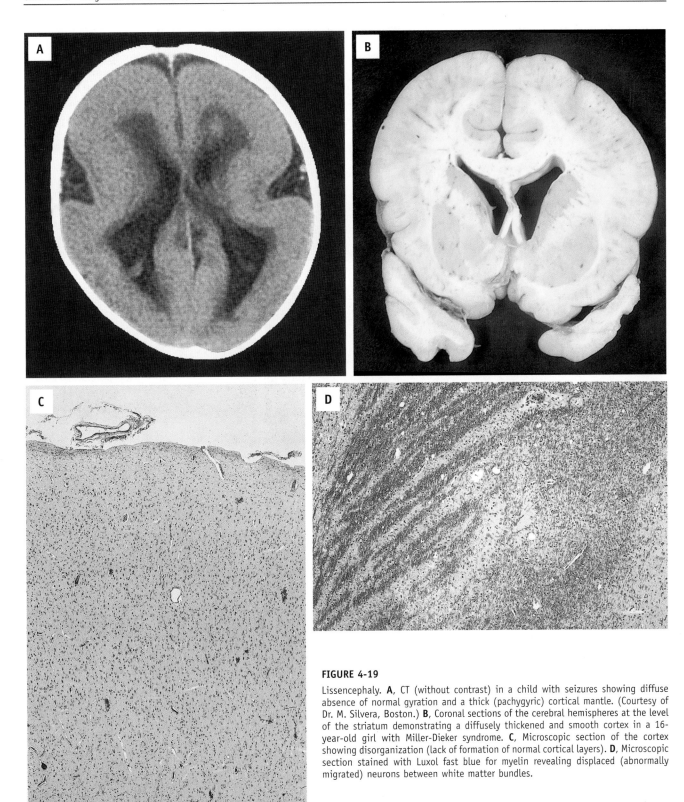

FIGURE 4-19

Lissencephaly. **A**, CT (without contrast) in a child with seizures showing diffuse absence of normal gyration and a thick (pachygyric) cortical mantle. (Courtesy of Dr. M. Silvera, Boston.) **B**, Coronal sections of the cerebral hemispheres at the level of the striatum demonstrating a diffusely thickened and smooth cortex in a 16-year-old girl with Miller-Dieker syndrome. **C**, Microscopic section of the cortex showing disorganization (lack of formation of normal cortical layers). **D**, Microscopic section stained with Luxol fast blue for myelin revealing displaced (abnormally migrated) neurons between white matter bundles.

the adult pattern of secondary and tertiary (i.e., named) gyri (Fig. 4-20). Cortical dysplasia is usually a unifocal disorganization of neurons that often have characteristic cytologic abnormalities (Fig. 4-21). Neuronal heterotopias are misplaced collection of neurons, usually in the white matter periventricular regions beneath the ependyma (periventricular nodular heterotopia [Fig. 4-22]) or along the pial surface (subarachnoid glioneuronal heterotopia) (Fig. 4-23).

Clinically, *type I lissencephaly* is most recognizable as the Miller-Dieker syndrome. Affected individuals have a characteristic facies, including bitemporal hollowing, a short nose with a broad nasal bridge and upturned nares, long and thin upper lip, small chin, and often low-set and posteriorly rotated ears. Sporadic occurrence of the brain abnormality without the typical facies is known as "isolated lissencephaly sequence." Type I lissencephaly is manifested in the neonatal period as

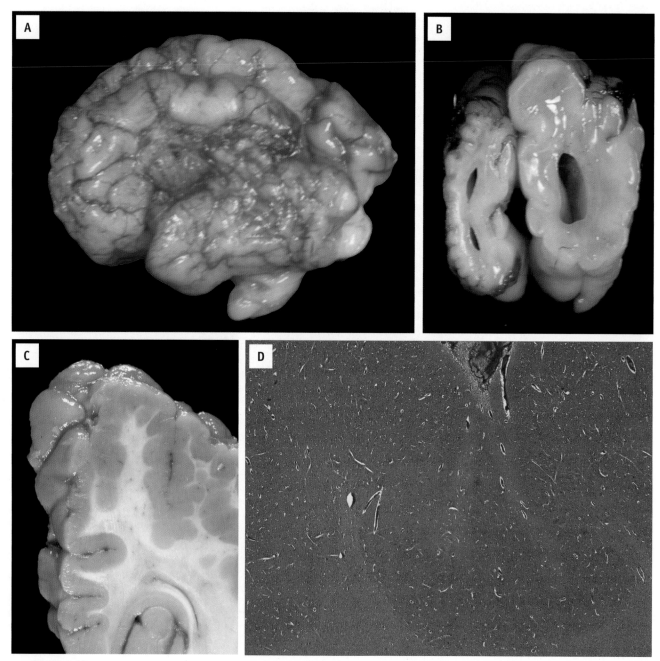

FIGURE 4-20

Polymicrogyria. **A**, Left lateral hemisphere of a 26-week-gestation stillborn fetus with abnormally small, complex gyri along the sylvian fissure (perisylvian polymicrogyria). **B**, Coronal section of the same specimen showing the small gyri on the surface of the hemisphere (*left*). **C**, Coronal section of the right parieto-occipital region from a child; note the polymicrogyric cortex in the *upper right* and contrast with the normal cortical ribbon in the *lower left*. **D**, Low-power photomicrograph of polymicrogyric cortex revealing the complex folding of the superficial layers of cortex.

marked hypotonia, followed later by permanent spastic quadriparesis. Seizures are characteristic and may be difficult to control; they may begin as neonatal seizures or as infantile spasms with myoclonic and tonic seizures that later lead to a Lennox-Gastaut situation with the additional occurrence of atonic seizures. Fast α- and β-activity mixed with high-amplitude slow activity is seen on the electroencephalogram. Mental and psychomotor retardation is usually profound. Cardiac anomalies occur in 20% to 25% of all cases and genital anomalies in approximately 70% of males.

The Miller-Dieker syndrome locus (*LIS1*) has been mapped to chromosome 17p13.3 and the gene identified. The gene encodes platelet-activating factor (PAF) acetylhydrolase-1, β1-subunit, an enzyme that inacti-

vates PAF. Studies in mice and cell culture systems show that PAF is involved in cytoskeletal dynamics and is required for neuronal migration. These data lend support to the hypothesis that deranged cell migration causes classic lissencephaly.

An X-linked form of lissencephaly is due to a mutation in the gene *XLIS* at Xq22.3-q23, which encodes the novel protein doublecortin (DCX). Males with *XLIS* mutations have a severe and usually lethal form of lissencephaly. In contrast, females with mutations have an apparent normal cortical ribbon, a band of white matter, and then a band of gray matter, with the remaining white matter underlying this second band of gray matter ("double cortex"). The normal cortical ribbon is thought to arise from cells that undergo lyonization of

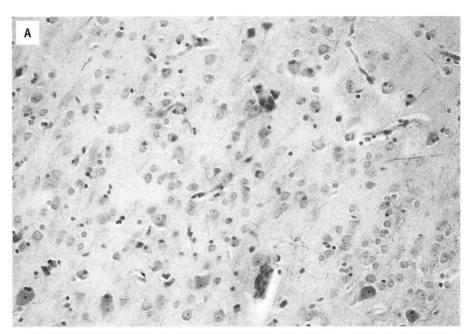

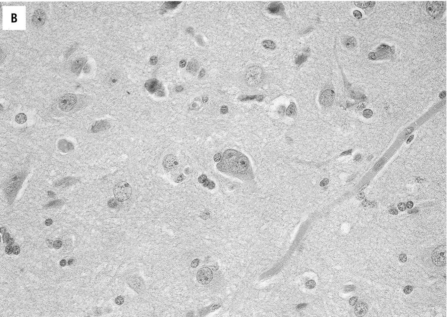

FIGURE 4-21

Cortical dysplasia. **A**, Histologic section stained with cresyl violet and Luxol fast blue showing disorganization of normal cortical architecture. **B**, Binucleated (dysplastic) neuron.   *Continued*

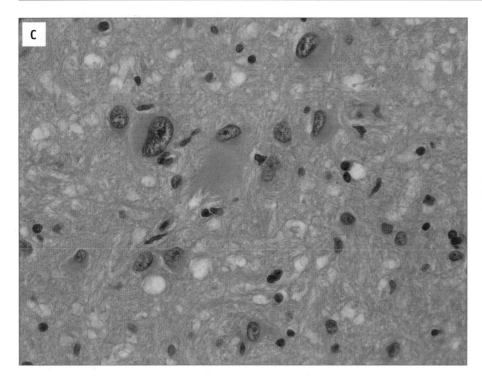

FIGURE 4-21, cont'd
C, Enlarged, bizarre cells with abundant eosinophilic cytoplasm ("balloon" cells).

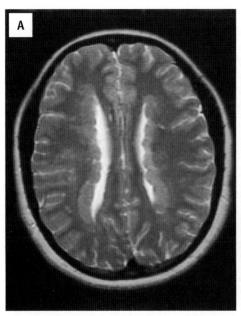

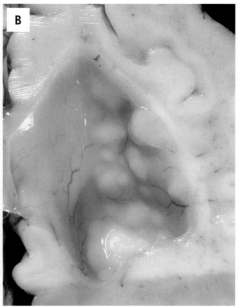

FIGURE 4-22

Periventricular nodular heterotopia. **A**, T2-weighted axial MRI of the hemispheres showing multiple nodules of heterotopic tissue with gray matter signal along both lateral ventricles. (Courtesy of Dr. L. Hsu, Boston.) **B**, View into the frontal pole of the lateral ventricle illustrating nodular protrusion of the heterotopia into the ventricular space. (Courtesy of Dr. U. De Girolami, from the collection of the late Dr. E. P. Richardson, Jr., Boston.)

the X chromosome harboring the mutant allele (i.e., from cells expressing the normal allele) and migrate normally to the cortical plate. Cells in which the normal allele is inactivated express the mutant gene, thereby failing to completely migrate, and form a band of gray matter within the cerebral white matter. Doublecortin is a microtubule-associated protein required for normal cell migration.

Type II ("cobblestone") lissencephaly is found in a group of disorders associated with congenital muscular dystrophy and often with eye abnormalities, including the Walker-Warburg syndrome (WWS), the Finnish "muscle-eye-brain" (MEB) disease of Santavuori, and Fukuyama's congenital muscular dystrophy (FCMD). WWS is the most severe and is associated with a high incidence of neonatal lethality. Inheritance is autosomal recessive, the syndrome being caused by a mutation in the gene for *O*-mannosyltransferase on 9q. The brain malformation may include not only the gyral abnormalities but also hydrocephalus, cerebellar hypoplasia

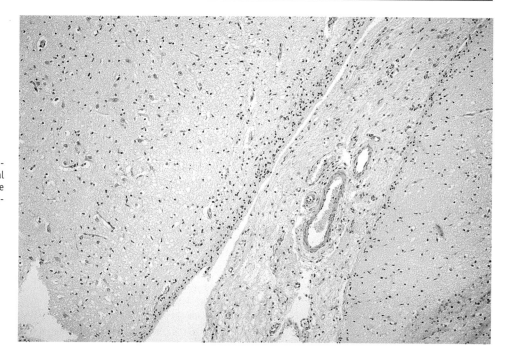

FIGURE 4-23

Subarachnoid glioneuronal heterotopia: histologic section of cerebral cortex with heterotopic tissue in the subarachnoid space surrounding subarachnoid vessels.

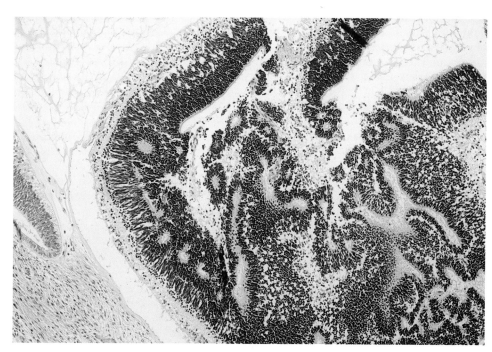

FIGURE 4-24

Retinal dysplasia: microscopic evidence of disorganization of retinal epithelium with the formation of rosettes and irregular papillary structures.

(sometimes Dandy-Walker malformation), occipital encephalocele, or any combination of these findings. Patients show profound hypotonia at birth. Retinal dysplasia (Fig. 4-24), anterior chamber malformations, cataracts, choroidal colobomas, optic nerve hypoplasia, and microphthalmos have been described. Serum creatine kinase levels are elevated as a result of the muscular dystrophy. Contractures may be present at birth (arthrogryposis multiplex congenita) or develop later.

MEB disease of Santavuori, a disease occurring largely in Finland, resembles WWS in many respects.

It is manifested at birth or in the first few months of life as hypotonia. Elevated serum creatine kinase is detected, usually by 1 year of age. Subsequent motor development is markedly delayed, and in fact, worsening of spasticity and contractures may occur into early childhood. Mental retardation and seizures are common. Retinal degeneration and optic atrophy are usual and may be accompanied by the eventual development of cataracts; congenital glaucoma has been described. The electroretinogram may become flattened, whereas visual evoked potentials tend to be progressively delayed and of abnormally high amplitude. The syndrome is due to mutations in the glycosyltransferase gene *POMGNT1* at 1p34-p33.

FCMD is quite common in Japan, where it is second only to Duchenne's muscular dystrophy as a cause of progressive motor disability in childhood. Outside Japan, however, it is exceedingly rare. In contrast to MEB disease and WWS, eye involvement, usually myopia and optic atrophy, is of lesser frequency and severity. Patients do demonstrate psychomotor retardation and progressive muscular weakness and contractures. Seizures occur in about half the patients. Linkage is to chromosome 9q31, and a novel gene has recently been identified.

Polymicrogyria arises in several settings, including conditions such as Zellweger's syndrome (an inherited disorder of peroxisome biogenesis) (Fig. 4-25) and disruptions (see Fig. 4-20; see also "Disruptions of Developing Gray and White Matter" later). Clinically, it is associated with seizures and mental retardation. Zellweger's syndrome is also associated with metabolic defects in hepatic and renal function related to failure of peroxisomal function, which is fatal in the second year of life.

Heterotopia can be sporadic, can be inherited as a simple mendelian trait, or can occur as part of a more complex syndrome. They may be asymptomatic, incidental findings on imaging or at autopsy, or they may be manifested as seizures, usually with onset in childhood. Focal, multifocal, or generalized seizures can occur; infantile spasms and the Lennox-Gastaut syndrome are seen with more extensive heterotopic gray matter deposits. Motor and cognitive deficits may coexist. The least severe clinical manifestations are seen when the abnormality is localized to the periventricular region (see Fig. 4-22), in contrast to those associated with subcortical band heterotopia. Two periventricular hetero-

topia syndromes are an autosomal recessive form that occurs with microcephaly and is associated with a mutation in the *ARFGEG2* gene and a second form that is X-linked in which women in affected families tend to have seizures or mental retardation, or both, and affected males are thought to not survive the embryonic period. Mutations in *filamin-A* have recently been identified as the cause of this latter disorder. Filamin-A appears to participate in communication between the cell surface and the cytoskeleton, again linking the cell migration defects to cytoskeletal anomalies.

As with heterotopia, the initial clinical manifestation of *cortical dysplasia* is usually a seizure in infancy, childhood, or adulthood. In infancy, the seizures can be focal or can start as infantile spasms. Later, the seizures may evolve to tonic seizures and drop attacks. Neonatal onset as early infantile epileptic encephalopathy has also been reported. Electroencephalographic findings are variable.

PATHOLOGIC FEATURES

Lissencephaly and pachygyria probably represent points on a spectrum, with lissencephaly referring to a diffuse bilateral abnormality (see Fig. 4-19) and pachygyria representing a focal or multifocal abnormality with similar gross and microscopic features (Fig. 4-26; see also Fig. 4-25). As mentioned earlier, at least two distinct types of *lissencephaly* exist. Classic (or *type I*) lissencephaly is the prototype pattern and is the form seen in the autosomal dominant Miller-Dieker syndrome, in addition to other autosomal recessive and X-linked forms. The distribution of cortical changes varies depending on the syndrome, with relative sparing of the frontal lobes in *LIS1* mutations versus sparing of the occipital lobes in *XLIS* mutations. Regardless of which lobe is involved, the affected cortex is extremely thick and overlies cerebral white matter, which is proportionally diminished in volume. Normally, the cerebral cortical architecture is made up of six layers and represents about a 10th of the total cerebral hemisphere thickness. In classic lissencephaly, in contrast, the cerebral cortex–to–white matter ratio is 4:1, with a cortical mantle consisting of four abnormal layers (see Fig. 4-19). Layer I is a relatively normal-appearing molecular layer, whereas layer II is a

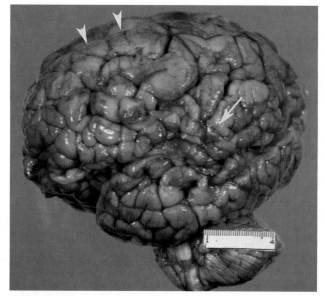

FIGURE 4-25

Zellweger's syndrome: lateral view of the brain showing complex, small gyri (polymicrogyria) along the sylvian fissure (*arrow*) with pachygyria along the parasagittal region (*top* of the hemisphere) (*arrowheads*).

NEURONAL MIGRATION DEFECTS—PATHOLOGIC FEATURES

Gross Findings

▶ Lissencephaly type I is characterized by complete or subtotal lack of gyri and sulci, except for the interhemispheric and sylvian fissures, as well as marked widening of cortical thickness and blurring of the gray-white distinction on cut surface; it has 4:1 ratio of gray to white matter

▶ X-linked lissencephaly has a "double cortex" appearance, with the broad band of subcortical heterotopic gray matter occupying the centrum ovale

NEURONAL MIGRATION DEFECTS—PATHOLOGIC FEATURES—cont'd

▶ Lissencephaly type II has a "cobblestone" appearance, with fine stippling of all or part of the surface of the cortex; on cut section it is of variable thickness, with a 1:1 ratio of gray to white matter and a nodular or scalloped gray-white junction

▶ Pachygyria is widening of some or most gyri, usually parasagittally

▶ Polymicrogyria is an increased number and complexity of tiny gyri, lending a "Moroccan leather" appearance, over all or part of the brain; it is usually perisylvian or at the edges of porencephalic (encephaloclastic) defects

▶ Zellweger's syndrome has both pachygyria and polymicrogyria

▶ Focal cortical dysplasia is a grossly visible localized expansion of gyrus, with blurring of the gray-white distinction on cut surface

▶ Heterotopic gray matter appears as "crust" along the pial surface, as a band or nodule in deep white matter, or as subependymal nodules protruding into the ventricle

Microscopic Features

▶ Lissencephaly type I and pachygyria are microscopically identical, with four layers in a vaguely "inside out" organization when compared with normal neocortex

▶ Type II has disorganized neurons, glia, vessels, and collagen in a crust-like layer over a discontinuous pial remnant and a deeper layer of disorganized neurons

▶ "Four-layered" polymicrogyria (seen in intrauterine disruptions) has a fused layer I with undulating, small complex gyri containing four layers of neurons lying beneath and essentially absence of the middle layers, thought to be due to ischemia; "unlayered" polymicrogyria is seen in Zellweger's syndrome

▶ Focal cortical dysplasia has disorganized groups of large, bizarre neurons, "balloon" cells with features of glia and neurons, and occasionally Rosenthal fibers and calcifications

▶ Heterotopia are collections of mature-appearing, but displaced, neurons seen as a band deep to the cortex (subcortical band heterotopia), along the pia/arachnoid (subarachnoid glioneuronal heterotopia), or as nodules in the deep white matter (periventricular nodular heterotopia)

Genetics

▶ Lissencephaly type I (Miller-Dieker syndrome) is caused by *LIS1* mutations at 17p13.3; it has autosomal dominant inheritance

▶ X-linked lissencephaly is caused by a mutation in the doublecortin gene at Xq22.3-q23

▶ Muscle-eye-brain disease is caused by loss-of-function mutations in the glycosyltransferase *POMGNT1* gene; the gene map locus is 1p34-p33

▶ Fukuyama's congenital muscular dystrophy with type II lissencephaly is caused by a mutation in the *fukutin* gene, which maps to chromosome 9

▶ Walker-Warburg syndrome is caused by a mutation in the gene for protein *O*-mannosyltransferase (*POMT1*) at 9q34.1, 9q31

▶ Some examples of bilateral perisylvian polymicrogyria appear to be X-linked and map to Xq28; a form associated with cerebellar ataxia maps to 16q12.2-21

▶ Zellweger's syndrome is caused by genes involved in peroxisome biogenesis, including peroxin (*PEX1*) (7q21), *PEX2* (8q), *PEX3* (6q), *PEX5* (chromosome 12), and *PEX6* (6p)

▶ Focal cortical dysplasia has been associated with loss of heterozygosity and sequence alterations leading to amino acid exchange in the gene product of the tuberous sclerosis gene *TSC1*

▶ Autosomal recessive periventricular heterotopia with microcephaly has been associated with a mutation in *ARFGEG2*, whereas the X-linked dominant form has been mapped to Xq28 and may be caused by a mutation in the *filamin-A* gene

Differential Diagnosis

▶ Pachygyria and polymicrogyria are components of several entities and must be considered in light of other brain and systemic findings, as well as the clinical and family history

▶ Focal cortical dysplasia is histologically similar to tuberous sclerosis but lacks the other multifocal CNS lesions and systemic findings

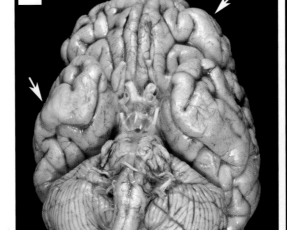
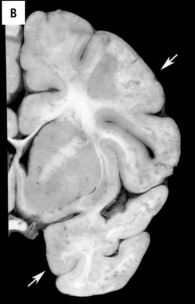

FIGURE 4-26

Pachygyria. **A**, Basal view showing thickening of the lateral frontal and inferior temporal lobe gyri bilaterally (*arrows*). **B**, Coronal section of the right hemisphere at the level of the striatum with a thick lateral frontal and inferior temporal cortex (*arrows*).

band of pyramidal neurons and layer III contains numerous myelinated fibers and fewer neurons and overlies a very thick layer of disorganized neurons in layer IV. The underlying white matter has decreased volume and occasionally contains single neurons or small heterotopia. Although other regions of the brain are usually spared in classic lissencephaly, anomalies in the cerebellum, the inferior olivary nuclei, and the corticospinal tracts have been described. The developmental timing of these malformations is believed to coincide with the interval during which neuronal progenitors leave the ventricular zone and migrate along radial glia to the cortical plate, between 10 and 20 gestational weeks.

In *type II lissencephaly*, seen in patients with WWS, MEB disease, and FCMD, the surface of the brain is less smooth than in type I lissencephaly and has a more irregular, "cobblestone" appearance. These cobblestone areas may alternate with regions of *pachygyria* (abnormally broad gyri) resembling those seen in type I lissencephaly. The brain may show other malformations, including agenesis of the corpus callosum and hindbrain malformations such as cerebellar dysplasia or Dandy-Walker malformation (see the section "Posterior Fossa Malformations" later). Microscopically, unlike the 4:1 ratio of cortex to white matter found in classic lissencephaly, the cobblestone form of lissencephaly has an approximately 1:1 ratio of cortex to white matter, with no evidence of lamination in the cortical layer. Instead, there appear to be two broad bands of neurons: the outer band is a disorganized layer intertwined with collagen and blood vessels of the pia/arachnoid, and the inner band is a disorganized group of neurons likely to be the remnants of the cortical plate. The appearance suggests a multifocal disruption of the pia-glia limitans that allows migrating neurons to flow past the normal pial surface and into the leptomeninges. The eye abnormalities include defects in the iris and other components of the uvea (coloboma) and retinal dysplasia (see Fig. 4-24).

Polymicrogyria is recognized macroscopically as fine stubbling on the surface of the brain (sometimes likened to "Moroccan leather") (see Fig. 4-20). This appearance is due to a disorganized confluence of small gyri that appear to be partially fused to one another. Microscopically, the small complex gyri undulate beneath a fused layer I. Unlike lissencephaly/pachygyria, the border between polymicrogyria and the adjacent normal cortex is quite distinct, and layer VI in normal cortex and the deepest layer of the polymicrogyric cortex are continuous. Based on these pathologic features, the timing of occurrence of polymicrogyria is generally thought to be later in neocortical development and arise from defects occurring between 17 and 25 or 26 weeks' gestation. Hypoxic-ischemic disruption of the intermediate layers of the cortex at this developmental interval could give rise to the observed changes (see "Disruptions of Developing Gray and White Matter" later).

Heterotopia consists of collections of disorganized neurons in inappropriate places. Heterotopia in the cerebral hemispheres can take on several patterns. It may occur as focal, isolated anomalies found incidentally on imaging or at autopsy or may have clinical mani-

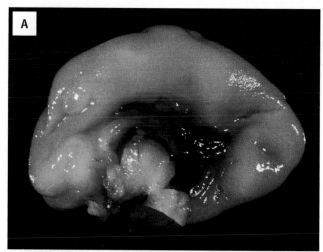

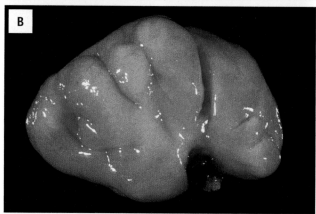

FIGURE 4-27

Aicardi's syndrome. **A**, Medial view of the right hemisphere from a 22-week-gestation fetus showing absence of the corpus callosum. **B**, On lateral view, abnormal cortical gyration is seen in the parietal region.

festations as described earlier. Occasionally, an isolated heterotopia or multifocal cerebral heterotopia in the deep white matter is associated with an overlying cortical malformation. Aicardi's syndrome has heterotopia as a constant feature, as well as agenesis or hypoplasia of the corpus callosum (discussed in the later section "Midline/Commissural Defects") and abnormal cortical gyration (Fig. 4-27). Retinal lacunae, cerebellar abnormalities, and hemivertebrae may also be found. Aicardi's syndrome appears to be an X-linked–dominant, male-lethal condition, so only girls are affected clinically by the infantile spasms and profound psychomotor retardation. Purkinje and granule cell heterotopia are another type of neuronal migration defect that may be extensive or, more commonly, limited and of no clinical significance (Fig. 4-28). The combination of heterotopic neurons admixed with fibrillary glial tissue is known as glioneuronal heterotopia and is often found in the leptomeninges overlying a cortical anomaly or around the base of the brain (see Fig. 4-23). The mislocalized tissue can form a radiographically and grossly identifiable plaque over the surface of the brain.

Focal cortical dysplasia is characterized grossly by local expansion of the cortical gyri with blurring of

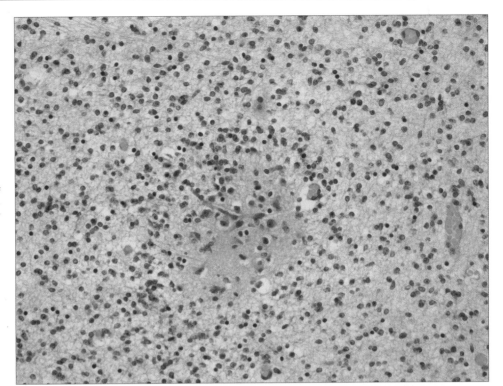

FIGURE 4-28

Cerebellar heterotopia: collection of small granule cells and large Purkinje-like neurons in the deep cerebellar white matter.

the border between the cerebral cortex and underlying white matter. Microscopically, the normal cytoarchitecture is disrupted by a disorganized array of cytologically atypical neurons, including binucleated forms, reactive glial cells, and "balloon cells" (cells with shared features of both neurons and astrocytes) (see Fig. 4-21). Immunohistochemically, the balloon cells may be nestin, glial fibrillary acidic protein (GFAP), or synaptophysin positive (or any combination of positivity), findings indicative of their immature or incompletely differentiated status. Microcalcifications may be seen in some cases. Since these lesions are often epileptogenic, they may be surgically removed to assist in the management of medically intractable seizures. Varying degrees of cortical disorganization can accompany hamartomas and low-grade neoplasms of childhood, such as dysembryoplastic neuroepithelial tumors and gangliogliomas.

RADIOLOGIC FEATURES

In type I lissencephaly, the normal gyral and sulcal pattern is effaced by a smooth agyric surface on CT (see Fig. 4-19) and MRI. The cerebral cortex is markedly thickened with variable preservation of the cerebral white matter. Often, on MRI a layer of white matter may focally separate a thin cortical layer from a deeper swath of gray matter representing arrested neurons. A diffuse pattern of such gray matter duplication ("double cortex") corresponds to the pathologic finding of subcortical band heterotopia. In so-called incomplete lissencephalies (with or without 17p mutations), pachy-

gyric and agyric areas may coexist along with shallow, vertical sylvian fissures. In X-linked lissencephaly, the posterior cerebral lobes are relatively spared, in contrast to the agyria and pachygyria anteriorly. Of course, care must be taken when reviewing prenatal MRI and ultrasonography because the cortex is normally free of convolutions until at least 18 gestational weeks.

In WWS and MEB disease (type II lissencephalies), hydrocephalus is seen frequently, as well as patchy white matter hyperintensity on T2-weighted MRI. The irregular, fine nodularity of the cortex at the gray-white junction corresponds to the cobblestone pattern seen on pathologic evaluation. In FCMD, MRI of the brain demonstrates areas of pachygyria and polymicrogyria, as well as regions of abnormal T2 signal in white matter. The white matter is hypodense on CT.

Periventricular nodular heterotopia appears as irregular nodules of gray matter signal intensity along the ventricular surfaces (see Fig. 4-22).

DIFFERENTIAL DIAGNOSIS

As mentioned earlier, the Miller-Dieker phenotype is distinguished from isolated lissencephaly sequence by the lack of distinctive facial features in the latter, although bitemporal hollowing and a small chin may be seen in some patients with isolated lissencephaly sequence. The distinction between these two entities is not entirely straightforward inasmuch as microdeletions detected by fluorescent in situ hybridization (FISH) have been seen in a significant number of patients with isolated lissencephaly sequence, thus suggesting a relationship to Miller-Dieker syndrome.

The differential diagnosis of the lissencephaly type II syndromes is complex, as reflected in the many essentially synonymous designations of these entities, including the MEB, HARD±E (hydrocephalus, agyria, retinal dysplasia, ± encephalocele), and CODM (congenital ocular dysplasia/muscular dystrophy) syndromes, which share phenotypic features. FCMD, despite many similar features, does not usually include the severe eye and brain anomalies found in WWS. If clinically important, distinction among these entities can be assisted by genetic studies.

Cortical anomalies recapitulating the syndromic features of lissencephaly, pachygyria, and polymicrogyria can be seen as components of several other entities. Specifically, Zellweger syndrome, a disorder of peroxisomal biogenesis characterized by neonatal hypotonia, facial dysmorphism, open fontanelles, and renal and hepatic abnormalities, has both lissencephalic/pachygyric and polymicrogyric cortical changes (see Fig. 4-25). The related peroxisomal disorders neonatal adrenoleukodystrophy, rhizomelic chondrodysplasia punctata, and bifunctional enzyme deficiency may show migrational abnormalities. The metabolic abnormalities glutaric aciduria type II, pyruvate dehydrogenase deficiency, nonketotic hyperglycemia, and sulfite oxidase deficiency/molybdenum cofactor deficiency are examples of other metabolic disorders that occasionally demonstrate cortical dysplasia.

Polymicrogyria may also occur in various settings, including lissencephaly type II conditions and the Aicardi, Neu Laxova, and Smith-Lemli-Opitz syndromes (see the earlier section "Holoprosencephaly Sequence"), thus reflecting the nonspecific nature of the malformation. In addition, polymicrogyria can occur in a variety of chromosomal abnormalities and in disruptions (see the corresponding sections later). Likewise, neuronal heterotopia and focal cortical dysplasia may accompany many of these same syndromes.

Both periventricular and subcortical band heterotopia can occur as X-linked inherited conditions, although they map to different regions on the X chromosome. In familial band heterotopia, affected females are found to have heterotopia and often seizures, whereas affected males show more severe brain malformations, including lissencephaly. This gender difference is thought to result from random X chromosome inactivation in females, in which full expression of the defect is prevented and a spectrum of developmental disturbances from focal heterotopia to lissencephaly can occur.

PROGNOSIS AND THERAPY

As mentioned earlier, eye involvement (myopia, infantile glaucoma, retinal and optic nerve hypoplasia, coloboma, and cataracts) is commonly seen, along with mental retardation and seizures, in patients with FCMD, MEB disease, and WWS. In FCMD, like other congenital dystrophies, the onset of marked diffuse weakness and hypotonia, facial weakness, and joint contractures is noted in the neonatal

period, with mortality approaching 50% in infancy. In WWS and MEB disease, mortality is also quite high in the first months of life. There are no specific therapies for any of the neuronal migration defects, although surgery to remove the localized malformation may be effective for seizure control in cases of focal cortical dysplasia.

MIDLINE/COMMISSURAL DEFECTS

CLINICAL FEATURES

Agenesis of the corpus callosum (whether *partial* or *complete*) is a relatively common malformation that may be isolated or associated with other brain or systemic anomalies (Figs. 4-29 to 4-31). It may occur sporadically or as part of a chromosome aberration syndrome such as trisomy 18. Familial cases have also been reported. When part of the X-linked–dominant Aicardi's syndrome (callosal agenesis or hypogenesis with or without interhemispheric cysts, focal cortical dysplasia or heterotopia, and chorioretinal lacunae [see Fig. 4-27]), infantile spasms may be seen. Aicardi's syndrome may also occur with Dandy-Walker or other cerebellar abnormalities (see the later section "Posterior Fossa Malformations") and delayed cerebral myelination. Callosal agenesis is the most common structural abnormality in fetal alcohol syndrome and is sometimes associated with severe midline facial defects as well. Some cases of callosal agenesis are incidental findings at autopsy in adults with no neurologic or developmental difficulties.

Absence of the septum pellucidum may occur as an isolated lesion or concurrent with anomalies of the optic system (*septo-optic dysplasia*) (Fig. 4-32). The former may be asymptomatic or, along with two thirds of septo-optic dysplasia cases, result in hypothalamic-pituitary axis endocrine dysfunction. This endocrine dysfunction can lead to small stature and hypothyroidism. Visual disturbances are due to reduced acuity related to the clinically detectable optic nerve hypoplasia. Nystagmus is occasionally a feature. *Cavum septi pellucidi* (Fig. 4-33) and *cavum vergae* are persistent separations between the rostral or caudal leaves of the septum, respectively, that usually fuse in the third trimester; these changes are generally incidental findings of no clinical significance.

RADIOLOGIC FEATURES

Since the corpus callosum develops rostrocaudally after the telencephalic commissural fibers cross over between the 11th and 20th weeks of gestation, this abnormality can be seen even in early prenatal ultrasonograms as a "bat wing" configuration of the ventricles. Prenatal MRI can readily illustrate the ventricular configuration (see Fig. 4-30) and, often, any associated structural brain and facial anomalies. In neonates and adults, MRI in the sagittal and coronal planes best demonstrates the

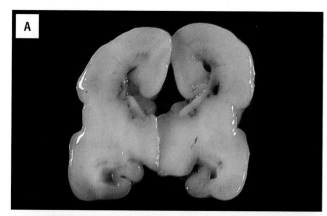

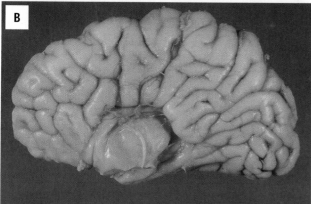

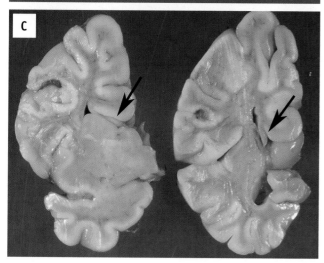

FIGURE 4-29

Complete agenesis of the corpus callosum. **A**, Coronal section from an 18-week-gestation fetus showing vertical ("bat wing") orientation of the lateral ventricles. **B**, Midsagittal section of the right hemisphere from an infant; note the appearance of radiating gyri resulting from absence of the cingulate gyrus and corpus callosum. **C**, Coronal section of the left lateral hemisphere illustrating the vertical ventricular profile and a Probst bundle (*arrow*).

optic system may be difficult to resolve. The septum pellucidum is absent on CT or MRI, and the third ventricle and foramen of Monro may be markedly enlarged.

PATHOLOGIC FEATURES

In total agenesis, the medial surface of the hemispheres shows secondary abnormalities characterized by absence of the pericallosal artery and replacement of the

abnormalities. An interhemispheric cyst, when present, has imaging qualities similar to those of CSF, along with a wall that may cause a mass effect on the adjacent cerebral hemispheres.

In septo-optic dysplasia, the optic canals may be small on CT or plain radiographs, although hypoplasia of the

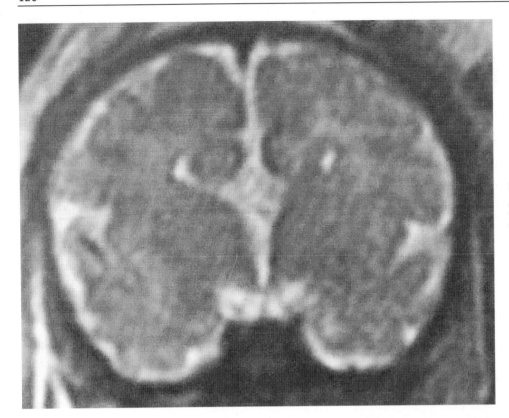

FIGURE 4-30

Agenesis of the corpus callosum: fetal MRI showing the "bat wing" ventricles. (Courtesy of Dr. D. Levine, Boston.)

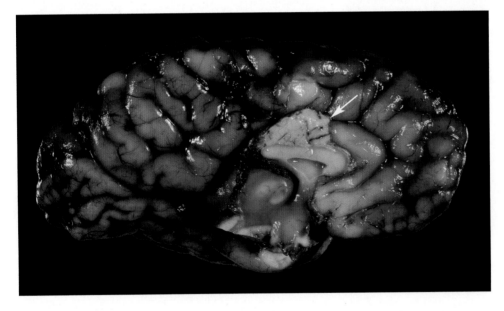

FIGURE 4-31

Partial agenesis of the corpus callosum: midsagittal view of the left hemisphere showing preservation of the rostrum of the corpus callosum, but absence of the body and genu, which have been replaced by a midline lipoma (*arrow*).

normal cingulate gyrus by perpendicular (often referred to as "radiating") gyri (see Fig. 4-29). On coronal sections, no crossing white matter fibers are seen, and the lateral ventricles have a vertical ("bat wing") orientation (see Fig. 4-29). This most severe form is due to total absence of callosal fibers or to their inability to cross the midline. In the latter circumstance, remnant callosal fibers form aberrant anteroposterior tracts known as Probst's bundles that lie lateral to the cingulate gyri along the medial aspects of the lateral ventricles (see Fig. 4-29). Partial agenesis of the corpus callosum is classically posterior, so there is a relatively normal genu and anterior body (see Fig. 4-31). Occasionally, the fornices (hippocampal commissures) or anterior commissure appears hypertrophic. Whether total or partial, callosal agenesis may be accompanied by lipomas, cysts, vascular anomalies, or calcifications along the medial aspect of the hemispheres.

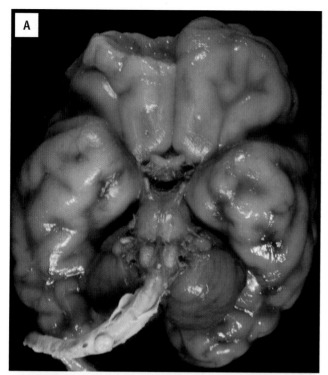

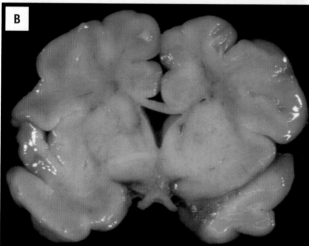

FIGURE 4-32

Septo-optic dysplasia. **A**, View of the base of the brain showing absence of the olfactory bulbs and tracts and very small optic nerves and chiasm. **B**, Coronal section of the hemispheres at the level of the optic chiasm revealing absence of the septum pellucidum, a condition lending a "monoventricle" appearance; the hypothalamus is hypoplastic.

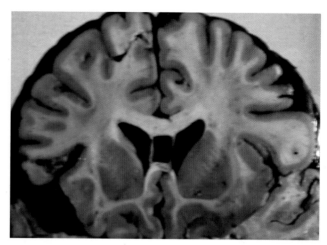

FIGURE 4-33

Cavum septi pellucidi. Note the widened leaves of the septum in this incidental example in an adult. (Courtesy of Dr. M. E. McLaughlin, Boston.)

MIDLINE/COMMISSURAL DEFECTS—PATHOLOGIC FEATURES

Gross Findings

▶ When the callosum is absent, the pericallosal artery and cingulate gyrus are also absent and replaced by "radiating gyri"
▶ Coronal sections of callosal agenesis show the vertical "bat wing" configuration of the lateral ventricles and a Probst bundle (noncrossing fibers aggregated in an anteroposteriorly directed fascicle at the superomedial edge of the hemisphere)
▶ Lipomas, cysts, or calcifications may be present medially in the interhemispheric fissure
▶ In septo-optic dysplasia, absence of the septum pellucidum leads to a "pseudo-monoventricular" appearance with a rounded outline and a thin corpus callosum
▶ Cavum septi pellucidi and cavum vergae are persistent separations between the anterior and posterior leaves of the septum, respectively

Microscopic Features

▶ A Probst bundle consists of axons with variable myelination; otherwise, callosal agenesis has no specific microscopic features
▶ In septo-optic dysplasia, the optic nerves and tracts may be hypoplastic, with reduced numbers of axons and hypomyelination, hypoplasia of the lateral geniculate nucleus, and disorganization of the hypothalamus

Genetics

▶ Callosal agenesis has diverse genetic causes and may be autosomal dominant, recessive, or X-linked
▶ The Aicardi syndrome gene map locus is Xp22
▶ *HEXS1* mutations are found in some cases of septo-optic dysplasia; the gene map locus is 3p21.2-p21.1

Differential Diagnosis

▶ In fetal brain specimens, artifactual tearing of the callosum may mimic agenesis, and the septum pellucidum is normally cavum (fusing near term or even after birth)
▶ Closed head injury can cause tearing, separation, or fenestration of the septum pellucidum

Cavum septi pellucidi and cavum vergae are seen in fetuses as developmentally normal midline cavities (the former is rostral and the latter is caudal) lying between the two leaves of the septum (see Fig. 4-33). They tend to become obliterated toward term but persist postnatally in a minority of individuals. Complete agenesis of the septum pellucidum results in a "pseudo-monoventricle" because of marked expansion of the foramen of Monro and third ventricle. In septo-optic dysplasia (see Fig. 4-32), there may be gross or microscopic dysplasia of the hypothalamus, in addition to the absent septum pellucidum; hypoplasia of the optic nerves, chiasm, and tracts; and hypoplasia of the lateral geniculate nucleus.

DIFFERENTIAL DIAGNOSIS

In fetal specimens from the late second trimester, the corpus callosum is very easily torn artifactually while removing the brain; however, the ventricles should lack the slight expansion and vertical orientation of those in callosal agenesis. In addition, the presence of a cingulate sulcus, which is visible by 19 gestational weeks, should serve to indicate that the corpus callosum was present in situ.

Isolated absence of the septum pellucidum is rare and should thus prompt careful examination to detect commonly associated abnormalities such as arrhinencephaly or limited forms of holoprosencephaly, callosal agenesis, or abnormalities of the optic system. Occasionally, long-standing hydrocephalus may result in separation of the previously fused leaves of the septum pellucidum or in fenestration or loss of the septum pellucidum. Wide (>1 cm) separation of the two leaves has been seen in boxers and is presumed to be a result of multiple blows to the head.

PROGNOSIS AND THERAPY

Since isolated callosal agenesis may be asymptomatic and only incidentally discovered, the other neuropathologic abnormalities associated with the lesion determine the clinical course, which as mentioned earlier for Aicardi's syndrome can include seizures, mental retardation, and visual abnormalities. Patients with septo-optic dysplasia characterized by only limited optic hypoplasia and midline defects have a better developmental prognosis than do those with more extensive anomalies.

POSTERIOR FOSSA MALFORMATIONS

CLINICAL FEATURES

Hindbrain malformations account for a significant proportion of all CNS anomalies and may be encountered anytime from midgestation through young adulthood. The use of second-trimester ultrasonography for dating and monitoring of asymptomatic pregnancies has led to prenatal detection of posterior fossa abnormalities, primarily Dandy-Walker malformations, and an increased incidence of these findings among abortuses. Historically, the scheme of classification of posterior fossa

---

POSTERIOR FOSSA MALFORMATIONS—FACT SHEET

Definition

▶ Aplasia is complete absence (very rare)
▶ Hypoplasias include
  ▶ Dandy-Walker malformation, or absence of the cerebellar vermis (partial or complete) with cystic dilatation of the fourth ventricle
  ▶ Joubert's syndrome (absent vermian foliation and apposition of the cerebellar hemispheres at the midline)
  ▶ Rhombencephalosynapsis (fusion of the cerebellar hemispheres and dentate across the midline)
▶ Disorganizations (possible migration defects) include
  ▶ Lhermitte-Duclos disease (also called dysplastic gangliocytoma of the cerebellum; aberrant organization and thickening of the folia)
  ▶ Cerebellar polymicrogyria (irregular fusion of the cerebellar folia)
  ▶ Purkinje/granule cell heterotopia (aberrant migration of cerebellar cortical neurons to cerebellar white matter)
▶ Displacements include
  ▶ Chiari I (cerebellar tonsils displaced below the foramen magnum)
  ▶ Chiari II (cerebellar vermis displaced below the foramen magnum, along with hindbrain crowding and anomalies of the brain stem, associated with myelomeningocele) (see the section "Neural Tube Defects")
▶ Destructive/degenerative lesions such as cerebellar ataxias (see Chapter 6) and ischemia of the posterior circulation (see the section "Disruptions of Developing Gray and White Matter" and Chapter 2)
▶ Aqueductal malformations include stenosis, atresia, and dysplasia as components of other malformations or occlusions related to disruptions, infections, or neoplasia

Gender Distribution

▶ Although most posterior fossa malformations do not have a gender predilection, Lhermitte-Duclos disease affects males somewhat more often, and X-linked aqueductal stenosis occurs only in males

Clinical Features

▶ Mental retardation occurs in 25% to 50% of patients with Dandy-Walker malformation; cerebellar ataxia and hydrocephalus are also seen
▶ Joubert's syndrome and rhombencephalosynapsis are characterized by intermittent hyperpnea, eye movement abnormalities, ataxia, and mental retardation
▶ Isolated cerebellar polymicrogyria and cerebellar cortical heterotopia are usually asymptomatic
▶ Lhermitte-Duclos disease causes symptoms of increased intracranial pressure
▶ Aqueductal stenosis results in hydrocephalus

Radiologic Features

▶ Dandy-Walker malformation includes cystic expansion of the fourth ventricle, upward displacement of the tentorium, and a defect in the midline of the cerebellum, visible on midsagittal CT or MRI, even prenatally
▶ Chiari I malformation shows displacement of the tonsils into the foramen magnum on CT or MRI, along with compression of the caudal brain stem/rostral cervical spinal cord and shortening of the clivus

▶ Midline abnormalities on neuroimaging correspond to the gross findings seen in Joubert's syndrome, rhombencephalosynapsis, and Lhermitte-Duclos disease (see the "Pathologic Features" box)

▶ The hydrocephalus of aqueductal stenosis is variably severe, with transependymal flow of CSF and flattening and thinning of the cerebral mantle seen on neuroimaging

Prognosis and Treatment

▶ For Dandy-Walker complex, up to 40% die (often because of associated systemic malformations) in early life, with 75% of survivors having cognitive deficits

▶ Joubert's syndrome and rhombencephalosynapsis also have a high incidence of death in the infantile period, with mental retardation and ataxia in survivors

▶ Lhermitte-Duclos disease may be occult until late childhood or early adulthood, when surgical decompression becomes necessary; it is a component of Cowden's disease (see the later section "Familial Malformations/Tumor Syndromes")

▶ Chiari I and II malformations may require surgical release of cord tethering (see the earlier section "Neural Tube Defects")

▶ Aqueductal stenosis necessitates shunting of the resulting hydrocephalus; associated malformations may dictate the clinical course

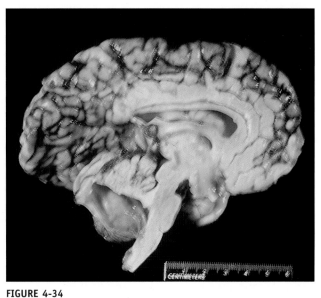

FIGURE 4-34

Dandy-Walker malformation: midsagittal section from a term infant specimen showing absence of the inferior vermis and cystic expansion of the fourth ventricle (partial or variant malformation).

anomalies was that of Chiari, in which type I is chronic cerebellar tonsillar herniation, with ataxia causing referral to the surgeon for release of a "tethered" cord, a condition not generally seen by the neuropathologist. Type II (also known as the Arnold-Chiari malformation) is displacement of pegs of cerebellar vermis below the level of the foramen magnum and is associated with an open neural tube defect, usually lumbosacral myelomeningocele (discussed earlier under "Neural Tube Defects"). Type III is quite rare and refers to a posterior cervico-occipital encephalocele, and type IV is a deficiency of the vermis, better known as Dandy-Walker syndrome. In general, current neuropathologic usage refers only to types I and II. A more workable categorization recognizes five groups: *aplasias*; *hypoplasias*, including Dandy-Walker malformation, Joubert's syndrome, and rhombencephalosynapsis; *disorganizations*, including migration defects; *displacements*, including Chiari I and II malformations; and *destructive/degenerative lesions*. In this section, only the hypoplasias, disorganizations, and displacements are discussed. In addition, *aqueductal malformations* are discussed for the sake of completeness.

Clinically, in patients with the Dandy-Walker malformation (the typical example of *hypoplasia* [Figs. 4-34 to 4-36]), mental retardation is seen in 25% to 50% of patients surviving to childhood. Cerebellar nystagmus and gait disturbance are less common. Progressive symptoms of hydrocephalus usually require shunting. A host of other nonspecific neurobehavioral symptoms may develop. It must be emphasized, however, that the main clinical significance of the Dandy-Walker malformation is its high frequency (around 70%) of concurrence with other cerebral and visceral anomalies, such as congenital heart disease and renal abnormalities,

which tend to determine the individual prognosis. Associated karyotypic abnormalities have included complete or partial trisomies of chromosomes 21, 18, 13, and 11 (see the later section on trisomies) and aberrations of chromosome 5. Most instances are sporadic, although familial occurrence is documented in approximately 2% of cases. Association with maternal *cis*-retinoic acid medication has raised speculation that interference with homeobox gene expression may be the mechanism of the hindbrain malformation.

Patients with Joubert's syndrome or rhombencephalosynapsis (Fig. 4-37) (forms of midline cerebellar disorganization described later) show intermittent hyperpnea, abnormal eye movements, ataxia, and mental retardation; some patients also have renal abnormalities and retinal dysplasia (see Fig. 4-24).

Minor *migrational defects* such as microscopic cerebellar cortical heterotopia (see Fig. 4-28) are extremely common and thought to be of no clinical consequence. However, macroscopic disorganization of the cerebellar cortex, including so-called cerebellar polymicrogyria and Lhermitte-Duclos disease (dysplastic gangliocytoma of the cerebellum), are less frequently encountered. The former probably originates in the manner of cerebral cortical polymicrogyrias, either genetically determined or secondary to an insult at the critical point of cell migration leading to disturbed architecture (Fig. 4-38). In Lhermitte-Duclos disease, one cerebellar hemisphere is hypertrophic, with thickened folia containing large displaced dysplastic neurons, some with features of Purkinje cells. Affected patients have signs of increased intracranial pressure. Half the patients with Lhermitte-Duclos disease have Cowden's disease, an autosomal dominant condition (see "Familial Malformations/Tumor Syndromes" later).

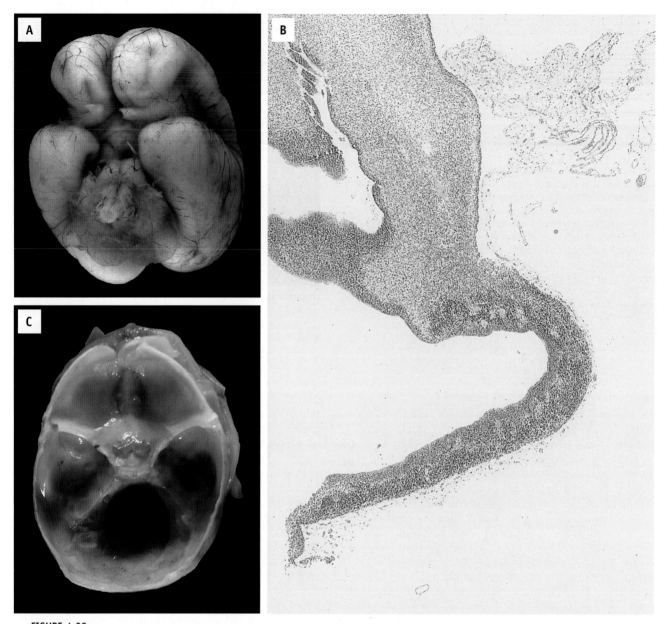

FIGURE 4-35

Dandy-Walker malformation. **A**, Basal view of the brain from a late second-trimester fetus. Note the clear membrane of a cyst beneath the caudal aspect of the brain stem. **B**, Histology of the cyst membrane, which consists of disorganized immature central neuroglial tissue and arachnoid overlying the dilated fourth ventricle. **C**, Base of the skull from the same fetus showing an enlarged, bowl-shaped posterior fossa.

In posterior fossa anomalies characterized by *displacement*, Chiari I malformations (Fig. 4-39) are manifested as ataxia in childhood or early adulthood and may require neurosurgical release of a tethered cord (see "Neural Tube Defects" earlier). Type II encompasses a significant proportion of abortuses, often identified antenatally because of the distal neural tube defect. Clinically, a Chiari II malformation may be manifested as lower brain stem and cranial nerve dysfunction. Dysphagia leading to feeding difficulties, drooling, nasal regurgitation, stridor, vocal cord paralysis, and life-threatening apneic spells can occur. Cyanotic episodes are ominous and carry considerable mortality. Nystagmus, retrocollis, and opisthotonos can be seen. Later

occurrence of the Chiari II malformation may, in addition, include loss of head control, new weakness in the arms, and increasing spasticity leading to quadriparesis (see "Neural Tube Defects" earlier).

RADIOLOGIC FEATURES

Many of the posterior fossa abnormalities are readily visualized on routine neuroimaging, including prenatal ultrasonography and fetal MRI (see Fig. 4-36). Partial or complete absence of the cerebellar vermis with cystic

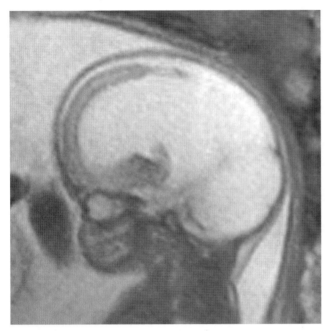

FIGURE 4-36

Dandy-Walker malformation: fetal MRI, sagittal view, illustrating a cystic fourth ventricle and elevation of the tentorium. (Courtesy of Dr. D. Levine, Boston.)

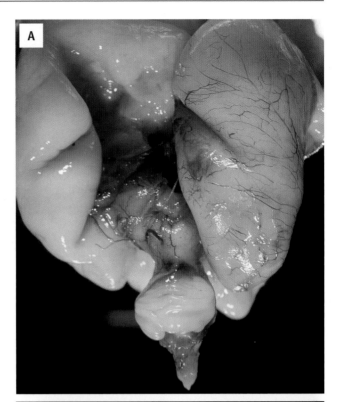

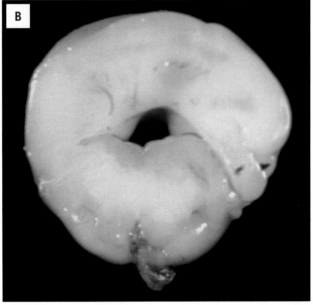

FIGURE 4-37

Rhombencephalosynapsis. **A**, Dorsal aspect of the brain revealing the small, knob-like cerebellum. **B**, On axial section, the cerebellum has deficient hemispheres that are poorly distinguished from the midline vermis.

expansion of the fourth ventricle, an enlarged posterior fossa, and an elevated tentorium (Dandy-Walker complex) are visible on midsagittal views by CT or MRI. Chiari I malformation is seen in the midsagittal plane as displacement of the tonsils into the foramen magnum (on MRI or CT), as well as compression of the inferior medulla by the odontoid and shortening of the clivus (best seen on CT). Spine imaging in patients with Chiari I malformation often demonstrates syringomyelia or hydromyelia (discussed in the section "Neural Tube Defects"). Chiari II malformations are also described in the earlier section "Neural Tube Defects." Joubert's syndrome shows nearly complete absence of the vermian foliation, an enlarged superior cerebellar peduncle on sagittal views, deficiency of the dorsal aspect of the midbrain, and apposition of the cerebellar hemispheres along the midline. Rhombencephalosynapsis features fusion of the cerebellar hemispheres and dentate nuclei across the midline with absence of the vermis.

PATHOLOGIC FEATURES

True *aplasia* of the cerebellum is exceedingly rare, and most such reported cases are thought to instead represent massive disruptions. Alternatively, it may be an embryonic lethal phenotype.

Hypoplasias and *displacements* represent the bulk of the posterior fossa abnormalities seen. The best-known example of cerebellar hypoplasia is the Dandy-Walker malformation, or the occurrence of partial (see Fig. 4-

34) or complete (see Fig. 4-35) agenesis of the vermis with cystic dilatation of the fourth ventricle. An enlarged, bowl-shaped posterior fossa (see Fig. 4-35), an elevated tentorium cerebelli, and hydrocephalus are usual associated features. The constellation was recognized in 1914 by Dandy and Blackfan, who attributed the expanded fourth ventricle to atresia of the foramina

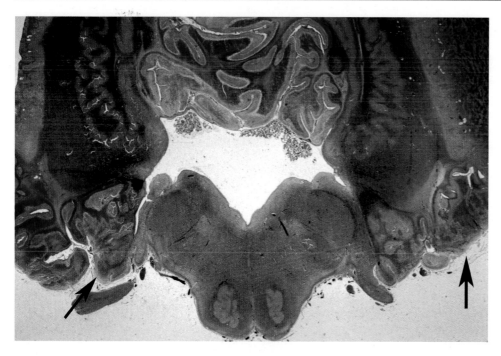

FIGURE 4-38

Cerebellum with dysplasia: transilluminated whole-mount axial section of the cerebellum and medulla demonstrating cerebellar polymicrogyria (*arrows*). (Courtesy of Dr. U. De Girolami, from the collection of the late Dr. E. P. Richardson, Jr., Boston.)

of Luschka and Magendie with secondary accumulation of CSF because of outflow obstruction. The occasional lack of hydrocephalus, as would be expected in foraminal atresia, and the demonstration of foraminal patency in some cases, as well as the embryologic observation that the foramen of Magendie is normally closed through the fourth month of gestation, have called that theory into question, however. Whatever the actual mechanism, the Dandy-Walker malformation must arise during the interval in which the cerebellum, pons, and medulla oblongata become differentiated from the middle and hindbrain segments of the neural tube, which are first visible at about 4 postovulatory weeks.

A membranous edge of the transverse crease above the pontine flexure (the anterior medullary velum) extends caudally to cover the fourth ventricle by 8 weeks. Cell migration from the rhombic lip and subsequent proliferation give rise to the recognizable contour of the cerebellum, which fully covers the fourth ventricle by 16 weeks. Thus, macroscopically and ultrasonographically detectable anomalies can be appreciated by this time. Studies in chick and mouse mutants have implicated the patterning influence of genes homologous to the homeobox genes *engrailed* in *Drosophila* and *En* in mice. In mice, the initial targeted gene disruptions of *En1*, an earlier-acting gene, showed missing colliculi and

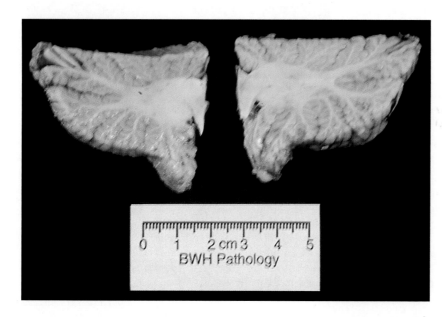

FIGURE 4-39

Chiari I malformation: bisected cerebellum from a young adult with elongation of the cerebellar tonsils resulting from displacement into the foramen magnum.

POSTERIOR FOSSA MALFORMATIONS—PATHOLOGIC FEATURES

Gross Findings

▶ Dandy-Walker malformation includes partial (75% of cases) or complete agenesis of the vermis, along with cystic dilatation of the fourth ventricle, elevation of the tentorium, a bowl-shaped posterior fossa, and hydrocephalus

▶ In Joubert's syndrome, the vermian lobules and superior cerebellar peduncles are hypoplastic

▶ Rhombencephalosynapsis has fusion of dentate nuclei across the midline, often with other supratentorial midline abnormalities (see the earlier section "Midline/Commissural Defects")

▶ In Lhermitte-Duclos disease, the cerebellar folia of one hemisphere are expanded and cause a mass effect

▶ Chiari I malformation has displacement of the cerebellar tonsils into the foramen magnum, whereas Chiari II malformation has displacement of the vermis and inferior cerebellum associated with myelomeningocele and hydrocephalus (see the earlier section "Neural Tube Defects")

▶ Aqueductal stenosis causes often dramatic third and lateral ventricular expansion, "pseudopolymicrogyria," and white matter volume loss with thinning of the corpus callosum

Microscopic Features

▶ The cyst covering the dilated fourth ventricle in Dandy-Walker malformation is made up of ependyma and glia apposed to pia-arachnoid, sometimes with disorganized cerebellar cortex at the margins

▶ Joubert's syndrome is characterized by disorganization of the hypoplastic, fused vermian lobules, cerebellar cortical heterotopia, and sometimes dysplasia of brain stem nuclei

▶ Rhombencephalosynapsis may also have cerebellar cortical heterotopia and disorganization along with a single midline dentate nucleus

▶ Lhermitte-Duclos disease shows an "inside-out" cerebellar cortical arrangement consisting of myelinated fibers along the surface and enlarged, dysplastic ganglion cells in the center of the hypertrophic folia

▶ Chiari I and II malformations both demonstrate disorganization of the displaced cerebellar tissue (see also "Neural Tube Defects")

▶ Aqueductal stenosis may be due to forking or fenestration of the aqueduct or occlusion by subependymal glial tissue (scar), hemosiderotic or necrotic debris, tumor, or inflammation, depending on the underlying cause; the atrophic deep hemispheric white matter may be gliotic and hypomyelinated from pressure effects

Genetics

▶ Although many posterior fossa malformations may be familial, the genetic basis for most remains undefined

▶ Lhermitte-Duclos disease is associated with Cowden's syndrome and is due to mutations in PTEN/MMAC1, located on 10q23 (see the section "Familial Malformation/Tumor Syndromes")

Differential Diagnosis

▶ Destructive lesions of the cerebellum (hemorrhages, infarcts) may mimic Dandy-Walker malformation on neuroimaging but are distinctive on pathologic examination

▶ Joubert's syndrome and rhombencephalosynapsis share similar features but are distinguished by superior cerebellar peduncle hypoplasia in the former and midline dentate fusion in the latter

▶ Lhermitte-Duclos disease may be clinically mistaken for tumor and eventuate in biopsy for diagnosis

cerebellum, thus suggesting a transcriptional role. In *En2* nulls, only subtle foliation defects were seen, consistent with an influence of that gene on later cerebellar development. Subsequently, En1 was shown to be a homeodomain-containing transcription factor defining cellular entry into the cerebellar lineage. Both En1 and En2 are under control of homologues of the paired box–containing genes *Pax2*, *Pax5*, and *Pax8* and the wingless gene *Wnt-1*. As expected, Wnt-1 and Pax5 nulls demonstrated complete cerebellar aplasia. A minority of Pax5 heterozygotes were missing the inferior colliculi and had disrupted vermian development. Interestingly, in recently generated transgenic mice ectopically overexpressing En1, cystic malformations of the posterior lobules of the vermis develop, along with dilatation of the fourth ventricle and postnatal hydrocephalus. In one study of developing human cerebellum at 18 to 21 weeks' gestational age, En1 and En2 gene expression was reflected in RNA in situ hybridization signals. These signals were strongest in the cerebellar granule cells, the white matter of the vermis and flocculus, and the inferior olive, as well as the caudal brain stem nuclei, locations corresponding to structures originating in the rhombic lip. These investigations may eventually contribute to our understanding of the pathogenesis of the Dandy-Walker anomaly.

Pathologically, about 25% of Dandy-Walker cases have complete absence of the vermis (the remainder being partial, or the so-called Dandy-Walker variant). The cyst can vary in size and is composed of an inner, often atrophic ependymal layer apposed to a glial and pia/arachnoid layer (see Fig. 4-35). Disorganized cerebellar cortical tissue may be present at the edge. Associated cerebral malformations have included cerebral gyral abnormalities, heterotopias, agenesis of the corpus callosum, aqueductal forking or stenosis, and occipital encephalocele.

Another well-described, although rare cerebellar hypoplasia is Joubert's syndrome, in which the cerebellar vermian lobules are small or absent and accompanied by heterotopia of cerebellar cortical cells and marked hypoplasia of the superior cerebellar peduncles. Abnormalities of brain stem nuclei are variable features. An entity known as rhombencephalosynapsis demonstrates fusion of the dentate nuclei across the midline of the cerebellum (see Fig. 4-37) and frequent association with supratentorial commissural defects.

Displacements of cerebellar tissue include Chiari I and Chiari II (Arnold-Chiari) malformations. In the former, tonsillar tissue is chronically herniated below the level of the foramen magnum (see Fig. 4-39), whereas the latter has caudally malpositioned vermian structures (see Fig. 4-7). Both have small posterior fossae, considered a primary mesenchymal defect in type I and a consequence of the distal spinal dysraphism (usually lumbosacral myelomeningocele) in type II. The mechanism of development of the posterior fossa abnormality in Chiari II malformation is thought to be secondary to the caudal neural tube defect (see the earlier section "Neural Tube Defects"). This theory is supported somewhat by study of splotch mice, which have recessively inherited neural tube defects with leakage of

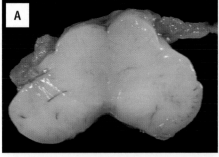

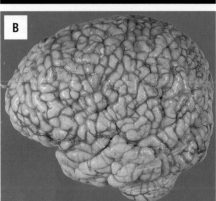

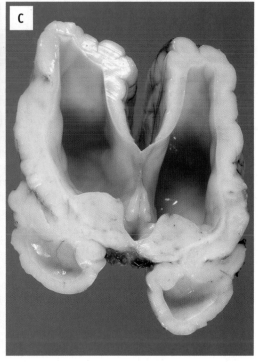

FIGURE 4-40

X-linked aqueductal stenosis. **A**, Axial section of the midbrain showing absence of the aqueduct. **B**, Left lateral view of the brain in this patient demonstrating "pseudopolymicrogyria," or the appearance of complex gyri resulting from the marked ventricular expansion during cortical development. **C**, A coronal section through the hemispheres at the level of the temporal poles demonstrates the hydrocephalus.

CSF leading to transient fourth ventricular collapse. The failure of distention of the ventricular system then results in underdevelopment of the posterior fossa mesenchymal structures. Unfortunately, this model does not completely correlate with the human syndrome, which is sporadic except for rare association with trisomy 13 or 18. In humans, embryologic evidence supportive of this mechanism includes closure of the neural tube at an earlier stage than posterior fossa development and the fact that half of affected fetuses younger than 23 weeks' gestation lack hydrocephalus.

Disruptions and *degenerative* entities involving the posterior fossa are unusual and beyond the scope of this section.

Aqueductal malformations are of several types. *Dysplasia of the aqueduct* is often found in malformed brains, such as those with holoprosencephaly and Walker-Warburg syndrome. *Isolated aqueductal stenosis*, characterized by a reduced lumen only with no histologic changes of the aqueduct or abnormalities of the cerebellum and brain stem, is rare. *X-linked aqueductal stenosis* (Fig. 4-40) is associated with massive hydrocephalus causing macrocephaly, pyramidal tract abnormalities, and thumb deformities and is due to a mutation in the gene on Xq28 encoding the L1 cell adhesion molecule. *Occlusion of the aqueduct*, which may be infectious, neoplastic, or hemorrhagic, can result in triventricular hydrocephalus. In such cases, the lumen of the aqueduct is of normal size (or dilated) but is occluded by necrotic tissue, inflammatory debris, or hemorrhage from fetal or perinatal disruptions (see "Disruptions of Developing Gray and White Matter" later). Over time, the ependymal layer of the aqueduct, as well as elsewhere in the ventricular system, is

disrupted and replaced by reactive gliosis and hemosiderin deposits. Given the experimental induction of inflammation-free aqueductal stenosis with mumps virus in hamsters, the possibility of a viral origin of aqueductal stenosis in humans is also possible.

DIFFERENTIAL DIAGNOSIS

The main differential diagnosis of Dandy-Walker malformation is the sporadically occurring retrocerebellar cyst (Fig. 4-41), which can indent the inferior aspect of the cerebellar hemispheres and vermis and mimic vermian hypoplasia. A midsagittal section through the cyst and underlying cerebellum, however, should readily distinguish the two because with a retrocerebellar cyst, the vermis is distorted rather than frankly absent.

Distinction between type I and II Chiari malformations is made on the basis of a distal neural tube closure defect and displacement of vermian tissue in Chiari II; in Chiari I, only displacement of tonsillar tissue is present.

Joubert's syndrome may be difficult to distinguish radiographically and pathologically from the Dandy-Walker complex, except on the basis of the hypoplasia of the superior cerebellar peduncle seen in the former.

PROGNOSIS AND THERAPY

In the Dandy-Walker complex, the outcome is related to severity, with a poorer prognosis (40% mortality and cognitive deficits in 75% of those surviving) in patients

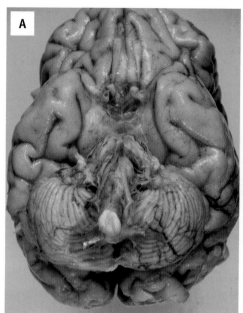
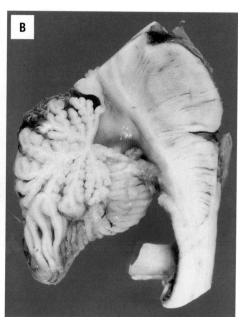

FIGURE 4-41

Retrocerebellar cyst. **A**, Basal view of the brain. Note the thin arachnoid cyst depressing the inferior aspect of the cerebellum. **B**, Midsagittal section through the vermis showing deformation of the folia of the cerebellar vermis, but no loss of vermian lobules.

in whom the complex is diagnosed in intrauterine or early postnatal life than in those in whom it is not diagnosed until childhood or later. Often, the prognosis is related more to the associated CNS or systemic abnormalities. Management of the hydrocephalus is usually the only treatment that can be offered. Patients with Joubert's syndrome and rhombencephalosynapsis have abnormal eye movement, ataxia, and mental retardation of variable clinical severity, although survival beyond infancy is unusual. Lhermitte-Duclos disease may require surgical decompression of the hypertrophic cerebellar folia to reduce symptoms of increased intracranial pressure. Patients who have Lhermitte-Duclos disease as a component of the Cowden syndrome are at risk for breast and other life-threatening malignancies (see "Familial Malformation/Tumor Syndromes" later).

For Chiari I and II malformations, surgical decompression by occipital craniectomy is frequently required, as mentioned earlier in "Clinical Features" in this section (also see the section "Neural Tube Defects").

DISRUPTIONS OF DEVELOPING GRAY AND WHITE MATTER

The foregoing sections have considered primarily abnormalities of development related to genetic or environmental influences on early organogenesis. The term "disruption" reflects a later (whether intrauterine or extrauterine) event that alters the configuration of previously normally developed structures. Disruptions often affect both gray (i.e., cerebral cortex, thalamus, and hippocampus) and white matter at the same time. However, their distinct neuropathologic patterns are discussed separately. This section discusses *gray matter*

injuries (porencephaly, perisylvian polymicrogyria, hydranencephaly, ulegyria, multicystic encephalomalacia, thalamic injury, and pontosubicular necrosis), *white matter damage* (periventricular leukomalacia), and *perinatal hemorrhage*. The vast majority of disruptions have in common some element or elements of decreased perfusion (ischemia) and low oxygen tension (hypoxia), phenomena that tend to occur together, particularly in a premature infant or a term infant with congenital heart or lung disease, and in practice they are referred to jointly by the commonly used term "hypoxia-ischemia."

DISRUPTIONS OF DEVELOPING GRAY MATTER

CLINICAL FEATURES

Encephaloclastic lesions of developing neocortex include infarcts, in which whole segments of cortex are lost, analogous to the situation in adults. When such an infarct is resorbed, a cystic cavity known as *porencephaly* results (Fig. 4-42). Occasionally, bilateral porencephaly arises in the region of the sylvian fissures, in the distribution of the middle cerebral arteries, and has been called "basket brain"; the cingulate gyri and medial hemispheric structures are preserved (corresponding to the "handle" of the basket), whereas the lateral parietal and frontal lobes are cystic bilaterally. A milder degree of bilateral middle cerebral artery hypoperfusion in utero is thought to result in *perisylvian polymicrogyria*, a condition called schizencephaly in the older literature (Fig. 4-43). The polymicrogyria in the perisylvian regions and found at the margins of some porencephalic

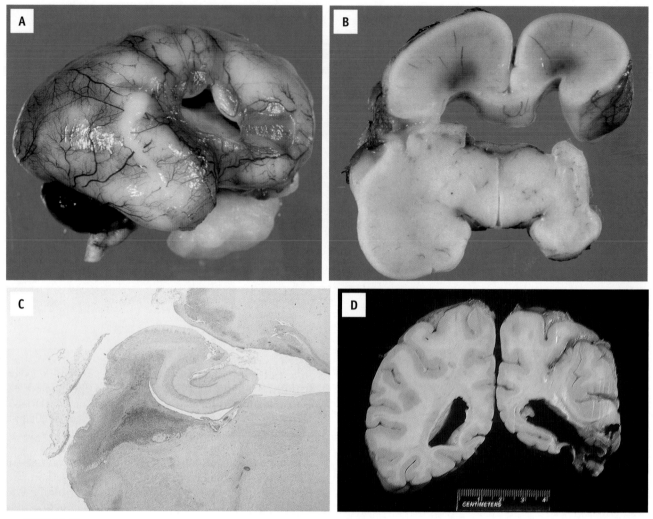

FIGURE 4-42

Porencephaly. **A**, Right lateral view of the brain of a 23-week-gestation fetus with a defect in the cerebral mantle in the region of the sylvian fissure. **B**, Coronal section of same case. Note the communication of the defect with the right lateral ventricle; a lesser degree of disruption is also present in the same region on the *left*. **C**, Microscopic section showing segmental loss of the cortical plate just lateral to the hippocampus (*left* side of the field). **D**, Coronal section of the parieto-occipital lobes from an older individual with a unilateral defect, also in communication with the lateral ventricle.

cysts is thought to be due to incomplete ischemia in the tissue lying near the defect. *Hydranencephaly* ("bubble brain") results from massive intrauterine hemispheric necrosis (Fig. 4-44). Various insults occurring at 22 to 27 weeks, including trauma, attempted abortion, TORCH infection, and household gas intoxication, have been correlated with hydranencephaly, although most antecedent events are unknown. Twin gestations are at increased risk for hydranencephaly, "basket brain," and perisylvian polymicrogyria, presumably because of altered hemodynamics in utero such as twin-twin transfusion. *Ulegyria* refers to focal hypoxic-ischemic injury to the cortex that does not result in frank cavitation but instead appears as neuronal loss, cortical atrophy, and gliosis at the depths of the sulci (Fig. 4-45). *Multicystic encephalomalacia* differs from porencephaly and hydranencephaly by the occurrence of innumerable cysts separated by glial septa that involve the cortex and white matter in all lobes (Fig. 4-46). These cystic areas evolve

from segmental infarcts, often with accompanying hemorrhage; lesser degrees of insult result in a horizontal loss of neurons known as laminar necrosis (see Fig. 4-46). Pontosubicular necrosis is a term describing an association between acute neuronal injury to the subiculum (and often the adjacent hippocampus) and the intralaminar nuclei of the basis pontis (Fig. 4-47). The combination of perinatal thalamic or basal ganglionic neuronal loss (or both) and gliosis is known as *status marmoratus* ("marbled state") (Fig. 4-48).

For all these lesions, the extent of destruction dictates the clinical picture. Hydranencephaly and "basket brain" are associated with spasticity, severe seizures, and vegetative signs; mortality in infancy is high. Head enlargement develops in longer-surviving infants as a result of scarring of the aqueduct leading to hydrocephalus. Porencephaly and ulegyria may result in hemiparesis, blindness, and seizures, depending on the cortical sites involved. Ulegyria may also be clinically

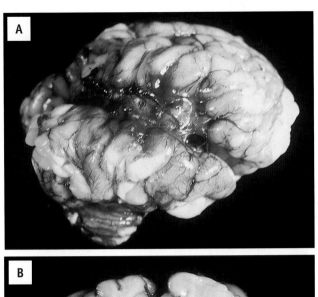

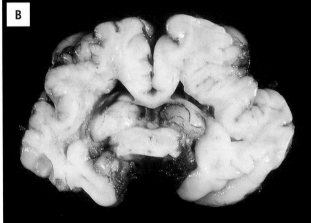

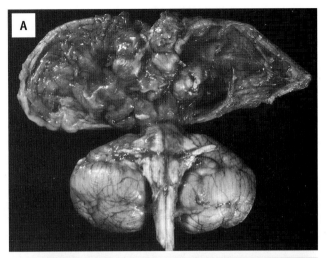

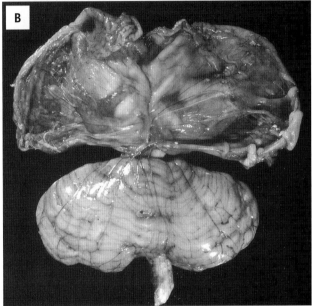

FIGURE 4-44

Hydranencephaly. **A** and **B**, Ventral and dorsal views of the brain, respectively. Note the subtotal loss of both cerebral hemispheres, represented only as a membranous remnant, with relative preservation of the brain stem and cerebellum. (Courtesy of Dr. U. De Girolami, from the collection of the late Dr. E. P. Richardson, Jr., Boston.)

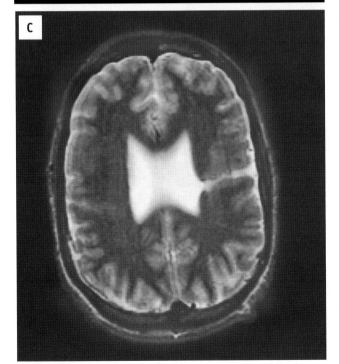

FIGURE 4-43

Perisylvian polymicrogyria ("schizencephaly"). **A**, Right lateral aspect of the brain demonstrating complex gyration along a broad perisylvian cleft. **B**, On coronal section at the level of the thalamus, polymicrogyric cortex lines the margins of the clefts bilaterally. **C**, Axial MRI demonstrating a cleft lined with irregular gray matter signal on the *left*; the *right* shows only the abnormal cortex without a cleft. (Courtesy of Dr. L. Hsu, Boston.)

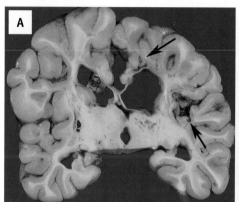

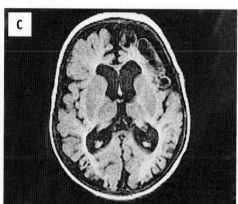

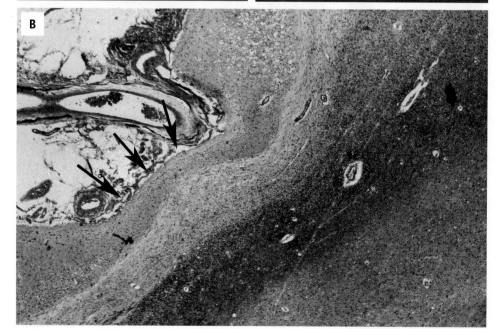

FIGURE 4-45

Ulegyria in multicystic encephalomalacia. **A**, Coronal section at the level
of the hippocampus showing multiple healed infarcts, often involving
the depths of the sulci (*arrows*), leading to a "mushroom"-like appearance
of adjacent preserved cortical segments. **B**, Histologic section of the
cortex at sulcal depth with marked
thinning and scarring (*arrows*).
C, Axial MRI showing multifocal loss
of cortical gray matter and underlying white matter in a 1-year-old
baby. (Courtesy of Dr. J. Soul,
Boston.)

DISRUPTIONS OF DEVELOPING GRAY MATTER—FACT SHEET

Definition

▶ Destructive, or encephaloclastic, lesions of gray matter include single or multiple localized infarcts of the cortex (porencephaly, multicystic encephalomalacia) or near-total loss of the hemispheres (hydranencephaly)

▶ Schizencephaly is bilateral perisylvian (middle cerebral artery territory) cortical loss bordered by polymicrogyria; severe cases lead to "basket brain" (bilateral porencephaly)

▶ Ulegyria is loss of cortex at the depths of the sulci

▶ Pontosubicular necrosis is concurrent neuronal necrosis in the basis pontis and subiculum

▶ Perinatal thalamic or basal ganglia injury (or both) results in status marmoratus

Incidence/Prevalence and Gender Distribution

▶ Very low birth weight infants (<1500 g) have a high risk for perinatal gray matter injury

Clinical Features

▶ Hydranencephaly and "basket brain" are characterized by spasticity, seizures, vegetative signs, hydrocephalus from aqueductal scarring, and high mortality in infancy

▶ Ulegyria, porencephaly, schizencephaly, and multicystic encephalomalacia are associated with focal motor deficits and blindness, the combination and severity depending on the cortical regions involved

▶ Pontosubicular necrosis often occurs with white matter injury in vulnerable premature infants (see later)

▶ Status marmoratus results in choreoathetosis, as well as the spasticity and motor deficits of cerebral palsy

Radiologic Features

▶ On CT, porencephaly has a smooth-walled, unenhancing cavity from the ventricle to the subarachnoid space that is bounded by tissue with white matter signal intensity

▶ Schizencephaly is bilateral perisylvian clefts or depressions bounded by nodular or polymicrogyric gray matter signal on neuroimaging

▶ "Basket brain" and multicystic encephalomalacia have variably sized, irregular cavities, sometimes containing blood products or other debris, with adjacent cortical thinning and white matter hypointensity on MRI

▶ Hydranencephaly on MRI has complete absence of the cerebral mantle, except sometimes in the posterior inferior occipital lobes and inferior medial frontal lobes; the brain stem may be atrophic

▶ Ulegyria appears as preserved gyral crests, loss of sulcal cortex, and abnormal signal of the underlying white matter

▶ Early thalamic/basal ganglionic injury has high attenuation on CT; it eventuates in patchy hyperintensity and volume loss on MRI as status marmoratus develops

Prognosis and Treatment

▶ The most severe lesions (hydranencephaly, "basket brain," and multicystic encephalomalacia) are associated with high mortality in infancy

▶ Localized porencephaly, schizencephaly, and ulegyria often require anticonvulsant treatment or even surgical resection of areas causing refractory epilepsy

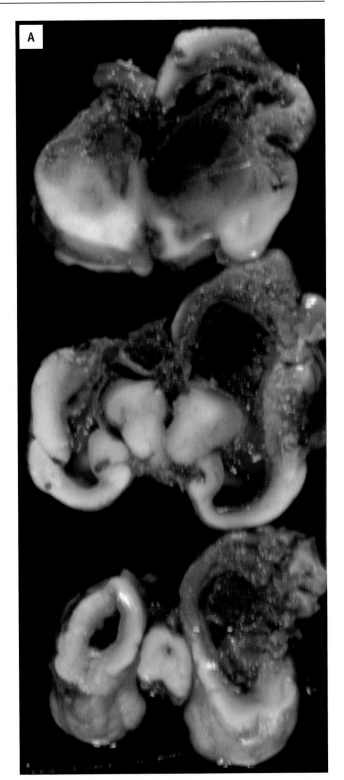

FIGURE 4-46

Cortical infarcts. **A,** Coronal sections through the hemispheres of a 30-week-gestation premature infant surviving several days. Note the broad segments of cortical discoloration, softening, and hemorrhage.

Continued

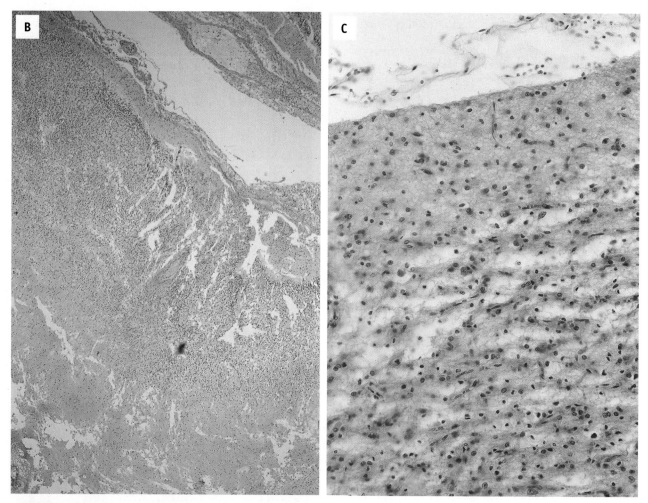

FIGURE 4-46, cont'd

B, Microscopic section of an acute infarct involving the full cortical thickness. **C**, Focally, necrosis and beginning gliosis involve only the deeper layers of the cortex ("laminar necrosis").

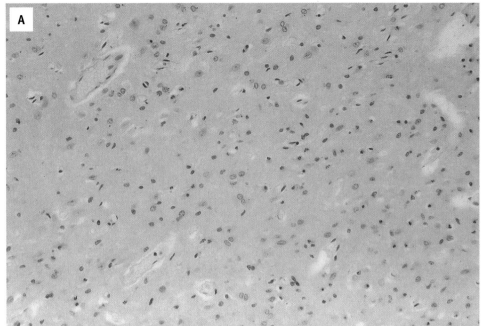

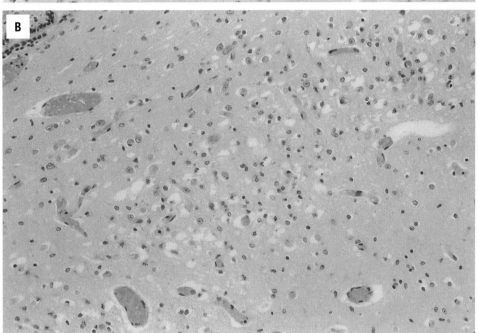

FIGURE 4-47

Pontosubicular necrosis. **A** and **B**, Histology of the basis pontis and subiculum, respectively. Both sites show individual neuronal necrosis characterized by hypereosinophilia of the cytoplasm and nuclear condensation.

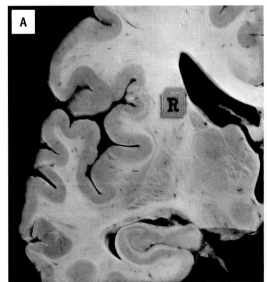

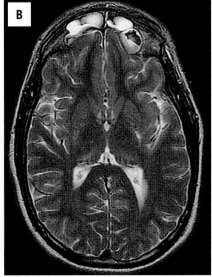

FIGURE 4-48

Status marmoratus. **A**, Coronal section of the right ("R") hemisphere. Note the marbled gray/white appearance of both the thalamus medially and the putamen laterally. (Courtesy of Dr. U. De Girolami, from the collection of the late Dr. E. P. Richardson, Jr., Boston.) **B**, MRI of a 14-year-old child surviving hypoxia-ischemia at birth. The patchy T2 hyperintensity in the basal ganglia and thalamus corresponds to scarring and neuronal loss. (Courtesy of Dr. M. Silvera, Boston.)

silent. Pontosubicular necrosis, seen more frequently in premature infants, is highly associated with white matter injury (periventricular leukomalacia, discussed later). The clinical features accompanying status marmoratus classically include static (nonprogressive) bilateral choreoathetosis, motor and intellectual retardation, spastic diplegia, and sometimes epilepsy, all of which fall under the rubric of "cerebral palsy."

RADIOLOGIC FEATURES

Porencephaly is visible on CT or MRI as a unilateral, smooth-walled, unenhancing cavity that usually extends from the lateral ventricle to the subarachnoid space. In general, the cyst lacks any internal structure and is bounded by tissue with white matter signal intensity. Schizencephaly, in contrast, is a cleft, typically perisylvian and bilateral, bordered by polymicrogyric or nodular tissue with gray matter signal characteristics (see Fig. 4-43). Basket brain appears on CT or MRI as bilaterally symmetric (middle cerebral artery distribution), irregularly shaped cavities that may have thin septations traversing the cavities, as well as evidence of debris, blood products, or both. The appearance is similar to that in multicystic encephalomalacia, in which the cavities may occur anywhere in the hemispheres and represent sequelae of partial asphyxia. On MRI, multicystic encephalomalacia is characterized by cortical thinning with hypointensity of the underlying white matter and hyperintensity of the glial strands between and across the cystic cavities.

Hydranencephaly may be difficult to distinguish from severe untreated hydrocephalus by CT; MRI can delineate a thin rim of compressed parenchyma in hydrocephalus, however. By MRI, the cerebral hemispheres may be nearly completed replaced by CSF, except in the most posterior inferior occipital lobes and the most inferior medial aspects of the frontal lobes. The diencephalon and cerebellum may be relatively spared, but the brain stem is often atrophic.

Ulegyria is detectable as a mushroom-shaped preservation of the crests of gyri in the face of atrophy of the cortex along the depths of the sulci. By MRI, the underlying white matter has signal characteristics of gliosis.

Thalamic injury in the perinatal period is appreciable as high attenuation on CT, a finding suggestive of hemorrhage or calcification. Later, patchy hyperintensity on spin-echo MRI corresponds to status marmoratus (see Fig. 4-48). Recently, survivors of prematurity have been found to have decreased thalamic volume on quantitative MRI.

PATHOLOGIC FEATURES

Porencephaly refers macroscopically to loss of cortical tissue extending from the brain surface to the ventricle. As mentioned earlier, these cavities are usually found in the sylvian region unilaterally. The margins are

---

DISRUPTIONS OF DEVELOPING GRAY MATTER— PATHOLOGIC FEATURES

Gross Findings

▶ Anomalous gyral architecture, usually polymicrogyria, may be seen at the edges of porencephalic defects and along the perisylvian clefts or depressions of schizencephaly
▶ Hydranencephaly shows subtotal replacement of the cerebral hemispheres by a thin membrane with relative preservation of the diencephalon; the descending corticospinal tracts are markedly atrophic
▶ Multicystic encephalomalacia has numerous, often wedge-shaped defects of cortical gray and white matter that may contain debris or be bounded focally by chalky calcifications
▶ Ulegyria has a mushroom-like appearance because of atrophy of the cortex at the depths of the suci
▶ Injury to the thalamus and basal ganglia result in a reticulated pattern of scarring grossly resembling marble (status marmoratus)
▶ Pontosubicular necrosis is not grossly identifiable unless very severe

Microscopic Features

▶ Acute injury to the cortex appears as apoptosis or necrosis in the deep cortical layers (laminar necrosis), sometimes with disruption of layer I astrocytes and endothelial cells leading to superficial hemorrhage; with resolution of injury, macrophages and reactive astrocytes predominate, with eventual evolution to a glial scar or cysts
▶ Polymicrogyria associated with gray matter injury occurring before 24 weeks' gestation may be four layered or unlayered (see "Neuronal Migration Defects" earlier)
▶ Porencephaly, multicystic encephalomalacia, ulegyria, and the occasional cortical remnants in hydranencephaly are bordered by gliotic tissue, sometimes with calcifications, and by hypomyelinated white matter; disorganized nodules of gray matter may be identified microscopically as well if the insult occurred before the third trimester
▶ Pontosubicular necrosis shows neuronal apoptosis (nuclear fragmentation) or hypereosinophilia of the cytoplasm with nuclear shrinking ("red" neurons) in the intralaminar pontine neurons of the basis pontis and in the subiculum, between CA1 of the hippocampus and the entorhinal cortex; in surviving infants, these areas later show neuronal loss and gliosis
▶ Thalamic/basal ganglia injury consists of patchy neuronal necrosis with eventual glial scarring and aberrant myelination leading to status marmoratus
▶ Neuronal injury at any gray matter site may be reflected as mineralization (or ferrugination) of neuronal cell bodies, axons, or both

Immunohistochemical Features

▶ Macrophages responding to gray matter injury are detectable by immunostaining for CD68 or leukocyte common antigen
▶ Gliosis in any of these patterns of injury can be highlighted by immunostaining for GFAP

Differential Diagnosis

▶ *Toxoplasma*, rubella, cytomegalovirus, or herpesvirus (TORCH) infections or trauma may mimic hypoxia-ischemia–induced gray matter injury
▶ Leigh's disease (mitochondrial complex deficiency) may mimic hypoxic-ischemic lesions of the brain stem and basal ganglia

smooth and may have an anomalous gyral architecture, either polymicrogyria or gyri radiating outwardly from the lips of the defect (see Fig. 4-43). Rarely, vascular occlusion or atresia of the major cerebral artery branch or branches on the affected side or sides can be identified. The basal ganglia, cerebellum, and brain stem are usually spared, although descending white matter tracts may be secondarily atrophic. The anomalous gyral architecture and general lack of significant glial scarring on microscopic examination are consistent with an intrauterine insult occurring after neuroblast migration and during gyration (i.e., after 20 to 24 weeks).

Microscopically, the acute phase of injury is marked by apoptosis (death of individual cells) or as broad zones of necrosis of neurons in the middle and deeper layers of the cortex (laminar necrosis) (see Fig. 4-46). In severe cases, all layers of the cerebral cortex suffer neuronal loss (see Fig. 4-46) and are replaced by reactive gliosis. Large lesions may grossly resemble fused gyri (pachygyria) or ill-developed, disorganized sulci (polymicrogyria) (discussed earlier). Cortical cytoarchitecture and connectivity are disrupted in this process and may appear microscopically disorganized as either unlayered or four-layered polymicrogyria. Unlayered polymicrogyria displays a festoon-like, chaotic pattern of neuronal orientation, whereas four-layered polymicrogyria is characterized by a superficial acellular molecular layer (layer I) that infolds and fuses to produce a microsulcus, a second cellular layer consisting of neuronal types normally belonging to cortical laminae II and III, a third layer devoid of neurons that contains mostly glial cells, and a fourth layer contiguous with normal layer VI of the adjacent cortex. This microscopic appearance, along with the fact that it tends to border porencephalic defects, suggests that four-layered polymicrogyria may be a sequela of laminar necrosis of layers IV and V that is caused by early ischemic, toxic, or infectious injury. Healed lesions may also have fibroblastic proliferation in the subarachnoid space.

So-called pseudopolymicrogyria (see Fig. 4-40) may be seen in cases of severe congenital hydrocephalus. In this setting, the increased sulcation is believed to allow increased surface area for cortical neuronal organization, thereby somewhat overcoming the loss of sulcal depth in the thinned cerebral mantle. The numbers and organization of cortical layers are preserved, however.

Since the areas involved in *hydranencephaly* (see Fig. 4-44) are often in the distribution of the carotid arteries, the inferior temporal and occipital lobes tend to be preserved. The basal ganglia and thalamus are variably affected, but the descending tracts are always atrophic. Microscopically, the membranous remnants of disrupted brain tissue are made up of reactive astrocytes, fibroblasts and collagen, and subarachnoid vessels, sometimes with hemosiderosis and macrophages.

In *multicystic encephalomalacia* (see Fig. 4-45), microscopic evidence of resolved infarction and hemorrhage, including macrophages and hemosiderin, accompanies the marked gliosis and suggests an insult in the perinatal period (i.e., late gestation to early infancy). Multicystic encephalopathy may be encountered in infectious encephalopathy secondary to cytomegalovirus,

toxoplasmosis, and *Listeria*. As with porencephaly and hydranencephaly, associated events have included maternal suicide attempts and parturition-related complications such as cord prolapse.

Ulegyria demonstrates atrophy, often with complete loss of cortical neurons, at the depths of the sulci with relative sparing of the crests of the gyri. The scarring at the depth of the sulcus and sparing of the gyral crest result in a "mushroom"-like appearance of the gyrus on cross section (see Fig. 4-45). Ulegyric lesions have very well defined borders and may include discrete islands of preserved neurons within the lesion. Given their localization to end-arterial zones, they have been considered sequelae of hypoperfusion.

Pontosubicular necrosis (see Fig. 4-47) is a lesion that tends to occur in premature rather than in term infants because of the particular vulnerability of these gray matter regions to hypoxia-ischemia in the developing brain, for reasons unknown. In contrast, the neurons of Sommer's sector in the hippocampus are more vulnerable in term babies. Pontosubicular necrosis is highly associated with white matter necrosis, as discussed later. Microscopically, hypereosinophilic ("red") neurons as well as apoptotic (fragmented) nuclei are scattered throughout the intralaminar pontine nuclei and subiculum. Examination at later times shows neuronal loss and prominence of reactive astrocytes.

In recent years, vulnerability of the thalamus to hypoxia-ischemia, especially in preterm babies, has been appreciated both on neuroimaging and at autopsy. Such injury, which consists acutely of neuronal apoptosis, may be quite subtle and easily overlooked. As the hypoxia-ischemia evolves, reactive gliosis arises, and focal glial scars with neuronal loss may be seen. Mineralization of adjacent neurons or vessels may occur. Similar injury may also be seen in the basal ganglia. In babies surviving a year or more, damage to the thalamus and basal ganglia may lead to a type of disturbed architecture known as *status marmoratus* (or *etat marbre*), in which aberrant myelination of disoriented axons and glial processes leads to a marbled gross appearance (see Fig. 4-48).

Experimental induction of porencephaly and hydranencephaly in puppies and fetal monkeys by carotid artery injection supports a vascular cause of these disruptions. Likewise, in utero infection by Akabane virus in goats and cattle has been clearly associated with hydranencephaly.

DIFFERENTIAL DIAGNOSIS

In practice, these lesions are distinctive, although some may occur together. Intrauterine infection by TORCH agents (toxoplasmosis, rubella, cytomegalovirus, and herpesviruses) can lead to neuronal loss, gliosis, and mineralization; however, periventricular calcifications and microglial nodules can be clues to the infectious nature of the lesion. In addition, the infectious agent may be visible on routine or specially stained sections.

LESIONS OF DEVELOPING WHITE MATTER

CLINICAL FEATURES

Periventricular leukomalacia (PVL) is the overall term for perinatal injury to white matter and consists of both focal and diffuse components. The most severe form has both focal necrosis with cystic degeneration (Figs. 4-49 to 4-51) and diffuse white matter gliosis (Fig. 4-52), whereas the mildest degree of involvement is characterized by only diffuse white matter gliosis. PVL is thought to be the consequence of ischemia, with or without reperfusion, and cytokine release potentiated by infection, and occurs with the highest frequency in premature infants (i.e., birth at <38 weeks) and term infants with cardiorespiratory abnormalities (i.e.,

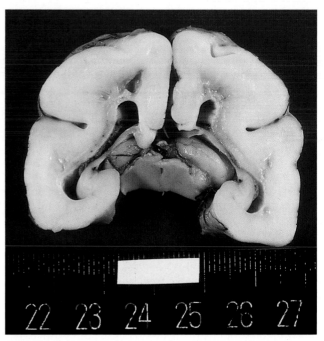

FIGURE 4-49

Periventricular leukomalacia: bilateral cavitating necrosis in the parietal lobes of a premature (28-week-gestation) infant surviving for 2 weeks.

DISRUPTIONS OF DEVELOPING WHITE MATTER—FACT SHEET

Definition

▶ PVL is injury to the deep periventricular white matter and consists of both focally necrotic and diffuse (non-necrotic) components
▶ Diffuse injury without focal necrosis is also called perinatal telencephalic leukoencephalopathy

Incidence/Prevalence

▶ The incidence of white matter injury is increased in premature infants born between 24 and 32 gestational weeks, especially those surviving more than a few days, and in infants with cardiorespiratory disturbance
▶ The prevalence in premature infants (<38 weeks' gestation) at autopsy is 25% to 75%

Clinical Features

▶ PVL results in myelination delay and deficiency, as well as permanent white matter loss in the focally necrotic areas; it affects projection fibers and causes the motor deficits of cerebral palsy (leg > arm > face) in 5% to 10% of survivors
▶ Half of very low birth weight (<1500 g) infants surviving to school age also have cognitive deficits
▶ Blindness results from involvement of the optic radiations in the parieto-occipital lobes

Radiologic Features

▶ Transcranial ultrasound detects the most severe cavitating lesions but is less sensitive in detecting diffuse injury
▶ MRI readily detects signal abnormalities acutely and over time:
  ▶ T2 hyperintensity
  ▶ Cysts or glial scars from the healed necrotic lesions
  ▶ Thinning of the corpus callosum and hydrocephalus ex vacuo

Prognosis and Treatment

▶ The prognosis is difficult to establish in the neonatal period, although Apgar scores of 0 to 3 in the first 20 minutes of life are associated with a high (>50%) incidence of death and, in survivors, a high (>50%) incidence of cerebral palsy
▶ Treatment is directed toward hemodynamic stabilization as a means of preventing the injury; specific therapies for established PVL, other than supportive and rehabilitative care, are lacking

---

congenital diaphragmatic hernia or cyanotic congenital heart disease). The especially vulnerable period is between 24 and 32 postconceptional weeks. Three phenomena are thought to underlie the risk for PVL: (1) the existence of "watershed" (end-vascular) zones in the developing periventricular white matter (rather than in the cortex as in adults); (2) the immaturity of the autoregulatory systems of the cerebral circulation such that drops in cerebral perfusion pressure are poorly compensated; and (3) the intrinsic susceptibility of developing oligodendrocyte precursors to free radical, glutamate, and cytokine injury.

Since myelination occurs for the most part after birth according to a well-described, fairly predictable sequence in the human fetus and infant, PVL results in myelination delay as well as permanent myelin deficiency, with or without appreciable loss of white matter volume. The latter occurs when frank necrosis affects projection axons in the deep white matter; clinically, such myelin deficiency leads to motor deficits known as cerebral palsy. Because PVL tends to affect the superior rather than the lateral projections in the corona radiata, children with cerebral palsy are likely to have greater involvement of the legs than the arms, a pattern known as spastic diplegia. Blindness results from necrosis and cavitation of the optic radiations in the parieto-occipital lobes, a site of predilection for PVL.

RADIOLOGIC FEATURES

Cystic lesions (the most severe form) are visible on transcranial ultrasonography (see Fig. 4-50); up to

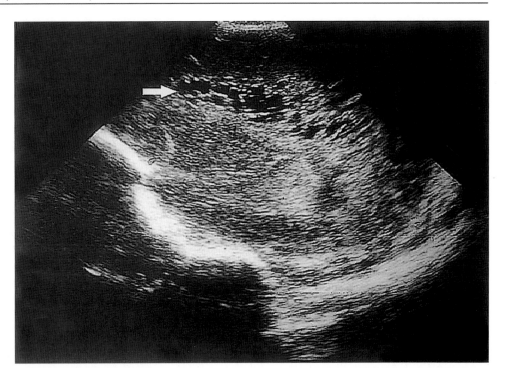

FIGURE 4-50

Periventricular leukomalacia: trans-fontanelle ultrasonogram (sagittal plane) showing spotty echolucencies (*arrow*) indicating cystic necrosis of white matter. (Courtesy of Dr. J. Soul, Boston.)

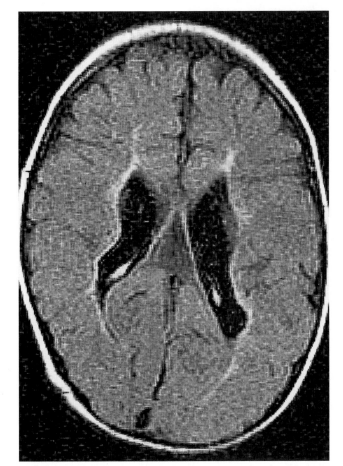

FIGURE 4-51

Periventricular leukomalacia. MRI in a 2-year-old with cerebral palsy shows thinning of the corpus callosum, increased T2 signal in the periventricular white matter and corona radiata, and mild expansion of the lateral ventricles. (Courtesy of Dr. J. Soul, Boston.)

70% of PVL lesions (primarily the diffuse, non-necrotic changes) are missed. MRI is a superior modality for detecting the signal abnormalities corresponding to acute injury to the white matter, but such studies may be difficult to obtain in an unstable premature infant. Later, myelination disruption appears as increased T2-weighted signal (see Fig. 4-51). Cystic cavities may be obvious on MRI, along with evidence of delayed or permanently deficient myelination as determined by signal characteristics. In children monitored over time by MRI, early cavitations may be replaced by glial scars with adjacent white matter hypomyelination and hydrocephalus ex vacuo, thus suggesting a capacity for remodeling in some lesions. The corpus callosum may remain markedly thin and the overall white matter volume reduced in severe cases, however.

PATHOLOGIC FEATURES

The mildest and possibly earliest manifestation of hypoxia-ischemia in the hemispheric white matter is characterized neuropathologically by duskiness and softening of the deep cerebral white matter and histologically by the occurrence of prominent, hypertrophic astrocytes, "acutely damaged glia" (pyknotic nuclei), capillary cell proliferation, and perivascular "globules" that may mineralize. This histologic picture has been termed perinatal telencephalic leukoencephalopathy (see Fig. 4-52). It shares many of the same features as the diffuse white matter gliosis component of PVL, which appears as a widespread proliferation of GFAP-positive cells (see Fig. 4-52) accompanying myelin pallor on Luxol fast blue stain. Diffuse gliosis may be seen alone or in conjunction with the focally necrotic lesions

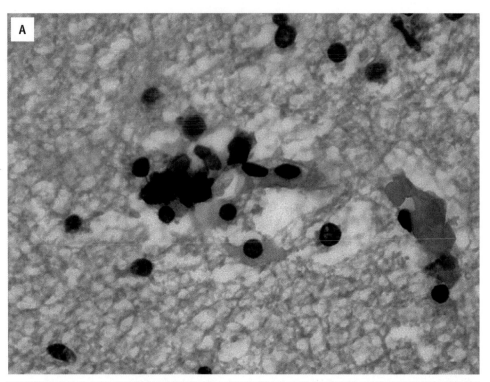

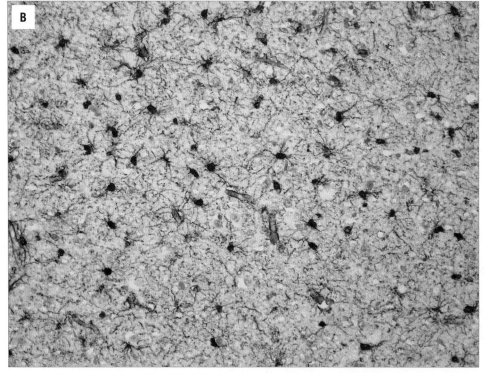

FIGURE 4-52

Periventricular leukomalacia. **A**, Diffuse white matter injury characterized by perivascular mineralization and prominent reactive-appearing astrocytes (perinatal telencephalic leukoencephalopathy). **B**, Immunostain for glial fibrillary acidic protein highlights numerous brown-staining reactive astrocytes.

of severe PVL (Figs. 4-53 and 4-54). These circumscribed regions of tissue loss, measuring 0.2 to 1.0 cm, usually occur within 1.5 cm of the ventricular wall in the hemispheric white matter. Generally, they are anterior to the frontal horns, lateral to the atria, or along the occipital horns. Within 3 to 8 hours of the inciting event, shrinkage of glial cell nuclei is accompanied by vacuolization, eosinophilia, and axon beading or swelling. Astroglial and capillary prominence develop by 12 hours after injury, followed by microglial proliferation progressing to macrophage infiltrates over the next few days. Mineralization of disrupted axons and necrotic glial cells and processes at the periphery of the lesion, with associated gliosis, occurs within days to weeks. If large enough, the area becomes cavitated as macrophages clear the necrotic debris (see Fig. 4-54);

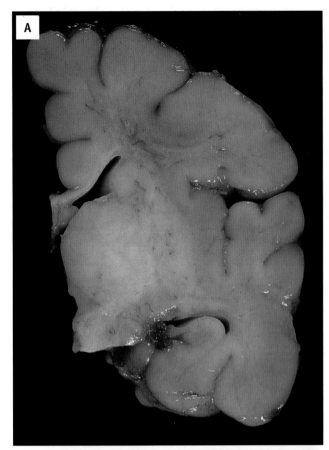

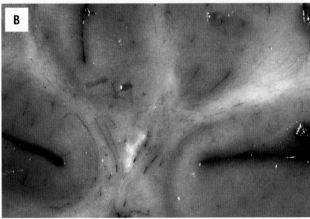

FIGURE 4-53

Periventricular leukomalacia. **A**, Coronal section of the right hemisphere at the level of the thalamus showing multiple tiny chalky spots of necrosis in the white matter at the angle of the lateral ventricle. **B**, Close-up view of chalky necrotic foci.

Prognosis and Therapy

In the premature nursery, the aim is to stabilize systemic blood pressure to sustain adequate cerebral perfusion, maintain adequate glucose levels, and control seizures. In children with PVL who survive the neonatal period and in whom the motor disorder of cerebral palsy eventually develops, supportive care and physical rehabilitation can be offered. Unfortunately, up to 50% of survivors of prematurity, with and without PVL, demonstrate cognitive delay, thus suggesting subtle cortical, thalamic, or hippocampal damage (or any combination of such damage). Research centered on the prevention of both white and gray matter injury by using free radical scavengers or glutamate antagonists, for example, is ongoing.

PERINATAL HEMORRHAGE

Clinical Features

The risk of hemorrhage in the neonatal brain is heightened by prematurity and its attendant vulnerability to

small cysts may remain after the area heals (Fig. 4-55). Because oligodendroglia are among the damaged elements whether in the focal or diffuse components, myelin delay or deficiency can occur and is visible as pallor on myelin-stained autopsy brain sections. If severe, the white matter volume is macroscopically reduced and is marked by hydrocephalus ex vacuo and thinning of the corpus callosum and descending tracts.

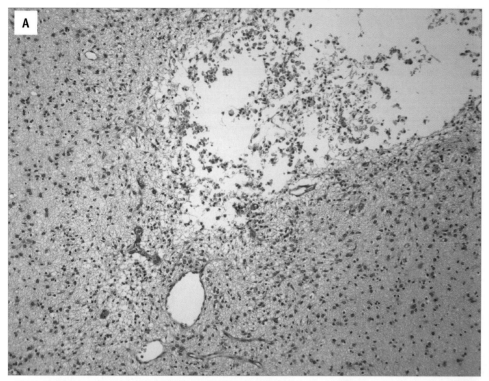

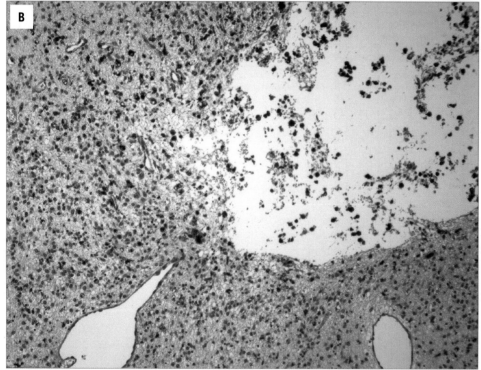

FIGURE 4-54

Periventricular leukomalacia. **A**, Microscopic section through a focally necrotic lesion demonstrating the loss of all cellular elements (cystic cavity), macrophage infiltrates, and reactive astrocytes at the edges. **B**, Immunohistochemical stain for the macrophage marker CD68 highlighting the abundant macrophage response (brown-stained cells).

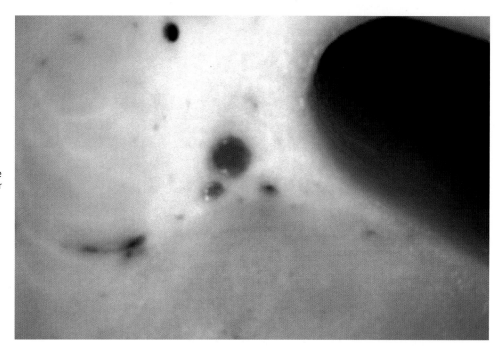

FIGURE 4-55

Periventricular leukomalacia: multiple cysts in periventricular white matter at the sites of healed necrosis.

PERINATAL HEMORRHAGE—FACT SHEET

Definition and Incidence/Prevalence

▶ Germinal matrix hemorrhages arise from periventricular germinal zones, with or without intraventricular hemorrhage (IVH)
   ▶ Highest incidence (approximately 19%) in infants born at less than 34 gestational weeks
▶ Cerebellar hemorrhage, with or without subarachnoid extension
   ▶ Incidence of 5% to 10% in neonatal intensive care autopsy series, higher in premature than in term infants
▶ Choroid plexus hemorrhage
   ▶ 1% of term babies and 50% of premature babies with germinal matrix hemorrhage

Clinical Features

▶ Acute germinal matrix hemorrhage:
   ▶ Alteration in level of consciousness, hypotonia, abnormal eye movements, respiratory disturbance
   ▶ In severe cases with IVH and parenchymal venous infarction, catastrophic deterioration to stupor or coma, increased intracranial pressure, brain stem dysfunction, seizures, flaccid quadriparesis
▶ Cerebellar hemorrhage: signs of brain stem compression, CSF obstruction
▶ Choroid plexus hemorrhage: asymptomatic unless causing large IVH

Radiologic Features

▶ Germinal matrix hemorrhage detectable by transcranial ultrasound, CT, or MRI:
   ▶ Grade I: limited to the germinal matrix
   ▶ Grade II: rupture of blood from the germinal matrix into the ventricles, without ventricular expansion
   ▶ Grade III: IVH with ventricular enlargement
   ▶ Grade IV: IVH and hemorrhage into hemispheric parenchyma (so-called periventricular venous infarct)
▶ Cerebellar and subarachnoid hemorrhages best detected by CT, although may be missed if not large

Prognosis and Treatment

▶ Grades III and IV IVH have 74% mortality and, in survivors, high morbidity, including shunt dependence for hydrocephalus resulting from scarring of CSF outflow tracts and resorption sites
▶ Cerebellar hemorrhage in premature babies has very high mortality, with survivors affected by motor deficits, ataxia, tremor, and hypotonia

---

hypoxia-ischemia. The periventricular gray matter in utero is composed of immature cells (neuroblasts and glial progenitors), proliferation and migration of which peak between the 18th and 26th gestational week, as mentioned earlier. It is known by variable terms, such as germinal matrix, germinal zone, or ganglionic eminence. The vessels in this region are actively remodeling during the third trimester and have incompletely formed basal lamina and loosely interdigitated glial endfeet. For these reasons, they are thought to be vulnerable to any alterations in hemodynamics that lead to the development of *germinal matrix hemorrhages* (Fig. 4-56). If large, these hemorrhages can result in extensive destruction of necessary precursor cells, as well as adjacent mature structures such as the caudate and internal capsule, and can interrupt the overlying ventricular (ependymal) surface and give rise to *intraventricular hemorrhage* (Fig. 4-57) and its serious sequelae. Germinal matrix hemorrhages are most common in premature infants younger than 34 weeks' postconceptional (gestational plus postnatal) age, with approximately 19% affected. Grade I hemorrhage refers to hemorrhage limited to the germinal matrix, whereas grade II designates rupture of blood into the ventricles, although

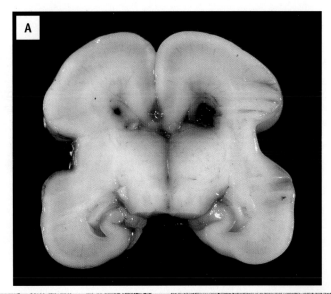

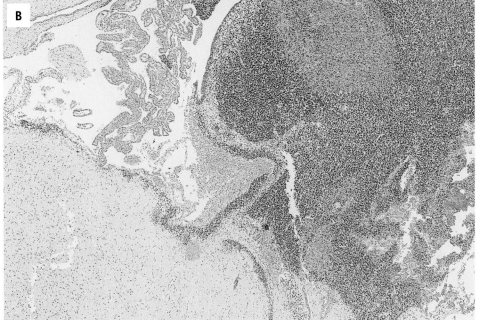

FIGURE 4-56

Germinal matrix hemorrhage. **A**, Focal, acute hemorrhage limited to the germinal matrix in a 20-week-gestation fetus. **B**, Acute extravasation of red cells into the cellular germinal matrix.

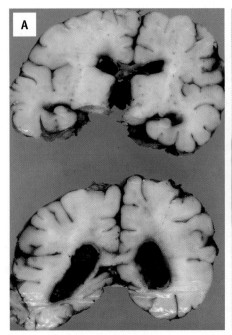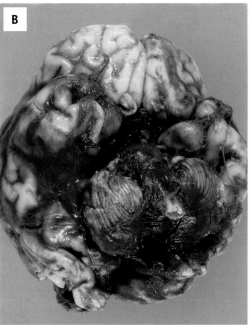

FIGURE 4-57

Germinal matrix hemorrhage with intraventricular extension. **A**, Coronal section of the hemispheres showing all ventricles distended by blood originating from the germinal matrix. **B**, Extension of blood from the ventricular system out of the lateral and medial foramina of the cerebellum and spreading diffusely in the subarachnoid space.

without an increase in ventricular size. Grade III is accompanied by ventricular enlargement, and grade IV involves the hemispheric parenchyma as part of a so-called venous infarct (Figs. 4-58 and 4-59). Mortality increases with increasing grade such that only 26% of infants with grade III or IV intraventricular hemorrhage survive and those who do have significant neurologic handicap.

The risk of hemorrhage at other sites in the CNS, although most commonly in the subarachnoid space, is also increased in preterm infants. In particular, hemorrhage of the superficial cerebellar cortex with extension into the posterior fossa subarachnoid space is occasionally seen in the premature nursery (occurring in 2% to 3%). Autopsy series of neonatal intensive care unit cases include 5% to 10% of such cases, however. In survivors of severe cerebellar hemorrhage, poor CSF resorption and hydrocephalus can eventually develop (Fig. 4-60).

The choroid plexus may be the site of acute hemorrhage in up to 1% of term babies and up to 50% of preterm babies with germinal matrix hemorrhage. The hemorrhage may be confined to the stroma of the choroid plexus or can extend into the ventricular space; the former causes no or only limited symptoms.

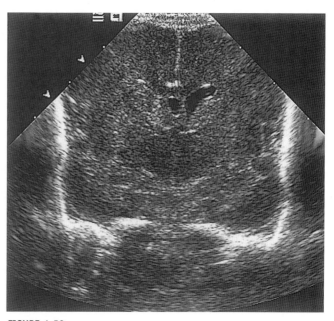

FIGURE 4-58

Germinal matrix hemorrhage: coronal transfontanelle ultrasonogram demonstrating bilateral acute germinal matrix hemorrhage and mild ventricular dilatation of the left ventricle (*right* side of the image). (Courtesy of Dr. J. Soul, Boston.)

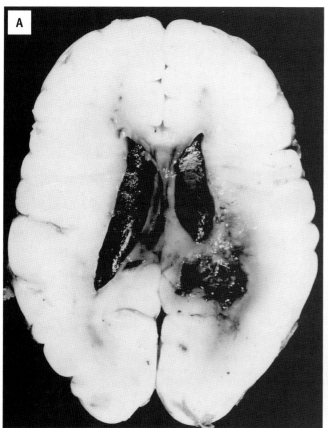

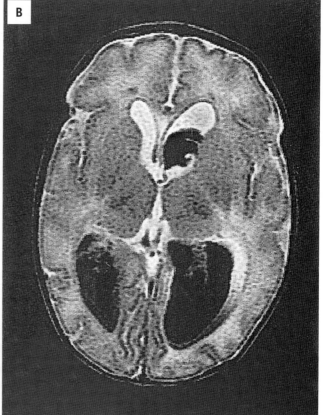

FIGURE 4-59

Periventricular hemorrhagic infarction. **A,** Axial section showing intraparenchymal hemorrhagic necrosis in the right parietal white matter and blood filling the lateral ventricles. (Courtesy of Dr. U. De Girolami, from the collection of the late Dr. E. P. Richardson, Jr., Boston.) **B,** MRI in a 28-week-gestation premature infant with a recent germinal matrix hemorrhage with ventricular extension and periventricular hemorrhagic infarction. (Courtesy of Dr. J. Soul, Boston.)

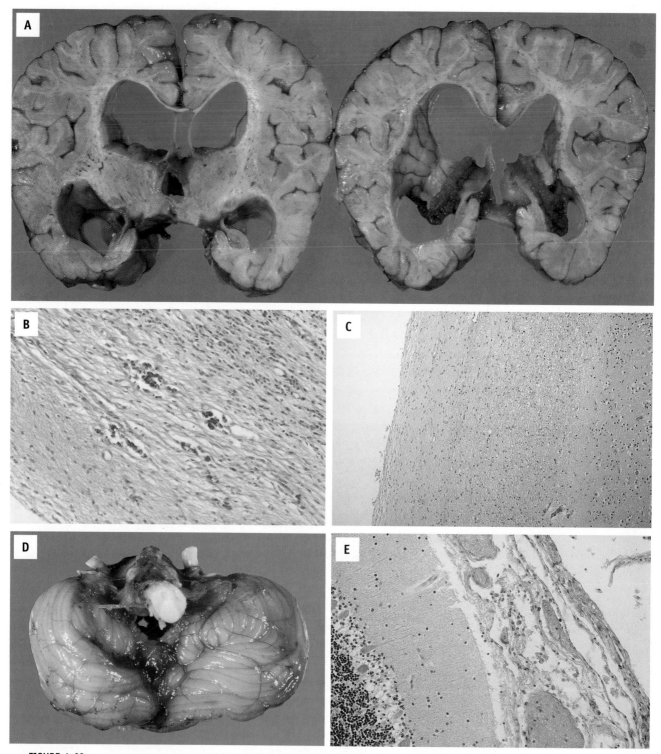

FIGURE 4-60

Hydrocephalus after intraventricular hemorrhage. **A**, Coronal section of the cerebral hemispheres with markedly expanded ventricles lined by rust-discolored ependyma from an 11-month-old former premature infant. **B**, Hemosiderin deposits and gliosis in the ventricle wall. **C**, Thinned cerebral mantle with pallor of white matter myelin (central blue band in this Luxol fast blue–stained section); the ventricular ependymal surface is on the *left* and the cortical ribbon on the *right*. **D**, Inferior view of the cerebellum with grossly visible hemosiderin staining of the arachnoid. **E**, Histologic section of hemosiderotic arachnoid overlying the cerebellar cortex.

RADIOLOGIC FEATURES

Germinal matrix hemorrhage is often first detected by transcranial ultrasound with the probe placed on the open anterior fontanelle (see Fig. 4-58). In grade IV lesions, ultrasonography reveals hypoechogenicity corresponding to acute hemorrhage. Confirmatory findings on CT or MRI are blood or blood products in the floor of the lateral ventricles, with or without extension into the ventricles or adjacent hemispheric parenchyma. Over time, the ventricles may become dilated (Fig. 4-61; see also Fig. 4-60).

Subarachnoid and cerebellar hemorrhages, if limited, may be missed by transcranial ultrasonography but can be readily detected by CT and MRI.

PATHOLOGIC FEATURES

Macroscopically, germinal matrix hemorrhages may range in size from a millimeter or two (see Fig. 4-56), to coalescent foci measuring several millimeters, to hematomas rupturing into the lateral ventricles and forming large blood casts of the entire ventricular system (see Fig. 4-57). The most severe may result in extrusion of blood through the foramina of Luschka and Magendie and pooling of subarachnoid blood around the base of the brain stem and anterior inferior portion of the cerebellum (see Fig. 4-57). As in the neocortical hemorrhagic disruptions described earlier, germinal matrix (or ganglionic eminence) hemorrhages arise by means of endothelial cell necrosis and vascular wall rupture. They begin as microscopic foci but can enlarge or become confluent and result in degeneration of radial glial fibers. Influx of macrophages and leukocytes eventually leads to resorption, often with residual periventricular cyst formation (Fig. 4-62). Hemosiderosis, gliosis, and rosette-like remnants of ependymal cells leave footprints of the previous insult. In noncavitating healed lesions, mineralization of cell bodies and processes may persist as markers of injury. In the case of the most extensive lesions, hemosiderosis and fibrosis may involve the aqueduct or the subarachnoid space, or both, and restrict the flow of CSF and cause hydrocephalus (see Fig. 4-60).

Cerebellar hemorrhages share many of the same pathologic features as subarachnoid hemorrhages, which can occur anywhere in the nervous system.

PROGNOSIS AND THERAPY

As mentioned earlier, the outcome of germinal matrix hemorrhage is influenced by its extent, with 67% of babies with grade I or II lesions surviving with a low incidence of long-term deficit. In contrast, those with grade III or IV lesions have higher mortality and significant morbidity related primarily to the location of the parenchymal injury, as well as the need for shunting of hydrocephalus.

PERINATAL HEMORRHAGE—PATHOLOGIC FEATURES

Gross Findings
- ▶ Germinal matrix hemorrhage:
  - ▶ Acute: range from a few millimeters to coalescent clots and massive rupture into the ventricles, with extension out of the fourth ventricular foramina to the basal subarachnoid space
  - ▶ Chronic: resorption of extravasated blood by macrophages resulting in glial-lined cysts in the floor of the lateral ventricles; thickening of the leptomeninges and scarring of CSF outflow tracts and sites of resorption resulting in hydrocephalus
- ▶ Periventricular hemorrhagic infarction: unilateral, roughly fan-shaped hemorrhage in deep white matter with softening and a dusky discoloration of the surrounding parenchyma; occur on the same side as large germinal matrix hemorrhage
- ▶ Cerebellar hemorrhage: usually unilateral, sometimes vermian, and ranging from focal subpial or subependymal clots to massive clots destroying cortex and causing a mass effect
- ▶ Choroid plexus hemorrhage: if large, may obscure normal architecture of the glomus of the choroid plexus and may fill the atrium of the lateral ventricle

Microscopic Features
- ▶ Acute hemorrhages:
  - ▶ Germinal matrix, deep white matter, cerebellum, or choroid plexus: extravasated red cells surrounding vessels with fibrinoid changes in the walls
  - ▶ Periventricular hemorrhagic infarction also shows parenchymal necrosis and occasional thrombosis of the parenchymal venules
- ▶ Chronic:
  - ▲ All sites: macrophages, hemosiderosis
  - ▶ Post-IVH with subarachnoid hemorrhage: disruption and scarring of the ependyma, fibrosis of the leptomeninges

Differential Diagnosis
- ▶ Trauma, vascular malformations, coagulopathy

HIPPOCAMPAL SCLEROSIS

CLINICAL FEATURES

Hippocampal sclerosis, also called mesial temporal or Ammon's horn sclerosis, refers to gliosis and neuronal loss in the hippocampus, particularly the region known as Sommer's sector, in association with long-standing seizure disorder. Since many seizure disorders may be due to developmental conditions, this entity is considered here.

Seizures are either "primary" (idiopathic) or "secondary" to a structural lesion such as a malformation, neoplasm, healed traumatic lesion, abscess, or parasitic infection. Any of these lesions may produce focal or generalized epileptic activity, depending on their site and size. In the clinical setting of complex partial seizures, it is unclear whether the hippocampal sclerosis is the cause or the consequence of seizure activity because it is often the only neuropathologic abnormality. Febrile

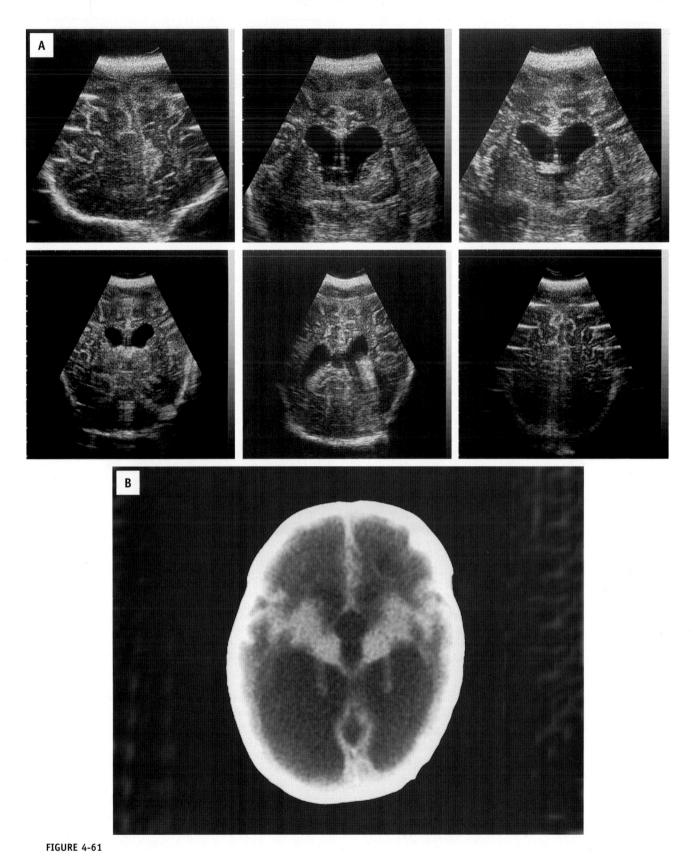

FIGURE 4-61

Hydrocephalus after intraventricular hemorrhage. **A**, Transfontanelle ultrasonogram (coronal view) from a premature infant. **B**, Axial computed tomographic scan of 11-month-old prematurely born baby with nonobstructive hydrocephalus.

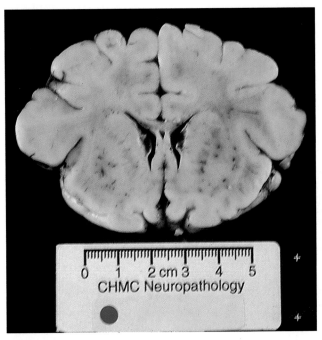

FIGURE 4-62

Germinal matrix cysts: short-term survivor of prematurity with bilateral cysts in the floor of the lateral ventricles corresponding to sites of resolved limited germinal matrix hemorrhages.

convulsions in infancy occur in 2% to 3% and predispose to the later development of epilepsy, which has a worldwide prevalence between 4 and 10 per 1000. A link between prolonged infantile febrile convulsions and the later development of chronic temporal lobe epilepsy and hippocampal sclerosis has been demonstrated. Successful treatment of some cases of medically intractable epilepsy by surgical resection of a sclerotic Ammon horn is further evidence that hippocampal sclerosis is in fact the causative lesion.

Genetic factors probably play a part in the development of hippocampal sclerosis. The lesion may be seen in several types of autosomal dominant neonatal or infantile convulsion syndromes (linked to 20q, 8q, 19q, 2q) and some childhood epilepsies with complex inheritance (linked to 15q). A polymorphism in the gene for the proinflammatory cytokine interleukin-1β is significantly associated with hippocampal sclerosis, thus suggesting that inflammatory responses may contribute to its pathogenesis.

RADIOLOGIC FEATURES

The neuroimaging findings depend on the underlying cause of the seizures (tumor, malformation, trauma, vascular disease, etc.). Mesial temporal sclerosis is detected on the basis of atrophy of Ammon's horn and accompanying dilation of the temporal horn of the lateral ventricle, findings that are typically unilateral (Fig. 4-63).

HIPPOCAMPAL SCLEROSIS—FACT SHEET

Definition

▶ Neuronal loss and gliosis in the CA1 and CA4 segments of the hippocampus
▶ Associated with long-standing seizure disorders of all causes

Incidence/Prevalence

▶ The prevalence of seizure disorders of all types (focal, generalized, complex partial) is 4 to 10 per 1000, with marked geographic variability
▶ Hippocampal sclerosis develops in a subset of patients with prolonged seizures, especially febrile convulsions in infancy

Gender and Age Distribution

▶ The prevalence of epilepsy of all types is slightly higher in males
▶ Incidence of epilepsy of all types:
  ▶ Highest in the neonatal period because of febrile convulsions; occurs in 2% to 3% of babies
  ▶ Decreases after infancy, rises after 60 years of age

Clinical Features

▶ Hippocampal sclerosis is often the only structural abnormality in complex partial seizures

Radiologic Features

▶ Depends on the nature of the lesion causing the seizures (tumor, trauma, vascular malformation, metabolic disorder, focal cortical dysplasia, etc.)
▶ In seizures without a detectable structural cause, mesial temporal sclerosis, visible as atrophy of the mesial temporal lobe with expansion of the temporal horn of the lateral ventricle, may be the only finding

Prognosis and Treatment

▶ Mesial temporal lobectomy is effective in pharmacoresistant cases
▶ The risk of accidental as well as sudden unexpected death is increased in epilepsy patients in general

---

PATHOLOGIC FEATURES

The typical macroscopic appearance of hippocampal sclerosis is unilateral atrophy and uniform white coloration of the hippocampal formation, with loss of the gray-white distinction (see Fig. 4-63). This appearance can be appreciated at autopsy and in mesial temporal lobectomies performed for control of medically refractory seizures. The temporal horn of the lateral ventricle is typically enlarged as a result of the loss of adjacent tissue. Microscopically, the loss of pyramidal and dentate layer neurons may be profound, particularly in Sommer's sector (CA1) and the end-folium (CA4), and can be highlighted by immunohistochemical stains for astrocytes (GFAP) (see Fig. 4-63). Dispersion or discontinuity of the dentate granule cell layer has also been described. Mineralization may be seen, especially in long-standing lesions. Atrophy of the white matter

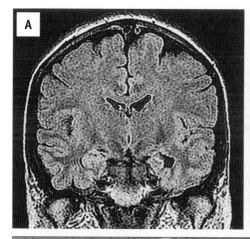

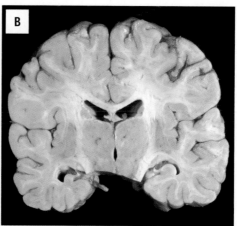

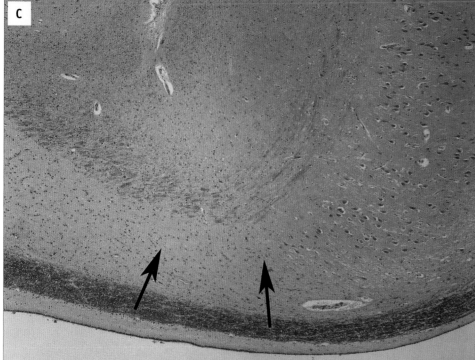

FIGURE 4-63

Mesial temporal sclerosis. **A** and **B**, MRI (Courtesy of Dr. L. Hsu, Boston) and a gross coronal section, respectively, showing atrophy of the left hippocampus and enlargement of the temporal horn of the lateral ventricle. **C**, Histologic section of the hippocampus with complete neuronal loss in the CA1 segment (*arrows*).

efferents (the alveus and fimbria, as well as the fornix) may be visible grossly and microscopically.

DIFFERENTIAL DIAGNOSIS

Microscopically, the pattern of scarring may be reminiscent of that seen after hypoxia-ischemia (i.e., after cardiac arrest), a clinical history of which should be obtainable.

PROGNOSIS AND THERAPY

Anticonvulsant drugs are the first line of therapy for partial complex and other types of seizures. If such drugs fail to adequately prevent or reduce the number of seizures, surgical en bloc resection of the anterior mesial temporal lobe and amygdala is successful in up to 80% of cases. The increased risk of premature death in patients with seizure disorders is attributed to accidents, drowning, and sudden, unexpected death presumably caused by cardiorespiratory compromise during or after an unwitnessed seizure.

TRISOMY DEFECTS

Trisomies affecting the nervous system include trisomy 21 (Down syndrome), trisomy 18, trisomy 13 (Patau's syndrome), and trisomy 9.

HIPPOCAMPAL SCLEROSIS—PATHOLOGIC FEATURES

Gross Findings
- ▶ Unilateral atrophy of the hippocampus with expansion of the temporal horn of the lateral ventricle

Microscopic Features
- ▶ Neuronal loss and gliosis in CA1, CA4, and sometimes CA3
- ▶ Disruption or dispersion of the dentate granule cell layer
- ▶ Mineralization in long-standing cases
- ▶ Atrophy of the hippocampal projections

Immunohistochemical Features
- ▶ Gliosis can be highlighted by GFAP immunostain

Genetics
- ▶ Neonatal and infantile febrile seizures linked to 20q, 8q, 19q
- ▶ Childhood epilepsies have complex inheritance linked to 15q

Differential Diagnosis
- ▶ Hypoxic-ischemic injury, such as after cardiac arrest

CLINICAL FEATURES

Seen in 1 in 1000 live births, *Down syndrome* (*trisomy 21*) is clinically characterized by microcephaly and mental retardation, both of which range from mild to severe. Five percent to 10% of cases may suffer seizure disorder. The typical clinical and pathologic changes of Alzheimer's disease universally develop in individuals with Down syndrome beginning in the fourth decade. Affected children also have a high incidence of congenital cardiac defects, duodenal atresia, and later development of acute leukemias.

In *trisomy 18* (also known as *Edwards' syndrome*), which occurs in 1 in 5000 live births, the clinical picture is one of dolichocephaly with malformed ears, micrognathia, deficient philtrum, midline facial clefts, and clinodactyly. Ophthalmologic defects include short palpebral fissures, microphthalmos, and corneal opacities. Genitourinary and cardiac anomalies are frequent. Affected individuals have severe mental retardation related to cerebral dysgenesis (described later).

Patau's syndrome (*trisomy 13*) occurs in approximately 1 in 6000 live births and is typified by microcephaly, severe mental delay, and abnormal facies, including absence of the eyebrows and shallow supraorbital ridges, as well as a cleft palate, low-set malrotated ears, and cardiac malformations. Ocular defects such as microphthalmos or anophthalmia and coloboma are frequent. Holoprosencephaly is the main neuropathologic hallmark (see the earlier section "Holoprosencephaly Sequence") and occurs in up to 80% of patients; callosal agenesis or Dandy-Walker complex occurs in many of the remainder.

The clinical features of the rarer *trisomy 9* include micrognathia, microcephaly, wide cranial sutures,

---

TRISOMY DEFECTS—FACT SHEET

Definition
- ▶ The most common human trisomies arise from chromosomal nondisjunction and generate an extra copy of chromosome 9, 13, 18, or 21
- ▶ Each may have extra-CNS manifestations as well

Incidence/Prevalence
- ▶ Trisomy 21: 1 per 1000 live births
- ▶ Trisomy 18: 1 per 5000 live births
- ▶ Trisomy 13: 1 per 6000 live births

Clinical Features
- ▶ All are characterized by microcephaly and mental retardation; trisomy 13 and trisomy 18 have a high incidence of holoprosencephaly (see "Holoprosencephaly Sequence," earlier)
- ▶ Trisomy 21 (Down syndrome): seizure disorder in 5% to 10%; Alzheimer's disease develops in all patients surviving to the fourth to fifth decade; also, cardiac defects, leukemia, duodenal atresia
- ▶ Trisomy 18 (Edwards' syndrome): dolichocephaly, malformed ears and facial features, ophthalmologic defects; also, genitourinary and cardiac defects
- ▶ Trisomy 13 (Patau's syndrome): abnormal facies, ocular defects, callosal agenesis, Dandy-Walker complex (see earlier)
- ▶ Trisomy 9: abnormal facies, microcephaly, wide cranial sutures, cardiac anomalies, fixed or dislocated joints, renal and genitourinary abnormalities

Radiologic Features
- ▶ Trisomy 21: subtle abnormalities, including brachycephaly, narrow superior temporal gyrus, small cerebellum; calcifications of the basal ganglia seen on ultrasonography and CT
- ▶ Trisomy 13: imaging of holoprosencephaly, callosal agenesis, hippocampal dysplasia with expansion of the temporal horns of the lateral ventricles, or posterior fossa malformation as previously described
- ▶ Trisomy 18: cerebral gyral pattern anomalies, pontocerebellar hypoplasia, hippocampal dysplasia, and callosal agenesis on MRI
- ▶ Trisomy 9: hippocampal dysplasia, cystic dilatation of the fourth ventricle

Prognosis and Treatment
- ▶ All trisomies cause mental retardation of varying degrees
- ▶ Seizures require medical and rarely surgical therapy
- ▶ The overall prognosis depends on associated systemic abnormalities, especially cardiac

---

low-set ears, deep-set eyes with narrow palpebral fissures, cardiac anomalies, fixed or dislocated joints, renal and genitourinary abnormalities, and intrauterine growth retardation.

RADIOLOGIC FEATURES

Down syndrome may have only subtle neuroimaging abnormalities, such as brachycephaly, a narrow superior temporal gyrus, and a small cerebellum. Calcifications of the basal ganglia along the lenticulostriate vessels have been described on both ultrasonography and CT. Atlantoaxial subluxation is found in 10% to 22% of patients with Down syndrome and predisposes them, along with structural abnormalities of the odontoid process, to spinal cord injury.

In trisomy 13, the neuroradiologic findings of holoprosencephaly, callosal agenesis, or posterior fossa malformation are identical to those previously described in the corresponding sections. In trisomy 18, anomalies in the cerebral gyral pattern, pontocerebellar hypoplasia, and callosal agenesis are well seen on MRI, as discussed in earlier sections. Hippocampal dysplasia with expansion of the temporal horns of the lateral ventricles, seen in both trisomy 18 and trisomy 9, is also easily identified on MRI. Cystic dilatation of the fourth ventricle is a nearly universal finding in trisomy 9.

PATHOLOGIC FEATURES

Macroscopically, the brain of an individual with *Down syndrome* is small and weighs significantly less than normal for age (micrencephaly). The foreshortened frontal lobes lend a "globular" appearance to the brain (Fig. 4-64). The cerebellum may be disproportionately small. The superior temporal gyrus has been described as narrow or short in some cases. Despite these fairly consistent overt gross changes, routine microscopic techniques are unable to detect any abnormalities. By specialized techniques such as Golgi impregnation, cytoarchitectural abnormalities, including fewer and shorter dendrites, have been described in cerebral corti-

---

TRISOMY DEFECTS—PATHOLOGIC FEATURES

Gross Findings

▶ For all trisomies, the brain is small (micrencephaly), with foreshortened frontal lobes and a small cerebellum
▶ In trisomy 21, the superior temporal gyrus is narrow or short
▶ Holoprosencephaly (as described earlier) occurs in trisomy 18 or 13
▶ Trisomy 9 has incomplete rotation of the hippocampus, pachygyria, callosal agenesis, Dandy-Walker malformation or cystic dilatation of the fourth ventricle (or both)

Microscopic Features

▶ In all trisomies, disturbances in cortical lamination and heterotopia of neurons in the basal forebrain, brain stem, and cerebellum (especially in trisomy 18) have been identified
▶ Trisomy 9 shows disorganization of the hippocampus and simplification of the inferior olive
▶ The neurofibrillary tangles and senile plaques of Alzheimer's disease develop in aged patients with Down syndrome

Genetics

▶ Complete autosomal trisomies, as well as mosaic forms, can give rise to these clinical entities

---

cal neurons. In some cases, disturbances in cortical lamination have been identified. Mineralization of lenticulostriate vessels may be seen (see Fig. 4-64). In aged patients with Down syndrome, the neurofibrillary tangles and senile plaques of Alzheimer's disease are readily identified.

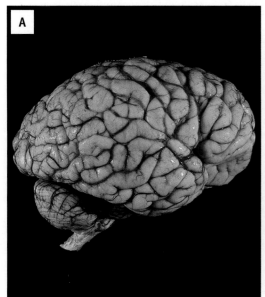
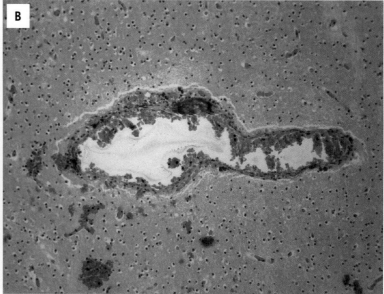

FIGURE 4-64

Trisomy 21. **A,** View of the right lateral aspect of the brain revealing a foreshortened, slightly "globular" appearance of the hemispheres, a very narrow and short superior temporal gyrus, and a small cerebellum. **B,** Microscopic section of the basal ganglia. The vessels have mural and perivascular mineral deposits.

When holoprosencephaly occurs in trisomy 18 or 13, the macroscopic and histologic changes are as described earlier. These trisomies may also show (either isolated or in addition to the forebrain defects) evidence of neuronal migration defects, including malposition (heterotopia) of neurons in the basal forebrain, brain stem, and cerebellum (see Figs. 4-23 and 4-28). Thickening of the dorsal limb of the inferior olive or the dentate (dentato-olivary dysplasia) is well recognized, especially in trisomy 18.

Trisomy 9 is typified by pachygyria, callosal agenesis, and Dandy-Walker malformation in some instances. Any of the trisomies may cause hippocampal maldevelopment (Fig. 4-65).

DIFFERENTIAL DIAGNOSIS

Clearly, none of the features described are unique (i.e., pathognomonic) for each trisomy, so complete evaluation of all CNS and systemic lesions is necessary to arrive at an accurate diagnosis in the absence of cytogenetic data.

PROGNOSIS AND THERAPY

Life span in each trisomy is highly dependent on the presence or absence of associated anomalies of the heart or other major organ systems. Seizure disorder in Down syndrome is usually well controlled medically, and survival into adulthood and old age is fairly common. As mentioned earlier, Alzheimer's disease with its attendant morbidity and mortality develops in virtually all patients older than 35 years with Down syndrome.

FAMILIAL MALFORMATION/TUMOR SYNDROMES

These syndromes are wide ranging in their phenotypes and include entities called phacomatoses (neurofibromatosis types 1 and 2, tuberous sclerosis, von Hippel–Lindau disease, Sturge-Weber syndrome, ataxia-telangiectasia, neurocutaneous melanosis, and basal cell nevus or Gorlin's syndrome) in the older literature. They, along with the familial retinoblastoma syndrome, Cowden's disease, Li-Fraumeni syndrome, and Turcot's syndrome, are discussed separately.

NEUROFIBROMATOSIS TYPE 1

CLINICAL FEATURES

Neurofibromatosis type 1 (NF1) is a fairly common autosomal dominant condition (occurring in 1 in 3000 to 5000 persons) in which numerous cutaneous and deep neurofibromas arise along with typical café au lait spots on the skin and Lisch nodules on the iris. Plexiform neurofibromas (Fig. 4-66), malignant peripheral

FIGURE 4-65

Trisomy 13: hippocampal dysplasia. Note the disordered, looped curves of the hippocampus, as well as heterotopic nodules (*arrowheads*) and subarachnoid glioneuronal tissue (*arrow*).

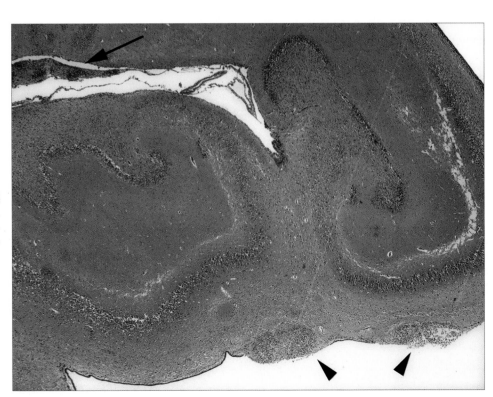

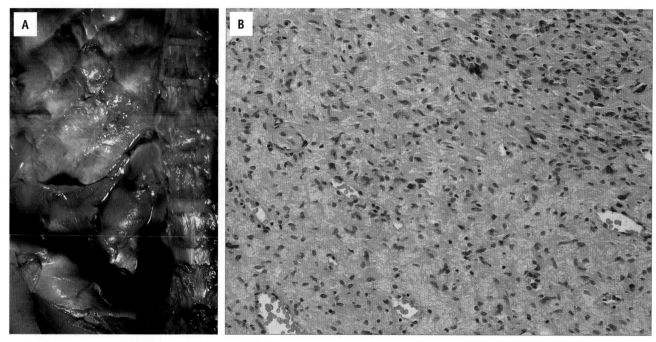

FIGURE 4-66

Neurofibromatosis type 1. **A**, View of the right retroperitoneum and thorax (the vertebral column is on the *right*) showing massive, sausage-like expansion of all intercostal nerves by plexiform neurofibromas. **B**, Section of a neurofibroma made up of spindle cells.

NEUROFIBROMATOSIS TYPE 1—FACT SHEET

Definition and Clinical Features

▶ See Table 4-1
▶ Seizures and cognitive delay are common
▶ Hydrocephalus may be related to aqueductal stenosis
▶ Extraneural tumors occurring at a higher than expected frequency in NF1 patients include pheochromocytomas, intestinal carcinoid tumors, rhabdomyosarcomas of soft tissue, and juvenile chronic myeloid leukemia

Incidence/Prevalence

▶ 1 in 3000 to 5000

Radiologic Features

▶ "NF spots" (nonenhancing, T2-bright areas) in the white matter of the cerebral hemispheres, brain stem, and cerebellum beginning around 2 to 3 years of age, increasing in number and dimensions until the second decade, and then disappearing by the age of 20
▶ Berry aneurysms and cerebral vascular dysplasia on angiography
▶ Optic gliomas, diffuse astrocytomas, and peripheral nerve tumors have imaging characteristics identical to those of sporadic tumors.
▶ On plain radiographs, bony abnormalities may involve the orbits, sphenoid wings, and vertebral column (causing scoliosis)

Prognosis and Treatment

▶ The prognosis depends on the evolution of central and peripheral nervous system neoplasms, which may require aggressive therapy
▶ Seizures are managed medically and hydrocephalus by ventricular shunting

nerve sheath tumors, optic or hypothalamic system gliomas (Fig. 4-67), or diffuse astrocytomas are sources of morbidity and mortality in affected individuals. Seizures may be idiopathic or associated with structural lesions detectable on neuroimaging (see the next section). Some affected persons have cognitive delay, and some have hydrocephalus related to aqueductal stenosis. Extraneural tumors occurring at a higher than expected frequency in NF1 patients include pheochromocytomas, intestinal carcinoid tumors, rhabdomyosarcomas of soft tissue, and juvenile chronic myeloid leukemia. Diagnostic criteria for NF1 are listed in Table 4-1. The gene for NF1 is located on chromosome 17q12 and codes for a protein known as neurofibromin, which is part of the family of Ras guanosine triphosphatase–activating proteins.

RADIOLOGIC FEATURES

By neuroimaging, NF1 patients may have numerous "NF spots" (white matter vacuolizations) in the white matter of the cerebral hemispheres, brain stem, and cerebellum. These spots are nonenhancing, T2-bright areas found in more than 75% of children with NF1 beginning around 2 to 3 years of age; they increase in number and dimensions until the second decade and then disappear by the age of 20 years. Berry aneurysms as well as intimal proliferation (dysplasia) of cerebral blood vessels may be visible on angiographic studies. The optic gliomas, diffuse astrocytomas, and peripheral nerve tumors arising in these individuals have imaging

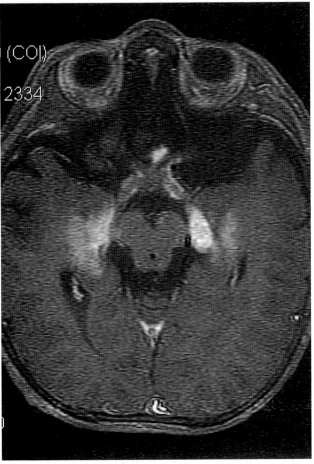

FIGURE 4-67

Neurofibromatosis type 1: MRI (T1 weighted with gadolinium contrast) of the brain showing bilateral thickening and enhancement of the optic nerves and chiasm, as well as abnormal signal in the optic radiations, typical of an optic pathway glioma. (Courtesy of Dr. M. Silvera, Boston.)

TABLE 4-1
Diagnostic Criteria for Neurofibromatosis Type 1 (Two or More of the Listed Features)
At least 6 café au lait spots >5 mm in diameter in prepubertal individuals or >15 mm in postpubertal individuals
At least 2 neurofibromas of any type or 1 plexiform neurofibroma
Axillary and/or inguinal freckling
Optic nerve glioma
Dysplasia of the sphenoid wing or thinning of the cortex of a long bone
First-degree relative with NF1 by these criteria

characteristics identical to those in non-NF patients, except that NF patients tend to have bilateral optic system and chiasmatic involvement (see Fig. 4-67). On plain radiographs, bony abnormalities may involve the orbits and sphenoid wings, as well as the vertebral column, which can be associated with scoliosis.

PATHOLOGIC FEATURES

Peripheral neurofibromas are of three types (nodular, diffuse, or plexiform). The nodular types have a globular outline and are well circumscribed, whereas the diffuse types are irregular swellings that lack a definite border grossly. Plexiform neurofibromas follow the course of involved cutaneous or deep nerves and have a worm- or rope-like appearance. All are spindle cell tumors of variable cellularity, usually with a densely packed fascicular appearance (see Fig. 4-66), but sometimes with a loose, myxoid background. Occasional preserved myelinated axons from the involved nerve may traverse the tumor. The nodular type has a fine con-

nective tissue capsule, which allows for ready excision; however, the diffuse and plexiform variants may infiltrate extensively into adjacent normal tissue. In NF1 patients, these neoplasms have a propensity for progression from benign tumors of cosmetic importance to aggressive, life-threatening malignant peripheral nerve sheath tumors. Evolution to malignancy is heralded clinically by rapid growth and pathologically by the presence of detectable mitotic activity in the tumor spindle cells, as well as nuclear pleomorphism, regional necrosis, and invasion of contiguous tissues. Immunohistochemically, peripheral nerve sheath tumors, whether benign or malignant, demonstrate reactivity for the neural crest marker S-100 protein; malignant peripheral nerve sheath tumors may lose immunoreactivity, however, so only scattered individual cells may be highlighted by the stain, in contrast to the high degree of staining in neurofibromas.

The optic system tumors and diffuse astrocytomas of NF1 are identical macroscopically and microscopically to those seen in non-NF patients. The tissue substrate for the "NF spots" identified on neuroimaging is intramyelinic edema, thus suggesting transiently disordered myelination.

NEUROFIBROMATOSIS TYPE 1—PATHOLOGIC FEATURES

Gross and Microscopic Findings
► Peripheral neurofibromas (nodular, diffuse, or plexiform types) and the optic system tumors and diffuse astrocytomas of NF1 are identical macroscopically and microscopically to those seen in non-NF patients
► "NF spots" identified on neuroimaging correspond to intramyelinic edema, thus suggesting transiently disordered myelination

Genetics
► The gene for NF1 is on chromosome 17q12 and codes for neurofibromin

DIFFERENTIAL DIAGNOSIS

The main differential diagnostic consideration of an excised peripheral neurofibroma is a schwannoma or other spindle cell neoplasm. Since schwannomas are also S-100 immunoreactive, one must rely on the finding of interstitial axons (detectable on silver impregnations such as Bodian stains or by immunohistochemistry for neurofilament protein) in neurofibromas and on the gross appearance of a fusiform expansion of the nerve (more usual for neurofibromas) versus the extrafascicular, "stuck-on" appearance of schwannomas. Generally, in patients with all the stigmata of NF1 (see Table 4-1), such differentiation is not a problem.

PROGNOSIS AND THERAPY

Treatment of NF1 is aimed at control of the CNS neoplasms. Surveillance of the MRI "bright spots" is necessary to ensure that an evolving astrocytoma is not missed. Peripheral neurofibromas are problematic because of their sheer number, and the diffuse and plexiform types are problematic because of the widespread involvement of normal nerve and surrounding connective tissue. Since excision of all such lesions is impossible, watchfulness for signs of malignant transformation, such as rapid growth, is instead necessary for early surgical control. Seizures are managed medically and hydrocephalus by ventricular shunting as necessary. The life span of NF1 patients is extremely variable and parallels the penetrance and severity of the many manifestations of the disease; however, the appearance of malignant peripheral nerve sheath tumors considerably worsens survival.

NEUROFIBROMATOSIS TYPE 2

CLINICAL FEATURES

Neurofibromatosis type 2 (NF2; also known as central neurofibromatosis) has an autosomal dominant inheritance, with affected individuals demonstrating schwannomas, particularly bilateral vestibular tumors, meningiomas, gliomas (Fig. 4-68), and less commonly, cerebral calcifications and cataracts. Sporadic cases occur. Table 4-2 lists the diagnostic criteria. An earlier-onset phenotype known as the Wishart type is manifested by multiple tumor types, whereas a later-onset phenotype shows bilateral vestibular tumors only (Gardner type). Clinical symptoms related to these findings are no different from those in non-NF2 patients. Occasionally, the syndrome is not suspected until workup for one neoplasm (e.g., vestibular schwannoma) discloses occult lesions of other types (e.g., multiple meningiomas) because in contrast to NF1, cutaneous stigmata are generally lacking. There are rare patients,

---

TABLE 4-2

Diagnostic Criteria for Neurofibromatosis Type 2

Bilateral vestibular schwannomas

or

A first-degree relative with NF2 *and*

One vestibular schwannoma *or*

Two of the following: meningioma, schwannoma of another nerve, glioma of any type, posterior subcapsular lens opacity, or cerebral calcification

or

Two of the following:

    One vestibular schwannoma

    Multiple meningiomas

    Schwannoma of another nerve, glioma of any type, subcapsular lens opacity, or cerebral calcification

---

however, who have cutaneous schwannomas that may be plexiform. Seizures may arise in association with meningioangiomatosis, a characteristic hamartomatous lesion of the superficial cerebral cortex. The gene for NF2 is on chromosome 22q12 and encodes a cytoskeletal protein known as merlin (also called schwannomin); the gene is thought to function as a tumor suppressor gene.

RADIOLOGIC FEATURES

NF2 is characterized on neuroimaging by the neoplasms mentioned (see Fig. 4-68). The occasional appearance of syringomyelia is thought to be secondary to the intraspinal or nerve root neoplasms. Calcifications of

---

NEUROFIBROMATOSIS TYPE 2—FACT SHEET

Definition and Clinical Features

▶ See Table 4-2

▶ Earlier-onset phenotype associated with multiple tumor types (Wishart type)

▶ Later-onset phenotype associated with bilateral vestibular tumors only (Gardner type)

▶ Seizures may arise in association with meningioangiomatosis, a hamartomatous lesion of the superficial cerebral cortex

Radiologic Features

▶ Vestibular schwannomas and meningiomas are multiple but are otherwise similar to those seen sporadically

▶ Syringomyelia may arise from compression of the cord by central or peripheral neoplasms

▶ Calcifications of the cerebral and cerebellar cortices, periventricular regions, and choroid plexus

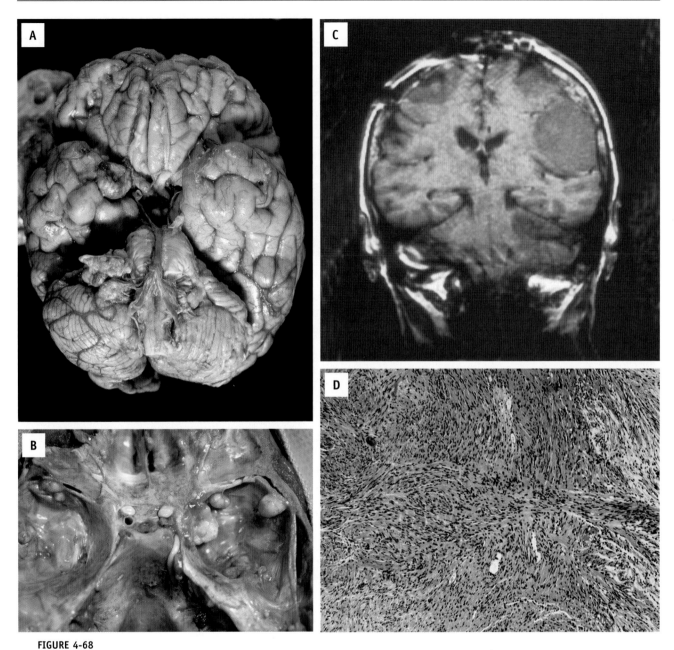

FIGURE 4-68

Neurofibromatosis type 2. **A**, Ventral aspect of the brain showing an acoustic schwannoma at the right cerebellopontine angle, as well as meningiomas over the right medial temporal lobe and right lateral frontal lobe (the latter with attached dura). **B**, Skull base from the same patient showing multiple meningiomas. **C**, Computed tomographic scan of the same patient demonstrating the large right frontal meningioma and right acoustic schwannoma. **D**, Microscopic section of an acoustic schwannoma demonstrating compact fascicles of tumor cells on the left (Antoni A areas) alternating with looser arrangements of cells (Antoni B areas) on the right.

the cerebral and cerebellar cortices, periventricular regions, and choroid plexus may be identified.

PATHOLOGIC FEATURES

In NF2, the vestibular schwannomas are largely indistinguishable from the sporadically occurring tumors (see Fig. 4-68), but some have been described as having a more lobular appearance with greater cellularity.

Grossly, schwannomas tend to be circumscribed nodules arising from the covering of the nerve, although fusiform expansion of nerves is seen, especially in the confines of the spinal canal and neural foramina. Rarely, growth of peripheral schwannomas occurs in an unusual plexiform pattern, analogous to the plexiform neurofibromas of NF1. Microscopically, schwannomas have a biphasic pattern of densely packed spindle cells in a fascicular pattern (so-called Antoni A areas) alternating with zones of looser tumor tissue (Antoni B areas) (see Fig. 4-68). Collagenized vascular walls, hemosiderin deposits, and interstitial foamy macrophages are considered markers of chronicity and degeneration in these lesions, which are generally slow growing. Immunohistochemically, schwannomas are S-100 positive.

The meningiomas and gliomas, including diffuse astrocytomas of the hemispheres or brain stem, pilocytic astrocytomas, and most frequently, ependymomas of the spinal cord, are grossly and microscopically identical to those seen in non-NF2 patients. Like the meningeal and Schwann cell neoplasms, the glial tumors may be multiple. A typical, although not pathognomonic lesion of NF2 is meningioangiomatosis, a plaque-like cortical mass of meningothelial and fibroblast-like spindle cells growing along and around small penetrating vessels (Fig. 4-69), some of which may appear disorganized and ectatic, similar to a vascular malformation. "Schwannosis" may be seen as a proliferation of Schwann cells at spinal dorsal root entry zones, with or without an adjacent schwannoma of the root. The brain may harbor microscopic collections of S-100 protein– and focally GFAP-immunopositive glia called glial hamartias in the cortex, basal ganglia, thalamus, and cerebellum (Fig. 4-70). Neuropathologic descriptions of the calcifications seen on neuroimages have not been reported.

DIFFERENTIAL DIAGNOSIS

The unusual plexiform schwannomas seen in the setting of NF2 have been confused with the plexiform neurofibromas of NF1 on the basis of their similar gross and light microscopic characteristics. However, as in nodular versions of these tumors, the presence of scattered neurofilament-immunoreactive axons within a given tumor serves to reinforce its identity as a neurofibroma. The distinction is important because plexiform schwannomas have a much lower rate of transformation to malignancy than plexiform neurofibromas do.

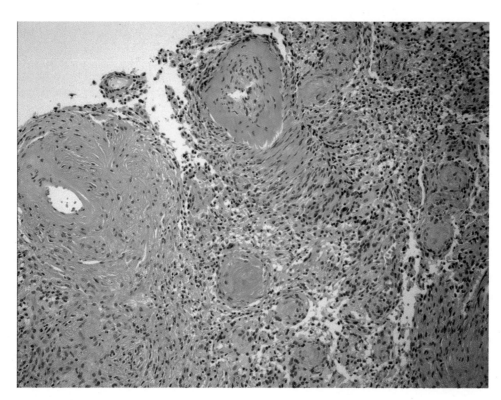

FIGURE 4-69

Neurofibromatosis type 2: meningioangiomatosis characterized by dense collagen and meningothelial cell proliferation surrounding small vessels in the subarachnoid space.

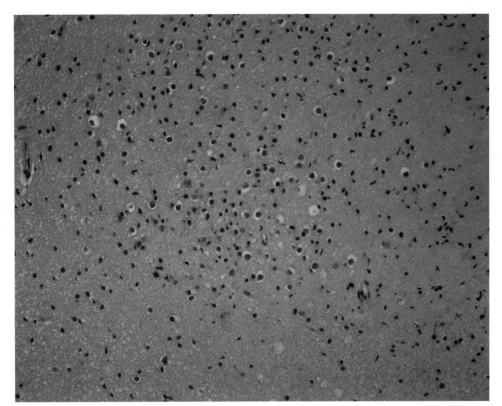

FIGURE 4-70

Neurofibromatosis type 2. A glial hamartia such as this one, made up of small, round, granular or oligodendroglia-like cells, may be scattered throughout the brain.

PROGNOSIS AND THERAPY

As in NF1, the prognosis for individuals with NF2 is quite variable, even within affected families; it is largely determined by the grade and extent of the glial and meningeal tumors because vestibular schwannomas by themselves are rarely fatal. Hearing loss, however, is a common outcome.

TUBEROUS SCLEROSIS

CLINICAL FEATURES

Tuberous sclerosis is an autosomal dominant complex with numerous CNS abnormalities, including cortical and subcortical hamartomas, subependymal glial nodules (Fig. 4-71), and subependymal giant cell astrocytomas. Cutaneous angiofibromas of the face ("adenoma sebaceum"), shagreen patches and ash-leaf spots of the skin, subungual fibromas, cardiac rhabdomyomas, intestinal hamartomatous polyps, and renal angiomyolipomas are among the extraneural lesions of tuberous sclerosis. The diagnostic criteria are outlined in Table 4-3. The typical cortical tubers may give rise clinically to seizures, including infantile spasms; mental retardation is common. Signs of increased intracranial pressure may herald the growth of subependymal giant

---

TUBEROUS SCLEROSIS—FACT SHEET

Definition and Clinical Features

▶ See Table 4-3
▶ Cutaneous angiofibromas of the face ("adenoma sebaceum"), shagreen patches and ash-leaf spots of the skin, subungual fibromas, cardiac rhabdomyomas, intestinal hamartomatous polyps, renal angiomyolipomas
▶ Seizures, including infantile spasms
▶ Subependymal giant cell astrocytomas may block the foramen of Monro and cause hydrocephalus and increased intracranial pressure

Incidence/Prevalence

▶ 1 in 6000 live births

Radiologic Features

▶ By transfontanelle ultrasonography, hyperechoic tubers and subependymal nodules are noted in the neonatal period
▶ T1-weighted MRI shows enhancing subependymal hamartomas, whereas the cortical tubers are seen even without contrast
▶ CT demonstrates calcification of tubers and subependymal hamartomas

Prognosis and Treatment

▶ Seizures may be refractory to medical treatment and require surgery
▶ Hydrocephalus may require placement of a ventricular shunt
▶ Subependymal giant cell astrocytomas can recur and lead to death

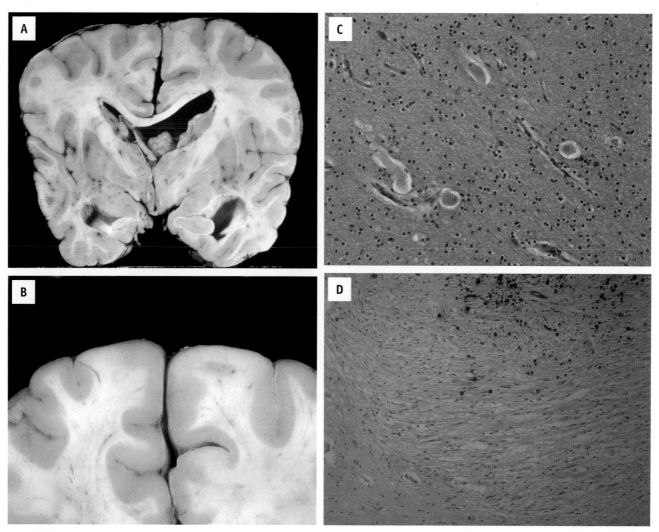

FIGURE 4-71

Tuberous sclerosis. **A**, Coronal section of the cerebral hemispheres disclosing multiple subependymal nodules/giant cell tumors in the floor of the lateral ventricles, as well as enlarged gyri. (Courtesy of Dr. U. De Girolami, from the collection of the late Dr. E. P. Richardson, Jr., Boston.) **B**, Close-up view of a cortical tuber showing expansion of the gyrus and blurring of the gray-white junction. **C**, Histology of a cortical tuber. Scattered enlarged "balloon" cells are seen in the disorganized cortex, as well as in hypomyelinated white matter (Luxol fast blue–stained section). **D**, Subependymal nodule showing calcification and enlarged, bizarre cells.

cell astrocytomas because the foramen of Monro may become blocked and give rise to hydrocephalus. The disease has been associated with mutations in two genes, *TSC1* (on chromosome 9q34) and *TSC2* (on 16p13.3), the latter coding for a protein called tuberin, which is important in cell cycle regulation and differentiation. The incidence is approximately 1 in 6000 live births.

RADIOLOGIC FEATURES

Because the typical tubers and subependymal hamartomas are present early in life, a diagnosis can be made significantly before development of the skin manifestations in the second decade. In fact, transfontanelle ultrasonography can detect the hyperechoic tubers and subependymal nodules in the neonatal period. By postcontrast T1-weighted MRI the subependymal

hamartomas are enhanced, whereas the cortical tubers are seen even without contrast. CT demonstrates calcification of both types of lesions.

PATHOLOGIC FEATURES

The cortical tubers of tuberous sclerosis have a characteristic gross appearance consisting of expansion of a gyrus or group of adjacent gyri and loss of the gray-white distinction (see Fig. 4-71). The subependymal hamartomas (see Fig. 4-71) resemble "candle gutterings," or droplets of wax, along the floors of the lateral ventricles and may have chalky yellow-white calcium deposits. Subependymal giant cell tumors are larger nodules of confluent, granular tissue that expand to fill the lateral ventricle; they often cause a mass effect on the surrounding tissues and even a midline shift.

TABLE 4-3

Diagnostic Criteria for Tuberous Sclerosis

Definitive: 1 primary feature, 2 secondary features, *or* 1 secondary plus 2 tertiary features

Provisional: 1 secondary and 1 tertiary feature *or* 3 tertiary features

Suspect: 1 secondary feature *or* 2 tertiary features

Primary features: facial angiofibromas, multiple subungual fibromas, cortical tuber,* subependymal nodule or giant cell tumor,* multiple retinal nodules, multiple calcified exophytic subependymal nodules by neuroimaging

Secondary features: affected first-degree relative, cardiac rhabdomyoma(s), retinal achromia, cortical tuber(s) by neuroimaging, noncalcified subependymal nodules by neuroimaging, shagreen patch, forehead plaque, pulmonary lymphangioleiomyomatosis,* renal angiomyolipoma, renal cysts*

Tertiary features: hypomelanotic macules, "confetti" skin lesions, renal cysts by imaging, dental enamel pits, hamartomatous rectal polyps,* bone cysts by imaging, pulmonary lymphangioleiomyomatosis by imaging, cerebral white matter heterotopia by neuroimaging, gingival fibromas, hamartomas of other organs,* infantile spasms

---

*Histologically confirmed.

TUBEROUS SCLEROSIS—PATHOLOGIC FEATURES

Gross and Microscopic Findings

▶ Cortical tubers show gross expansion of a gyrus or group of adjacent gyri and loss of gray-white distinction; microscopically, expansion and disorganization of the cortical layers are evident, with bizarre cells having both neuronal (ganglion cell) and glial characteristics

▶ Subependymal hamartomas are nodules along the floor of the lateral ventricles and may have chalky yellow-white calcium deposits

▶ Subependymal giant cell tumors fill the lateral ventricle and cause a mass effect

▶ Both subependymal hamartomas and giant cell tumors have enlarged, bizarre cells with abundant eosinophilic cytoplasm and nuclei with prominent nucleoli; the latter are more densely cellular and may have necrosis

Genetics

▶ Autosomal dominant inheritance
▶ Mutations in two genes, *TSC1* (on chromosome 9q34) and *TSC2* (on 16p13.3)

Differential Diagnosis

▶ Tubers resemble focal cortical dysplasia (see earlier)

Microscopically, the tubers show expansion and disorganization of the cortical layers, with many scattered bizarre cells having both neuronal (ganglion cell) and glial characteristics (see Fig. 4-71). The tubers are in many ways indistinguishable from the sporadically occurring isolated nodules of focal cortical dysplasia associated with epilepsy (see the earlier section "Neuronal Migration Defects"). For example, some balloon cells may show immunostaining for NeuN, neurofilament protein, or synaptophysin (neural markers), and some stain with GFAP (an astrocytic marker). They may also stain with nestin (a marker of glioneuronal precursor cells), thus suggesting an arrest in maturation. Microscopic hamartomatous aggregates of these dysplastic glioneuronal cells may also occur in the deep white matter. Macroscopically normal-appearing cortex may show microscopic disorganization consisting of altered lamination of neurons. Mineralization of tubers, subependymal glial nodules (see Fig. 4-71), and subependymal giant cell astrocytomas may be seen on histologic evaluation.

DIFFERENTIAL DIAGNOSIS

As mentioned earlier, a cortical tuber may be histologically indistinguishable from focal cortical dysplasia. Its accompaniment by cutaneous stigmata and neuroimaging evidence of other typical tuberous sclerosis lesions allows resolution of the differential diagnosis.

PROGNOSIS AND THERAPY

The morbidity in patients with tuberous sclerosis relates primarily to seizures, which may be difficult to treat medically, and to the hydrocephalus caused by the subependymal glial nodules and astrocytomas, which may require placement of a ventricular shunt. Even though subependymal giant cell astrocytomas are histologically benign, they tend to recur and ultimately lead to death in a proportion of tuberous sclerosis patients. As in all brain tumor patients treated with radiotherapy, complications such as white matter necrosis or late development of radiation-induced second malignancies can occur.

VON HIPPEL–LINDAU DISEASE

CLINICAL FEATURES

An autosomal-dominant condition, von Hippel–Lindau (vHL) disease is typified by cystic capillary hemangioblastomas (Fig. 4-72) of the cerebellum and retina, clear cell carcinomas of the kidney, and less frequently, pheochromocytomas and pancreatic or inner ear neoplasms. The diagnostic criteria for vHL disease are listed in Table 4-4. Initial manifestation in the second or third decade is usually related to the retinal angiomas, which

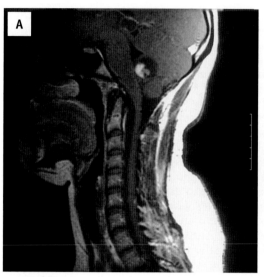 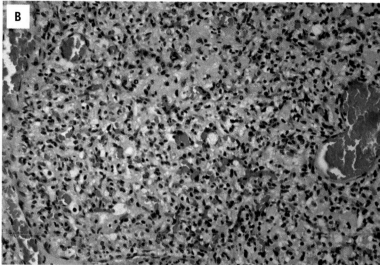

FIGURE 4-72

von Hippel–Lindau disease. **A,** Sagittal MRI of the posterior fossa and spine showing a large cyst in the right cerebellar hemisphere with an enhancing mural nodule and a smaller enhancing nodule in the lower cervical spine, consistent with multiple hemangioblastomas. (Courtesy of Dr. L. Hsu, Boston.) **B,** Hemangioblastoma of the cerebellum featuring stromal cells with foamy cytoplasm between fine capillaries.

can hemorrhage and result in retinal detachment and uveitis. Eye pain and visual loss may be significant, even with very small angiomas. Eventually, hemangioblastomas arise (earlier in vHL than in non-vHL patients) and are heralded clinically by ataxia and headache. They may be multiple and may involve other sites besides the cerebellum (e.g., brain stem, spinal cord). As in sporadic cases, hemangioblastomas may cause polycythemia through their elaboration of erythropoietin. Endolymphatic sac tumors can cause hearing loss. The *VHL* gene is on chromosome 3p25-26 and appears to have a tumor suppressor function.

VON HIPPEL–LINDAU DISEASE—FACT SHEET

Definition and Clinical Features

▶ See Table 4-4
▶ Cystic capillary hemangioblastomas of the cerebellum and retina, clear cell carcinomas of the kidney, pheochromocytomas, pancreatic or inner ear neoplasms
▶ Retinal angiomas can hemorrhage and result in retinal detachment and uveitis
▶ Hemangioblastomas cause ataxia and headache, may be multiple, and may involve the brain stem and spinal cord; they may cause polycythemia from the secretion of erythropoietin

Radiologic Features

▶ Hemangioblastomas are identical to those occurring sporadically but may be multiple and involve sites in addition to the cerebellum

Prognosis and Treatment

▶ Significant mortality associated with the multiple and frequently recurring hemangioblastomas
▶ Visual loss from the retinal lesions

RADIOLOGIC FEATURES

The hemangioblastomas of vHL disease are identical on neuroimaging to those occurring sporadically, although they may be multiple and involve sites in addition to the cerebellum (see Fig. 4-72). Spinal lesions may have an associated syrinx.

PATHOLOGIC FEATURES

Macroscopically, the capillary hemangioblastomas of vHL disease may, as in sporadic cases, arise as a mural nodule in a smooth-walled cyst, whether in the cerebellum, brain stem, or spinal cord. They may also be noted as small nodules on the meninges at any point in the neuraxis. Rare examples of other central neoplasms, including ependymoma, medulloblastoma, and choroid plexus papilloma, have been described in vHL disease. The retinal angiomas are histologically identical to the central capillary hemangioblastomas (see Fig. 4-72).

TABLE 4-4

Diagnostic Criteria for von Hippel–Lindau Disease

Capillary hemangioblastoma of the cerebellum or retina
     and
Renal cell carcinoma, pancreatic islet cell tumor, endolymphatic sac tumor, *or* pheochromocytoma, *or*
Family member with vHL disease

VON HIPPEL–LINDAU DISEASE—PATHOLOGIC FEATURES

Gross and Microscopic Findings

▶ Hemangioblastomas arise as a mural nodule in a smooth-walled cyst or as small nodules on the meninges at any point in the neuraxis
▶ Retinal angiomas and CNS capillary hemangioblastomas are histologically identical to those occurring sporadically

Genetics

▶ The VHL gene is on chromosome 3p25-26
▶ Autosomal dominant inheritance

Differential Diagnosis

▶ Hemangioblastomas resemble metastatic renal cell carcinoma

The stromal cells contain lipid (detectable on frozen sections by staining with oil red O). Immunohistochemically, hemangioblastoma cells are of uncertain derivation or differentiation because they may be positive for GFAP and neuron-specific enolase.

DIFFERENTIAL DIAGNOSIS

The histologic appearance of capillary hemangioblastomas is similar enough to clear cell carcinoma of the kidney that occasional difficulty can arise in evaluating a resected brain mass from a vHL patient with a known renal cell carcinoma. Immunohistochemistry may assist in some cases inasmuch as renal cell carcinoma tends to be more strongly positive than hemangioblastoma for the epithelial markers epithelial membrane antigen and cytokeratin.

PROGNOSIS AND THERAPY

Patients with vHL disease have significant mortality associated with the multiple and frequently recurring hemangioblastomas and require close clinical surveillance by neuroimaging starting at a young age. Visual loss from the retinal lesions can lead to blindness.

STURGE-WEBER SYNDROME

CLINICAL FEATURES

Also known as encephalofacial angiomatosis, Sturge-Weber syndrome is diagnosed by the presence of angiomatosis of the skin overlying the face and the eye and extending to involve the leptomeninges of the brain (Fig. 4-73). The facial lesion can involve one or more divisions of the trigeminal nerve. Neonatal and infantile development may be normal until the onset of infantile spasms and later evolution to focal or generalized seizures, which can be difficult to control with medication. Mental deficiencies become evident, and hemiparesis is seen ultimately in 30% of patients. Rarely, the lesion is bilateral.

RADIOLOGIC FEATURES

By MRI with contrast administration, innumerable enhancing vessels occupy the subarachnoid space, usually over the sylvian region. The glomus of the choroid plexus may be enlarged on the same side of the lesion. In older subjects, atrophy and calcification of the underlying cortex may be seen easily on CT.

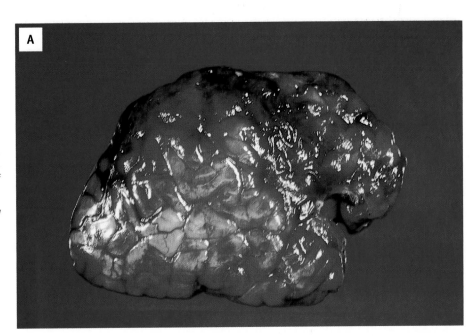

A

FIGURE 4-73
Sturge-Weber encephalofacial angiomatosis. **A**, Corticectomy specimen from the right hemisphere showing a dense mat of tangled vessels over the entire surface, particularly prominent over the sylvian fissure. *Continued*

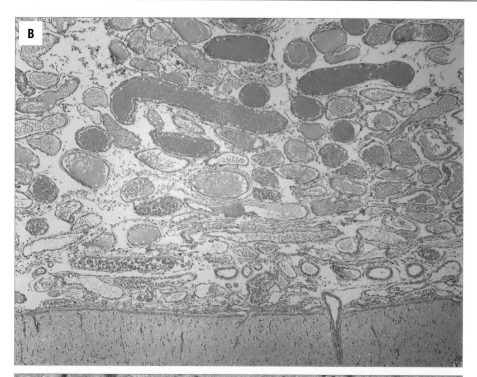

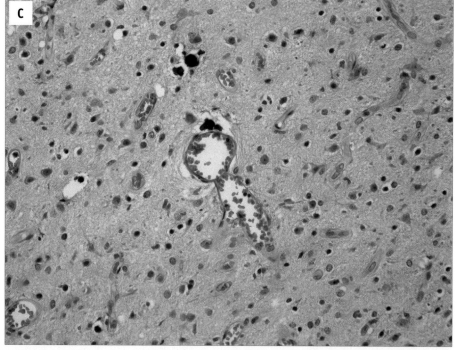

FIGURE 4-73, cont'd
B, Microscopy of the subarachnoid vessels.
C, Perivascular calcifications and gliosis in
the underlying cortex.

PATHOLOGIC FEATURES

Multiple thin-walled, ectatic vessels cover the pial
surface in a disorganized mat (see Fig. 4-73). The lesion
is thought to arise developmentally from persistence of
the primordial vascular channels normally seen only
between the 4th and 8th weeks of embryonic life. Microscopically, vessels penetrating into the cerebral cortex
may have thickened walls with "droplet" calcifications,
along with atrophy and gliosis of adjacent parenchyma

(see Fig. 4-73). Calcifications also arise in the subjacent
white matter.

DIFFERENTIAL DIAGNOSIS

Although the lesion over the brain surface somewhat
resembles an arteriovenous malformation, a true arteriovenous anastomosis is not present. The vessels are
small caliber and lack evidence of flow at high (arterial)

STURGE-WEBER SYNDROME—FACT SHEET

Definition and Clinical Features

▶ Angiomatosis of the skin overlying the face and the eye and extending to involve the leptomeninges of the brain
▶ Facial lesion involving one or more divisions of the trigeminal nerve
▶ Infantile spasms and later evolution to focal or generalized seizures; can be difficult to control with medication
▶ Mental deficiencies, hemiparesis are common

Radiologic Features

▶ By MRI with contrast, innumerable enhancing vessels occupy the subarachnoid space over the sylvian region, with enlargement of the glomus of the choroid plexus
▶ Eventually, atrophy and calcification of the underlying cortex may be seen on CT

Prognosis and Treatment

▶ Refractory seizures may require surgical management in the form of hemispherectomy (corticectomy)
▶ Bilateral involvement of the brain is associated with a poor prognosis
▶ Plastic facial surgery may be necessary

---

pressure. In addition, arteriovenous malformations are not associated with angiomatosis of the facial skin and soft tissue, the other hallmark of Sturge-Weber syndrome.

PROGNOSIS AND THERAPY

As mentioned earlier, patients tend to have mental retardation and seizures of variable severity. Refractory seizures may require surgical management in the form of hemispherectomy (corticectomy) (see Fig. 4-73). Such radical surgery is more successful and less morbid when undertaken early in life. Hemiparesis may develop spontaneously and worsen with time, or it may develop after hemispherectomy for seizure control. Bilateral involvement of the brain is associated with a poor prognosis. Occasionally, plastic facial surgery may be neces-

---

STURGE-WEBER SYNDROME—PATHOLOGIC FEATURES

Gross and Microscopic Findings

▶ Multiple thin-walled, ectatic vessels cover the pial surface
▶ Microscopically, penetrating vessels may have thickened walls with calcifications, and the cortex shows atrophy and gliosis of adjacent parenchyma

Genetics

▶ Not defined

Differential Diagnosis

▶ Arteriovenous malformations, although they lack facial involvement

---

sary in involved sites such as the eyelids or lips, which can undergo secondary ulceration or trauma.

ATAXIA-TELANGIECTASIA

CLINICAL FEATURES

This autosomal recessive disorder is marked by cerebellar degeneration, immunodeficiency, tumor diathesis, and sensitivity to radiation. It occurs in 1 in 40,000 births and results from a mutation in the *ATM* gene located on 11q22-23. The gene is important in DNA repair. Mucocutaneous and conjunctival telangiectases (Fig. 4-74) become detectable by 3 or 4 years of age, at which time ataxia has already begun to be apparent. Loss of speech, myoclonus, and choreoathetosis ultimately develop, as do serious sinonasal and pulmonary infections related to impaired immune function, including reduced levels of IgA and IgG. Catastrophic intracranial bleeding can occur (see Fig. 4-74). In longer-surviving individuals, hematologic and solid malignancies develop in 10% to 15%.

RADIOLOGIC FEATURES

Cerebellar cortical atrophy affecting the vermis to a greater degree than the hemispheres may be visible on CT or MRI. Secondary dilatation of the fourth ventricle and sulcal prominence may be noted. Acute intra-

---

ATAXIA-TELANGIECTASIA—FACT SHEET

Definition and Clinical Features

▶ Cerebellar degeneration, immunodeficiency, tumor diathesis, sensitivity to radiation
▶ Mucocutaneous and conjunctival telangiectases, loss of speech, myoclonus, choreoathetosis
▶ Serious sinonasal and pulmonary infections are related to impaired immune function

Incidence/Prevalence

▶ 1 in 40,000 births

Radiologic Features

▶ Cerebellar cortical atrophy affecting the vermis is visible on CT or MRI
▶ Secondary dilatation of the fourth ventricle may be noted
▶ Acute intraparenchymal hemorrhages are visible, although the causative telangiectases are not

Prognosis and Treatment

▶ Wheelchair required by the end of the first decade because of ataxia
▶ Bacterial and viral respiratory tract infections are chronic
▶ Catastrophic intracranial bleeding can occur
▶ In longer-surviving individuals, hematologic and solid malignancies develop in 10% to 15%

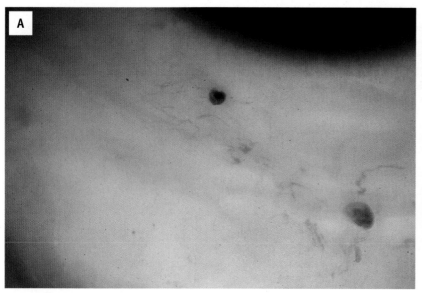

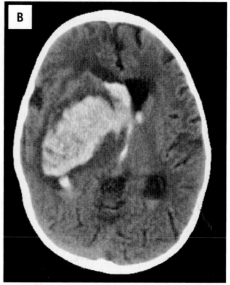

FIGURE 4-74

Ataxia-telangiectasia. **A**, Conjunctival telangiectases. (Courtesy of Dr. M. E. McLaughlin, Boston.) **B**, MRI of a patient suffering a massive intra-cerebral hemorrhage. (Courtesy of Dr. M. Silvera, Boston.)

parenchymal hemorrhages may be variable in size; the causative telangiectases are not usually discernible by neuroimaging (see Fig. 4-74).

PATHOLOGIC FEATURES

Cerebellar cortical atrophy may be seen grossly as decreased cerebellar weight with wide separation of the folia. Microscopically, the atrophy is characterized by loss of Purkinje and granule cells, as well as Bergmann gliosis and thinning of the molecular layer with corresponding atrophy of the inferior olive. There have been reports of Lewy body–like inclusions in the substantia nigra, posterior column degeneration, and anterior horn cell loss.

ATAXIA-TELANGIECTASIA—PATHOLOGIC FEATURES

Gross and Microscopic Findings

▶ Cerebellar cortical atrophy (decreased cerebellar weight with wide separation of the folia) is seen grossly
▶ Microscopically, loss of Purkinje and granule cells, Bergmann gliosis and thinning of the molecular layer, atrophy of the inferior olive
▶ Cytomegaly and nuclear atypia in the anterior pituitary and peripheral nerve
▶ Depletion of lymphoid tissues such as the thymus and lymph nodes and dilated vascular channels in the skin and conjunctiva

Genetics

▶ Mutation in the *ATM* gene located on 11q22-23
▶ Autosomal recessive inheritance

Differential Diagnosis

▶ Inherited spinocerebellar degeneration

Vascular telangiectases may be difficult to find in the CNS, even when death is due to massive intraparenchymal hemorrhage. Cytomegaly and nuclear atypia have been seen in many tissues, including the anterior pituitary, and in Schwann cells of peripheral nerves. There may be depletion of lymphoid tissue such as the thymus and lymph nodes, in addition to the dilated vascular channels in the skin and conjunctiva (see Fig. 4-74).

PROGNOSIS AND THERAPY

Most affected children require the use of a wheelchair by the end of the first decade because of ataxia. Therapy is centered on prevention of complications of bacterial and viral respiratory tract infections, which are usually chronic. As mentioned previously, intracranial bleeding and the development of malignancies impose significant limits on the quality and length of life of these patients.

COWDEN'S DISEASE

CLINICAL FEATURES

Cowden's disease, an autosomal dominant condition, is characterized by verrucous skin changes, cobblestone papules of the oral cavity, multiple trichilemmomas, colonic hamartomatous polyps, thyroid nodules, and an increased risk for breast cancer. The defective gene, *PTEN/MMAC1*, is located on chromosome 10q23 and encodes a protein that regulates phosphatidylinositol 3′-kinase, which is involved with growth control, cell migration, and cell survival. The CNS lesion is known as Lhermitte-Duclos disease (or dysplastic gangliocytoma) (Fig. 4-75) and is often seen in patients with Cowden's disease. Clinically, affected individuals have cerebellar signs and symptoms, primarily ataxia or increased intracranial pressure from a mass effect in the posterior fossa. Lhermitte-Duclos disease, which usually comes to attention in the third or fourth decade, may be the first manifestation of the syndrome and should prompt surveillance for systemic lesions, especially breast malignancy. About half of patients with Lhermitte-Duclos disease have Cowden's disease. These patients may also have mental retardation or epilepsy.

RADIOLOGIC FEATURES

Neuroimaging of the cerebellum in Cowden's disease may identify the typical folial thickening and T2 hyperintensity, which can at times mimic an enhancing malignancy

(see Fig. 4-75). The lesion usually involves one hemisphere, sometimes the vermis, and is only rarely bilateral.

PATHOLOGIC FEATURES

The hallmark of Lhermitte-Duclos disease (a feature of Cowden's disease) is coarsening and expansion of the folia on the surface of the affected cerebellar hemisphere (the lesion is nearly always unilateral). On cut section, the gray-white distinction between the cerebellar cortical layers and the underlying folial and deep hemispheric white matter may be blurred. The dentate nucleus may also be obscured. Histologically, a loosely "inside-out" pattern of organization may be appreciated, with enlarged ganglion cells resembling Purkinje cells and small neurons resembling granule cells in the deep aspect of the folia, as well as disoriented myelinated

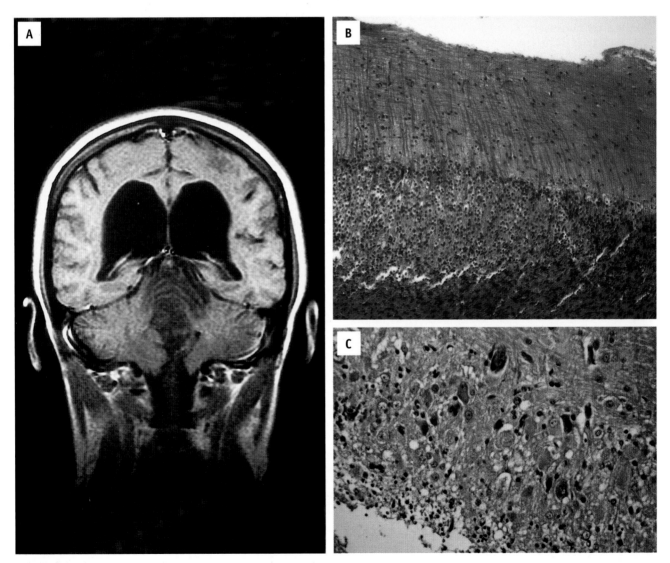

FIGURE 4-75

Lhermitte-Duclos disease. **A**, Coronal MRI of the cerebellum, which has markedly thickened folia in the midline and a mass effect causing hydrocephalus. (Courtesy of Dr. L. Hsu, Boston.) **B**, Cerebellar cortex with abnormal myelinated fibers (*blue*) in the molecular layer (Luxol fast blue stain for myelin). **C**, Bizarre, Purkinje-like cells in the deep aspect of the thickened folia.

COWDEN'S DISEASE—FACT SHEET

Definition and Clinical Features

▶ Verrucous skin changes, cobblestone papules of the oral cavity, multiple trichilemmomas, colonic hamartomatous polyps, thyroid nodules, and an increased risk for breast cancer

▶ CNS lesion known as Lhermitte-Duclos disease (or dysplastic gangliocytoma of the cerebellum)

▶ Affected individuals present with cerebellar signs and symptoms, such as ataxia or increased intracranial pressure from a mass effect in the posterior fossa, in the third or fourth decade

▶ About half of patients with Lhermitte-Duclos disease have Cowden's disease

▶ Patients with Cowden's disease may also have mental retardation or epilepsy

Radiologic Features

▶ Expansion of the cerebellar folia with T2 signal abnormality, usually unilateral

▶ A mass effect may obstruct the fourth ventricle and lead to hydrocephalus

Prognosis and Treatment

▶ Surgery may be necessary to remove abnormal tissue and relieve the mass effect

▶ Recurrences are rare, and no adjuvant therapy is needed

▶ Surveillance is required for associated malignancies such as breast cancer

---

fibers running along the surface (see Fig. 4-75). Large, dysplastic-appearing ganglion cells, isolated and in small groups, may also occupy any layer. The lesion may be hamartomatous (malformative) rather than neoplastic given its very low mitotic rate, although lesions occasionally do grow or recur. Other CNS lesions in Cowden's disease include megalencephaly and heterotopia (as discussed elsewhere in this chapter).

COWDEN'S DISEASE—PATHOLOGIC FEATURES

Gross and Microscopic Findings

▶ Folia thickening and distortion, blurring of gray-white distinction grossly

▶ Microscopically, "inside-out" pattern of organization with enlarged ganglion cells resembling Purkinje cells and small neurons resembling granule cells in the deep aspect of the folia, as well as disoriented myelinated fibers running along the surface

Genetics

▶ The defective gene, *PTEN/MMAC1*, is located on chromosome 10q23 and encodes a protein that regulates phosphatidylinositol 3′-kinase

▶ Autosomal dominant inheritance

Differential Diagnosis

▶ On small biopsy specimens, the lesion may resemble ganglioglioma

---

DIFFERENTIAL DIAGNOSIS

Lhermitte-Duclos disease may be confused with a neoplasm such as ganglioglioma on small surgical biopsy specimens, which may be undertaken occasionally if neuroimaging is indeterminate.

PROGNOSIS AND THERAPY

Surgical removal of the Lhermitte-Duclos lesion can resolve the cerebellar ataxia or mass effect; recurrences are rare.

NEUROCUTANEOUS MELANOSIS

CLINICAL FEATURES

This syndrome is defined as diffuse melanocytosis (proliferation of melanocytes in the leptomeninges) and giant or multiple congenital nevi of the skin, including the congenital nevus of Ota. The cutaneous nevi are usually midline and often involve the head and back of the neck, with the most extensive lesions covering the back and buttocks as well. Approximately 10% of patients with large congenital nevi also have leptomeningeal melanocytosis, whereas 25% of individuals with meningeal lesions have pigmented lesions on the skin, including giant nevi. These conditions have been proposed to represent "nevomelanocytic neurocristopathies," or developmental abnormalities of the neural crest. A responsible gene has not been identified.

NEUROCUTANEOUS MELANOSIS—FACT SHEET

Definition and Clinical Features

▶ Diffuse proliferation of melanocytes in the leptomeninges, giant or multiple congenital nevi of the skin, including the congenital nevus of Ota

▶ Cutaneous nevi are usually midline and often involve the head and back

▶ Ten percent of patients with large congenital nevi also have leptomeningeal melanocytosis, whereas 25% of individuals with meningeal lesions have pigmented lesions on the skin, including giant nevi

Radiologic Features

▶ Diffuse membranous or plaque-like thickening and enhancement of the leptomeninges

Prognosis and Treatment

▶ Diffuse melanocytosis may cause hydrocephalus and cranial and spinal nerve root symptoms

▶ Primary leptomeningeal melanoma may arise and has same poor prognosis as metastatic melanoma to the CNS

RADIOLOGIC FEATURES

By neuroimaging, diffuse membranous or plaque-like thickening and enhancement of the leptomeninges are evident. Short–repetition time/short–echo time MRI sequences reveal hyperintensity, which is thought to be indicative of melanin deposits.

PATHOLOGIC FEATURES

On gross examination of the brain, spinal cord, or both, a dense black-brown discoloration overlies the affected surfaces and may lead to internal hydrocephalus because of interference with CSF resorption and circulation over the base of the brain. Smaller, localized lesions may be nodular (melanocytomas) or plaque-like. Microscopically, melanocytosis has cytologic features resembling those of cutaneous nevi, with polygonal cells having prominent nucleoli and cytoplasmic melanin. These cells generally remain localized to the leptomeninges, although they may penetrate down the Virchow-Robin perivascular spaces in the superficial cortex or subpial zones of the brain stem and spinal cord. Primary malignant melanomas of the leptomeninges (Fig. 4-76) have cytologic atypia and invasion, just as in their cutaneous counterparts. Like cutaneous melanocytic lesions, CNS melanocytosis shows immunohistochemical reactions for S-100 protein and HMB-45; the cells are negative for keratins or other epithelial or glial markers. Electron microscopy demonstrates typical melanosomes, premelanosomes, or both.

NEUROCUTANEOUS MELANOSIS—PATHOLOGIC FEATURES

Gross and Microscopic Findings

▶ Dense black-brown discoloration overlying the affected surfaces grossly
▶ Smaller, localized lesions may be nodular (melanocytomas) or plaque-like
▶ Microscopically, melanocytosis resembles cutaneous nevi, with polygonal cells having prominent nucleoli and cytoplasmic melanin
▶ Primary malignant melanoma of the leptomeninges shows cytologic atypia and invasion
▶ Immunohistochemically, cells are positive for S-100 protein and HMB-45 and are negative for keratins or other epithelial or glial markers
▶ Electron microscopy demonstrates melanosomes

Genetics

▶ Not defined

Differential Diagnosis

▶ Pigmented nerve sheath tumors of the spinal nerve root can mimic a melanocytoma
▶ Distinction between a localized meningeal melanocytoma and primary or metastatic melanoma relies on the finding of cytologic features of malignancy, including invasion, mitoses, necrosis

---

DIFFERENTIAL DIAGNOSIS

Pigmented nerve sheath tumors, if localized to the portion of nerve root just adjacent to the cord, could mimic a melanocytoma. Distinction between diffuse melanocytosis and primary malignant melanoma of the

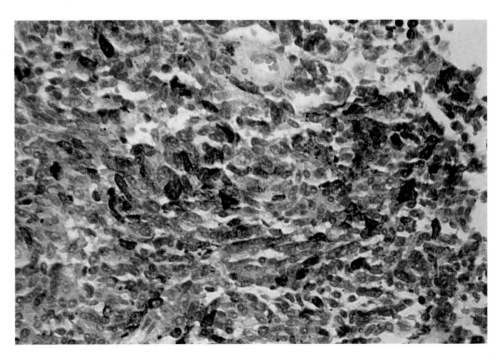

FIGURE 4-76
Neurocutaneous melanosis: primary leptomeningeal melanoma arising in a patient with diffuse leptomeningeal melanocytosis. Note the abundant melanin pigment produced by cells with large nuclei and prominent nucleoli.

leptomeninges can be quite difficult on small biopsy samples. Likewise, distinction between a localized meningeal melanocytoma and primary or metastatic melanoma relies on the finding of cytologic features of malignancy, as well as perhaps a high proliferative index in the latter.

PROGNOSIS AND THERAPY

Despite the challenge in making a distinction between diffuse melanocytosis and primary leptomeningeal melanoma, the clinical outcomes of both are poor. The former leads to hydrocephalus, which can be quite difficult to control, and cranial and spinal nerve root symptoms can be debilitating. Malignant melanoma, whether nodular or diffuse, carries the same ominous prognosis as it does outside the CNS because of its relative resistance to both chemotherapy and radiotherapy.

FAMILIAL RETINOBLASTOMA

CLINICAL FEATURES

Retinoblastomas arising in both eyes, whether synchronously or metachronously, signify a familial tumor syndrome with germline mutations of the *RB* gene. Although "familial," most germline mutations in fact arise sporadically, with only 10% of cases demonstrating autosomal dominant inheritance. Individuals with the *RB* mutation have retinoblastomas earlier in life (usually within the first year), often have multifocal

retinal tumors, and also have a high risk for the later development of pineoblastoma (resulting in so-called trilateral retinoblastoma). In addition, osteosarcomas may arise either within or outside the radiation fields.

Infants and children up to the age of 3 years may present with a "white pupil" (leukocoria) that leads to ophthalmologic examination and subsequent CNS imaging. Older children may complain of pain in the eye or decreased vision.

RADIOLOGIC FEATURES

On CT, retinoblastomas are noted as calcified masses in the globe, usually posteriorly along the retinal margin. They tend to enhance after contrast administration. Spread along the optic nerve can be detected, somewhat better by MRI than by CT. Trilateral retinoblastoma has imaging characteristics as described for pineoblastoma.

PATHOLOGIC FEATURES

Macroscopically, the tumor is visible as a fluffy, white to tan mass occupying the vitreous (Fig. 4-77). Occasionally, streak-like extension of tumor along the ciliary body or iris may occur, and rarely, tumor may be exophytic beyond the confines of the globe. Microscopically, retinoblastoma arises from the nuclear layers of the retina and may spread as contiguous layers or as discrete foci to other points on the retinal surface. The tumor has the classic features of "small blue cells," often arranged in Flexner-Wintersteiner rosettes (with a central lumen) or Homer Wright rosettes (with central fibrillarity) (see Fig. 4-77). Mitoses and necrotic foci may be common. Like other primitive neuroectodermal

---

FAMILIAL RETINOBLASTOMA—FACT SHEET

Definition and Clinical Features
▶ Retinoblastomas arising in both eyes ("white pupil" or leukocoria), whether synchronously or metachronously, usually within the first year of life
▶ May have multifocal retinal tumors and also a high risk for later development of pineoblastoma ("trilateral retinoblastoma")
▶ Osteosarcomas may arise either within or outside the radiation fields

Radiologic Features
▶ On CT, retinoblastomas are enhancing calcified masses in the globe
▶ Spread along the optic nerve can be detected by MRI
▶ Trilateral retinoblastoma has imaging characteristics as described for pineoblastoma

Prognosis and Treatment
▶ Early enucleation can be curative in up to 95% of cases of isolated retinoblastoma, although invasion of the optic nerve, choroid, and extraocular soft tissues has a very low cure rate
▶ Bilateral or "trilateral" retinoblastoma has a high rate of mortality by the end of the first decade of life

---

FAMILIAL RETINOBLASTOMA—PATHOLOGIC FEATURES

Gross and Microscopic Findings
▶ Macroscopically, the tumor is a white-tan mass filling the vitreous; rarely, exophytic beyond the globe
▶ Microscopically, retinoblastoma arises from the nuclear layers of the retina and is made up of "small blue cells" in sheets and in Flexner-Wintersteiner rosettes (with a central lumen) or Homer Wright rosettes (with central fibrillarity)
▶ Mitoses and necrosis common
▶ Immunohistochemically positive for neural markers (neuron-specific enolase, NeuN, synaptophysin) or occasionally GFAP
▶ The pineal tumor of trilateral retinoblastoma is indistinguishable from sporadic pineal parenchymal tumors

Differential Diagnosis
▶ Rhabdomyosarcoma involving the orbit

Genetics
▶ Germline mutations of the *RB* gene on 13q14

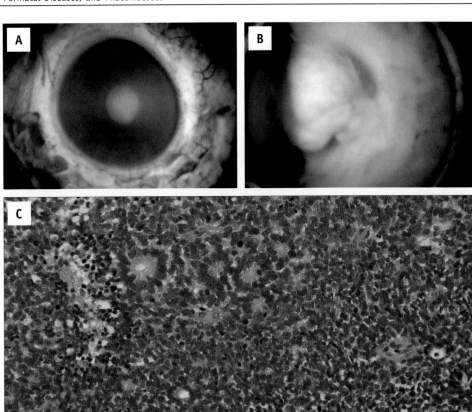

FIGURE 4-77

Retinoblastoma. **A**, Enucleation specimen with leukocoria (white visible through the pupil). **B**, Sagittal section through the eye globe (lens on the *left*) revealing a white, lobulated tumor mass arising from the retina and nearly filling the posterior chamber. (Courtesy of Dr. E. Bundock, Boston.) **C**, Histologic section showing residual retina (bottom of the field) and a "small blue cell" appearance of the tumor with numerous rosettes and focal necrosis.

tumors to which retinoblastoma is analogous, tumor cells may be stained immunohistochemically for neural markers (neuron-specific enolase, NeuN, synaptophysin) or occasionally GFAP. Spread along the optic nerve and into the choroid and extraocular soft tissues indicates a high stage of disease.

The pineal tumor of trilateral retinoblastoma has features resembling those of intraocular retinoblastoma and pineoblastoma (i.e., a poorly differentiated, aggressive, "small blue cell" tumor).

DIFFERENTIAL DIAGNOSIS

The differential diagnosis is limited because of the fairly classic gross and histologic features; however, occasional confusion can arise with other "small blue cell" tumors of childhood that can involve the orbital contents, such as embryonal rhabdomyosarcoma. The latter expresses markers of muscle, such as desmin or myoglobin, and lack neural or glial markers.

PROGNOSIS AND THERAPY

Invasion of the optic nerve, choroid, and extraocular soft tissues is associated with a very low cure rate. Enucleation before such spread, however, can be curative in up to 95% of cases of isolated retinoblastoma. In contrast, bilateral or "trilateral" retinoblastoma has a high rate of mortality by the end of the first decade of life because of the difficulty of resection of pineal tumors, the high incidence of subarachnoid spread of "small blue cells," and the frequent occurrence of osteosarcomas.

LI-FRAUMENI SYNDROME

CLINICAL FEATURES

This autosomal dominant disorder results in numerous primary neoplasms in childhood or early adult life. A wide

---

LI-FRAUMENI SYNDROME—FACT SHEET

Definition and Clinical Features

▶ See Table 4-5
▶ Numerous primary neoplasms in childhood or early adult life, including astrocytomas, medulloblastomas, cerebral hemispheric primitive neuroectodermal tumors, choroid plexus and ependymal tumors, meningiomas and schwannomas, sarcomas of bone and soft tissues, breast cancer, and with a lesser frequency, leukemia, visceral epithelial malignancies, and adrenocortical carcinoma

Radiologic Features

▶ CNS tumors are identical on neuroimaging to those arising sporadically

Prognosis and Treatment

▶ For each tumor, the prognosis and treatment are similar to that of the sporadically occurring counterpart; however, the overall survival of patients with multiple tumors is reduced

---

TABLE 4-5

Diagnostic Criteria for Li-Fraumeni Syndrome

For the full syndrome (all of the listed features):

  Sarcoma before age 45

  First-degree relative with any tumor before age 45

  Another first- or second-degree relative with cancer before age 45 or sarcoma at any age

For the variant:

  Three separate primary cancers, one arising before age 45

      or

  Childhood cancer or Li-Fraumeni–related tumor before age 45

      and

  First- or second-degree relative with any cancer arising before age 60

---

variety of brain tumors, including astrocytomas, medulloblastomas, cerebral hemispheric primitive neuroectodermal tumors, choroid plexus and ependymal tumors, meningiomas, and schwannomas, have been reported to occur in affected families. In addition, affected individuals are at high risk for the development of sarcomas of bone and soft tissue, breast cancer, and with a lesser frequency, leukemia, visceral epithelial malignancies, and adrenocortical carcinoma. Diagnostic criteria for both the full-blown syndrome and the variant condition are listed in Table 4-5. Most patients with Li-Fraumeni syndrome have a germline mutation in *TP53*, a tumor suppressor gene. In Li-Fraumeni kindreds, as in sporadic populations, there is a bimodal distribution of CNS tumors such that medulloblastomas, peripheral neuroectodermal tumors, and choroid plexus carcinomas tend to develop in children whereas astrocytomas develop in adults.

RADIOLOGIC FEATURES, PATHOLOGIC FEATURES, DIFFERENTIAL DIAGNOSIS, AND PROGNOSIS AND THERAPY

The neuroimaging, neuropathology, and treatment of tumors in patients with Li-Fraumeni syndrome are not

different from those arising sporadically in the general population. In Li-Fraumeni syndrome, gliomas may be multicentric, a more ominous factor. In addition, surveillance for the development of initial or additional tumors may be intensified in members of these families.

TURCOT'S SYNDROME

CLINICAL FEATURES

In this syndrome, medulloblastomas or high-grade gliomas arise along with adenomatous polyps and carcinomas of the colon. Type 1 Turcot's syndrome encompasses glioblastomas in patients without familial adenomatous polyposis and with or without hereditary non–polyposis-associated colorectal carcinoma; these families have germline mutations of DNA mismatch repair genes, such as *hMLH1*, *hMSH2*, or *hPMS2*. Glioblastomas may develop at an overall younger age

---

LI-FRAUMENI SYNDROME—PATHOLOGIC FEATURES

Gross and Microscopic Findings

▶ Depending on the tumor, identical to sporadic forms
▶ Gliomas may be multicentric, an unusual feature in patients without Li-Fraumeni syndrome

Genetics

▶ Autosomal dominant disorder caused by a germline mutation for *TP53*, a tumor suppressor gene

---

TURCOT'S SYNDROME—FACT SHEET

Definition and Clinical Features

▶ Medulloblastomas or high-grade gliomas arise along with adenomatous polyps and carcinomas of the colon
  ▶ Type 1: glioblastomas in patients without familial adenomatous polyposis (FAP) and with or without hereditary non–polyposis-associated colorectal carcinoma; glioblastomas arise at a younger age than in sporadic cases
  ▶ Type 2: medulloblastomas in individuals with FAP

Radiologic Features, Prognosis and Treatment

▶ Brain tumors are identical to those arising sporadically and are treated in the same manner

---

TURCOT'S SYNDROME—PATHOLOGIC FINDINGS

Gross and Microscopic Findings
▶ Identical to sporadically occurring medulloblastomas and gliomas

Genetics
▶ Type 1: germline mutations of the DNA mismatch repair genes *hMLH1*, *hMSH2*, or *hPMS2*
▶ Type 2: germline mutations of the *APC* gene

GORLIN'S SYNDROME—PATHOLOGIC FEATURES

Gross and Microscopic Findings
▶ Identical to the lesions seen sporadically

Genetics
▶ Inherited in an autosomal dominant fashion
▶ Germline mutation in *PTCH* on chromosome 9q22.3

---

than in sporadic cases. In type 2, individuals with familial adenomatous polyposis (germline mutations of the *APC* gene) present with medulloblastomas.

RADIOLOGIC FEATURES, PATHOLOGIC FEATURES, DIFFERENTIAL DIAGNOSIS, AND PROGNOSIS AND THERAPY

The tumors arising in Turcot's syndrome do not show apparent differences from those occurring spontaneously and are treated similarly.

GORLIN'S SYNDROME

CLINICAL FEATURES

Gorlin's syndrome, also known as the nevoid basal cell carcinoma syndrome, is, like many of the familial tumor conditions, inherited in an autosomal dominant fashion. In addition to the multiple cutaneous basal cell carcinomas arising initially in childhood, these patients also demonstrate odontogenic keratocysts of the jaws, palmar and plantar dyskeratoses, skeletal malformations, and ovarian fibromas. Medulloblastomas, intracranial calcifications (particularly of the falx cerebri), macrocephaly (see the relevant section), agenesis of the corpus callosum (see the earlier section "Midline/Commissural Defects"), congenital hydrocephalus, and meningiomas are among the CNS manifestations that have been described. Other neoplasms reported in association with Gorlin's syndrome include melanomas, leukemias and lymphomas, and breast and lung carcinomas. The syndrome results from a germline mutation in *PTCH* on chromosome 9q22.3; 40% of cases represent new mutations (i.e., without a previous family history).

RADIOLOGIC FEATURES, PATHOLOGIC FEATURES, DIFFERENTIAL DIAGNOSIS, AND PROGNOSIS AND THERAPY

The medulloblastomas occurring in patients with Gorlin's syndrome tend to be the desmoplastic subtype, but otherwise are not distinguishable on neuroimaging or neuropathology from their sporadic counterparts. Radiotherapy for medulloblastomas has been associated with subsequent accelerated appearance and growth of cutaneous basal cell carcinomas in the radiation field.

GORLIN'S SYNDROME—FACT SHEET

Definition and Clinical Features
▶ Also called nevoid basal cell carcinoma syndrome because of multiple cutaneous basal cell carcinomas arising starting in childhood
▶ Odontogenic keratocysts of the jaws, palmar and plantar dyskeratoses, skeletal malformations, ovarian fibromas, medulloblastomas, intracranial calcifications, macrocephaly, agenesis of the corpus callosum, congenital hydrocephalus, and meningiomas may develop
▶ Less common neoplasms include melanomas, leukemias and lymphomas, and breast and lung carcinomas

Radiologic Features, Prognosis and Treatment
▶ Imaging and treatment modalities for lesions of Gorlin's syndrome are the same as those in patients without Gorlin's syndrome

---

SUGGESTED READINGS

General

Barkovich A: Pediatric Neuroimaging, 3rd ed. Philadelphia, Lippincott Williams &Wilkins, 2000.
Encha-Razavi F, Folkerth R, Harding B: Congenital malformations and perinatal diseases. In Gray F, De Girolami U, Poirier J (eds): Escourolle & Poirier Manual of Basic Neuropathology, 4th ed. Philadelphia, Butterworth Heinmann, 2004, pp 249-267.
Freide R: Developmental Neuropathology, 2nd ed. Berlin, Springer-Verlag, 1989.
Graham DI, Lantos PL: Greenfield's Neuropathology, 7th ed. London, Arnold, 2002.
Jones K: Smith's Recognizable Patterns of Human Malformations, 4th ed. Philadelphia, WB Saunders, 1988.
Online Mendelian Inheritance in Man: http://www.ncbi.nlm.nih.gov/entrez/query.fcgi?db = OMIM
Stevenson R, Hall J, Goodman R: Human Malformations and Related Anomalies. New York, Oxford University Press, 1993.

Microcephaly/Macrocephaly

Stevenson D, Sunshine P: Fetal and Neonatal Brain Injury, 2nd ed. New York, Oxford University Press, 1997.
Volpe JJ: Neurology of the Newborn, 4th ed. Philadelphia, WB Saunders, 2001.

Neural Tube Closure Defects

Czeizel AE, Dudas I: Prevention of the first occurrence of neural-tube defects by periconceptional vitamin supplementation. N Engl J Med 1992;327:1832-1835.

Gilbert JN, Jones KL, Rorke LB, et al: Central nervous system anomalies associated with meningomyelocele, hydrocephalus, and the Arnold-Chiari malformation: Reappraisal of theories regarding the pathogenesis of posterior neural tube closure defects. Neurosurgery 1986;18:559-564.

Golden JA, Chernoff GF: Multiple sites of anterior neural tube closure in humans: Evidence from anterior neural tube defects (anencephaly). Pediatrics 1995;95:506-510.

Herman JM, McLone DG, Storrs BB, Dauser RC: Analysis of 153 patients with myelomeningocele or spinal lipoma reoperated upon for a tethered cord. Presentation, management and outcome. Pediatr Neurosurg 1993;19:243-249.

Rauzzino M, Oakes WJ: Chiari II malformation and syringomyelia. Neurosurg Clin N Am 1995;6:293-309.

Holoprosencephaly Sequence

Ming JE Muenke M: Holoprosencephaly: From Homer to Hedgehog. Clin Genet 1998;53:155-163.

Porter JA, Young KE, Beachy PA: Cholesterol modification of hedgehog signaling proteins in animal development. Science 1996;274:255-259.

Roessler E, Belloni E, Gaudenz K, et al: Mutations in the human Sonic Hedgehog gene cause holoprosencephaly. Nat Genet 1996;14:357-360.

Neuronal Migration Defects

Feng Y, Walsh CA: Protein-protein interactions, cytoskeletal regulation and neuronal migration. Nat Rev Neurosci 2001;2:408-416.

Mochida GH, Walsh CA: Genetic basis of developmental malformations of the cerebral cortex. Arch Neurol 2004;61:637-640.

Midline/Commissural Defects

Davila-Gutierrez G: Agenesis and dysgenesis of the corpus callosum. Semin Pediatr Neurol 2002;9:292-301.

Jellinger K, Gross H, Kaltenback E, Grisold W: Holoprosencephaly and agenesis of the corpus callosum: Frequency of associated malformations. Acta Neuropathol (Berl) 1981;55:1-10.

Rosser TL, Acosta MT, Packer RJ: Aicardi syndrome: Spectrum of disease and long term prognosis in 77 females. Pediatr Neurol 2002;27:343-346.

Posterior Fossa Malformations

Golden JA, Rorke LB, Bruce DA: Dandy-Walker syndrome and associated anomalies. Pediatr Neurosci 1987;13:38-44.

Hatten ME, Heintz N: Mechanisms of neural patterning and specification in the developing cerebellum. Annu Rev Neurosci 1995;18:385-408.

Morgan JI, Smeyne RJ: Transgenic approaches to cerebellar development. Perspect Dev Neurobiol 1997;5:33-41.

Disruption of Developing Gray and White Matter and Perinatal Hemorrhage

Kinney HC, Back SA: Human oligodendroglial development: Relationship to periventricular leukomalacia. Semin Pediatr Neurol 1998;5:180-189.

Kinney HC, Haynes RL, Folkerth RD: White matter lesions in the perinatal period. In Golden JA, Harding BN (eds): Pathology and Genetics: Acquired and Inherited Diseases of the Developing Nervous System. Basel, ISN Neuropath Press, 2004, pp 156–170.

Leviton A, Gilles FH: Acquired perinatal leukoencephalopathy. Ann Neurol 1984;16:1-8.

Marin-Padilla M: Developmental neuropathology and impact of perinatal brain damage. I: Hemorrhagic lesions of neocortex. J Neuropathol Exp Neurol 1996;55:758-773.

Skullerud K, Skjaeraasen J: Clinicopathological study of germinal matrix hemorrhage, pontosubicular necrosis, and periventricular leukomalacia in stillborn. Childs Nerv Syst 1988;4:88-91.

Stevenson D, Sunshine P: Fetal and Neonatal Brain Injury, 2nd ed. New York, Oxford University Press, 1997.

Volpe JJ: Neurobiology of periventricular leukomalacia in the premature infant. Pediatr Res 2001;50:553-562.

Hippocampal Sclerosis

Blumcke I, Thom M, Wiestler OD: Ammon's horn sclerosis: A maldevelopmental disorder associated with temporal lobe epilepsy. Brain Pathol 2002;12:199-211.

Lewis DV, Barboriak DP, MacFall JR, et al: Do prolonged febrile seizures produce medial temporal sclerosis? Hypotheses, MRI evidence, and unanswered question. Prog Brain Res 2002;135:263-278.

Trisomy Defects

Golden JA, Schoene WC: Central nervous system malformations in trisomy 9. J Neuropathol Exp Neurol 1993;52:71-77.

Lubec G, Engidawork E: The brain in Down syndrome (trisomy 21). J Neurol 2002;249:1347-1356.

Familial Malformation/Tumor Syndromes

Ball S, Arolker M, Purushotham AD: Breast cancer, Cowden disease and PTEN-MATCHS syndrome. Eur J Surg Oncol 2001;27:604-606.

Barbagallo JS, Kolodzieh MS, Silverberg NB, Weinberg JM: Neurocutaneous disorders. Dermatol Clin 2002;20:547-560.

Classon M, Harlow E: The retinoblastoma tumour suppressor in development and cancer. Nat Rev Cancer 2002;2:910-917.

Clifford SC, Maher ER: Von Hippel-Lindau disease: Clinical and molecular perspectives. Adv Cancer Res 2001;82:85-105.

Comi AM: Pathophysiology of Sturge-Weber syndrome. J Child Neurol 2003;18:509-516.

Hamilton SR, Liu B, Parsons RE, et al: The molecular basis of Turcot's syndrome. N Engl J Med 1995;332:839-847.

Kandt RS: Tuberous sclerosis complex and neurofibromatosis type 1: The two most common neurocutaneous diseases. Neurol Clin 2003;21:983-1004.

Kimmelman A, Liang BC: Familial neurogenic tumor syndromes. Hematol Oncol Clin North Am 2001;15:1073-1084.

Kleihues P, Cavenee WK: Pathology and Genetics of Tumours of the Nervous System. Lyon, France, IARC Press, 2000.

Manfredi M, Vescovi P, Bonanini M, Porter S: Nevoid basal cell carcinoma syndrome: A review of the literature. Int J Oral Maxillofac Surg 2004;33:117-124.

Marsh D, Zori R: Genetic insights into familial cancers—update and recent discoveries. Cancer Lett 2002;181:125-164.

Narayanan V: Tuberous sclerosis complex: Genetics to pathogenesis. Pediatr Neurol 2003;29:404-409.

Perlman S, Becker-Catania S, Gatti RA: Ataxia-telangiectasia: Diagnosis and treatment. Semin Pediatr Neurol 2003;10:173-182.

Shibata D, Aaltonen LA: Genetic predisposition and somatic diversification in tumor development and progression. Adv Cancer Res 2001;80:83-114.

Tucker T, Friedman JM: Pathogenesis of hereditary tumors: Beyond the "two-hit" hypothesis. Clin Genet 2002;62:345-357.

Varley JM: Germline TP53 mutations and Li-Fraumeni syndrome. Hum Mutat 2003;21:313-320.

5 Dysmyelinating and Demyelinating Disorders

B. K. Kleinschmidt-DeMasters • Jack H. Simon

OVERVIEW OF LEUKODYSTROPHIES

Leukoencephalopathies, white matter disorders evident on neuroimaging and histologic examination, can be due to a wide variety of causes, including nutritional conditions, infections, toxins, mitochondrial disorders, and vascular causes. The term "leukodystrophy" is usually confined to progressive diseases of myelin/myelin-forming cells with an underlying genetic cause and frequently with lysosomal and peroxisomal defects. The term "dysmyelinating" is also applied to leukodystrophies to indicate that the myelin that is formed is often not metabolically and functionally correct from the onset.

Today, leukodystrophies are most frequently diagnosed premortem by the clinical history; physical examination; neuroimaging studies; biochemical analysis of blood, urine, and cerebrospinal fluid; and nerve conduction studies. They rarely come to biopsy as they did in the 1950s and 1960s when definitive laboratory testing was unavailable. Brain biopsy is generally undertaken only if the disorder cannot be diagnosed by these other means, such as in Alexander's disease. By the time the pathologist encounters patients at the end stage of disease, at autopsy, the diagnosis has usually been well established.

In the uncommon cases in which the diagnosis has not been made in life, the diagnostic considerations for the pathologist revolve around other inherited disorders of white matter or multiple sclerosis (MS). In select instances, the differential diagnosis may include vitamin deficiencies (e.g., vitamin B_{12} deficiency), toxic conditions (e.g., solvent vapor/toluene leukoencephalopathy), metabolic disorders (e.g., central pontine myelinolysis), viral diseases (e.g., progressive multifocal leukoencephalopathy, subacute sclerosing panencephalitis, human immunodeficiency virus [HIV] leukoencephalopathy), hypoxic-ischemic disorders (carbon monoxide poisoning, hypoxic-ischemic hemorrhagic leukoencephalopathy), vascular diseases (CADASIL [cerebral autosomal dominant arteriopathy with subcortical infarcts and leukoencephalopathy]), and radiation/chemotherapy-induced white matter damage. Patient age, clinical history, laboratory studies, and additional special studies for viruses usually can quickly eliminate these other causes.

For clinicians, there are a few distinguishing features in the early phases of leukodystrophies. Variants of adrenoleukodystrophy and metachromatic leukodystrophy can develop from childhood to young adulthood, whereas Canavan's disease and Krabbe's disease are virtually always clinically evident in the early infant period.

Magnetic resonance imaging (MRI) can suggest the diagnosis based on a predilection for anterior cerebral involvement in metachromatic leukodystrophy and Alexander's disease. In contrast, posterior cerebral involvement of the parieto-occipital lobe white matter is characteristic of adrenoleukodystrophy and Krabbe's disease. Relative sparing of the arcuate fibers (U-fibers) helps distinguish several of the inherited leukodystrophies from MS, which often involves the arcuate fibers, but it is not generally helpful in the early stages of the disorder. Cystic changes in white matter can be seen in the infantile forms of Alexander's disease. Such changes, however, must be distinguished from large Virchow-Robin spaces, which can occur incidentally or as a result of hypertension. In general, leukodystrophies are characterized by bilateral symmetry of the lesions, although asymmetric changes can be seen in the early phases of leukodystrophies, especially adrenoleukodystrophy.

For the pathologist, a full general autopsy with complete neuropathologic examination, including removal of the spinal cord and sampling of the peripheral nerves, is recommended for cases that come to autopsy. Identification of abnormalities outside the central nervous system (CNS) can be helpful in corroborating the diagnosis. Adrenoleukodystrophy and metachromatic leukodystrophy both show accumulation of abnormal material within the cytoplasm of cells in systemic organs. Metachromatic leukodystrophy and Krabbe's disease are both characterized by involvement of the peripheral nervous system. The adult variants of adrenoleukodystrophy may manifest the brunt of the damage in the spinal cord and also demonstrate mild and variable changes in the peripheral nervous system. In contrast, histopathologic findings are confined to the CNS in Alexander's, Canavan's, and Pelizaeus-Merzbacher diseases.

ADRENOLEUKODYSTROPHY

CLINICAL FEATURES

Adrenoleukodystrophy is the most common inherited leukodystrophy. Clinically, three distinct manifestations of this X-linked disorder can be seen. The most frequent

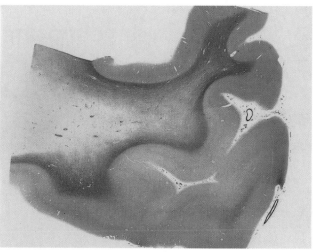

FIGURE 5-1

Adrenoleukodystrophy may be characterized by patchy myelin loss in early or less severe examples of the disease, but there is still relative sparing of myelin near the junction of gray and white matter (arcuate fibers, U-fibers) on this Luxol fast blue–periodic acid–Schiff (PAS)–stained whole-mount section.

ADRENOLEUKODYSTROPHY—FACT SHEET

Definition

▶ Inherited, X-linked, progressive peroxisomal disorder of myelin/myelin-producing cells caused by a deficiency of adrenoleukodystrophy protein (ALDP) and accumulation of very long chain fatty acids (VLCFAs)

Incidence and Location

▶ Disease incidence, 1 per 21,000 males; combined female and male incidence, 1 per 16,800 in the United States, nearly equivalent to phenylketonuria
▶ Involves the central nervous system and some visceral organs (adrenocortical fasciculata-reticularis zone, Leydig cells of the testis)
▶ Peripheral nervous system involvement mild and variable

Gender and Age Distribution

▶ Adrenomyeloneuropathy (40% to 45% of cases): young, adult male onset
▶ Childhood cerebral type (35% of cases): boys 4 to 8 years of age
▶ Primary adrenocortical insufficiency/Addison's disease (30% of cases): male children; adrenomyeloneuropathy may develop during adulthood
▶ Heterozygote female carriers: middle-aged onset in women

Clinical Features

▶ Adrenomyeloneuropathy: most common variant, progressive paraparesis, sphincter disturbances slowly progressive over decades; 25% to 40% may proceed to cerebral involvement and symptoms with a rapid downhill course after that point
▶ Childhood cerebral type: most severe variant, with deficits in cognition, vision, hearing, later motor disturbances; death in 2+ years
▶ Primary adrenocortical insufficiency: most common inherited form of Addison's disease, primary adrenal insufficiency
▶ Heterozygote female carriers: a third to half with mild adrenomyeloneuropathy, only 1% with adrenal insufficiency

Radiologic Features

▶ Confluent symmetric white matter lesions in the parieto-occipital lobes that advance in a caudal-rostral and outward progression, often across the splenium of the corpus callosum
▶ The margin and leading edge of a lesion typically show contrast enhancement
▶ Pontomedullary corticospinal tract involvement is common

Prognosis and Treatment

▶ Bone marrow transplantation most effective therapy for cerebral forms but must be used in early stages of the disease
▶ Dietary use of Lorenzo's oil in asymptomatic individuals (no benefit in patients with neurologic symptoms)
▶ Lovastatin, 4-phenylbutyrate are new therapeutic approaches
▶ Adrenal hormone replacement does not alter the neurologic course of disease

---

is adrenomyeloneuropathy (40% to 45% of cases), which affects young adult men. The childhood cerebral type (35% of cases) is the second most frequent and affects boys 4 to 8 years of age. Some children present with primary adrenal insufficiency (Addison's disease), but adrenomyeloneuropathy or cerebral demyelination develops later in life (Figs. 5-1 and 5-2). Heterozygote female carriers may also have mild symptoms of adrenomyeloneuropathy. Patients with cerebral types of the disease show deficits in cognition, hearing, and vision and die within a few years. Patients with adrenomyeloneuropathy experience progressive paraparesis and slowly progressive sphincter disturbances. Some patients have adrenocortical insufficiency.

PATHOLOGIC FEATURES

Except for the early predominance of posterior lobe involvement, the pattern at autopsy in advanced stages of disease is not particularly characteristic, although sparing of the arcuate fibers (U-fibers) may be seen. Demyelination is usually confluent and symmetric (Fig. 5-3). The signature histologic feature of adrenoleukodystrophy is its involvement of both CNS and selected systemic organ sites, including the adrenocortical fasciculata-reticularis zone and Leydig cells of the testis. In these areas, the cell cytoplasm contains linear, lamellar inclusions that grotesquely expand the cytoplasmic volume. In the brain, however, more macrophages contain bubbly myelin degradation products, which can overshadow the lamellar inclusions. Macrophages with myelin breakdown products generally show periodic acid–Schiff (PAS)-positive cytoplasmic staining, whereas those with lamellar inclusions show little or no

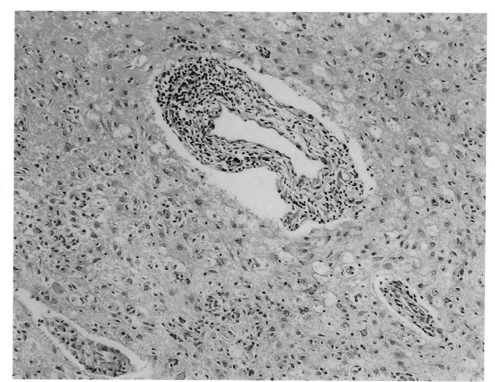

FIGURE 5-2

Adrenoleukodystrophy typically shows prominent perivascular lymphocytic inflammation in areas of active demyelination, coupled with hypercellularity as a result of numerous macrophages and reactive astrocytes.

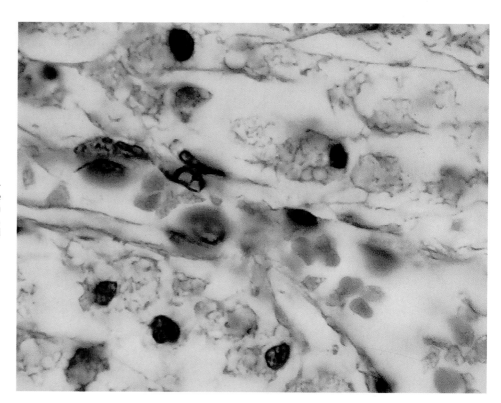

FIGURE 5-3

In adrenoleukodystrophy, macrophages within actively demyelinative lesions often predominantly contain bubbly myelin degradation products, not the pathognomonic striated lamellar material.

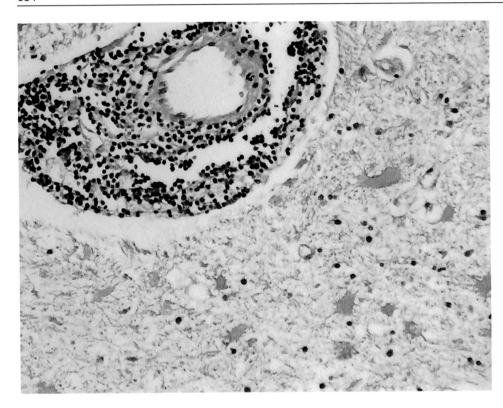

FIGURE 5-4
Adrenoleukodystrophy in the central, older portions of large demyelinative lesions may be characterized by few macrophages, but prominent reactive astrocytes and perivascular non-neoplastic lymphocytic cuffing are present.

ADRENOLEUKODYSTROPHY—PATHOLOGIC FEATURES

Gross Findings
► Confluent symmetric lesions in the parieto-occipital lobes that advance in a caudal-rostral progression
► Brownish discoloration and depression of the cerebral white matter, corpus callosum, posterior limb internal capsule, and optic system fibers
► Arcuate fibers relatively spared

Microscopic Features
► Childhood cerebral form: inflammatory demyelinating process with prominent perivascular lymphocytic cuffing by T cells and, to a lesser extent, B cells
► Numerous vacuolated macrophages that contain PAS-positive myelin debris
► Scattered macrophages with cytoplasm containing striated and cleft-like material; the amount of PAS positivity is inversely correlated with the striated (VLCFA material) content
► Reactive astrocytosis in demyelinated white matter
► Adrenocortical fasciculata-reticularis zone expanded by cells containing eosinophilic, cytoplasmic, lamellar, or striated material
► Adults with adrenomyeloneuropathy show myelin pallor and axonal loss in the ascending posterior columns (especially the gracile fasciculus) and descending corticospinal tracts, with little or no perivascular inflammation
► An inflammatory demyelinating process in the cerebrum will develop in some patients with adrenomyeloneuropathy
► Apoptosis of oligodendrocytes has been identified

Ultrastructural Features
► Macrophages contain either myelin debris and lipid droplets or the more specific lamellar-lipid profiles of VLCFAs

Immunohistochemical Features
► Lymphocytes at the edge of lesions are predominantly CD8 immunoreactive
► Astrocytes and macrophages may show tumor necrosis factor-α and interleukin-1 immunoreactivity

Genetics
► X-linked
► The gene for X-linked adrenoleukodystrophy maps to Xq28
► The gene codes for the peroxisomal membrane protein ALDP
► More than 400 mutations identified (mutations updated at *www.x.ald.nl*)
► No genotype-phenotype correlation

Differential Diagnosis
► Other inherited leukodystrophies
► Multiple sclerosis
► Progressive multifocal leukoencephalopathy

PAS-positive staining. The signature histologic feature of the cerebral lesions is the presence of intense, non-neoplastic perivascular lymphocytic cuffing composed predominantly of T cells (Fig. 5-4). Myelopathy is characterized by either no inflammation or only occasional perivascular lymphocytes. The spinal cord shows tract degeneration with axon and myelin loss in the ascending posterior columns and descending corticospinal tracts, most severe in the cervical cord. Peripheral nerve damage is variable and mild and always lacks inflammation. Skin may show hyperpigmentation as a result of Addison's disease (Figs. 5-5 to 5-7).

DIFFERENTIAL DIAGNOSIS

Although distinguishing adrenoleukodystrophy from most cases of typical relapsing-remitting MS is not problematic, MS with onset in early childhood can be severe, show confluent demyelination, and be associated with perivascular lymphocytes. Hence, the single leukodystrophy most confused with MS is adrenoleukodystrophy. It is of historical interest that although Schilder originally described three cases of inflammatory leukodystrophy between 1912 and 1924, in retrospect one was adrenoleukodystrophy, whereas the others were severe acute MS and subacute sclerosing panencephalitis, thus underscoring the overlapping features of several types of inflammatory white matter disorders.

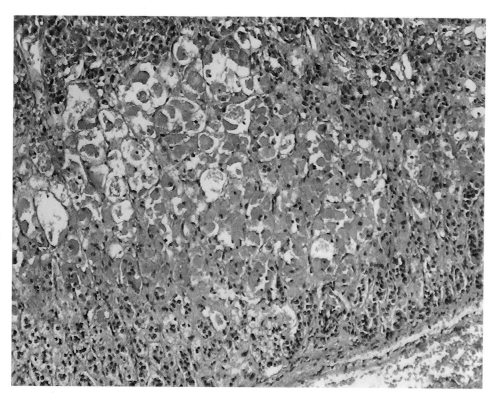

FIGURE 5-5
Adrenoleukodystrophy causes changes in systemic organs, with the adrenocortical cells in the fasciculata-reticularis zones showing severe distortion because of storage of eosinophilic cytoplasmic material.

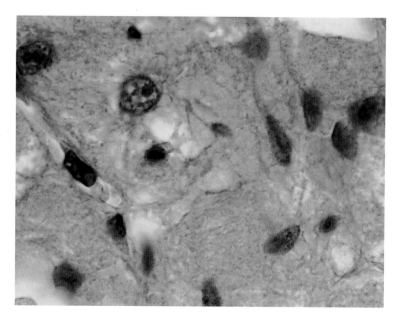

FIGURE 5-6
Adrenoleukodystrophy is caused by the accumulation of very long chain fatty acids and produces storage of characteristic, striated, lamellar cytoplasmic material in the central nervous system (CNS) and select systemic organ sites, seen here at high power in cells of the adrenocortical fasciculata-reticularis zones.

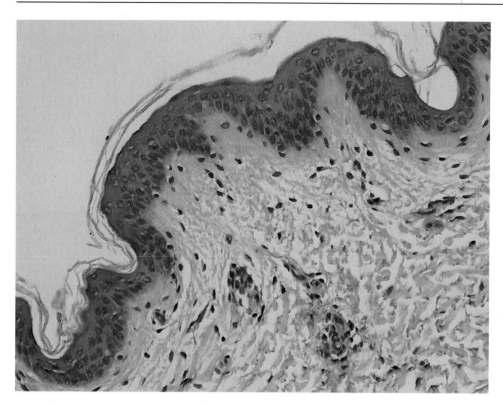

FIGURE 5-7
Adrenoleukodystrophy may be manifested as Addison's disease and show hyperpigmentation of the skin.

METACHROMATIC LEUKODYSTROPHY

CLINICAL FEATURES

Metachromatic leukodystrophy is an autosomal recessive disorder that occurs in three different forms: a late

---

METACHROMATIC LEUKODYSTROPHY—FACT SHEET

Definition

▶ Inherited, autosomal recessive, progressive storage disorder of myelin-producing cells usually caused by a deficiency of the lysosomal enzyme arylsulfatase A and the accumulation of sulfatide

Incidence and Location

▶ Deficiency of the lysosomal enzyme arylsulfatase A has an estimated incidence of 1 per 40,000 to 100,000
▶ Multiple sulfatase deficiency, only 50+ reported cases
▶ Deficiency of saposin D is least frequent cause of sulfatide accumulation
▶ Involves the central and peripheral nervous systems, as well as some visceral organs (renal tubules, gallbladder)

Gender and Age Distribution

▶ Late infantile form: onset at 1 to 3 years of age
▶ Juvenile/adolescent form: onset in late childhood/early teens
▶ Adult form: onset in the 20s to 30s

Clinical Features

▶ Late infantile form: most common variant; ataxia, dysarthria, dysphagia, loss of walking, vision, hearing, cognition; death in several years
▶ Juvenile/adolescent form: symptoms as above, but slower progression
▶ Adult form: behavior changes, psychosis, inappropriate behavior, frontal lobe syndrome with emotional lability and altered judgment, dementia in end stages

Radiologic Features

▶ Computed tomography (CT) and MRI show nonenhancing lesions, particularly of the deep white matter
▶ Preferential involvement of the frontal lobes; may show posterior progression
▶ Lesions usually bilateral, symmetric or nearly symmetric, and confluent; generally sparing the subcortical U-fibers
▶ The cerebellum may be involved, but less so than supratentorially
▶ Cerebral atrophy in advanced stages of disease
▶ In adrenomyeloneuropathy, cerebral white matter lesions are often present

Prognosis and Treatment

▶ Bone marrow transplantation for patients with mild nervous system involvement or for at-risk, asymptomatic relatives
▶ Bone marrow transplantation does not influence peripheral nervous system involvement
▶ Gallbladder surgery may be required for occasional patients with sulfatide-containing gallstones

infantile type with onset at 1 to 3 years of age, a juvenile adolescent type with onset in late childhood or the early teens, and an adult form that usually develops in the 20s or 30s. The clinical features are significantly different in the late infantile and the adult forms. The late infantile form is characterized by ataxia, dysarthria, dysphagia, cognitive problems, and death within several years. In contrast, individuals with the adult form often have striking behavioral changes and psychosis as a result of the frontal lobe predominance of involvement. The clinical diagnosis is frequently delayed in the adult form.

PATHOLOGIC FEATURES

Except for the early predominance of frontal lobe involvement, the pattern at autopsy in advanced stages

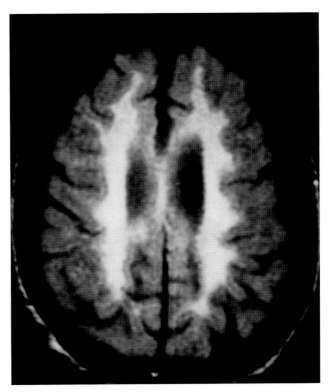

FIGURE 5-8

Metachromatic leukodystrophy in advanced stages demonstrates severe, diffuse ventricular white matter hyperintensity and lateral ventricular enlargement on magnetic resonance imaging (MRI). (Courtesy of Dr. Christopher Filley.)

METACHROMATIC LEUKODYSTROPHY—PATHOLOGIC FEATURES

Gross Findings
- Confluent symmetric lesions with brownish discoloration of white matter
- Cerebral atrophy and hydrocephalus ex vacuo in late stages of the disease
- Cerebellum and brain stem affected and atrophic

Microscopic Features
- The central and peripheral nervous systems show severe demyelination with accumulation of metachromatic material in macrophages
- Metachromatic material is pink on toluidine blue staining and brown on cresyl violet staining at acid pH
- No lymphocytic perivascular cuffing
- Reactive astrocytosis
- Metachromatic granules found in macrophages of the lymph nodes and spleen and the epithelium of renal tubules, gallbladder, adrenal medulla, sweat glands, bile duct, and pancreatic islets

Ultrastructural Features
- Macrophages contain storage material with alternating electron-dense and electron-lucent lamellar structures in a herringbone pattern

Immunohistochemical Features
- No specific immunohistochemical features

Genetics
- Autosomal recessive
- The gene for arylsulfatase A maps to 22q13
- 40+ mutations identified
- Homozygosity for mutations abolishes enzyme function completely and causes the infantile forms
- Missense mutations leave 3% to 5% of normal enzyme activity but cause the adult forms of disease
- Patients who are heterozygous for a null mutation plus a mild missense mutation may have a juvenile phenotype

Differential Diagnosis
- Other inherited leukodystrophies
- Multiple sclerosis

---

of disease is not particularly characteristic, although sparing of the arcuate fibers (U-fibers) may be seen. Demyelination is usually confluent and symmetric (Fig. 5-8). The signature feature is that metachromatic leukodystrophy shows accumulation of metachromatic material in the brain, peripheral nerves, and widespread visceral sites, including the epithelium of the gallbladder, bile ducts, and renal tubules (Fig. 5-9). In the brain, there is severe demyelination unassociated with inflammation (Fig. 5-10). Macrophages contain abundant PAS-positive material in the cytoplasm, but it is only on staining for metachromatic material that the diagnosis can be made on tissue. When toluidine blue staining is performed, the metachromatic material is pink, and when acidic cresyl violet is used, the material is brown. Metachromasia refers to the fact that the original blue color of the dye has been changed ("meta") to a different color as a result of the presence of sulfatide-containing material.

DIFFERENTIAL DIAGNOSIS

Because of the lack of inflammation and symmetry, this leukodystrophy is not usually confused with severe acute MS (Figs. 5-11 and 5-12). If a full autopsy is performed, systemic involvement can be recognized. Cases with brain-only examination may prompt concern about a variety of other rare inherited leukodystrophies unless staining for metachromatic material is undertaken.

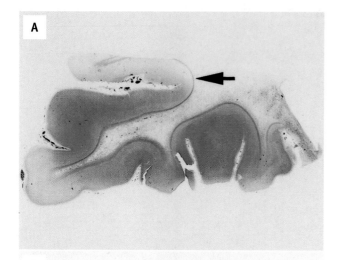

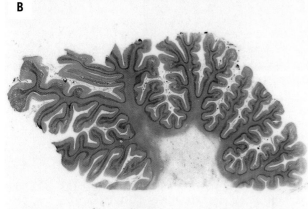

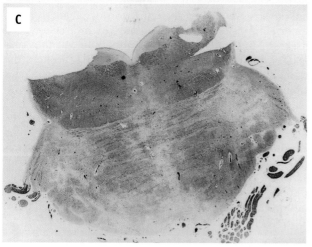

FIGURE 5-9

Metachromatic leukodystrophy at autopsy shows sparing of subcortical myelin (**A**, *arrow*, Luxol fast blue–PAS stain) even when the rest of the myelin is severely depleted; involvement extends beyond the cerebral hemispheric white matter into the cerebellar white matter (**B**) and brain stem (pons, **C**).

GLOBOID CELL LEUKODYSTROPHY (KRABBE'S DISEASE)

CLINICAL FEATURES

Krabbe's disease is an autosomal recessive disorder (Fig. 5-13). The overwhelming majority of patients with

---

GLOBOID CELL LEUKODYSTROPHY (KRABBE'S DISEASE)—FACT SHEET

Definition

▶ Inherited, autosomal recessive, progressive storage disorder of myelin-forming cells caused by a deficiency of the lysosomal enzyme galactosylceramidase (galactocerebrosidase β-galactosidase) and accumulation of psychosine (galactosylsphingosine)

Incidence and Location

▶ The infantile form has an estimated incidence of 1 per 100,000 to 200,000
▶ Involves the central and peripheral nervous systems

Gender and Age Distribution

▶ Infantile form: both sexes affected; infant is normal in first few months of life, followed by onset of symptoms at age 4 to 6 months
▶ Juvenile form: both sexes affected; onset at age 3 to 10 years
▶ Adult form: both sexes affected; onset usually in third to fifth decades

Clinical Features

▶ Infantile form: most common variant; hyperirritability, hypersensitivity to stimuli, some limb stiffness in the first few months of life, followed by severe mental deterioration, hypertonicity, optic atrophy; survival rare beyond 1½ years of age
▶ Juvenile form: progressive gait disturbance, spastic paraparesis, visual failure, dementia
▶ Adult form: slower progression of disease and patients may have normal life span; patients manifest progressive spastic paraparesis (pyramidal tract involvement may be asymmetric), limb weakness, and visual failure; intellectual function is usually intact; may have asymmetric neuropathy due to hypomyelination

Radiologic Features

▶ Confluent, symmetric periventricular lesions hyperintense on T2-weighted images and very rarely enhance
▶ On CT, lesions in deep gray matter and white matter may be hyperdense
▶ Cerebral atrophy in advanced disease stages

Prognosis and Treatment

▶ Bone marrow transplantation thus far has not altered the course of the infantile form
▶ Allogeneic hematopoietic stem cell transplants beneficial in a few patients with the juvenile form

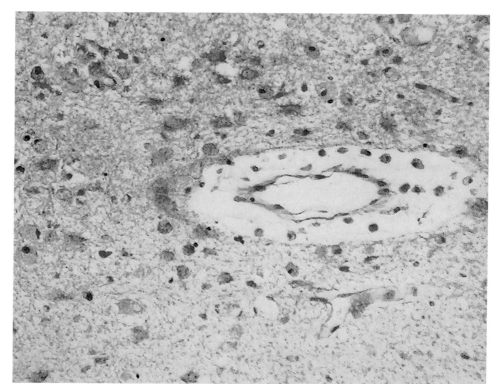

FIGURE 5-10

Metachromatic leukodystrophy features scattered macrophages within demyelinated areas, but no perivascular inflammation.

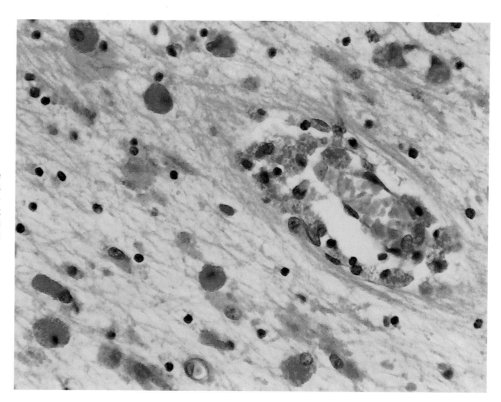

FIGURE 5-11

Metachromatic leukodystrophy, like most demyelinating disorders, shows macrophages that contain PAS-positive material; this stain does not help distinguish leukodystrophies from each other or from multiple sclerosis.

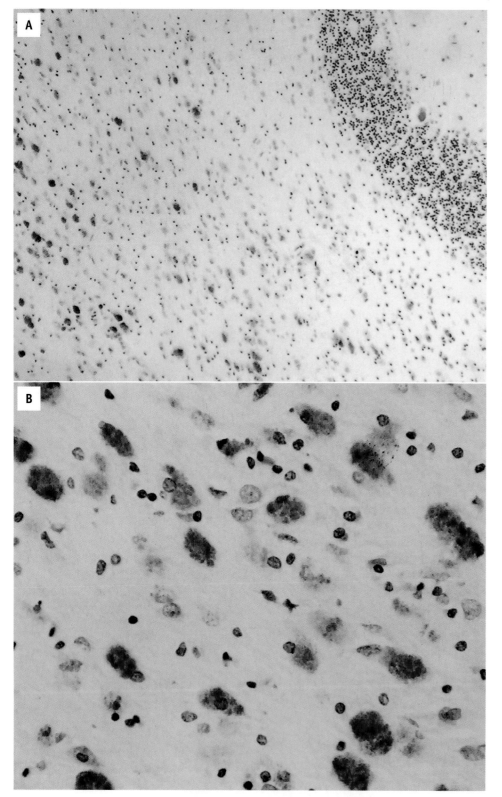

FIGURE 5-12
Metachromatic leukodystrophy can be distinguished from other leuko- dystrophies and multiple sclerosis by the use of acidic cresyl violet stain; this stain reveals, on low (**A**) and high (**B**) power, the brown, metachromatic cytoplasmic contents of macrophages, in contrast to the background blue stain of the dye.

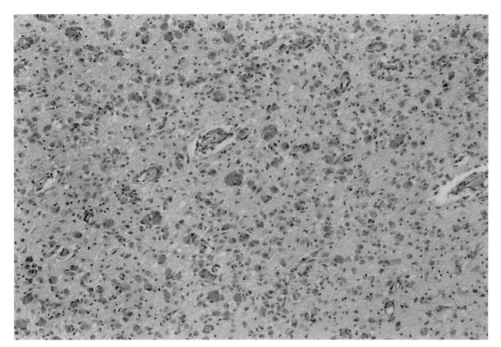

FIGURE 5-13
Krabbe's disease is now diagnosed by analysis for the defective enzyme, but before these laboratory tests were available, brain biopsies were conducted for diagnosis and the hypercellularity often simulated glioma.

globoid cell leukodystrophy are infants who acquire the disorder in the first year of life. Children are usually normal immediately after birth, but then progressive mental deterioration, hypertonicity, and optic atrophy develop. Survival is rare beyond 2 years of age. More recently, a rare adult form with slower progression has been recognized.

PATHOLOGIC FEATURES

Globoid cell leukodystrophy involves both the central and peripheral nervous systems, but no visceral organs (Fig. 5-14). Large confluent, nearly total demyelination in the CNS is present at the end stage of disease. The most characteristic histologic features are the presence of clusters of globoid cells (Fig. 5-15), which are

---

GLOBOID CELL LEUKODYSTROPHY (KRABBE'S DISEASE)— PATHOLOGIC FEATURES

Gross Findings
- ▶ Confluent symmetric demyelination with discolored, rubbery white matter
- ▶ Cerebral atrophy in the infantile form
- ▶ Peripheral nerves may be enlarged and firm

Microscopic Features
- ▶ Severe, nearly total myelin loss with relative sparing of subcortical arcuate fibers
- ▶ Characteristic multinucleated cells known as globoid cells arranged in clusters, especially around blood vessels
- ▶ Globoid cells represent mononuclear phagocytes that become multinucleated in response to phagocytosis of galactocerebroside; contain PAS-positive material
- ▶ Oligodendrocytes greatly decreased, with reactive astrocytosis
- ▶ Peripheral nerves show fibrosis, fibroblast proliferation, segmental demyelination, onion bulb formation, and perivascular PAS-positive macrophages

Ultrastructural Features
- ▶ Macrophages contain elongated tubular inclusions

Immunohistochemical Features
- ▶ No specific immunohistochemical features

Genetics
- ▶ Autosomal recessive
- ▶ Gene mapped to 14q25-31
- ▶ 65+ mutations described
- ▶ All adult forms have missense mutations at the 5′ end of the gene
- ▶ Genotype-phenotype correlations affected by polymorphisms

Differential Diagnosis
- ▶ Other inherited leukodystrophies
- ▶ Multiple sclerosis

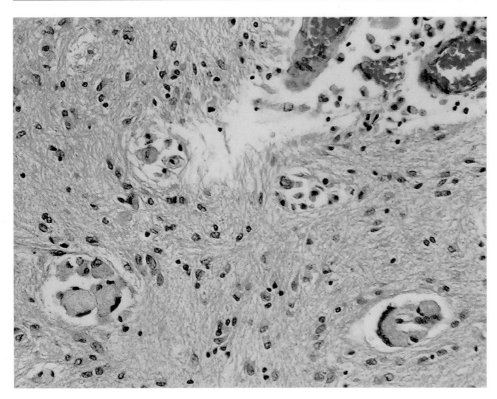

FIGURE 5-14
Krabbe's disease shows mononuclear and multinuclear bloated macrophages, but no perivascular lymphocytic inflammation in the demyelinated areas.

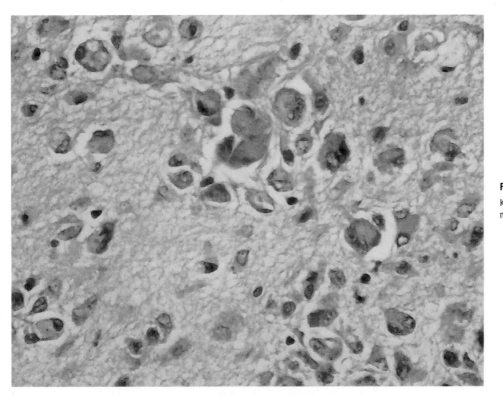

FIGURE 5-15
Krabbe's disease contains clusters of multinucleated "globoid cells."

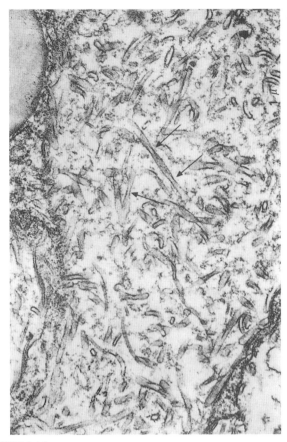

FIGURE 5-16

Krabbe's disease on electron microscopy shows accumulation of characteristic slender tubules (*arrows*) within the cytoplasm of macrophages. (Courtesy of Dr. Richard Prayson.)

multinucleated phagocytes. These cells represent phagocytosis of other mononuclear phagocytes in response to the galactocerebroside product that accumulates within them. Minimal lymphocytic inflammation is present. Oligodendrocytes are generally severely depleted. Peripheral nerves show fibroblastic proliferation, segmental demyelination, and accumulation of perivascular PAS-positive macrophages (Fig. 5-16).

DIFFERENTIAL DIAGNOSIS

Given the distinctive histologic features, usually little else enters the differential diagnosis. Some pathologists have noted that HIV leukoencephalopathy can also have multinucleated giant cells and could potentially be a diagnostic consideration. However, in cases of Krabbe's disease, the clustering and number of multinucleated giant cells greatly exceed that seen in HIV leukoencephalopathy, and the myelin loss is several-fold more severe.

ALEXANDER'S DISEASE

CLINICAL FEATURES

Alexander's disease is a dominant disorder but has so many new mutations that the inheritance pattern mimics a sporadic condition. It has infantile, juvenile, and adult forms, with the latter sometimes localized. Infants with the disease show developmental delay, megalencephaly, seizures, and progressive psychomotor retardation with spasticity and quadriparesis (Fig. 5-17). The infantile form is of greatest importance to pathologists because occasionally, the disorder comes to

---

ALEXANDER'S DISEASE—FACT SHEET

Definition
▶ Autosomal dominant, progressive disorder of astrocytes, usually caused by new mutations in the gene for glial fibrillary acid protein (GFAP); the disease is characterized by an excess of GFAP, diffuse or focal demyelination, and abundant Rosenthal fibers

Incidence and Location
▶ Rare
▶ Involves the CNS

Gender and Age Distribution
▶ Infantile form: onset in the first or second year of life, death 1 to 10 years after onset
▶ Juvenile form: both sexes affected; onset in older childhood
▶ Adult form: both sexes affected; onset in third to sixth decades but may manifest subtle symptoms earlier in life

Clinical Features
▶ Infantile form: developmental delay, megalencephaly, seizures, progressive psychomotor retardation, spasticity, quadriparesis
▶ Juvenile form: affected individuals more likely to exhibit bulbar signs; may not be significantly retarded and often do not have megalencephaly
▶ Adult form: signs are variable and can mimic multiple sclerosis; may manifest bulbar signs (dysphagia, dysphonia, dysarthria), hyperreflexia, dysautonomia, ataxia, sleep apnea; tendency for disease to affect medulla in particular and may lead to palatal myoclonus

Radiologic Features
▶ Extensive white matter involvement with frontal lobe predominance
▶ May be associated with cyst formation
▶ Arcuate fibers involved
▶ White matter may appear swollen with broadening of gyri
▶ Lesions often show a periventricular rim of low T2 and high T1 signal intensity
▶ Mild signal changes and swelling in the basal ganglia and thalamus; involvement of the brain stem and cerebellum

Prognosis and Treatment
▶ No specific therapy

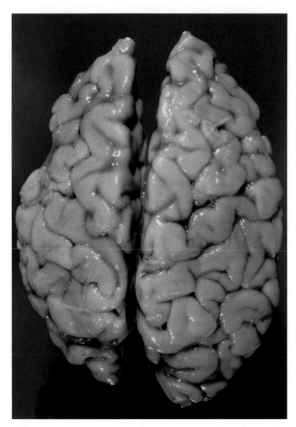

FIGURE 5-17
Alexander's disease, infantile form, may show macrocephaly and broadening of the gyri on gross brain examination. (Courtesy of Dr. Richard Prayson.)

surgical biopsy, since no systemic tests are available (Figs. 5-18 and 5-19).

PATHOLOGIC FEATURES

On biopsy specimens from patients with the infantile form, astrocytes may contain minute, eosinophilic, refractile intracytoplasmic bodies that represent pre-Rosenthal fibers. These fibers can be brought out with trichrome stain and immunostaining for glial fibrillary acidic protein. Few, if any, well-developed Rosenthal fibers may be present on biopsy material. However, by the time the patient comes to autopsy, the signature histologic feature is the presence of myriad elongated, sausage-shaped, refractile eosinophilic Rosenthal fibers (Figs. 5-20 and 5-21). These fibers are easily recognized on routine hematoxylin-eosin stain and are diffusely distributed throughout the brain in gray and white matter, but they particularly cluster in subpial and perivascular areas (Fig. 5-22). The disorder involves only the CNS. In infantile variants of Alexander's disease, deposition of Rosenthal fibers is associated with severe myelin loss and even cavitation of white matter. Occasional adult forms with more localized disease may show little or no myelin damage.

ALEXANDER'S DISEASE—PATHOLOGIC FEATURES

Gross Findings
▶ Infantile forms may show yellow-tan discoloration, gelatinous consistency, and even cyst formation in white matter
▶ Brain enlargement in early phases of the disease
▶ Cerebral atrophy in advanced disease stages
▶ Cortical gray matter, brain stem, and cerebellum usually preserved

Microscopic Features
▶ Striking accumulation of Rosenthal fibers
▶ Severe demyelination in the infantile forms, sometimes with cavitation
▶ Innumerable eosinophilic, elongated or rounded (in cross section), refractile Rosenthal fibers in white matter, especially in subpial and perivascular locations
▶ Inflammation and macrophage accumulation in some infantile cases
▶ Infantile forms show swollen astrocytes containing small cytoplasmic, eosinophilic hyaline granules representing miniature Rosenthal fibers
▶ Juvenile forms have less demyelination

Ultrastructural Features
▶ Rosenthal fibers composed of amorphous electron-dense material surrounded by 10-nm intermediate filaments

Immunohistochemical Features
▶ Rosenthal fibers usually stain poorly in the center, but the edges may be positive for β-crystallin, glial fibrillary acidic protein (GFAP), ubiquitin, and 27-kd heat shock protein

Genetics
▶ Most cases are caused by new mutations in the parental germline or the fetus and account for the majority of cases described as having a sporadic inheritance pattern
▶ The gene is autosomal dominant and acts as dominant negative
▶ Mutations in the gene for GFAP are responsible for the majority of cases

Differential Diagnosis
▶ Other inherited leukodystrophies

DIFFERENTIAL DIAGNOSIS

The profusion of Rosenthal fibers greatly exceeds that seen in neoplasms. Tumors that typically contain Rosenthal fibers include pilocytic astrocytomas, subependymomas, pleomorphic xanthoastrocytomas, and ganglion cell tumors, but they are not usually difficult to distinguish from Alexander's disease (Fig. 5-23). Histologically, however, the Rosenthal fibers are identical in both neoplastic and non-neoplastic conditions. On biopsy specimens, the aforementioned caveat should be remembered, namely, that the astrocytes may contain miniature intracytoplasmic pre-Rosenthal fibers rather than well-formed elongated structures.

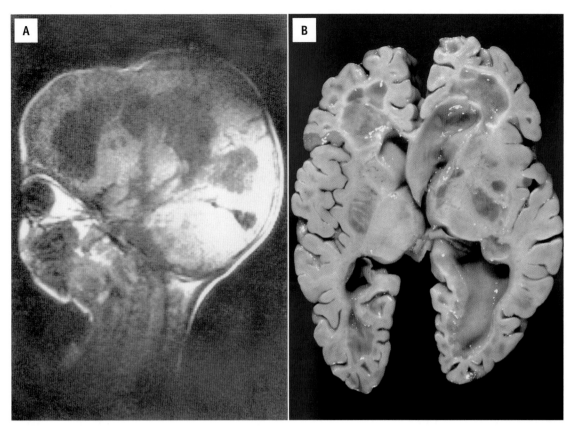

FIGURE 5-18

Alexander's disease, infantile form, often shows severe cystic change in white matter, most prominent in frontal lobes, on both premortem neuroimaging studies (**A**) and at autopsy (**B**, same child). (Courtesy of Dr. Richard Prayson.)

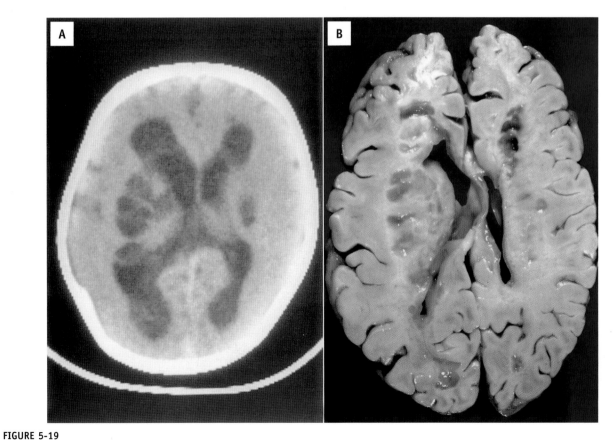

FIGURE 5-19

Alexander's disease, infantile form, illustrates the ease of detection for white matter diseases afforded by premortem neuroimaging studies, as well as the exquisite correlation that can be made between neuroimaging (**A**) and autopsy (**B**) findings.

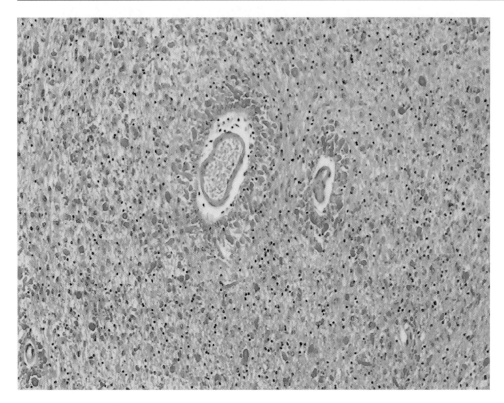

FIGURE 5-20

Alexander's disease manifests the characteristic histologic feature of massive Rosenthal fiber accumulation in central nervous system (CNS) sites, especially within the white matter and in perivascular locations.

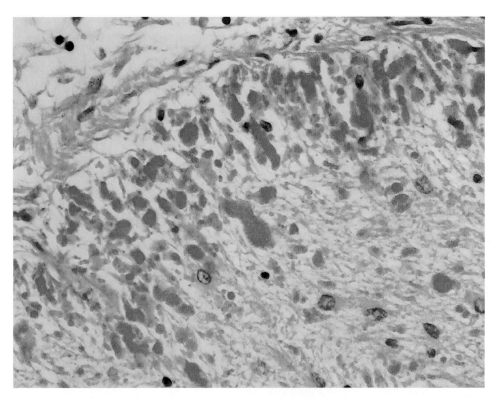

FIGURE 5-21

Alexander's disease is characterized by sausage-shaped, densely eosinophilic Rosenthal fibers in subpial locations; these fibers are histologically identical to the Rosenthal fibers seen in tumors or non-neoplastic chronic gliotic conditions, but they are many-fold more numerous, particularly in subpial and perivascular areas, in Alexander's disease than in neoplasms.

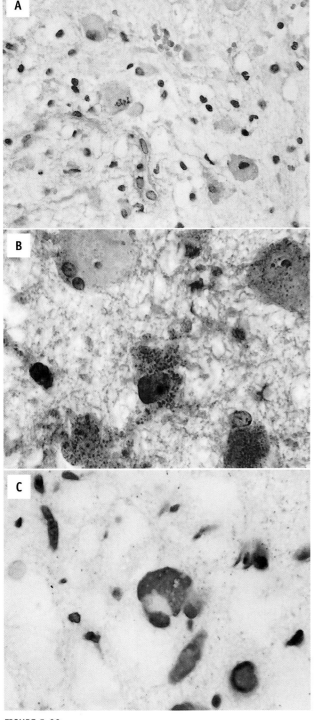

FIGURE 5-22

Alexander's disease still occasionally comes to biopsy, and infantile forms show a subtle intracytoplasmic accumulation of pre-Rosenthal material rather than the easily detectable, innumerable, seemingly "extracytoplasmic" Rosenthal fibers seen in later stages of the disease. These bloated astrocytes may be mistaken for macrophages on hematoxylin-eosin stain (**A**), but trichrome stain (**B**) brings out the speckled intracytoplasmic densities, and immunostaining for glial fibrillary acidic protein (**C**) clarifies their astrocytic nature.

CANAVAN'S DISEASE

CLINICAL FEATURES

Canavan's disease is a rare autosomal recessive disorder that is seen in the Ashkenazi Jewish population and much less frequently in non-Jewish groups. The most severe type is the infantile form, which has symptom onset very early in life, between the age of 10 weeks and 4 months. Canavan's disease is characterized by poor visual fixation and tracking, poor sucking, poor head control, and feeding difficulties. Survival is months to years and is variable.

CANAVAN'S DISEASE—FACT SHEET

Definition
▶ Inherited, autosomal recessive disorder of myelin/myelin-producing cells caused by a deficiency of the enzyme aspartoacylase and accumulation of *N*-acetylaspartate

Incidence and Location
▶ Most frequent in the Ashkenazi Jewish population, with a carrier frequency of 1 per 37.7 and an estimated disease frequency of 1 per 5000
▶ Canavan's disease is much less frequent in non-Jewish populations
▶ Involves the CNS

Gender and Age Distribution
▶ Infantile form: onset of symptoms between 10 weeks and 4 months
▶ Exceptional cases affect older children

Clinical Features
▶ Infantile form: poor visual fixation and tracking, poor sucking, irritability, poor head control, macrocephaly (>90th percentile), feeding difficulties, seizures; survival months to years
▶ Children may have sensorineural hearing loss because of alterations in the organ of Corti

Radiologic Features
▶ Proton nuclear magnetic resonance spectroscopy shows marked elevation of *N*-acetylaspartate in the brain
▶ MRI shows symmetric, diffuse, low signal intensity on T1-weighted images and high signal intensity on T2-weighted images
▶ U-fibers characteristically involved; relative sparing of the internal capsule
▶ Multiple cysts may be individually resolved
▶ Small ventricles initially; later, cerebral atrophy with ventricular enlargement

Prognosis and Treatment
▶ No specific therapy

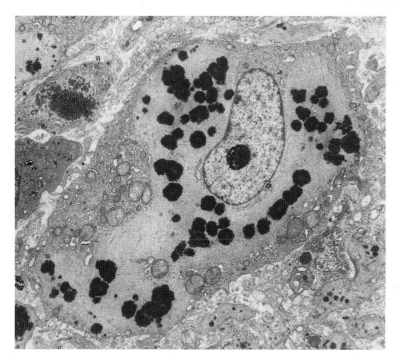

FIGURE 5-23
Alexander's disease, infantile form, on electron microscopy shows electron-dense, amorphous pre-Rosenthal material within the cytoplasm of astrocytes. (Courtesy of Dr. Gary Mierau.)

PATHOLOGIC FEATURES

Features of macrocephaly are striking in the early phases of the disease, but by the time the child comes to autopsy, brain weight may have normalized because of widespread cerebral atrophy. The disorder is confined to the CNS. The signature histologic feature is widespread vacuolization, usually in the subcortical white matter. More central areas of the white matter are totally devoid of myelin (Fig. 5-24). No inflammation is seen.

CANAVAN'S DISEASE—PATHOLOGIC FEATURES

Gross Findings
► Enlarged brain size
► Brain weight increased by 50% or more in the first 2 years of life
► Late in disease, brain weight decreases to near-normal levels
► Softening and gray-brown discoloration of white matter, including arcuate fibers, corpus callosum, internal capsules
► Preservation of cortical gray matter, basal ganglia, brain stem

Microscopic Features
► Widespread vacuolization especially severe at the cortical gray-white matter junction, with central white matter showing severe absence of myelin
► Oligodendrocytes and axons relatively preserved
► No inflammation
► Macrophages virtually absent, mild astrocytosis

Ultrastructural Features
► Electron microscopy shows that vacuoles are due to splitting of myelin lamellae at the intraperiod line
► Large vacuoles are electron lucent and "empty"
► Cortical cell bodies and astrocytic processes are severely swollen and contain elongated mitochondria with abnormal cristae

Immunohistochemical Features
► Myelin basic protein lines vacuoles

Genetics
► Autosomal recessive
► The gene codes for aspartoacylase, an enzyme necessary for the catabolism of N-acetylaspartate and N-acetylaspartoglutamate
► The gene maps to 17p13-ter
► Two mutations predominate in Jewish populations; mutations differ in non-Jewish populations
► No genotype-phenotype correlation

Differential Diagnosis
► Other inherited leukodystrophies

DIFFERENTIAL DIAGNOSIS

Other inherited leukodystrophies might be considerations, but the vacuolization of white matter is striking and distinctive in this disorder.

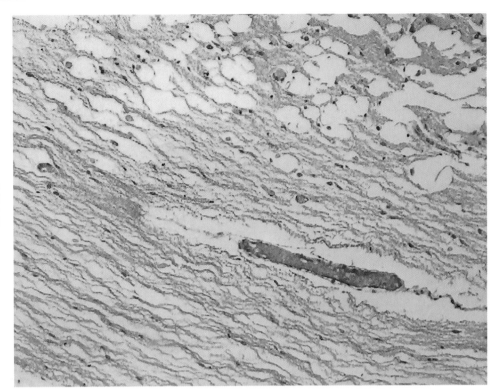

FIGURE 5-24
Canavan's disease demonstrates severe, nearly total absence of myelin, with characteristic vacuolization of myelin in the subcortical areas.

PELIZAEUS-MERZBACHER DISEASE

CLINICAL FEATURES

This rare X-linked disorder can have a fetal, young infant, or teenage onset in boys. Occasionally, neurologic symptoms also develop in female heterozygotes. Infants show abnormal eye movements with the first few months of life, followed by psychomotor deterioration, pyramidal tract signs, dystonia, and ataxia. Laryngeal stridor is seen. Older patients have mild spastic paraparesis that is slowly progressive over a period of decades.

PELIZAEUS-MERZBACHER DISEASE—FACT SHEET

Definition
▶ Inherited, X-linked recessive, progressive disorder of central myelin caused by a deficiency in proteolipid protein

Incidence and Location
▶ Rare
▶ Involves the CNS

Gender and Age Distribution
▶ Classic (type I), male: onset before 1 year of age
▶ Connatal (type II), male: fetal onset
▶ Transitional (type III), male: early teens

Clinical Features
▶ Classic (type I): presence of abnormal eye movements within the first few months of life, followed by psychomotor deterioration, bilateral pyramidal tract signs, dystonia, and ataxia by 2 years of age; laryngeal stridor is frequent
▶ Connatal (type II): reduction in intrauterine movements, congenital laryngeal stridor, severe psychomotor retardation
▶ Transitional (type III): mild spastic paraparesis slowly progressive over decades; ataxia and cognitive dysfunction in the late stage (X-linked spastic paraplegia type 2 and Pelizaeus-Merzbacher disease are allelic)
▶ Neurologic symptoms may develop in female heterozygotes

Radiologic Features
▶ MRI shows poor myelin formation when compared with age-matched controls
▶ Islands of very limited myelination; rarely, a diffuse "tigroid" pattern with islands of myelination as a striking manifestation
▶ White matter shows widespread high signal on T2-weighted images

Prognosis and Treatment
▶ No specific therapy

PATHOLOGIC FEATURES

Brain weight is considerably reduced, and the brain shows severe demyelination in early-onset forms; damage is confined to the CNS. The signature histologic feature is the presence of patchy, preserved islands of myelin, especially around blood vessels, in a so-called tigroid pattern. There is no inflammation.

PELIZAEUS-MERZBACHER DISEASE—PATHOLOGIC FEATURES

Gross Findings

► Brain weight reduced by a third to a half
► Cerebral white matter shows grayish discoloration
► Some sparing of arcuate fibers
► Optic nerves and brain stem, cerebellar, and spinal cord white matter atrophic

Microscopic Features

► Severe myelin loss in the deep cerebral white matter in the connatal form
► Patchy tigroid appearance of myelin damage because of preservation of perivascular islands of white matter
► Oligodendrocytes severely decreased, with apoptosis
► Increased astrocytosis
► Peripheral and cranial nerves intact in all forms because of the presence of different myelin structural protein in peripheral myelin (PMP-22)

Ultrastructural Features

► Almost no electron microscopic information available

Immunohistochemical Features

► No specific immunohistochemical features

Genetics

► X-linked recessive
► The gene maps to Xq22
► The gene codes for proteolipid protein (PLP), the main membrane protein of central myelin
► 40 different mutations identified, the most frequent of which leads to duplication of the *PLP* gene (two thirds of cases have duplications; the remainder are point mutations)
► Strong genotype-phenotype correlation, with duplications associated with a milder phenotype
► The classic form shows PLP accumulation in endoplasmic reticulum because of protein misfolding
► The severe connatal form shows PLP plus additional related protein (DM-20) accumulation in endoplasmic reticulum

Differential Diagnosis

► Other inherited leukodystrophies

DIFFERENTIAL DIAGNOSIS

Other early-onset inherited leukodystrophies may be considerations in some cases, particularly metachromatic leukodystrophy if staining for metachromasia is not undertaken. Diagnostic considerations in older patients with spastic paraparesis include various spinal cord degenerative diseases.

MULTIPLE SCLEROSIS

CLINICAL FEATURES

MS is one of the most frequent causes of acquired disability in young persons. Patients manifest variable neurologic signs and symptoms disseminated in time (defined as two or more sets of symptoms 30 + days apart) and space (two separate locations in the brain/spinal cord), without other identifiable causation. Early in the disease, paresthesias (numbness and tingling), monocular loss of vision, gait problems, weakness, double vision, urinary urgency or frequency, and constipation are characteristic. Cognitive dysfunction and fatigue are not uncommon, even in the relapsing stages of disease. Seizures and hearing loss are rare. The disease is typically initially relapsing and remitting, but more than half the patients eventually enter a secondary progressive stage with few relapses but cumulative deficits over time. At 15 years, 50% of patients require the use of a gait aid, and at 20 years, 50% use a wheelchair. About 10% to 15% of patients have "benign" MS with rare attacks and few cumulative deficits, although cognitive deficits may be present. Approximately 5% have rapidly progressive disease.

MULTIPLE SCLEROSIS—FACT SHEET

Definition

► Acquired, usually progressive chronic inflammatory disorder of the CNS that causes multiple demyelinating lesions "in space and time"; unknown cause

Incidence and Location

► Incidence of 8500 to 10,000 new cases per year in the United States
► The incidence increases with distance from the equator; high-incidence areas include the United Kingdom, Iceland, Canada, Australia, and the United States
► Demyelination confined to the CNS

Gender and Age Distribution

► Approximately three fourths of patients present between the ages of 15 and 45 years
► About two thirds of cases occur in women

MULTIPLE SCLEROSIS—FACT SHEET—cont'd

Clinical Features

▶ Relapsing-remitting type: 85% of cases; sporadic attacks with new or worsened symptoms over a period of 2 to 10 days and variable improvement over 1 to 6 months
▶ Primary progressive type: 15% of cases; progressive disease from the onset, without true relapses
▶ Secondary progressive: conversion to progressive disease in approximately 50% of relapsing-remitting patients
▶ Most patients have clinically isolated syndromes
▶ Cerebrospinal fluid usually shows a mild elevation in protein and lymphocytes, but glucose is always normal; most cases have oligoclonal bands

Radiologic Features

▶ Periventricular and, to a lesser extent, peripheral white matter T2-hyperintense lesions
▶ Supratentorial ovoid-shaped lesions
▶ Frequent cerebellar and brain stem surface lesions
▶ T1-weighted images often show "black holes," which represent focal areas of more severe injury
▶ Atrophy may be apparent early, as indicated by enlarged sulci, thinning of the corpus callosum, and widening of the third ventricle

Prognosis and Treatment

▶ The prognosis is variable, but at 15 years about 50% require a gait aid, and at 20 years about 50% need a wheelchair
▶ 10% to 15% have "benign" MS with rare attacks and little accumulated disability, although some may have important cognitive dysfunction
▶ 5% of patients have rapidly progressive disease
▶ Treatment includes medication for fatigue, spasticity, urinary and sexual dysfunction, pain, and depression
▶ Immunotherapies include corticosteroid for relapse, Betaseron (interferon beta-1b), Avonex (interferon beta-1a), Copaxone (glatiramer acetate), and Rebif (interferon beta-1a); secondary progressive disease is also treated with mitoxantrone

PATHOLOGIC FEATURES

Gross findings in patients with long-standing disease include mild to moderate cerebral atrophy and hydrocephalus ex vacuo. The optic nerves and chiasm may be grossly atrophic, and superficial plaques may be evident on the surface of the brain stem and corpus callosum or

MULTIPLE SCLEROSIS—PATHOLOGIC FEATURES

Gross Findings

▶ Patients with long-standing disease often have cerebral atrophy and hydrocephalus ex vacuo
▶ The optic nerves and chiasm may be grossly atrophic
▶ Superficial plaques may be evident on the surface of the brain stem and corpus callosum or lining the walls of the lateral ventricles
▶ Coronal sections show sharply outlined, gray-glistening patches of myelin loss, most of which range from 2 to 10 mm in diameter
▶ Predilection for demyelinative lesions to involve the periventricular/subependymal, perivenular, subpial, and gray-white junction locations

▶ The cerebrum, cerebellum, brain stem, spinal cord, and optic nerve/chiasm are variably involved, with at least two thirds of cases showing plaques in the cerebral, optic nerve, and spinal cord sites

Microscopic Features

▶ Subpial plaques are often wedge shaped, with a broad base adjacent to the subarachnoid space
▶ Periventricular lesions are variably coalescent
▶ Plaques involving gray matter (cortex, thalamus, basal ganglia, cerebellar cortex, gray matter of the spinal cord) are best seen with myelin stains
▶ Plaque activity is divided into active and inactive based on the presence or absence of macrophages; acute demyelination in lesions is characterized by the presence of macrophages that contain myelin debris stained with Luxol fast blue (LFB), and subacute activity in plaques is characterized by the presence of macrophages containing PAS-stained material; in most chronic plaques, any activity is confined to the perimeter of the plaque; very remote/chronic inactive plaques are devoid of any significant residual macrophages
▶ In acute MS, large numbers of LFB-positive macrophages are present throughout the plaque
▶ Remote plaques show severe loss of oligodendrocytes in the center of lesions and variable astrocytosis
▶ Remote plaques have variable numbers of perivascular lymphocytes and plasma cells
▶ Shadow plaques represent remyelinated lesions
▶ Axonal loss is present even in the early inflammatory stages; early oligodendrogliopathy may be more important than previously recognized

Ultrastructural Features

▶ Electron microscopy shows active breakdown of myelin initiated by macrophages that endocytose lysed myelin lamellae
▶ Oligodendrocytes occasionally have degenerative or apoptotic features
▶ No viral particles seen on electron microscopy

Immunohistochemical Features

▶ In actively demyelinating lesions, macrophages exhibit enhanced immunoreactivity for HLA-DR antigens and surface IgG
▶ Active lesions may show macrophages with immunostaining for MRP-14, a marker of early activation

Genetics

▶ In most populations, disease is associated with HLA-DR15 (a split of DR2)
▶ Concordance rate of 30% in monozygotic twins, 2% in dizygotic twins and siblings

Differential Diagnosis

▶ The clinical differential diagnostic list is broad and includes inherited leukodystrophies, viral diseases of central white matter (e.g., progressive multifocal leukoencephalopathy), nutritional/metabolic white matter disorders (e.g., vitamin B_{12} deficiency, central pontine myelinolysis), toxin exposure (solvent vapor abuse), and hypoxic-ischemic leukoencephalopathy (carbon monoxide, anoxic events)
▶ For pathologists who usually encounter disease at autopsy in patients with chronic, long-standing disease, the repetitive pattern of demyelinative lesions involving the characteristic periventricular, optic nerve/chiasm, spinal cord, and especially the perivenular sites makes gross diagnosis possible in the vast majority of cases

lining the walls of lateral ventricles when viewed from the mesial aspect. Coronal sections in typical relapsing-remitting MS reveal sharply outlined, gray-glistening patches of myelin loss, most of which range from 2 to 10 mm in diameter. These plaques show variable coalescence. Plaques in gray matter are not uncommon, but they may be more difficult to detect on the gross specimen and by MRI than white matter plaques. Active or acute plaques may be ill defined on the gross specimen, especially on freshly cut, unfixed brain. The plaque distribution pattern is virtually pathognomonic for the disease, with demyelinative lesions in periventricular/subependymal, perivenular, subpial, and gray-white junction locations (Figs. 5-25 and 5-26). Although the cerebrum, cerebellum, brain stem, spinal cord, and optic nerve/chiasm are variably involved, at least two thirds of patients have plaques in three of the sites: the cerebrum, optic nerve, and spinal cord.

Microscopically, plaques near the ventricles are immediately adjacent to the ependymal lining (Figs. 5-27 to 5-31). Subpial plaques are often wedge shaped, with the broad base adjacent to the subarachnoid space. Plaques at autopsy are usually either chronic active or chronic inactive. "Activity" is based on the presence or absence of macrophages. Chronic inactive plaques show hypocellularity, severe loss of oligodendrocytes, and astrocytosis, but no macrophages. Chronic inactive plaques may have variable numbers of perivascular lymphocytes and plasma cells. Chronic active plaques generally have hypocellular centers and PAS-positive macrophages confined to the edge of a large, otherwise inactive plaque

(Figs. 5-32 to 5-34). Acute demyelination is rarely seen in autopsy specimens, whereas in biopsy specimens of acute tumefactive demyelinating lesions, acute activity is often seen (Figs. 5-35 to 5-37). Acute myelin breakdown is characterized by the presence of macrophages that contain Luxol fast blue (LFB)-positive myelin debris.

DIFFERENTIAL DIAGNOSIS

The differential diagnosis premortem is broad and includes infections, infiltrative tumors, vitamin B_{12}

Text continued on p. 207

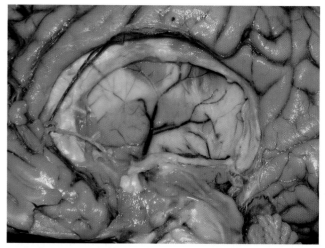

FIGURE 5-26

Multiple sclerosis at autopsy, as seen from the mesial aspect of the gross brain, may manifest ventricular enlargement, thinning of the corpus callosum, and brown-gray, well-demarcated plaques in the callosum and periventricular regions.

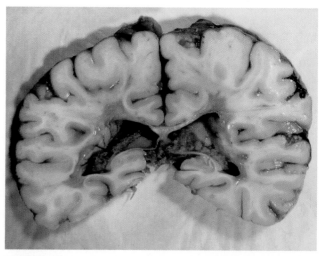

FIGURE 5-27

Multiple sclerosis at autopsy, on coronal sections, often shows relative symmetry of the demyelinative lesions, as illustrated by these confluent, bilateral, periventricular plaques. Note the linear plaque in the left cerebral white matter extending at right angles from the ventricular surface.

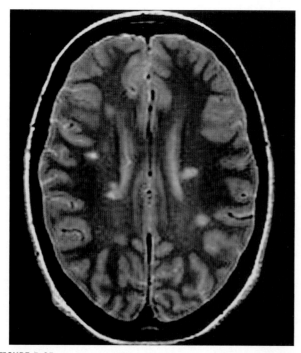

FIGURE 5-25

Multiple sclerosis on magnetic resonance imaging typically shows T2-hyperintense lesions in the periventricular and peripheral white matter; note that several periventricular lesions have an ovoid shape that extends at right angles to the ventricular surface.

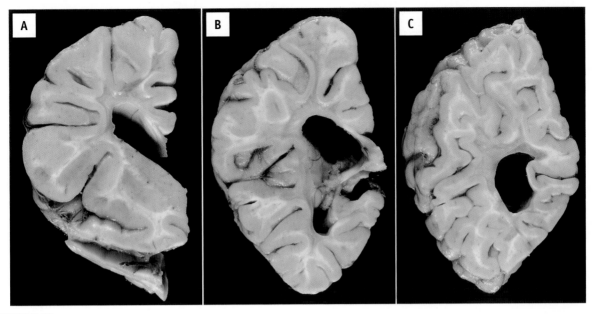

FIGURE 5-28

A-C, Multiple sclerosis at autopsy, on coronal sections, often demonstrates plaques that are immediately juxtaposed to the ventricular surface; they are depressed and associated with hydrocephalus ex vacuo. Note the more subtle plaques near the gray-white matter junctions (**A**).

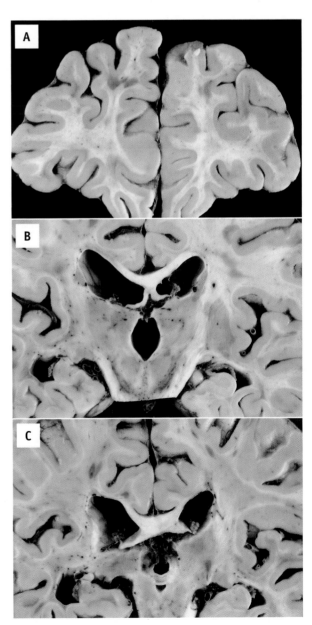

FIGURE 5-29

A-C, Multiple sclerosis at autopsy, on coronal sections, infrequently shows a predominance of plaques in the peripheral white matter and deep gray matter rather than the periventricular regions.

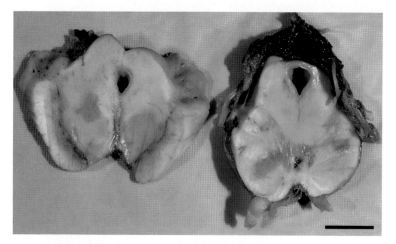

FIGURE 5-30

Multiple sclerosis at autopsy may manifest grossly visible plaques in brain stem sites, in this case associated with enlargement of the aqueduct of Sylvius.

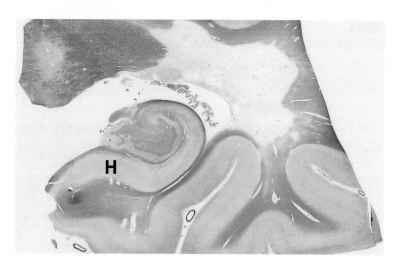

FIGURE 5-31

Multiple sclerosis is often associated with periventricular plaques near the temporal horn of the ventricle at the level of the hippocampus (H); note the characteristic sharp demarcation of the lesion from the surrounding white matter on this Luxol fast blue–PAS–stained whole-mount section.

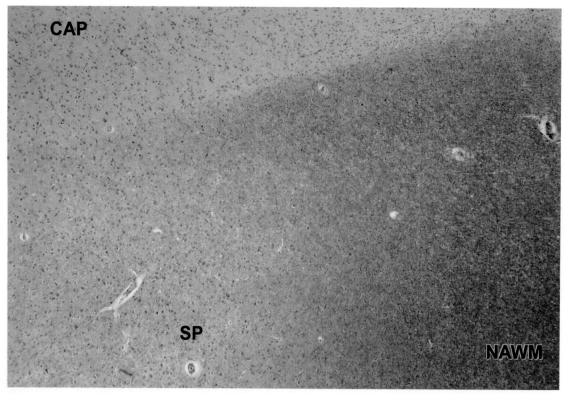

FIGURE 5-32

Multiple sclerosis may show complex lesions with a chronic active plaque (CAP) adjacent to a partially remyelinated, less well demarcated shadow plaque (SP) when compared with normal-appearing white matter (NAWM) (Luxol fast blue–PAS stain).

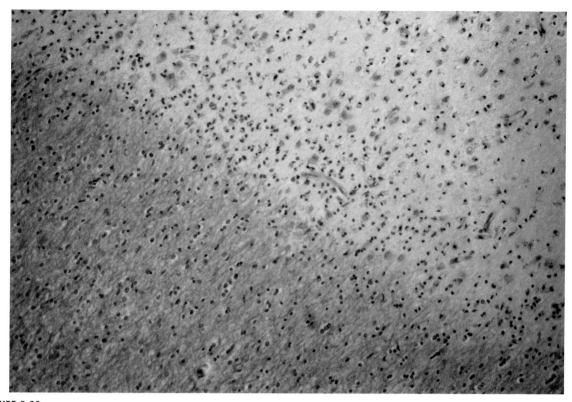

FIGURE 5-33

At autopsy, multiple sclerosis may show a few (or many) chronic active plaques with hypocellular centers, but hypercellularity at the perimeter (Luxol fast blue–PAS stain).

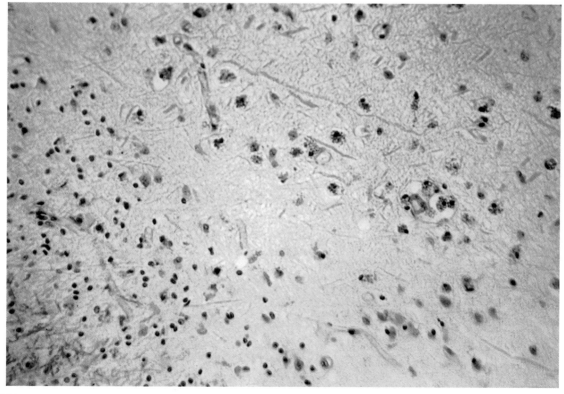

FIGURE 5-34

Chronic active plaques of multiple sclerosis are characterized by the presence of PAS-positive macrophages (Luxol fast blue–PAS stain).

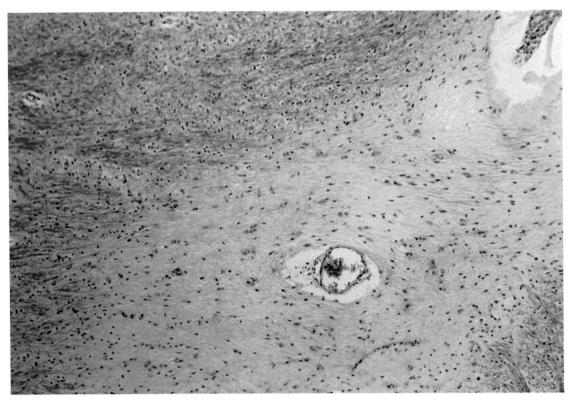

FIGURE 5-35
Multiple sclerosis plaques may have a perivenular location in small lesions (Luxol fast blue–PAS stain).

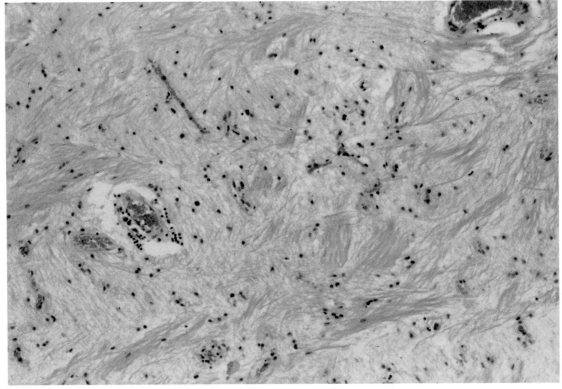

FIGURE 5-36
Multiple sclerosis at autopsy usually shows predominantly chronic inactive (remote) plaques that are hypocellular and devoid of macrophages.

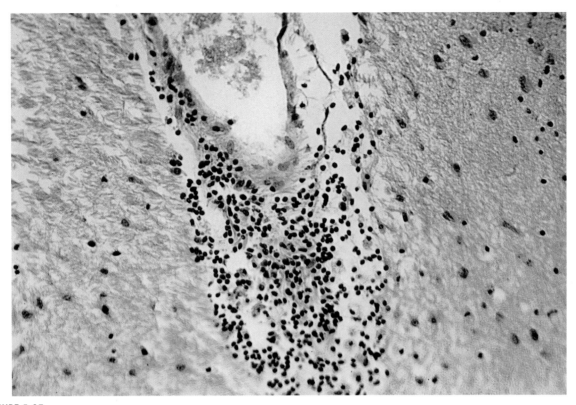

FIGURE 5-37

At autopsy, multiple sclerosis generally has relatively limited lymphocytic inflammation, but perivascular non-neoplastic lymphocytes (T and B cells), plasma cells, and a few macrophages can be seen in the center of old, inactive lesions.

deficiency, acute disseminated encephalomyelitis (ADEM), and several neurodegenerative diseases. At autopsy, the pattern of lesions is usually sufficiently distinctive to make the diagnosis of MS, even when little corroborating clinical information is available (Fig. 5-38). In young patients with large coalescent lesions of cerebral white matter, Schilder's disease, adrenoleukodystrophy, or other inherited leukodystrophies may be considerations.

OVERVIEW OF MULTIPLE SCLEROSIS VARIANTS

Several unusual demyelinating conditions were described 100 years ago around the turn of the last century. All except Devic's disease were considered by the original authors to represent rare, acute, or severe variants of MS. These disorders are known today mostly by eponymic designations. The first to be described was Devic's disease (1894, neuromyelitis optica), followed shortly thereafter by Marburg's disease (1906, acute MS, "encephalitis periaxialis diffusa"), Schilder's disease (1912, recognized as a childhood variant of Marburg's encephalitis periaxialis diffusa by Schilder), and Baló's disease (1928, "encephalitis periaxialis concentrica," concentric sclerosis). Baló

himself considered his "disease" to be similar to Marburg's and Schilder's disorders.

Other workers, however, almost immediately raised doubts about whether Devic's, Marburg's, Schilder's, and Baló's diseases represented unique, separate demyelinating disorders or MS variants as the original authors had contended. Since several of these original papers were only single case reports, it took some time before sufficient numbers of patients were accrued (with tissues studied by neuropathologists at autopsy) to put these disorders in proper perspective. Adding to the confusion was the fact that Schilder himself subsequently reported two more children with acute demyelinating disorders that he also thought represented acute childhood MS. Later review, however, revealed that he had actually reported three patients with three separate diseases, one showing acute MS and the other two manifesting adrenoleukodystrophy and subacute sclerosing panencephalitis.

Today, there are valid differences of opinion regarding how rigidly these terms, especially "Devic" and "Baló," should be applied. It has been debated whether the appellation "Devic's disease" should be used exclusively for patients with pure spinal cord and optic nerve/chiasm involvement or can be applied to MS patients in whom the initial manifestation was severe optic nerve or spinal cord disease, or both, but later in the course of the disease pathologically proven demyelinative plaques developed in other CNS sites. It has also

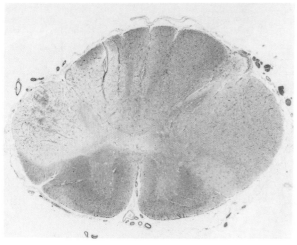

FIGURE 5-38

Multiple sclerosis at autopsy usually shows spinal cord involvement, although it may be more evident on stained sections of myelin than grossly. Note how plaques have their broad base on the subpial surface and show no respect for the spinal cord tracts or gray matter. Also note the darker staining of peripheral myelin (and the lack of peripheral nerve involvement) in this thoracic cord section (Luxol fast blue–PAS stain).

been debated whether "Baló's disease" should be confined to the original use of the term, which required widespread multiple concentric ring formation throughout cerebral hemispheres, as documented at autopsy, or may also be used when the concentric ring formation is minimally or focally present by neuroimaging studies in a single large acute demyelinating lesion. Finally, some clinicians favor the use of "Devic's disease" to indicate certain stereotypic sites of involvement, irrespective of coexistent disorders, rather than to denote a specific disease process. An example would be the use of "Devic's disease" for spinal cord and optic nerve lesions in patients with systemic lupus erythematosus or cancer.

Currently, most neuropathologists and neuroradiologists accept three of these disorders as variants of MS and have re-embraced the original authors' findings. Marburg's disease (acute MS), Schilder's disease (large coalescent, usually childhood MS with exclusive cerebral hemispheric involvement), and Baló's disease (alternating concentric rings of myelin loss and preservation in MS) are considered MS variants. Devic's disease still prompts debate. When it occurs as a variant of MS, it appears to lie on the severe end of the MS spectrum and to have a predilection for certain Asian populations.

All these MS variants are rare. They may be difficult, if not impossible, to diagnose by clinical and neuroimaging features in the early phases of the disease. The initial clinical manifestation is usually severe and rapidly progressive. Tumors or infectious disease may be in the differential diagnosis. Usually, evolution of clinical features over time, biopsy, or even autopsy is necessary to provide the final, accurate classification. Treatment decisions are more often empirical rather than based on a specific diagnosis. Despite these difficulties, from a research perspective, as "outliers" these MS variants do provide important material with which to address questions related to varied host response, barriers to remyelination, and issues regarding new hypotheses of MS pathogenesis.

DEVIC'S NEUROMYELITIS OPTICA (DEVIC'S DISEASE)

CLINICAL FEATURES

The key clinical features are acute visual loss, often bilateral, and acute transverse myelitis. Visual symptoms usually precede spinal symptoms, but the reverse is not uncommon. In patients initially seen with visual system difficulties, transverse myelitis characteristically develops within a few weeks, with severe paraplegia, sensory loss at a distinct level, and sphincter disturbances. Fixed weakness from the onset, rather than improvement over time after the initial event, is the typical course. The interval separating the visual and spinal syndromes may be hours, days, or weeks, but in most cases it is within 3 months. However, cases with a 2 or more year separation have been described. The clinical course is variable. The disorder may be monophasic without recurrent attacks (but with fixed deficits), or the patient may experience multiple severe relapses with stepwise neurologic deterioration. Devic's disease may also follow an acute progressive and fatal course, with patients suffering respiratory failure and death related to cervical myelitis. Rarely, there can be complete clinical recovery without relapse. The prognosis is poor in comparison to classic MS, with most patients having severe visual loss or an inability to ambulate without assistance within 5 years of onset.

PATHOLOGIC FEATURES

In patients dying in early phases of the disease, the cord may be swollen, similar to a tumor, whereas in late stages, there may be considerable shrinkage of the cord and cavitation because of the tissue destruction. Devic's disease is histologically characterized by considerably greater loss of axons than is seen in typical MS, along with necrotizing demyelination and cavitation in the spinal cord and optic nerves (Fig. 5-39). The tissue involvement often extends over numerous spinal cord segments (Fig. 5-40). Devic's disease may be characterized by a greater B-cell component, more prominent eosinophilic and neutrophilic infiltrates, complement activation, and vascular fibrosis, all rare in typical MS, along with more MS-like features, including T-cell infiltrates and the presence of macrophages. Depending on how one defines the entity, the remainder of the CNS shows little or no demyelinative disease.

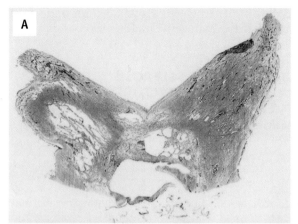

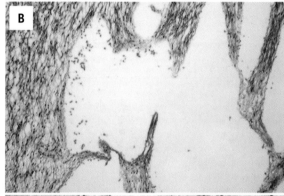

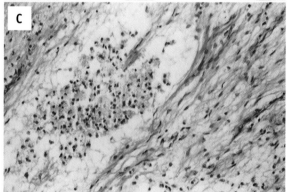

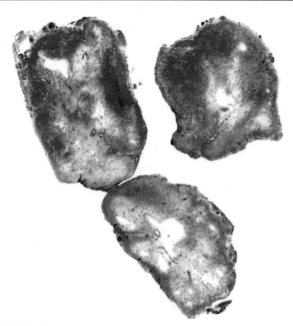

FIGURE 5-40

Devic's disease at autopsy may also manifest severe necrotic lesions in the spinal cord. Contrast these with the spinal cord lesions of typical multiple sclerosis in Figure 5-38 (Luxol fast blue–PAS stain).

▶ The spinal cord and optic nerve are exclusively affected in pure cases; cases showing overlap with MS also have lesions in typical MS sites such as the periventricular cerebral areas and the brain stem and at the gray-white matter junction
▶ Demyelination confined to the CNS

Gender and Age Distribution

▶ In Japanese cases, women are affected four times more frequently than men, with the average age of onset being 34 years and the mean duration of disease being 5 years

Clinical Features

▶ Unlike typical MS, the course is often rapidly progressive, and cerebrospinal fluid may contain neutrophils and markedly elevated protein levels
▶ Oligoclonal bands are absent in most cases
▶ The clinical course varies, with either monophonic disease without recurrent attacks but with fixed deficits, multiple severe relapses with stepwise neurologic deterioration, or an acute progressive course with respiratory failure and death from cervical myelitis

Radiologic Features

▶ Unlike typical MS, cranial MRI is almost always normal at initial evaluation
▶ The spinal cord initially tends to be enlarged and swollen
▶ Spinal cord lesions often exceed three cord segments in length and show full-thickness involvement of the cord
▶ Absence of brain lesions in pure forms

Prognosis and Treatment

▶ Poor, with most patients having severe visual loss or inability to ambulate without assistance by 5 years
▶ Treatment differs from that of typical MS
▶ Azathioprine may be the treatment of choice; plasma exchange and steroid therapy are also used; patients with anticardiolipin antibodies are also treated with antiplatelet and anticoagulant drugs

FIGURE 5-39

Devic's disease at autopsy shows exclusive or predominant involvement of the optic chiasm and spinal cord; note the highly destructive lesions in the optic chiasm on a whole-mount section (**A**), the obvious axonal loss (**B**, Bodian stain for axons), and cavitary lesions containing macrophages (**C**).

NEUROMYELITIS OPTICA (DEVIC'S DISEASE)—FACT SHEET

Definition

▶ Acute, severe necrotizing disorder of the spinal cord and optic nerves/chiasm; debated whether the disease is a separate entity or a form of MS; unknown cause

Incidence and Location

▶ Constitutes a greater proportion of MS cases in Japan, China, and other Asian countries, thus suggesting that genetic factors play a role

---

**NEUROMYELITIS OPTICA (DEVIC'S DISEASE)—
PATHOLOGIC FEATURES**

Gross Findings

▶ Swollen cord in patients who die in acute phases of the disease
▶ Tissue damage involves multiple cord segments
▶ In late stages of the disease the cord may show atrophy and cavitation

Microscopic Features

▶ Cavitary lesions may contain sheets of macrophages and an absence of axons
▶ Some cases show greater B-cell, eosinophil, and neutrophil inflammatory components than typical MS does
▶ The optic nerve may have cavitary lesions or less destructive focal or diffuse demyelination

Ultrastructural Features

▶ No specific features

Immunohistochemical Features

▶ No specific features

Genetics

▶ Increased incidence in Asian populations

Differential Diagnosis

▶ Devic's disease should be distinguished from cases with isolated necrotic cord lesions (acute necrotic myelopathy), which have been associated with systemic lupus erythematosus, lymphoproliferative disorders, acute hemorrhagic leukoencephalitis, postinfectious encephalomyelitis, and carcinoma of the lung
▶ Devic's disease–like pathology may be seen with autoimmune and connective tissue diseases such as systemic lupus erythematosus and Sjögren's syndrome; clinicians and pathologists differ regarding whether these cases should be called Devic's disease or whether cases with additional MS lesions should be called Devic's disease
▶ Devic's disease should be distinguished from subacute necrotizing myelopathy caused by vascular malformations of the spinal cord (Foix-Alajouanine syndrome)
▶ The finding of additional demyelinative lesions in characteristic MS locations in some patients makes a strong argument that some cases of Devic's disease are a variant of MS with a predominance of severe spinal cord and optic nerve/chiasm involvement

---

DIFFERENTIAL DIAGNOSIS

Depending on the initial manifestation (spinal or optic), the differential diagnosis by imaging consists of (for spinal manifestations) transverse myelitis, ADEM, including postvaccination, viral, and other infectious causes, and neoplasm. An abnormal brain MRI scan with typical demyelinating lesions in the cerebral hemispheres, cerebellum, and brain stem and consistent laboratory findings makes MS more likely. Vascular insults and collagen vascular disease are not always separable from Devic's disease without supporting laboratory or historical information. In patients with optic neuritis, especially if unilateral, imaging findings are nonspecific,

and the differential diagnosis will include optic neuritis from MS if the brain MRI findings are positive.

ACUTE MULTIPLE SCLEROSIS (MARBURG TYPE), INCLUDING ACUTE TUMEFACTIVE DEMYELINATING LESIONS PROMPTING BIOPSY

CLINICAL FEATURES

Rarely, an acute, idiopathic, inflammatory demyelinating disease may be relatively unresponsive to conventional

---

ACUTE MULTIPLE SCLEROSIS (MARBURG TYPE)—FACT SHEET

Definition

▶ Acute, idiopathic, inflammatory demyelinating disease with death usually ensuing 1 to 6 months after clinical onset; the disorder is thought to represent acute MS

Incidence and Location

▶ Less than 4% of patients die within 5 years of the onset of MS, and more rapidly fatal, Marburg-type cases are even rarer
▶ Cerebral hemispheric predilection for lesions, but the brain stem or optic nerves may also be involved
▶ Demyelination confined to the CNS

Gender and Age Distribution

▶ Occurs from childhood to adult ages; young adults are typical

Clinical Features

▶ Some workers limit the name "Marburg" to severe acute MS that is a monophasic illness with a fulminant clinical course and rapid demise
▶ Others use the term when patients with a more chronic MS course experience superimposed, acute severe exacerbations that result in rapid demise after the exacerbation
▶ Cerebrospinal fluid may not show oligoclonal bands

Radiologic Features

▶ Large, confluent lesions by MRI, usually involving the cerebral hemispheric white matter
▶ Lesions may show enhancement after the administration of MRI contrast agents
▶ Perilesional edema is often present
▶ Isolated lesions may simulate neoplasm
▶ Lesion distribution is similar to that of typical MS, although cases with plaques in restricted anatomic sites have been described

Prognosis and Treatment

▶ Poor; demise may occasionally occur within days or weeks of onset
▶ Most patients succumb within 1 to 6 months after clinical onset of the acute phase of illness
▶ Poorly responsive to corticosteroids (the first line of therapy)
▶ Patients with Marburg-type MS may benefit from plasma exchange
▶ Cases have also been described with response to combined corticosteroid and mannitol therapy

therapy (corticosteroids) and result in death or severe residual deficits, and it may then be classified as acute MS of the Marburg type. Death may occur in weeks to months, either from severe widespread cerebral lesions or from acute involvement of the lower brain stem or upper cervical cord. Patients who survive the acute phase may be left with significant deficits, or severe exacerbations may develop. Some patients who present with a large, acute, tumefactive demyelinative lesion that prompts biopsy later go on to exhibit a classic chronic relapsing/remitting course of typical MS (Figs. 5-41 and 5-42). These cases should perhaps not be considered "pure" Marburg-type MS, although at initial evaluation of the patient the outcome may not be at all clear. For the individual patient, the difficulty is that at initial clinical assessment there are no good predictors for whether a fulminant, rapidly fatal course will develop after biopsy, whether mild or severe MS will develop, or whether MS will even develop at all despite a several-year follow-up. It has been suggested that some patients with acute tumefactive demyelinating lesions prompting biopsy might actually have disorders intermediate between MS and large coalescent ADEM. Hence, the appellation "Marburg" is best applied to severe, acute MS that meets both the clinical and pathologic criteria for a monophasic illness and may best be defined by its malignant course and acute, severe demyelination. Recently,

Marburg-type MS has been hypothesized to be the result of a preexisting abnormality of myelin basic protein in a developmentally immature form. Alternatively, the Marburg type of demyelination may simply lie at the severe, acute end of the clinical spectrum of MS, possibly reflecting factors related to host response.

PATHOLOGIC FEATURES

Surgical and autopsy specimens contain demyelinative lesions (plaques) (Fig. 5-43) that are usually all of the same acute stage. At autopsy, the distribution of lesions is similar to typical MS, but there is a predilection for lesions to occur in the cerebral hemispheric white matter. Few, if any, older plaques are present, a finding paralleling the patient's rapid clinical downhill course. This situation is in contrast to typical relapsing-remitting MS, in which the demyelinative lesions at autopsy are usually remote or show differing ages of myelin breakdown, or both. Age of the demyelination can be assessed by several types of special stains, the most common of which is the histochemical stain for myelin (LFB) with a PAS counterstain. This stain allows distinction between very recently phagocytosed

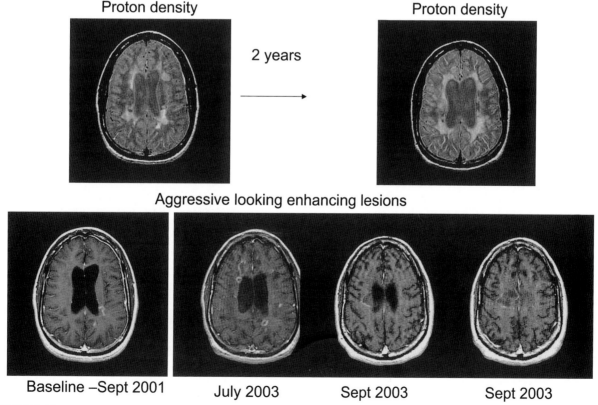

FIGURE 5-41

Acute multiple sclerosis may show rapid clinical and neuroimaging progression over a period of months or a few years on proton-density images (*top*) or contrast-enhanced T1-weighted images (*bottom*).

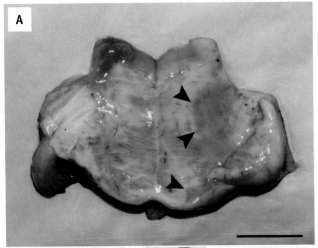

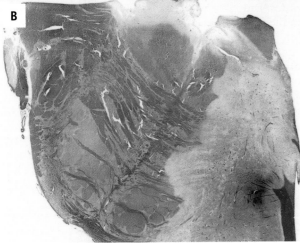

FIGURE 5-42
Acute multiple sclerosis at autopsy may show less well demarcated lesions, especially on unfixed brain cut fresh at the time of postmortem examination (**A**, *arrowheads*). In comparison, the lesion jumps out on myelin-stained whole-mount sections (**B**) (Luxol fast blue–PAS stain).

myelin within macrophages, which is as yet undigested and retains its LFB positivity, versus myelin that has been broken down to neutral lipids in macrophages (PAS positivity) as a result of a more advanced and sub-acute process. In the Marburg type of acute MS, abundant LFB-positive macrophages are seen throughout the hypercellular demyelinative lesions. When compared with the typical relapsing-remitting MS cases that come to autopsy, acute MS shows less chronic gliosis, more edema, and even partial bands of preserved myelin (see description of the Baló type later). More abundant perivascular inflammation than seen in typical MS may also be present.

DIFFERENTIAL DIAGNOSIS

The differential diagnosis at initial evaluation in-cludes ADEM, which may be favored by an appropriate

---

ACUTE MULTIPLE SCLEROSIS (MARBURG TYPE)— PATHOLOGIC FEATURES

Gross Findings
▶ Coronal sections show numerous white or yellow patches of myelin loss, in contrast to the depressed, gray-glistening appearance of remote lesions
▶ Acute lesions may not be as well demarcated as remote lesions
▶ Lesions occur in periventricular, brain stem, spinal cord, and optic nerve sites

Microscopic Features
▶ Plaques are hypercellular throughout the lesion and show severe loss of myelin and oligodendrocytes
▶ Macrophages contain Luxol fast blue–positive myelin debris indicative of acute, active myelin breakdown
▶ May see more abundant lymphocytes than in typical MS, but usually few plasma cells in true acute lesions
▶ Neutrophils are not seen
▶ Axons may be swollen and show retraction balls
▶ Subacute and chronic inactive lesions may also be present in some patients

Ultrastructural Features
▶ Oligodendrocytes are reduced in number and may show apoptosis
▶ Some cases have features of aberrant remyelination with redundant balls and loops of myelin

Immunohistochemical Features
▶ Acute lesions usually contain at least a small number of immunoreactive infiltrating T lymphocytes
▶ The earliest macrophages in lesions are derived from resident microglia and show immunohistochemical reaction for proliferation markers, but not MRP-14, an early marker of activated macrophages of blood monocyte origin that migrate into the lesion
▶ A few macrophages are immunoreactive for MRP-14
▶ During acute myelin breakdown, macrophages stain positively for surface IgG, activated complement, CD45, HLA-DR, and myelin proteins

Genetics
▶ No specific genetic features

Differential Diagnosis
▶ At initial evaluation, acute MS manifested as a single lesion may not be distinguishable from acute disseminated encephalomyelitis
▶ Inherited leukodystrophies, especially adrenoleukodystrophy

---

accompanying history of vaccination or recent viral or other infectious illness. If blood is present in the lesion on neuroimaging studies, acute hemorrhagic leukoencephalitis may also be a consideration; this disorder is generally thought to represent a hyperacute form of ADEM. Infectious and autoimmune disease can usually be excluded by clinical and laboratory features or by neuropathologic examination of a biopsy

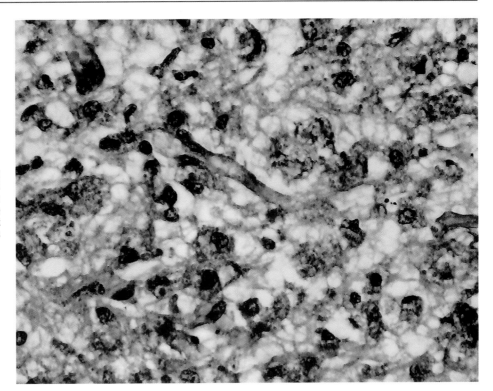

FIGURE 5-43

Acute multiple sclerosis is characterized by plaques with macrophages dispersed throughout the demyelinative lesion that contain Luxol fast blue–positive myelin debris, indicative of very recent myelin breakdown and phagocytosis (Luxol fast blue–PAS stain).

specimen or at autopsy. The difficulty with biopsies of tumefactive MS is that they may overlap with Marburg-type MS or be intermediate between ADEM and classic MS. Although classic ADEM is distinguishable from typical MS by the presence of multifocal, small perivenous demyelinative lesions in ADEM, this feature is not generally present in the large acute demyelinative lesions that prompt biopsy. There are no morphologic features in these biopsy specimens of single tumefactive demyelinative lesions that reliably predict whether MS will subsequently develop.

BALÓ'S CONCENTRIC SCLEROSIS

CLINICAL FEATURES

Baló's concentric sclerosis (BCS) might best be characterized as a relatively rare expression of pathology within the spectrum of MS. The original case of Baló was that of acute disease, with death within $3^{1}/_{2}$ months after onset in a 23-year-old man, which prompted Baló himself to consider the disorder that he described as a variant of acute MS. He named this process "encephalitis periaxialis concentrica," paralleling the name given several years earlier by Marburg to acute MS. The literature reflects two extremes of BCS: the earlier (pre-MRI neuroimaging) neuropathology literature is based primarily on autopsy material from patients after an acute, monophasic, fulminant disease process. In the autopsy

BCS series, disease typically progresses over a period of weeks to months, with severe disability or death as the typical outcome. Clinical symptoms typically include headache, aphasia, cognitive or behavioral dysfunction, seizures, or a combination of these factors. In contrast, the MRI-era literature tends to reflect a far greater range of disease, from focal BCS lesions coexisting with typical MS-like lesions, but it also acknowledges cases with a fulminant course ending in death. The more "benign" BCS has been described as monophasic, with resolution of the pathology and clinical findings over time, and as MS-like, with a multiphasic, but self-limited course that is responsive to therapy.

PATHOLOGIC FEATURES

BCS by definition shows a peculiar pattern of pathology in the cerebral hemispheric white matter that consists of a concentric, mosaic, or floral configuration of bands of relatively preserved myelin alternating with zones of demyelination. This pattern is visible on myelin-stained sections but is seen best when large tissue sections are available. Although the early literature emphasized BCS within the cerebral hemispheric white matter of the brain, this process also occurs within the optic chiasm and spinal cord, and BCS lesions can occur in the brain stem and cerebellum. Coexistence of BCS lesions with typical MS-like (nonconcentric) lesions has also been recognized. A Baló-like band pattern may likewise be seen along the periphery of acute MS plaques. The mechanism or mechanisms responsible for this peculiar pathology remain unknown despite several recently introduced and interesting theories.

DIFFERENTIAL DIAGNOSIS

Classic large and potentially mass-like BCS lesions may be confused with neoplasm or abscess. Follow-up neuroimaging studies usually clarify true demyelinating lesions as a resolving (nonmalignant) process. At autopsy, the feature of concentric "globe within a globe" bands of myelin loss and preservation is distinctive.

BALÓ'S CONCENTRIC SCLEROSIS—FACT SHEET

Definition
▶ Acute, idiopathic, inflammatory demyelinating disease closely related to the Marburg type of MS but is defined by the presence of concentric rings of intact normal white matter alternating with zones of demyelination ("concentric globe pattern"); the disorder is thought to represent a variant of acute MS

Incidence and Location
▶ The disease may be most common in Asian countries, especially the Philippines and China
▶ Demyelination confined to the CNS

Gender and Age Distribution
▶ Childhood to adult age range, 10 to 51 years
▶ Slightly more common in males

Clinical Features
▶ Patients may present with severe monophasic illness and have a fulminant course and rapid demise
▶ Symptoms in some cases are suggestive of a mass lesion
▶ Clinical features are similar to those of acute MS and typically include headache, aphasia, and cognitive or behavioral dysfunction
▶ Occasional patients may have increased intracranial pressure
▶ Rarely, the characteristic "concentric globe" pathologic pattern is recognized in patients with typical relapsing-remitting MS

Radiologic Features
▶ Lamellar lesions in isolation (classic) or rarely accompanying typical MS-like lesions
▶ Alternating zones of intensity on T1- and T2-weighted images
▶ The alternating zones may include contrast enhancement

Prognosis and Treatment
▶ Once thought to be fatal within 6 months to 2 years
▶ The advent of MRI diagnosis shows that some cases improve and are without relapses during 1- to 3-year follow-up intervals

---

BALÓ'S CONCENTRIC SCLEROSIS—PATHOLOGIC FEATURES

Gross Findings
▶ Multiple areas of gray discoloration throughout the white matter, especially of the cerebral hemispheres

Microscopic Features
▶ Concentric rings of alternating intact and absent myelin best appreciated with myelin stains
▶ The banding pattern is strikingly repetitive from case to case, with bands arranged in parallel waves and bands and with intact myelin almost always narrower than in those with myelin loss
▶ Fewer macrophages and more astrocytosis in the center of the rings
▶ The edges of lesions show bands of demyelination with numerous Luxol fast blue–containing macrophages, perivascular lymphocytes, and enlarged astrocytes
▶ A peculiar feature is the presence of cells containing clusters of dark nuclei, which represents endocytosis of oligodendrocytes by astrocytes

Ultrastructural Features
▶ Redundant whorls of myelin suggesting aberrant remyelination

Immunohistochemical Features
▶ One recent study showed loss of immunostaining for myelin-associated glycoprotein (but preservation of staining for myelin basic protein) in bands of intact myelin not yet infiltrated by macrophages

Genetics
▶ No specific genetic predisposition identified

Differential Diagnosis
▶ Overlaps with other forms of acute MS clinically, but the neuroimaging and histologic features are distinctive

---

SCHILDER'S DISEASE

CLINICAL FEATURES

Schilder's disease, also known as diffuse myelinoclastic sclerosis, is a rare demyelinating disorder for which the clinical and MRI appearance may overlap with inherited metabolic disorders of myelin, particularly adrenoleukodystrophy. A practical definition proposed by Poser (1985) includes the following components: (1) a subacute or chronic myelinoclastic disorder with one or two roughly symmetric plaques at least 2×3 cm in two of three dimensions; (2) involvement of the centrum semiovale; (3) these being the only lesions based on clinical, paraclinical, or imaging findings; and (4) exclusion of adrenoleukodystrophy. Normal ratios of VLCFAs and absence of involvement of the peripheral nervous system exclude adrenoleukodystrophy.

SCHILDER'S DISEASE—FACT SHEET

Definition

▶ Cases of MS in which the large single or multiple inflammatory demyelinating lesions develop acutely in one or both cerebral hemispheres

---

Incidence and Location

▶ Rare
▶ "Pure" cases show only cerebral hemispheric white matter involvement, usually bilateral
▶ "Transitional" cases also show additional brain stem, cerebellar, optic nerve/chiasm, and spinal cord lesions identical to those of typical MS
▶ Demyelination confined to the CNS
▶ Involvement of the peripheral nervous system should prompt concern about adrenoleukodystrophy

---

Gender and Age Distribution

▶ Childhood predominance in "pure" cases of disease in which only the cerebral hemispheres are involved
▶ "Transitional" cases show the same young to middle-age adult age range as typical MS does

---

Clinical Features

▶ The course may be progressive and fulminant, especially with "pure" forms
▶ Some patients have relapsing-remitting disease before the acute phase of MS ensues
▶ Headache, vomiting, seizures, visual problems
▶ Cerebrospinal fluid may be normal and have only a minor elevation in protein and cell count

---

Radiologic Features

▶ Large (often greater than 2 cm in diameter) bihemispheric cerebral white matter lesions
▶ Perilesional edema
▶ Lesions often show either diffuse or margin enhancement with gadolinium

---

Prognosis and Treatment

▶ Poor; most patients succumb within 1 to 2 years;. in general, early age at onset often results in severe neurologic deficits
▶ Treatment with corticosteroids and cyclophosphamide has been successful in some instances

---

Analogous to other MS variants, both "pure" forms and "transitional" forms have been described. "Pure" forms predominate in childhood and have plaques confined to the cerebral white matter. "Transitional" forms affect a broader age range of adolescents and adults and have large cerebral plaques combined with more typical MS plaques elsewhere. Disease duration is highly variable. In the 70 cases collected by Poser (1957), the mean duration was 6.2 years, with a range of 3 days to 45 years, but the duration was less than 1 year in 40%. The clinical course is diverse, but widespread white matter involvement usually produces subacute or chronic mental and neurologic deterioration, spastic paresis, convulsions, and involvement of vision and hearing. Pure psychiatric forms have been described. Increased intracranial pressure, headache, and vomiting may suggest a mass lesion.

PATHOLOGIC FEATURES

The defining feature of Schilder's disease is giant coalescent plaques of demyelination, usually involving the

---

SCHILDER'S DISEASE—PATHOLOGIC FEATURES

Gross Findings

▶ Large confluent lesions occupying a large percentage of cerebral white matter
▶ Acute lesions may not be as sharply demarcated from adjacent intact white matter as remote MS plaques are
▶ Demyelination often bilateral
▶ May or may show additional typical MS demyelinative lesions in the brain stem, spinal cord, cerebellum, or optic nerve/chiasm

---

Microscopic Features

▶ Acute demyelinative plaques with variable numbers of Luxol fast blue–containing macrophages indicative of acute myelin breakdown
▶ Some cases show extensive axonal loss resulting in cavitation
▶ Few older lesions
▶ Lymphocytic inflammation variable in amount and can be absent

---

Ultrastructural Features

▶ Oligodendrocytes are reduced in number and may show apoptosis
▶ Some cases have features of aberrant remyelination with redundant balls and loops of myelin

---

Immunohistochemical Features

▶ Acute lesions usually contain at least a small number of immunoreactive infiltrating T lymphocytes
▶ The earliest macrophages in lesions are derived from resident microglia and show immunohistochemical reaction for proliferation markers, but not MRP-14, an early marker of activated macrophages of blood monocyte origin that migrate into the lesion
▶ A few macrophages are immunoreactive for MRP-14
▶ During acute myelin breakdown, macrophages stain positively for surface IgG, activated complement, CD45, HLA-DR, and myelin proteins

---

Genetics

▶ No known genetic predisposition

Differential Diagnosis

▶ Must be distinguished from adrenoleukodystrophy, subacute sclerosis panencephalitis
▶ Inherited leukodystrophies

---

majority of the bilateral cerebral hemispheric white matter. Frank necrosis and cavitation may also occur. Histologically, the features of Schilder's disease are nearly identical to other forms of acute MS. Demyelinative lesions may be filled with macrophages containing LFB—evidence of acute myelin breakdown.

DIFFERENTIAL DIAGNOSIS

Myelinoclastic diffuse sclerosis remains a rare disorder with few cases meeting rigorous diagnostic criteria. Cases coming to biopsy must be distinguished from tumor, abscess, or ADEM based on histologic assessment. As expected, the differential diagnosis for Schilder's disease is similar to that for other acute forms of MS such as the Marburg type. An additional disorder in the differential diagnosis in children and adolescents is adrenoleukodystrophy.

ACUTE DISSEMINATED ENCEPHALOMYELITIS

CLINICAL FEATURES

ADEM is a monophasic, acute demyelinating disorder characterized by small perivascular sleeves of myelin loss widely disseminated throughout the brain and spinal cord (Fig. 5-44). Synonymous terms include perivenous encephalomyelitis, postinfectious encephalomyelitis, and postvaccinal encephalomyelitis. It was originally described after smallpox vaccinations. The disease was later identified after measles, mumps, rubella, varicella, and vaccinia infections. Today, it usually occurs in children after a nonspecific upper respiratory illness. Patients have an abrupt onset of headaches and fever approximately 2 to 12 days after the onset of their infection (or immunization). Recovery is generally rapid, and patients are seldom left with residual neurologic deficits.

PATHOLOGIC FEATURES

Grossly, the brain may be swollen. The signature feature is seen only microscopically and consists of narrow cuffs or sleeves of myelin loss around small veins. Veins may be severely congested. A few lymphocytes are usually present within the meninges, but in general, microglial clusters and neuronophagia (indicative of ongoing viral infection and tissue damage) are no longer present. The cellular infiltrates in demyelinated areas are composed chiefly of macrophages rather than lymphocytes.

ACUTE DISSEMINATED ENCEPHALOMYELITIS—FACT SHEET

Definition

▶ Monophasic, acute demyelinating disorder characterized by small perivascular sleeves of myelin loss widely disseminated throughout the brain and spinal cord along with associated perivascular mononuclear cell infiltrates

Incidence and Location

▶ Originally described after smallpox vaccinations
▶ Later identified after measles, mumps, rubella, varicella, or vaccinia infections
▶ Today usually occurs after a nonspecific upper respiratory illness
▶ The incidence after measles is 1 per 1000 cases
▶ Maximally involves the lower part of the spinal cord, brain stem, and cerebral white matter
▶ Demyelination confined to the CNS

Gender and Age Distribution

▶ Usually affects children and young adults

Clinical Features

▶ The interval from the onset of infection or immunization to neurologic symptoms is 2 to 12 days
▶ Clinical onset of symptoms is usually abrupt
▶ Often show headache and fever
▶ Clinical symptoms are progressive over a several-day period and may include aseptic meningitis, transverse myelitis, encephalomyelitis, or bilateral optic neuritis
▶ Varicella especially characterized by cerebellar involvement
▶ Recovery rapid starting within a week after onset and usually without residual neurologic deficit

Radiologic Features

▶ Cannot reliably distinguish ADEM from acute MS by initial neuroimaging features, especially in children
▶ Relatively monophasic course (relatively rare new lesions after 6 months) as compared with MS
▶ Relative sparing of normal-appearing white matter by magnetization transfer imaging in ADEM as compared with MS

Prognosis and Treatment

▶ Most cases now nonfatal
▶ Fatality rate historically highest after measles infection and smallpox vaccination

---

Unlike typical MS, lesions are all of the same age.

DIFFERENTIAL DIAGNOSIS

The differential diagnosis for the pathologist centers around acute MS and acute hemorrhagic leukoencephalitis.

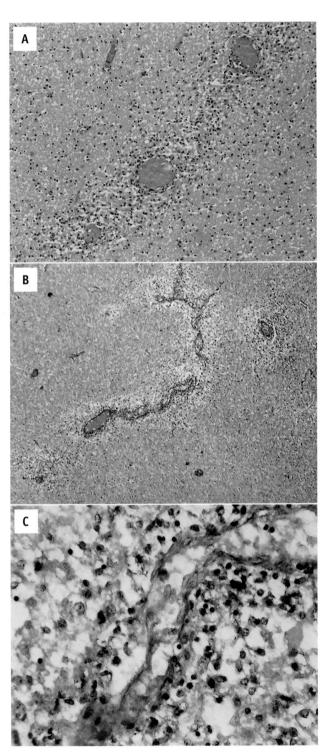

FIGURE 5-44

Acute disseminated encephalomyelitis shows hypercellular perivenular lesions (**A**), with demyelination best appreciated on Luxol fast blue–PAS staining (**B**), and perivascular lymphocytes and macrophages (**C**, Luxol fast blue–PAS stain).

ACUTE DISSEMINATED ENCEPHALOMYELITIS— PATHOLOGIC FEATURES

Gross Findings

▶ Patients dying in acute phases of the disease have a swollen brain and spinal cord
▶ Demyelination cannot usually be seen grossly

Microscopic Features

▶ Characteristic narrow cuffs or sleeves of myelin loss around small veins
▶ Cellular infiltrates in demyelinated areas are composed of chiefly macrophages rather than lymphocytes
▶ Small veins may be packed with red blood cells
▶ Perivascular hemorrhage may be seen but is less conspicuous than in acute hemorrhagic leukoencephalitis
▶ A mild number of lymphocytes in the meninges is typical
▶ Usually, microglial clusters and neuronophagia (indicative of ongoing viral infection and tissue damage) are no longer present
▶ Unlike typical MS, lesions are all of the same age

Ultrastructural Features

▶ No specific features

Immunohistochemical Features

▶ No specific features

Genetics

▶ No known genetic predisposition

Differential Diagnosis

▶ Acute MS
▶ Acute hemorrhagic leukoencephalitis
▶ Acute necrotizing myelopathy
▶ Rare patients have a recurrent or progressive course that can be distinguished from typical MS only by the confinement of demyelination to perivenous locations in ADEM

ACUTE HEMORRHAGIC LEUKOENCEPHALITIS (HURST'S DISEASE)

CLINICAL FEATURES

This disorder is a rare, fulminant form of ADEM, with numerous perivascular hemorrhages as a result of more severe vascular injury. Both children and adults can be affected. The disease is manifested by an abrupt onset of fever, neck stiffness, seizures, and focal signs. About half the patients have an antecedent upper respiratory tract illness 2 to 12 days before onset, similar to ADEM. The outcome is usually thought to be fatal, but in recent years, an increasing number of reports of patients who have survived have appeared in the literature.

ACUTE HEMORRHAGIC LEUKOENCEPHALITIS (HURST'S DISEASE)—FACT SHEET

Definition

▶ Hyperacute, fulminant form of acute disseminated encephalomyelitis with numerous perivascular hemorrhages because of more severe vascular injury

Incidence and Location

▶ Rare, although possible increased incidence in Japan and Taiwan
▶ Cerebral hemispheric white matter predominantly affected
▶ Involvement of the spinal cord uncommon, in contrast to acute disseminated encephalomyelitis

Gender and Age Distribution

▶ Childhood and young adult ages

Clinical Features

▶ Abrupt onset of fever, neck stiffness, seizures, focal signs
▶ In about half the cases there is an antecedent upper respiratory tract illness 2 to 12 days before onset, similar to acute disseminated encephalomyelitis
▶ Cerebrospinal fluid shows increased protein, pleocytosis with chiefly neutrophils, and often red blood cells
▶ Peripheral neutrophilic leukocytosis may also be seen
▶ Recent reports have suggested specific infectious agents linked to Hurst disease

Radiologic Features

▶ Cerebral swelling and hemorrhage
▶ Confluent nonenhancing lesions predominantly affect cerebral white matter
▶ Lesions may be asymmetric
▶ Lesions are larger, with more edema and mass effect, than those of acute disseminated encephalomyelitis
▶ Relative sparing of the cortex and basal ganglia

Prognosis and Treatment

▶ Usually considered fatal in the older literature, but recent studies have reported an improved prognosis

PATHOLOGIC FEATURES

Grossly, the brain is swollen and edematous, and herniations are frequent. The signature pathologic feature is the presence of multiple petechial and larger hemorrhages throughout the cerebral white matter, sometimes with associated large areas of necrosis. The basal ganglia are usually spared. Except for a recent case report of Hurst's disease with marked spinal cord involvement, the cord is spared. Microscopically, "ring and ball"

hemorrhages surround necrotic venules, which show fibrinoid vascular necrosis, fibrin exudates, and neutrophilic debris. Perivenous demyelination is seen but may be overshadowed by the perivenous hemorrhages.

DIFFERENTIAL DIAGNOSIS

Both acute fat embolism to the brain and hypoxic-ischemic leukoencephalopathy can cause widespread white matter hemorrhages. Staining for fat globules (by oil red O or Sudan black B stains) within the small vessels will make the diagnosis of fat embolism. Acute hemorrhagic leukoencephalitis (Fig. 5-45) and acute disseminated encephalitis are also differential diagnostic considerations.

ACUTE HEMORRHAGIC LEUKOENCEPHALITIS (HURST'S DISEASE)—PATHOLOGIC FEATURES

Gross Findings

▶ The brain is swollen and edematous, and herniations are frequent
▶ Multiple petechial and larger hemorrhages, sometimes with associated large areas of necrosis, seen throughout the cerebral white matter
▶ Basal ganglia, cerebral cortex usually intact

Microscopic Features

▶ "Ring and ball" hemorrhages surround necrotic venules
▶ Venules show fibrinoid vascular necrosis, fibrin exudates, and neutrophilic debris
▶ Neutrophilic inflammation contrasts with the lymphocytic inflammation of acute disseminated encephalomyelitis
▶ Perivenous demyelination is seen but may be overshadowed by the perivenous hemorrhages

Ultrastructural Features

▶ No specific features

Immunohistochemical Features

▶ No specific features

Genetics

▶ No known genetic predisposition, but at least one sibship has been described with disease

Differential Diagnosis

▶ Cerebral fat embolism
▶ Acute disseminated encephalomyelitis
▶ Hypoxic-ischemic hemorrhagic leukoencephalopathy

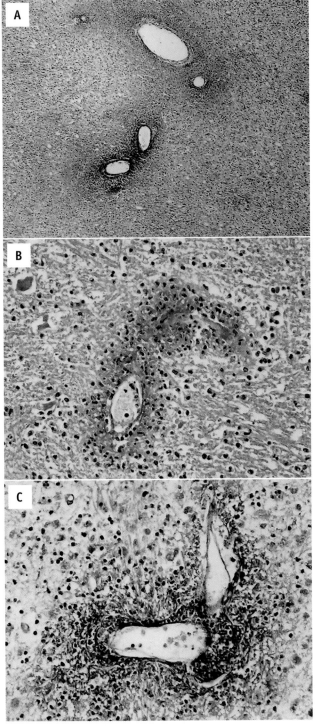

FIGURE 5-45

Acute hemorrhagic leukoencephalitis shows perivenular myelin loss (**A**), as well as more diffuse myelin pallor, but in contrast to acute disseminated encephalomyelitis, the vessels show necrosis and neutrophilic debris (**B**) and fibrinoid necrosis (**C**, dark purple material, Luxol fast blue–PAS stain).

SUGGESTED READINGS

Adrenoleukodystrophy

Bernal OG, Lenn N: Multiple cranial nerve enhancement in early infantile Krabbe's disease. Neurology 2000;54:2348-2349.

Bezman L, Moser AB, Raymond GV, et al: Adrenoleukodystrophy: Incidence, new mutation rate, and results of extended family screening. Ann Neurol 2001;49:512-517.

Chen X, DeLellis RA, Hoda SA: Adrenoleukodystrophy. Arch Pathol Lab Med 2003;127:119-120.

Feigenbaum V, Gelot A, Casanova P, et al: Apoptosis in the central nervous system of cerebral adrenoleukodystrophy patients. Neurobiol Dis 2000;7:600-612.

Luda E, Barisone MG: Adult-onset adrenoleukodystrophy: A clinical and neuropsychological study. Neurol Sci 2001;22:21-25.

Maier EM, Kammerer S, Muntau AC, et al: Symptoms in carriers of adrenoleukodystrophy relate to skewed X inactivation. Ann Neurol 2002;52:683-688.

Maria BL, Deidrick KM, Moser H, Naidu S: Leukodystrophies: Pathogenesis, diagnosis, strategies, therapies, and future research directions. J Child Neurol 2003;18:578-590.

Moser HW: Pathogenesis, genetics, and therapies of leukodystrophies. In American Academy of Neurology Education Program Syllabus, 3BS.002-12-35, 2002.

Moser HW, Loes DJ, Melhem ER, et al: X-Linked adrenoleukodystrophy: Overview and prognosis as a function of age and brain magnetic resonance imaging abnormality. A study involving 372 patients. Neuropediatrics 2000;31:227-239.

Powers JM, DeCiero DP, Cox C, et al: The dorsal root ganglia in adrenomyeloneuropathy: Neuronal atrophy and abnormal mitochondria. J Neuropathol Exp Neurol 2001;60:493-501.

Powers, JM, DeCiero, DP, Ito, M, et al: Adrenomyeloneuropathy: A neuropathologic review featuring its noninflammatory myelopathy. J Neuropathol Exp Neurol 2000;59:89-102.

Powers JM, De Vivo DC: Peroxisomal and mitochondrial disorders. In Graham DI, Lantos PL (eds): Greenfield's Neuropathology, 7th ed. London, Arnold, 2002.

Raymond GV: Peroxisomal disorders. Curr Opin Neurol 2001;14:783-787.

Schmidt S, Traber F, Block W, et al: Phenotype assignment in symptomatic female carriers of X-linked adrenoleukodystrophy. J Neurol 2001;248:36-44.

Supornsilchai V, Wacharasindhu S, Desudchit T: Adrenal functions in children with adrenoleukodystrophy. J Med Assoc Thai 2002;85:S286-S292.

van Geel BM, Bezman L, Loes DJ, et al: Evolution of phenotypes in adult male patients with X-linked adrenoleukodystrophy. Ann Neurol 2001;49:186-194.

Metachromatic Leukodystrophy

Austin JH: Metachromatic form of diffuse cerebral sclerosis: I. Diagnosis during life by urine sediment examination. 1957. Neurology 1998;51:333-345.

Black DN, Taber KH, Hurley RA: Metachromatic leukodystrophy: A model for the study of psychosis. J Neuropsychiatry Clin Neurosci 2003;15:289-293.

Bradl M, Linington C: Animal models of demyelination. Brain Pathol 1996;6:303-311.

Estrov Y, Scaglia F, Bodamer OA: Psychiatric symptoms of inherited metabolic disease. J Inherit Metab Dis 2000;23:2-6.

Filley CM, Gross KF: Psychosis with cerebral white matter disease. Neuropsychiatry Neuropsychol Behav Neurol 1992;2:119-125.

Gieselmann V: Metachromatic leukodystrophy: Recent research developments. J Child Neurol 2003;18:591-594.

Gieselmann V, Zlotogora J, Harris A, et al: Molecular genetics of metachromatic leukodystrophy. Hum Mutat 1994;4:233-242.

Kaye EM: Update on genetic disorders affecting white matter. Pediatr Neurol 2001;24:11-24.

Rapola J: Lysosomal storage diseases in adults. Pathol Res Pract 1994;190:759-766.

Suzuki K, Suzuki K: Lysosomal diseases. In Graham DI, Lantos PL (eds): Greenfield's Neuropathology, 7th ed. London, Arnold, 2002.

Globoid Cell Leukodystrophy (Krabbe's Disease)

Bajaj NP, Waldman A, Orrell R, et al: Familial adult onset of Krabbe's disease resembling hereditary spastic paraplegia with normal neuroimaging. J Neurol Neurosurg Psychiatry 2002;72:635-638.

De Gasperi R, Gama Sosa MA, Sartorato E, et al: Molecular basis of late-life globoid cell leukodystrophy. Hum Mutat 1999;14:256-262.

Fu L, Inui K, Nishigaki T, et al: Molecular heterogeneity of Krabbe disease. J Inherit Metab Dis 1999;22:155-162.

Given CA 2nd, Santos CC, Durden DD: Intracranial and spinal MR imaging findings associated with Krabbe's disease: Case report. AJNR Am J Neuroradiol 2001;22:1782-1785.

Jardim LB, Giugliani R, Pires RF, et al: Protracted course of Krabbe disease in an adult patient bearing a novel mutation. Arch Neurol 1999;56:1014-1017.

Kaye EM: Update on genetic disorders affecting white matter. Pediatr Neurol 2001;24:11-24.

Krivit W, Shapiro EG, Peters C, et al: Hematopoietic stem-cell transplantation in globoid-cell leukodystrophy. N Engl J Med 1998;338:1119-1126.

Loes DJ, Peters C, Krivit W: Globoid cell leukodystrophy: Distinguishing early-onset from late-onset disease using a brain MR imaging scoring method. AJNR Am J Neuroradiol 1999;20:316-323.

Marks HG, Scavina MT, Kolodny EH, et al: Krabbe's disease presenting as a peripheral neuropathy. Muscle Nerve 1997;20:1024-1028.

Matsumoto R, Oka N, Nagahama Y, et al: Peripheral neuropathy in late-onset Krabbe's disease: Histochemical and ultrastructural findings. Acta Neuropathol 1996;92:635-639.

Sabatelli M, Quaranta L, Madia F, et al: Peripheral neuropathy with hypomyelinating features in adult-onset Krabbe's disease. Neuromuscul Disord 2002;12:386-391.

Suzuki K: Globoid cell leukodystrophy (Krabbe's disease): Update. J Child Neurol 2003;18:595-603.

Suzuki K, Suzuki K: Lysosomal diseases. In Graham DI, Lantos PL (eds): Greenfield's Neuropathology, 7th ed. London, Arnold, 2002.

Taniike M, Mohri I, Eguchi N, et al: An apoptotic depletion of oligodendrocytes in the twitcher, a murine model of globoid cell leukodystrophy. J Neuropathol Exp Neurol 1999;58:644-653.

Wenger DA, Rafi MA, Luzi P: Molecular genetics of Krabbe disease (globoid cell leukodystrophy): Diagnostic and clinical implications. Hum Mutat 1997;10:268-279.

Alexander's Disease

Brockmann K, Meins M, Taubert A, et al: A novel GFAP mutation and disseminated white matter lesions: Adult Alexander disease? Eur Neurol 2003;50:100-105.

Harding BN, Surtees R: Metabolic and neurodegenerative diseases of childhood. In Graham DI, Lantos PL (eds): Greenfield's Neuropathology, 7th ed. London, Arnold, 2002.

Jacob J, Robertson NJ, Hilton DA: The clinicopathological spectrum of Rosenthal fibre encephalopathy and Alexander's disease: A case report and review of the literature. J Neurol Neurosurg Psychiatry 2003;74:807-810.

Johnson AB, Brenner M: Alexander's disease: Clinical, pathologic, and genetic features. J Child Neurol 2003;18:625-632.

Kinoshita T, Imaizumi M, Miura Y, et al: A case of adult-onset Alexander disease with Arg416Trp human glial fibrillary acidic protein gene mutation. Neurosci Lett 2003;350:169-172.

Messing A, Brenner M: Alexander disease: GFAP mutations unify young and old. Lancet Neurol 2003;2:75.

Mignot C, Boespflug-Tanguy O, Gelot A, et al: Alexander disease: Putative mechanisms of an astrocytic encephalopathy. Cell Mol Life Sci 2004;61:369-385.

Namekawa M, Takiyama Y, Aoki Y, et al: Identification of GFAP gene mutation in hereditary adult-onset Alexander's disease. Ann Neurol 2002;52:779-785.

Probst EN, Hagel C, Weisz V, et al: Atypical focal MRI lesions in a case of juvenile Alexander's disease. Ann Neurol 2003;53:118-120.

Stumpf E, Masson H, Duquette A, et al: Adult Alexander disease with autosomal dominant transmission: A distinct entity caused by mutation in the glial fibrillary acid protein gene. Arch Neurol 2003;60:1307-1312.

Canavan's Disease

Harding BN, Surtees R: Metabolic and neurodegenerative diseases of childhood. In Graham DI, Lantos PL (eds): Greenfield's Neuropathology, 7th ed. London, Arnold, 2002.

Ishiyama G, Lopez I, Baloh RW, Ishiyama A: Canavan's leukodystrophy is associated with defects in cochlear neurodevelopment and deafness. Neurology 2003;60:1702-1704.

Marks HG, Caro PA, Wang ZY, et al: Use of computed tomography, magnetic resonance imaging, and localized ^{1}H magnetic resonance spectroscopy in Canavan's disease: A case report. Ann Neurol 1991;30:106-111.

Surendran S, Matalon KM, Tyring SK, Matalon R: Molecular basis of Canavan's disease: From human to mouse. J Child Neurol 2003;18:604-610.

Pelizaeus-Merzbacher Disease

Cassidy SB, Sheehan NC, Farrell DF, et al: Connatal Pelizaeus-Merzbacher disease: An autosomal recessive form. Pediatr Neurol 1987;3:300-305.

Haenggeli CA, Engel E, Pizzolata GP: Connatal Pelizaeus-Merzbacher disease. Dev Med Child Neurol 1989;31:803-807.

Harding BN, Surtees R: Metabolic and neurodegenerative diseases of childhood. In Graham DI, Lantos PL (eds): Greenfield's Neuropathology, 7th ed. London, Arnold, 2002.

Koeppen AH, Robitaille Y: Pelizaeus-Merzbacher disease. J Neuropathol Exp Neurol 2002;61:747-759.

Inoue K, Osaka H, Imaizumi K, et al: Proteolipid protein gene duplications causing Pelizaeus-Merzbacher disease: Molecular mechanism and phenotypic manifestations. Ann Neurol 1999;45:624-632.

Saugier-Veber P, Munnich A, Bonneau D, et al: X-linked spastic paraplegia and Pelizaeus-Merzbacher disease are allelic disorders at the proteolipid protein locus. Nat Genet 1994;6:257-262.

Seitelberger F: Neuropathology and genetics of Pelizaeus-Merzbacher disease. Brain Pathol 1995;5:267-273.

Multiple Sclerosis

Cannella B, Raine CS: The adhesion molecule and cytokine profile of multiple sclerosis lesions. Ann Neurol 1995;37:424-435.

Coyle P: Diagnosis and classification of inflammatory demyelinating disorders. In Burks JS, Johnson KP (eds): Multiple Sclerosis Diagnosis, Medical Management, and Rehabilitation. New York, Demos, 2000.

Gass A, Filippi M, Rodegher ME, et al: Characteristics of chronic MS lesions in the cerebrum, brain stem, spinal cord, and optic nerve on T1-weighted MRI. Neurology 1998;50:548-550.

Keegan M, Pineda AA, McClelland RL, et al: Plasma exchange for severe attacks of CNS demyelination: Predictors of response. Neurology 2002;58:143-146.

Lucchinetti C, Bruck W, Parisi J, et al: Heterogeneity of multiple sclerosis lesions: Implications for the pathogenesis of demyelination. Ann Neurol 2000;47:707-717.

Lycklama G, Thompson A, Filippi M, et al: Spinal-cord MRI in multiple sclerosis. Lancet Neurol 2003;2:555-562.

Noseworthy JH, Lucchinetti C, Rodriguez M, Weinshenker BG: Multiple sclerosis. N Engl J Med 2000;343:938-952.

Prineas JW, McDonald WI, Franklin RJM: Demyelinating diseases. In Graham DI, Lantos PL (eds): Greenfield's Neuropathology, 7th ed. London, Arnold, 2002.

Simon JH: Brain and spinal cord atrophy in multiple sclerosis. Neuroimaging Clin N Am 2000;10:753-770.

Traugott U, Reinherz EL, Raine CS: Multiple sclerosis. Distribution of T cells, T cell subsets and Ia-positive macrophages in lesions of different ages. J Neuroimmunol 1983;4:201-221.

Devic's Neuromyelitis Optica

Cree BA, Goodin DS, Hauser SL: Neuromyelitis optica. Semin Neurol 2002;22:105-122.

de Seze J, Lebrun C, Stojkovic T, et al: Is Devic's neuromyelitis optica a separate disease? A comparative study with multiple sclerosis. Mult Scler 2003;9:521-525.

de Seze J, Stojkovic T, Ferriby D, et al: Devic's neuromyelitis optica: Clinical, laboratory, MRI and outcome profile. J Neurol Sci 2002;197:57-61.

Devic E: Myelite subaigue compliquee de nevrite optique. Bull Med 1894;8:1033-1034.

Fardet L, Genereau T, Mikaeloff Y, et al: Devic's neuromyelitis optica: Study of nine cases. Acta Neurol Scand 2003;108:193-200.

Fazekas F, Offenbacher H, Schmidt R, Strasser-Fuchs S: MRI of neuromyelitis optica: Evidence for a distinct entity. J Neurol Neurosurg Psychiatry 1994;57:1140-1142.

Filippi M, Rocca MA, Moiola L, et al: MRI and magnetization transfer imaging changes in the brain and cervical cord of patients with Devic's neuromyelitis optica. Neurology 1999;53:1705-1710.

Karussis D, Leker RR, Ashkenazi A, Abramsky O: A subgroup of multiple sclerosis patients with anticardiolipin antibodies and unusual clinical manifestations: Do they represent a new nosological entity? Ann Neurol 1998;44:629-634.

Kuroiwa Y: Neuromyelitis optica (Devic's disease, Devic's syndrome). In Koetsier JC (ed): Handbook of Clinical Neurology, vol 3, Demyelinating Diseases. Amsterdam, Elsevier Science, 1985, pp 397-408.

Lucchinetti CF, Mandler RN, McGavern D, et al: A role for humoral mechanisms in the pathogenesis of Devic's neuromyelitis optica. Brain 2002;125:1450-1461.

Mandler RN, Ahmed W, Dencoff JE: Devic's neuromyelitis optica: A prospective study of seven patients treated with prednisone and azathioprine. Neurology 1998;51:1219-1220.

Mandler RN, Davis LE, Jeffery DR, Kornfeld M: Devic's neuromyelitis optica: A clinicopathological study of 8 patients. Ann Neurol 1993;34:162-168.

O'Riordan JI, Gallagher HL, Thompson AJ, et al: Clinical, CSF, and MRI findings in Devic's neuromyelitis optica. J Neurol Neurosurg Psychiatry 1996;60:382-387.

Weinshenker BG: Neuromyelitis optica: What it is and what it might be. Lancet 2003;361:889-890.

Wingerchuk DM, Hogancamp WF, O'Brien PC, Weinshenker BG: The clinical course of neuromyelitis optica (Devic's syndrome). Neurology 1999;53:1107-1114.

Wingerchuk DM, Weinshenker BG: Neuromyelitis optica: Clinical predictors of a relapsing course and survival. Neurology 2003;60:848-853.

Acute Multiple Sclerosis (Marburg Type)

Beniac DR, Wood DD, Palaniyar N, et al: Marburg's variant of multiple sclerosis correlates with a less compact structure of myelin basic protein. Mol Cell Biol Res Commun 1999;1:48-51.

Bitsch A, Wegener C, da Costa C, et al: Lesion development in Marburg's type of acute multiple sclerosis: From inflammation to demyelination. Mult Scler 1999;5:138-146.

Davie CA, Hawkins CP, Barker GJ, et al: Serial proton magnetic resonance spectroscopy in acute multiple sclerosis lesions. Brain 1994;117:49-58.

Giubilei F, Sarrantonio A, Tisei P, et al: Four-year follow-up of a case of acute multiple sclerosis of the Marburg type. Ital J Neurol Sci 1997;18:163-166.

Mehler MF, Rabinowich L: Inflammatory myelinoclastic diffuse sclerosis. Ann Neurol 1988;23:413-415.

Mendez MF, Pogacar S: Malignant monophasic multiple sclerosis or "Marburg's disease." Neurology 1988;38:1153-1155.

Poser CM: Diffuse-disseminated sclerosis in the adult. J Neuropathol Exp Neurol 1957;16:61-78.

Poser CM: Myelinoclastic diffuse sclerosis. In Koetsier JC (ed): Handbook of Clinical Neurology, vol 3, Demyelinating Diseases. Amsterdam, Elsevier Science, 1985, pp 419-428.

Prineas JW, McDonald WI, Franklin RJM: Demyelinating diseases. In Graham DI, Lantos PL (eds): Greenfield's Neuropathology, 7th ed. London, Arnold, 2002.

Weinshenker BG: Therapeutic plasma exchange for acute inflammatory demyelinating syndromes of the central nervous system. J Clin Apheresis 1999;14:144-148.

Wood DD, Bilbao JM, O'Connors P, Moscarello MA: Acute multiple sclerosis (Marburg type) is associated with developmentally immature myelin basic protein. Ann Neurol 1996;40:18-24.

Baló's Concentric Sclerosis

Baló J: Encephalitis periaxialis concentrica. Arch Neurol Psychiatry 1928;19:242-264.

Bolay H, Karabudak R, Tacal T, et al: Balo's concentric sclerosis. Report of two patients with magnetic resonance imaging follow-up. J Neuroimaging 1996;6:98-103.

Caracciolo JT, Murtagh RD, Rojiani AM, Murtagh FR: Pathognomonic MR imaging findings in Balo concentric sclerosis. AJNR Am J Neuroradiol 2001;22:292-293.

Chen CJ: Serial proton magnetic resonance spectroscopy in lesions of Balo concentric sclerosis. J Comput Assist Tomogr 2001;25:713-718.

Chen CJ, Chu NS, Lu CS, Sung CY: Serial magnetic resonance imaging in patients with Balo's concentric sclerosis: Natural history of lesion development. Ann Neurol 1999;46:651-656.

Chen CJ, Ro LS, Chang CN: Serial MRI in pathologically verified Balo concentric sclerosis. J Comput Assist Tomogr 1996;20:732-735.

Chen CJ, Ro LS, Wang LJ Wong YC: Balo's concentric sclerosis: MRI. Neuroradiology 1996;38:322-324.

Iannucci G, Mascalchi M, Salvi F, Filippi M: Vanishing Balo-like lesions in multiple sclerosis. J Neurol Neurosurg Psychiatry 2000;69:399-400.

Itoyama Y, Tateishi J, Kuroiwa Y: Atypical multiple sclerosis with concentric or lamellar demyelinated lesions: Two Japanese patients studied post mortem. Ann Neurol 1985;17:481-487.

Karaarslan E, Altintas A, Senol U, et al: Balo's concentric sclerosis: Clinical and radiologic features of five cases. AJNR Am J Neuroradiol 2001;22:1362-1367.

Kastrup O, Stude P, Limmroth V: Balo's concentric sclerosis: Evolution of active demyelination demonstrated by serial contrast-enhanced MRI. J Neurol 2002;249:811-814.

Kim MO, Lee SA, Choi CG, et al: Balo's concentric sclerosis: A clinical case study of brain MRI, biopsy, and proton magnetic resonance spectroscopic findings. J Neurol Neurosurg Psychiatry 1997;62:655-658.

Kuroiwa Y: Concentric sclerosis. In Koetsier JC (ed): Handbook of Clinical Neurology, vol 3, Demyelinating Diseases. Amsterdam, Elsevier Science, 1985, pp 409-417.

Louboutin JP, Elie B: Treatment of Balo's concentric sclerosis with immunosuppressive drugs followed by multimodality evoked potentials and MRI. Muscle Nerve 1995;8:1478-1480.

Lucchinetti C, Bruck W, Parisi J, et al: Heterogeneity of multiple sclerosis lesions: Implications for the pathogenesis of demyelination [see comment]. Ann Neurol 2000;47:707-717.

Moore GR, Berry K, Oger JJ, et al: Balo's concentric sclerosis: Surviving normal myelin in a patient with a relapsing-remitting clinical course. Mult Scler 2001;7:375-382.

Moore GR, Neumann PE, Suzuki K, et al: Balo's concentric sclerosis: New observations on lesion development. Ann Neurol 1985;17:604-611.

Ng SH, Ko SF, Cheung YC, et al: MRI features of Balo's concentric sclerosis. Br J Radiol 1999;72:400-403.

Prineas JW, McDonald WI, Franklin RJM: Demyelinating diseases. In Graham DI, Lantos PL (eds): Greenfield's Neuropathology, 7th ed. London, Arnold, 2002.

Sekijima Y, Tokuda T, Hashimoto T, et al: Serial magnetic resonance imaging (MRI) study of a patient with Balo's concentric sclerosis treated with immunoadsorption plasmapheresis. Mult Scler 1997;2:291-294.

Spiegel M, Kruger H, Hofmann E, Kappos L: MRI study of Balo's concentric sclerosis before and after immunosuppressive therapy. J Neurol 1989;236:487-488.

Schilder's Disease

Eblen F, Poremba M, Grodd W, et al: Myelinoclastic diffuse sclerosis (Schilder's disease): Cliniconeuroradiologic correlations. Neurology 1991;41:589-591.

Fernandez-Jaen A, Martinez-Bermejo A, Gutierrez-Molina M, et al: Schilder's diffuse myelinoclastic sclerosis. Rev Neurol 2001;33:16-21.

Kotil K, Kalayci M, Koseoglu T, Tugrul A: Myelinoclastic diffuse sclerosis (Schilder's disease): Report of a case and review of the literature. Br J Neurosurg 2002;16:516-519.

Kurul S, Cakmakci H, Dirik E, Kovanlikaya A: Schilder's disease: Case study with serial neuroimaging. J Child Neurol 2003;18:58-61.

Nejat F, Eftekhar B: Decompressive aspiration in myelinoclastic diffuse sclerosis or Schilder disease. Case report. J Neurosurg 2002;97:1447-1449.

Poser CM: Diffuse-disseminated sclerosis in the adult. J Neuropathol Exp Neurol 1957;16:61-78.

Poser CM: Myelinoclastic diffuse sclerosis. In Koetsier JC (ed): Handbook of Clinical Neurology, vol 3, Demyelinating Diseases. Amsterdam, Elsevier Science, 1985, pp 419-428.

Poser S, Luer W, Bruhn H, et al: Acute demyelinating disease. Classification and non-invasive diagnosis. Acta Neurol Scand 1992;86:579-585.

Prineas JW, McDonald WI, Franklin RJM: Demyelinating diseases. In Graham DI, Lantos PL (eds): Greenfield's Neuropathology, 7th ed. London, Arnold, 2002.

Valk J, van der Knaap MS: Multiple sclerosis, neuromyelitis optica, concentric sclerosis, and Schilder's diffuse sclerosis. In Valk J, van der Knaap MS (eds): Magnetic Resonance of Myelin, Myelination, and Myelin Disorders. Berlin, Springer-Verlag, 1995, pp 179-205.

Acute Disseminated Encephalomyelitis

Gallucci M, Caulo M, Cerone G, Masciocchi C: Acquired inflammatory white matter disease. Childs Nerv Syst 2001;17:202-210.

Giang DW, Poduri KR, Eskin TA, et al: Multiple sclerosis masquerading as a mass lesion. Neuroradiology 1992;34:150-154.

Hynson JL, Kornberg AJ, Coleman LT, et al: Clinical and neuroradiologic features of acute disseminated encephalomyelitis in children. Neurology 2001;56:1308-1312.

Kepes JJ: Large focal tumor-like demyelinating lesions of the brain: Intermediate entity between multiple sclerosis and acute disseminated encephalomyelitis? A study of 31 patients. Ann Neurol 1993;33:18-27.

Prineas JW, McDonald WI, Franklin RJM: Demyelinating diseases. In Graham DI, Lantos PL (eds): Greenfield's Neuropathology, 7th ed. London, Arnold, 2002.

Schwarz S, Mohr A, Knauth M, et al: Acute disseminated encephalomyelitis: A follow-up study of 40 adult patients. Neurology 2001;56:1313-1318.

Acute Hemorrhagic Leukoencephalitis (Hurst's Disease)

An SF, Groves M, Martinian L, et al: Detection of infectious agents in brain of patients with acute hemorrhagic leukoencephalitis. J Neurovirol 2002;8:439-446.

Brunn A, Nacimiento W, Sellhaus B, et al: Acute onset of hemorrhagic leukoencephalomyelitis (Hurst) in the spinal cord. Clin Neuropathol 2002;21:214-219.

Case records of the Massachusetts General Hospital. Weekly clinicopathological exercises. Case 1-1999. A 53 year-old man with fever and rapid neurologic deterioration. N Engl J Med 1999;340:127-135.

Gillies CG, Grunnet M, Hamilton CW: Tubular inclusions in macrophages in the brain of a patient with acute hemorrhagic leukoencephalitis (Weston-Hurst syndrome). Ultrastructural Pathol 1994;18:19-22.

Kuperan S, Ostrow P, Landi MK, Bakshi R: Acute hemorrhagic leukoencephalitis vs ADEM: FLAIR MRI and neuropathology findings. Neurology 2003;60:721-722.

Leake JA, Billman GF, Nespeca MP, et al: Pediatric acute hemorrhagic leukoencephalitis: Report of a surviving patient and review. Clin Infect Dis 2002;34:699-703.

McLeod DR, Snyder F, Bridge P, Pinto A: Acute hemorrhagic leukoencephalitis in male sibs. Am J Med Genet 2002;107:325-329.

Mizuguchi M: Acute necrotizing encephalopathy of childhood: A novel form of acute encephalopathy prevalent in Japan and Taiwan. Brain Dev 1997;21:138-139.

Pfausler B, Engelhardt K, Kampfl A, et al: Post-infectious central and peripheral nervous system diseases complicating *Mycoplasma pneumoniae* infection. Report of three cases and review of the literature. Eur J Neurol 2002;9:93-96.

Prineas JW, McDonald WI, Franklin RJM: Demyelinating diseases. In Graham DI, Lantos PL (eds): Greenfield's Neuropathology, 7th ed. London, Arnold, 2002.

Rosman NP, Gottlieb SM, Bernstein CA: Acute hemorrhagic leukoencephalitis: Recovery and reversal of magnetic resonance imaging findings in a child. J Child Neurol 1997;12:448-454.

6 Neurodegenerative Diseases

Elizabeth J. Cochran

In recent years, tremendous advances have been achieved in understanding the genetic and biochemical abnormalities of many neurodegenerative diseases. These advances have challenged traditional clinical pathologic classification of these entities and have resulted in clustering of various diseases, which were not previously known to be so related, under one general heading (i.e., multisystem atrophy and Parkinson's disease). The neurodegenerative diseases discussed in this chapter are classified in accordance with our current understanding of genetic and biochemical abnormalities. However, much is still not understood about these entities, and it is likely that these classifications will continue to evolve as additional discoveries unfold.

ALZHEIMER'S DISEASE

CLINICAL FEATURES

Although heterogeneous in clinical expression, the most common and typical symptoms of Alzheimer's disease (AD) are memory loss and cognitive dysfunction. Patients usually present with short-term memory impairment. Judgment and visuospatial impairment (getting lost, inability to deal with new situations, inability to dress oneself) may also occur early in the disease process. With disease progression, initial symptoms worsen and the ability to perform even the most basic activities of daily life is lost. Word-finding difficulties, psychiatric and behavioral disturbances, incontinence, and apraxia are likely to be seen. Finally, complete deterioration of cognition, loss of mobility with resulting limb rigidity, incontinence, and mutism develop.

Inheritance of AD is genetically complex but may be divided into three groups: (1) the largest group (75%) is composed of individuals with apparently sporadic disease, (2) the second group (23% to 24%) consists of patients with a history of affected relatives but in whom the disease appears to develop randomly, and (3) the last group (1% to 2%) has a prominent family history consistent with a mendelian inheritance pattern, typically autosomal dominant and highly penetrant. This group

ALZHEIMER'S DISEASE—FACT SHEET

Definition

▶ Most common cause of dementia, characterized pathologically by the presence of senile plaques and neurofibrillary tangles

Incidence and Prevalence

▶ Incidence increases with age: between 70 and 80 years—1 to 2 cases per 100 individuals per year; >80 years—2 to 8 cases per 100 individuals per year
▶ Prevalence: approximately 4 million individuals currently affected with AD in the United States
  ▶ Between 60 and 64 years—1%
  ▶ >85 years—40%

Gender and Age Distribution

▶ Higher prevalence in women possibly because of a higher percentage of women in older age groups (ratio of 1.2 to 1.5)
▶ Mean age at onset is 80 years
▶ Early-onset disease occurs at ages younger than 60 to 65 years (approximately 7% of all AD)

Clinical Features

▶ Most common symptoms are memory loss and cognitive dysfunction
▶ Usually present with short-term memory impairment
▶ May present with judgment and visuospatial impairment
▶ Slowly progressive
▶ Eventual complete deterioration of cognition, loss of mobility, rigidity, incontinence, and mutism

Radiologic Features

▶ MRI and non–contrast-enhanced CT show diffuse cortical atrophy, with more severe involvement of the mesial temporal lobe structures and ventricular dilatation

Prognosis and Treatment

▶ Average duration is 7 years (range, 2 to 18 years)
▶ Cholinesterase inhibitors may have a temporary stabilizing effect on deterioration

is referred to as familial AD. It is usually of early onset (<60 years). The age at onset of AD in the first and second groups is usually older than 60 years. At present, mutations in three genes (presenilin-1, presenilin-2, and amyloid precursor protein) have been identified in families with autosomal dominant AD. Most of the mutations described thus far are in the presenilin-1 gene on chromosome 14.

Multiple candidate genes with possible associations with late-onset AD have been identified, but no studies have consistently replicated these associations. The only late-onset risk factor definitely associated with AD, in addition to age, is the apolipoprotein ε4 genotype.

The presence of an apolipoprotein ε4 allele has been found to influence the risk for AD in a dose-dependent manner by decreasing the age at onset of disease. The apo ε4 allele is not necessary nor sufficient for the development of AD.

PATHOLOGIC FEATURES

GROSS FINDINGS

A decrease in brain weight is a usual, but inconstant, finding. More severe atrophy is evident in early-onset and familial AD. Gyral atrophy and ventricular dilatation are typically seen (Figs. 6-1 and 6-2). The mesial temporal lobe structures, including the temporal cortex, amygdala, entorhinal cortex, and hippocampus, are most affected. The next most affected are the frontal and parietal lobes with relative sparing of the occipital lobe. Lateral ventricular dilatation is present, often most severe in the temporal horn.

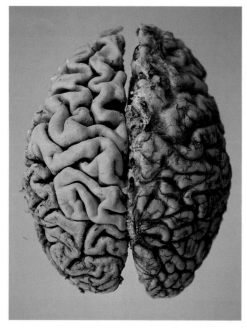

FIGURE 6-1

Gross photograph of the superior aspect of the brain of a patient with Alzheimer's disease. Note the cortical atrophy.

ALZHEIMER'S DISEASE—PATHOLOGIC FEATURES

Gross Findings

▶ Decreased brain weight
▶ Diffuse gyral atrophy and ventricular dilatation, with most severe involvement of the temporal cortex, amygdala, hippocampus, and entorhinal cortex and relative sparing of the occipital lobe

Microscopic Findings

▶ Diffuse and neuritic plaques found throughout the neocortex
▶ Neurofibrillary tangles most numerous in the hippocampus, amygdala, and entorhinal cortex, but usually also in the neocortex
▶ Neuritic plaque density and neurofibrillary tangle location and density used in the pathologic diagnosis

Ultrastructural Features

▶ Neuritic plaque exhibits the central core of the Aβ-amyloid protein, surrounded by distorted neurites usually containing paired helical filament–tau (PHF-tau)
▶ Neurofibrillary tangles are intraneuronal accumulations of PHF-tau

Genetics

▶ Most disease is sporadic
▶ Autosomal dominant early-onset AD is found in 1% to 2% of all AD
▶ Three genes have been identified that contain mutations in familial AD: presenilin-1, presenilin-2, and amyloid precursor protein
▶ The apolipoprotein ε4 allele confers an increased risk of AD by decreasing the age at disease onset

Immunohistochemical Features

▶ Neuritic and diffuse plaques and amyloid angiopathy immunoreact with antibodies to Aβ-amyloid protein
▶ Neurofibrillary tangles and neuritic plaques immunoreact with PHF-tau antibodies

Pathologic Differential Diagnosis

▶ Vascular dementia
▶ Diffuse Lewy body disease
▶ Frontotemporal lobar degeneration
▶ Creutzfeldt-Jakob disease

MICROSCOPIC FINDINGS

Essential findings are senile plaques and neurofibrillary tangles (NFTs). A senile plaque consists of an extracellular accumulation of Aβ-amyloid protein and, frequently, paired helical filament–tau (PHF-tau) protein in the neuropil of gray matter. Aβ-amyloid is derived from amyloid precursor protein, a membrane-spanning protein normally found in the brain. PHF-tau is an abnormally phosphorylated form of tau, a microtubule-associated protein. Several types of senile plaques occur, and subtypes vary in importance in the pathologic diagnosis of AD. Diffuse plaques are composed of Aβ-amyloid protein without PHF-tau and are frequently found in elderly individuals, usually without cognitive impairment. Neuritic plaques consist of Aβ-amyloid intermixed with thickened neurites (axons, dendrites)

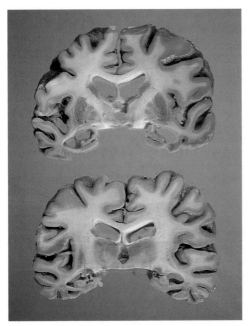

FIGURE 6-2

Coronal slice of the brain of a patient with Alzheimer's disease. Note the gyral atrophy and enlarged lateral ventricles, especially the temporal horns.

containing PHF-tau and have been found to correlate with the degree of cognitive impairment more closely than diffuse plaques do. For the purpose of diagnostic evaluation of the brain of a dementia patient, quantitation of the neuritic subtype is indicated. Neuritic plaques are seen with silver stains (Bielschowsky, Gallyas) or antibodies to PHF-tau protein (Fig. 6-3A and B). Diffuse plaques may also be identified with Bielschowsky stain, traditional amyloid stains such as Congo red and thioflavin S, and antibodies to Aβ-amyloid peptide (see Fig. 6-3C and D).

Senile plaques accumulate in the neocortex of the brain and are preferentially found initially in the associative cortices. The highest concentrations of plaques are found in cortical laminae II, III, and IV. A widely used method of determining the density of neuritic plaques is that created by the Consortium to Establish a Registry for Alzheimer's Disease (CERAD). An estimate of plaque density is determined by using a scale of 0 to 5. The plaques are examined at 100× in a field of approximately 1 mm². An estimate should be made of the region that appears to be most affected. The suggested cortical areas for evaluation are the midfrontal cortex, superior/middle temporal gyri, and inferior parietal cortex.

An NFT, in contrast to a senile plaque, is an intraneuronal aggregation of argyrophilic PHF-tau. NFTs are not easily discerned on hematoxylin-eosin staining. Silver stains (Bielschowsky, Gallyas, and Bodian), thioflavin S, or immunohistochemical staining with antibodies to tau protein is necessary for identification (Fig. 6-4). The shape of an NFT conforms to the shape of the neuronal cytoplasm that it occupies. Those in the cortex are usually flame shaped or triangular, and those

in the subcortical nuclei are typically globose and resemble a ball of yarn. Ultrastructural examination of NFTs has shown that they are composed of paired helical filaments, two filaments wound around each other with regular periodicity. Biochemical analysis of these filaments has shown they are abnormally phosphorylated tau protein. This PHF-tau is also found in the abnormal neurites of neuritic plaque. In addition to being deposited in plaques and NFTs, PHF-tau is found scattered throughout the gray matter in neuropil threads. NFTs, similar to senile plaques, are concentrated in specific cortical laminae: layers II and V of the association cortices and layers II and IV of the limbic cortex. However, in contrast to senile plaques, the distribution of NFTs occurs in a stereotypic pattern in AD patients and has been classified into six stages by Braak and Braak. In stages I and II, NFTs are found only in the transentorhinal cortex and hippocampus. Stage III shows an increased number of NFTs in the entorhinal cortex (Fig. 6-5) and still relatively sparse NFTs in the hippocampus and temporal cortex. Tangles increase in severity in stage IV. Stages V and VI are marked by progressively more widespread involvement of the neocortex by NFTs. NFTs have been found to correlate with the degree of cognitive impairment in AD patients.

Criteria for the pathologic diagnosis of AD have evolved over the past 25 years. Current guidelines, developed by a National Institute on Aging Reagan Consensus Conference in 1997, suggest the use of both neuritic plaques and NFTs in determining the likelihood of AD explaining a clinical diagnosis of dementia (Figs. 6-6 and 6-7). These criteria differ from previous criteria in that they do not modify the pathologic diagnosis based on the age or clinical diagnosis of the patient. According to the guidelines, a high likelihood of dementia being caused by AD exists when a CERAD frequent neuritic plaque score and a Braak stage of V/VI are found, an intermediate likelihood exists when a CERAD moderate neuritic plaque score and a Braak stage of III/IV are found, and a low likelihood exists when a CERAD sparse neuritic plaque score and a Braak stage of I/II are present.

Other pathologic findings in the brains of patients with AD are granulovacuolar degeneration, Hirano bodies, and cerebral amyloid angiopathy. Granulovacuolar degeneration occurs most commonly in the pyramidal neurons of the hippocampus and consists of a cytoplasmic vacuole containing a granule (Fig. 6-8). The granule is immunoreactive with antibodies to neurofilament, ubiquitin, tau, and tubulin. Hirano bodies are also found in the pyramidal neurons of the hippocampus and are cytoplasmic, eosinophilic, and usually rod-like (Fig. 6-9). They are composed of actin and appear paracrystalline ultrastructurally. Hirano bodies are immunoreactive for tau, Aβ-amyloid protein, and neurofilament. Both granulovacuolar degeneration and Hirano bodies are found in elderly nondemented individuals, the parkinsonian-dementia complex of Guam, and several other dementias, in addition to AD.

Deposition of Aβ-amyloid in the leptomeningeal and cortical small arteries and arterioles occurs in most

Text continued on p. 230

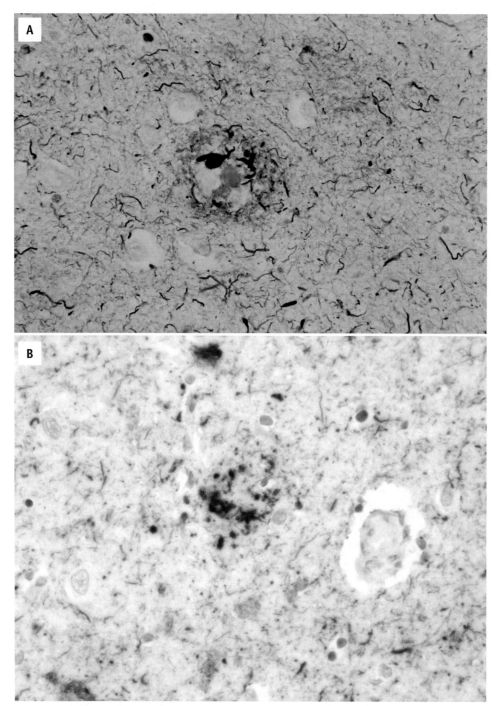

FIGURE 6-3
Senile plaques. **A**, Modified Bielschowsky–stained neuritic plaque. **B**, Tau-immunostained neuritic plaque.

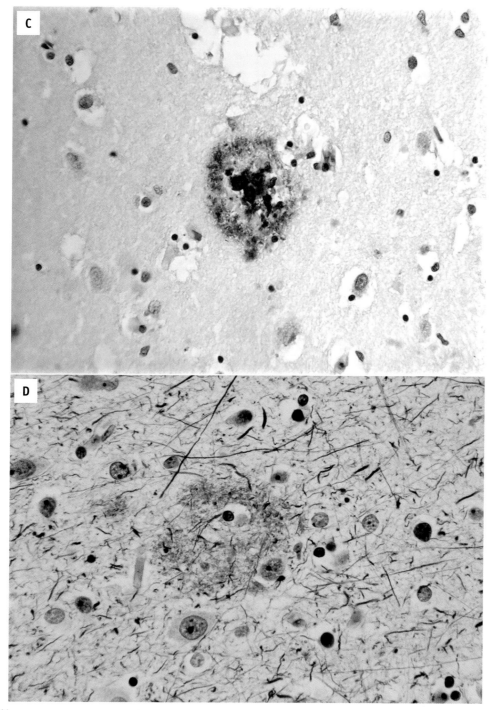

FIGURE 6-3, cont'd
C, Aβ-amyloid–immunostained plaque. **D**, Modified Bielschowsky–stained diffuse plaque.

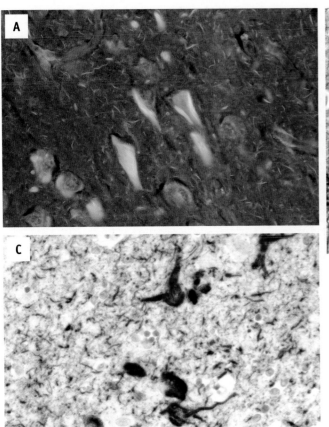

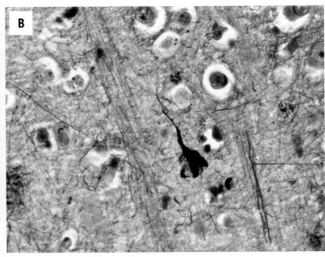

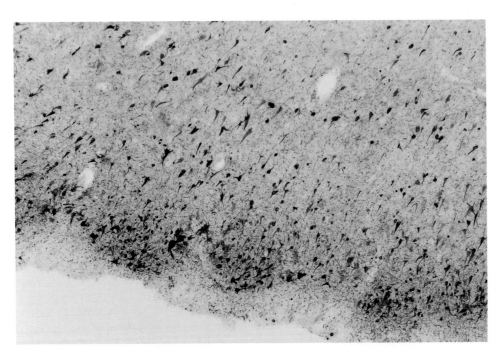

FIGURE 6-4

Neurofibrillary tangles. **A**, Thioflavin S–stained neurofibrillary tangles. **B**, Modified Bielschowsky–stained neurofibrillary tangle. **C**, Paired helical filament antibody–immunostained neurofibrillary tangle.

FIGURE 6-5

Paired helical filament antibody–immunostained neurofibrillary tangles in the entorhinal cortex. Note the dense clusters in layer II.

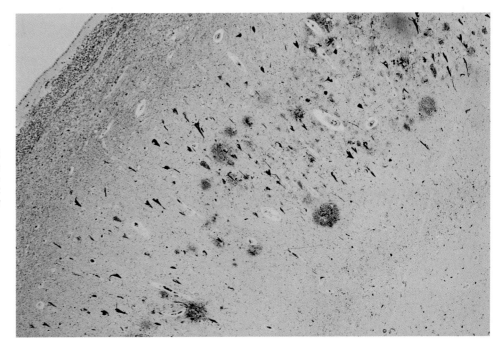

FIGURE 6-6

Alzheimer's disease. A modified Bielschowsky–stained section of the CA1 sector of the hippocampus contains a moderate density of neuritic plaques and frequent neurofibrillary tangles.

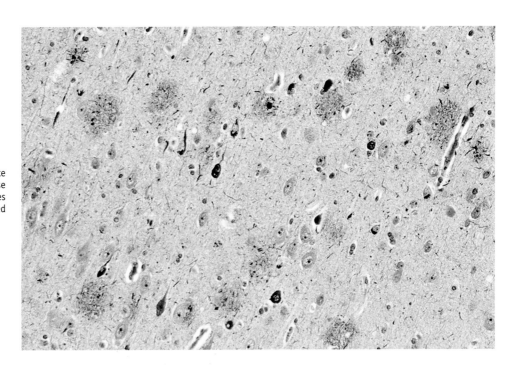

FIGURE 6-7

Alzheimer's disease. A moderate density of neuritic and diffuse plaques and neurofibrillary tangles is seen in the neocortex (modified Bielschowsky stain).

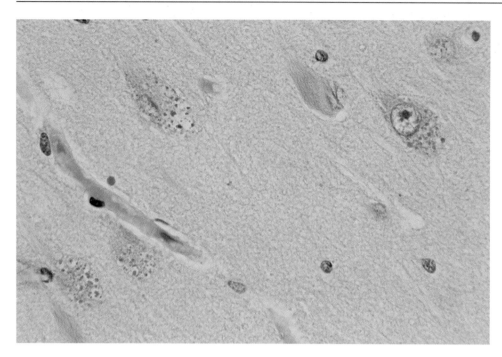

FIGURE 6-8

Granulovacuolar degeneration in multiple hippocampal neurons.

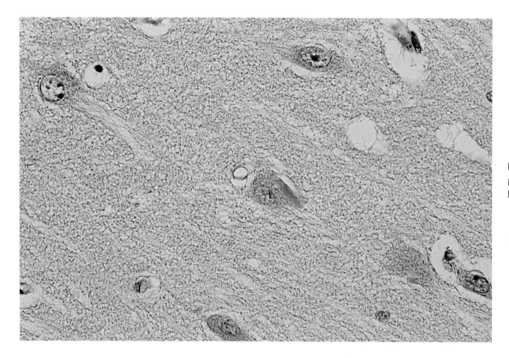

FIGURE 6-9

Hirano body in the cytoplasm of a hippocampal neuron.

individuals with AD (approximately 80%). It is associated with lobar hemorrhages and less commonly with infarcts. Aβ-amyloid protein is deposited external to the basal lamina in the media and adventitia (Fig. 6-10). It causes destruction of the muscular wall with a resultant "gun barrel" appearance of the vessels (Fig. 6-11). Aβ-amyloid almost never occurs in white matter, is preferentially deposited in the occipital lobe, and is also found in the cerebellum (Fig. 6-12).

ANCILLARY STUDIES

No established laboratory tests for AD currently exist. Blood tests (complete blood count, chemistry panels, thyroid function, and vitamin B$_{12}$ level) are performed to rule out other causes of dementia. A magnetic resonance imaging (MRI) scan is usually obtained, particularly in patients with atypical clinical symptoms.

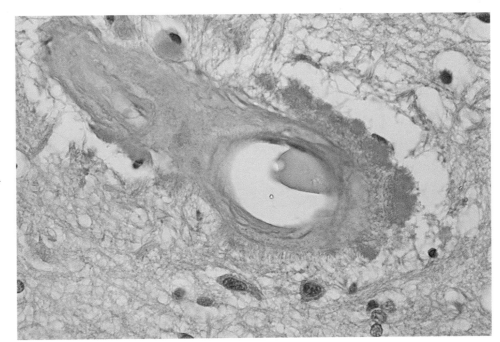

FIGURE 6-10

Cortical arteriole with amyloid deposition in the media and adventitia.

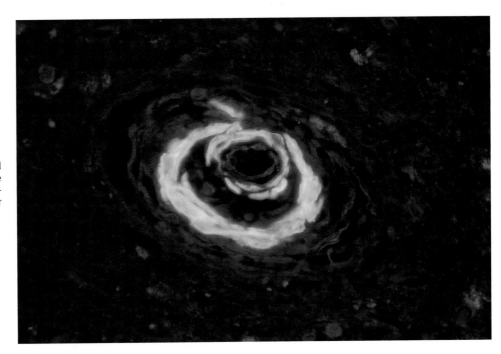

FIGURE 6-11

Cortical arteriole exhibiting amyloid deposition within its wall. Note the characteristic splitting of the arteriolar wall (thioflavin S stain under ultraviolet light).

Classically, it shows diffuse cortical atrophy with more severe involvement of the mesial temporal lobe structures and ventricular dilatation. In patients with strong family histories and onset of symptoms at an age younger than 60 years, genetic testing for one of the known mutations is indicated. Apolipoprotein ε4 allele testing may be performed, but the presence of an apo ε4 allele does not predict the development of AD. In patients with a clinical diagnosis of AD, it may marginally improve diagnostic accuracy.

DIFFERENTIAL DIAGNOSIS

Clinically, vascular dementia, dementia with Lewy bodies, frontotemporal dementias, and Creutzfeldt-Jakob disease are the most common dementias that should be considered in the differential diagnosis of AD, especially in the setting of an atypical clinical manifestation. Evaluation with MRI, cerebrospinal fluid analysis for elevated protein and 14-3-3 protein, and

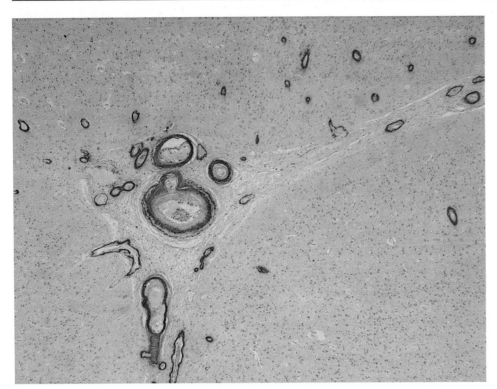

FIGURE 6-12
Leptomeningeal and cortical arterioles with Aβ-amyloid deposition within their walls (Aβ-amyloid immunostain).

electroencephalography (EEG) are tests that may help distinguish among these different entities. Pathologic examination is usually definitive. However, distinction from other neurodegenerative diseases in which NFTs or other abnormal tau deposits occur (progressive supranuclear palsy, corticobasal degeneration, frontotemporal lobar degeneration) may occasionally pose a problem. Although uncommon, AD and Creutzfeldt-Jakob disease or AD and frontotemporal lobar degeneration may both be found in the same patient. In addition, mixed dementias composed of the changes of AD and multiple infarcts or AD and diffuse Lewy body disease occur frequently.

PROGNOSTIC AND THERAPEUTIC CONSIDERATIONS

AD is a slowly progressive disease with an average duration of 7 years and a range of 2 to 18 years. At present, several medications are available that have a modest effect in stabilizing the clinical decline in AD patients. Because of the well-documented cholinergic deficit in AD, there has been a focus on development of cholinesterase inhibitors (donepezil, rivastigmine, galantamine). These drugs have produced temporary, but significant, slowing of symptom progression. Multiple other avenues of investigation for possible therapies reflect recent progress in understanding the pathogenesis of AD. Such therapies include nonsteroidal anti-inflammatory drugs, vitamin E, lipid-lowering medications, and vaccination with Aβ-amyloid peptide antibodies.

SYNUCLEINOPATHIES

The importance of α-synuclein protein in Parkinson's disease (PD) first became apparent with the discovery of a mutation in the α-synuclein gene on chromosome 4 in a kindred with the autosomal dominant form of PD. Although α-synuclein gene mutations have been found in only a few families, this discovery led to the identification of α-synuclein protein as an integral component of Lewy bodies, an essential neuropathologic finding in PD and dementia with Lewy bodies. The function of α-synuclein, a protein consisting of 127 to 140 amino acids, is incompletely understood. Subsequent to its discovery in Lewy bodies, it was also found to be deposited in the form of glial cytoplasmic inclusions in multiple system atrophy. The result of these discoveries led to the creation of a new category of neurodegenerative diseases, the synucleinopathies, defined by the deposition of α-synuclein as the primary neuropathologic finding in the brain.

LEWY BODY DISEASES

PARKINSON'S DISEASE

CLINICAL FEATURES

The peak onset of PD is between the ages of 55 and 65 years. The three classic features of PD are bradykinesia

PATHOLOGIC FEATURES

GROSS FINDINGS

Pallor of the substantia nigra and locus ceruleus are typically found at autopsy. Slight cortical atrophy and ventricular dilatation may also be present.

MICROSCOPIC FINDINGS

Severe loss of the melanin-containing, tyrosine hydroxylase–immunoreactive neurons of the substantia nigra pars compacta is typical of PD (Fig. 6-13). The neuronal loss is first seen in the ventrolateral portion of the substantia nigra, followed by the ventromedial and

or akinesia, cogwheel rigidity, and resting tremor. Tremor is frequently the initial symptom and is often asymmetric. A slow shuffling gait with a stooped posture and loss of arm swing, postural instability, and masked facies are also usually present.

Only a very small percentage of PD patients have been found to have a mendelian inheritance pattern. At least eight different familial forms of PD have been described. Park1 refers to the familial disease found in Italian and Greek kindreds and is associated with mutation of the α-synuclein gene on chromosome 4. Park2 refers to autosomal recessive juvenile-onset PD and is associated with a mutation in the *parkin* gene on chromosome 6. The *parkin* gene codes for a ubiquitin protein ligase. Mutations (partial deletions or point mutations) in the gene have been found to be responsible for approximately 50% of early-onset PD with autosomal recessive inheritance. Park5 is PD caused by a missense mutation in the ubiquitin–terminal hydroxylase L1 (*UCHL1*) gene on chromosome 4. Linkage studies have identified at least five other forms of PD linked to chromosomes on which specific genes have not yet been identified.

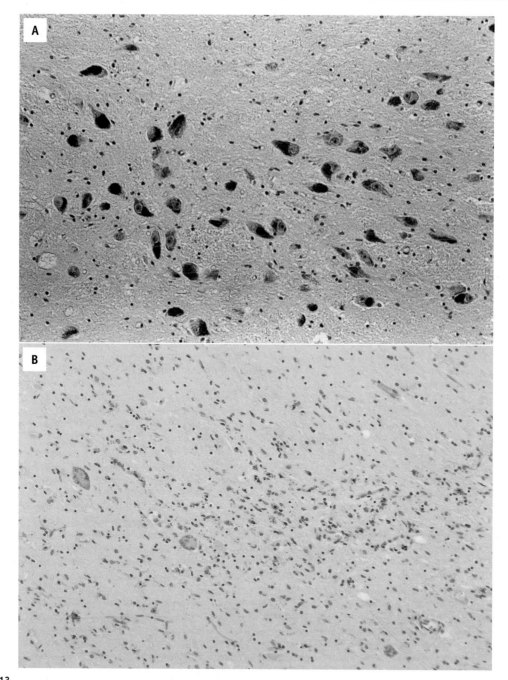

FIGURE 6-13

Parkinson's disease. **A**, Normal density of pigmented neurons in the substantia nigra. **B**, Decreased density of pigmented neurons as seen in Parkinson's disease. Note the pigment-laden macrophages.

dorsal areas. The result of the neuronal degeneration is dopaminergic denervation of the striatum. The ventro-lateral substantia nigra projects to the dorsal putamen; degeneration of this region of the nigra is seen in PD with predominantly akinetic-rigid symptomatology. In tremor-predominant PD, less severe total neuronal loss and less severe depletion of the lateral substantia nigra are evident. Neuronal loss in the substantia nigra stimulates reactive astrocytosis. In addition, melanin-laden macrophages and free pigment ("pigment incontinence") are also found in areas of neuronal loss.

Neuronal loss alone is not diagnostic of PD. The presence of Lewy bodies is necessary for definite diagnosis. Lewy bodies are intraneuronal cytoplasmic spherical inclusions ranging from 8 to 30 μm in diameter. They have hyaline eosinophilic cores surrounded by pale haloes (Fig. 6-14A). A single neuron may contain one or more Lewy bodies. They are ubiquitin, α-synuclein, and usually neurofilament immunoreactive. Antibodies to α-synuclein have been found to be more sensitive and specific markers of Lewy bodies than ubiquitin antibodies are. Electron microscopic examination shows

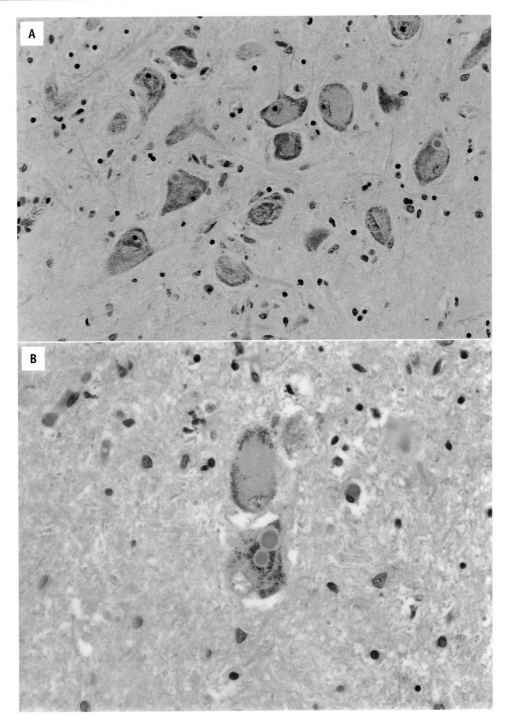

FIGURE 6-14

Parkinson's disease. **A**, Two neurons of the substantia nigra containing Lewy bodies. **B**, Lewy bodies in the cytoplasm of a nigral neuron adjacent to a neuron containing a large pale body.

radially arranged intermediate filaments (7 to 20 nm) associated with granular material and vesicular structures. Lewy bodies are also found in the locus ceruleus, nucleus basalis of Meynert, dorsal vagal nucleus, hypothalamus, olfactory bulb, Edinger-Westphal nucleus, raphe nuclei, intermediolateral cell column of the spinal cord, and autonomic ganglia.

Pale bodies are cytoplasmic areas of pallor also found in the pigmented neurons of the substantia nigra

(see Fig. 6-14B). Their immunostaining profile is similar to that of Lewy bodies, but their relationship to Lewy bodies remains unclarified. It has been hypothesized that pale bodies are precursors of Lewy bodies or that they develop in parallel with Lewy body formation.

Cortical Lewy bodies, in contrast to brain stem Lewy bodies, do not have a distinct halo. They are eosinophilic and usually round, are most frequently found in the lower cortical layers (V and VI), and are most numerous

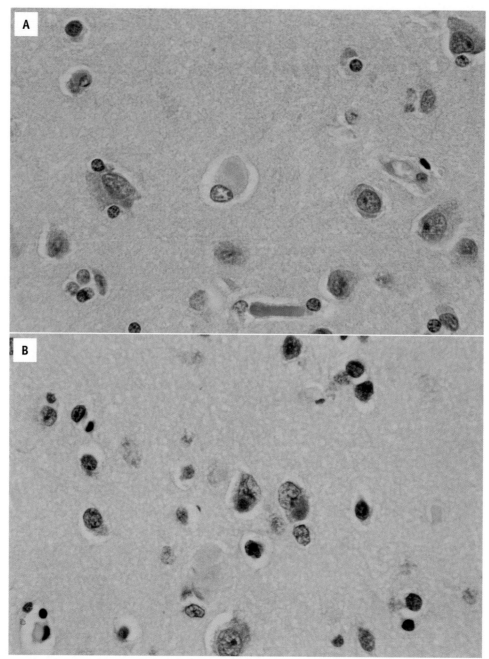

FIGURE 6-15

Cortical Lewy body in the superior temporal gyrus. **A**, Note the eosinophilic cytoplasmic inclusion without a halo. **B**, α-Synuclein–immunostained cortical Lewy bodies.

in the temporal, insular, and cingulate cortices. Cortical Lewy bodies are also ubiquitin and α-synuclein immunoreactive; the latter immunostaining aids in distinction from NFTs (Fig. 6-15). Cortical Lewy bodies are present in small numbers in virtually all cases of idiopathic PD with or without a history of dementia. Dementia is seen in approximately 50% of PD patients. Several issues remain to be definitively resolved regarding the histologic correlates of dementia in PD, including the relationship between PD and AD and the significance of cortical Lewy bodies, senile plaques, and NFTs in PD patients with and without dementia. A

recent study using α-synuclein immunohistochemistry to examine an autopsy group of PD patients with dementia showed that cortical Lewy bodies in significant density were present in 90%. In the remaining 10% of the patients with PD and dementia, no histologic correlate was found for the dementia. AD changes were found in addition to cortical Lewy bodies in 35% of the patients.

Dystrophic neurites (Lewy neurites) are found in brains of PD patients with dementia, as well as those with dementia and Lewy bodies. They are found in the CA2-CA3 sector of the hippocampus, accessory cortical nuclei of the amygdala, nucleus basalis of Meynert,

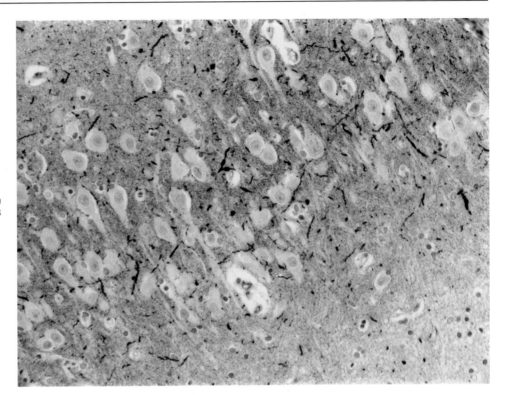

FIGURE 6-16

Lewy neurites immunostained with α-synuclein antibody in the CA2-CA3 sector of the hippocampus.

brain stem (substantia nigra, dorsal vagal nucleus), olfactory bulb, intermediolateral column of the spinal cord, and sympathetic and parasympathetic ganglia. The neurites are immunoreactive to α-synuclein, ubiquitin, and neurofilament (Fig. 6-16). Ubiquitin- and α-synuclein–immunoreactive glial cytoplasmic inclusions are also found in PD patients both without dementia and with dementia and Lewy bodies. They are found in the same areas as brain stem and cortical Lewy bodies.

ANCILLARY STUDIES

MRI and computed tomographic scans are usually normal in PD. No specific laboratory tests exist for PD.

DIFFERENTIAL DIAGNOSIS

Clinically, PD may be confused with progressive supranuclear palsy, multiple system atrophy, corticobasal degeneration, and dementia with Lewy bodies. Each may have significant clinical overlap with PD, but in their classic form, they exhibit distinct clinical signs. Progressive supranuclear palsy is often associated with impairment of upgaze, patients with multiple system atrophy may have ataxia or significant autonomic dysfunction, and corticobasal degeneration was originally reported with prominent apraxia. Dementia with Lewy bodies is typically manifested as dementia characterized by fluctuations in cognitive impairment and level of consciousness and hallucinations. Pathologically, all but dementia with Lewy bodies are quite distinct from PD.

PD and dementia with Lewy bodies may not be histopathologically distinguishable, and the two must be separated by review of the clinical findings, course, and neuropathology.

PROGNOSTIC AND THERAPEUTIC CONSIDERATIONS

Levodopa remains an important therapy for PD. Because of limitations in effectiveness with long-term use of levodopa, dopamine agonist therapy may be initiated at the time of diagnosis. Surgical treatments include thalamotomy for tremor and pallidotomy or ablation of the subthalamic nucleus for symptoms of PD and drug-induced dyskinesias. Placement of deep brain stimulators in the globus pallidus or subthalamus is also currently in use as an alternative to ablation of the nuclei, with less risk of adverse effects.

DIFFUSE LEWY BODY DISEASE

Multiple names have been attached to dementia associated with cortical and brain stem Lewy bodies. Most recently, "dementia with Lewy bodies" has been suggested as the preferred term because it identifies the distinctive clinical syndrome of dementia associated with fluctuating cognition, hallucinations, and Lewy bodies. Other names are Lewy body variant of Alzheimer's disease, diffuse Lewy body disease, and Lewy body dementia. In this chapter, the term diffuse Lewy body disease (DLBD) is used because it describes the pathologic findings without reliance on clinical information. DLBD is defined as the presence of cortical and brain stem Lewy bodies with or without changes associated with AD. In the absence of AD changes, the entity may more accurately be called pure DLBD. Patients with so-called pure DLBD are much less frequently encountered than are those with both diffuse Lewy bodies and AD-related changes. Kosaka has called DLBD with AD changes the common type of DLBD.

CLINICAL FEATURES

Age at onset is usually between 68 and 92 years. Characteristic clinical findings are fluctuations in cognitive impairment and level of consciousness. Visual hallucinations are found in the majority of patients. Up to 70% have parkinsonism characterized by bradykinesia, limb rigidity, and gait disorder. Tremor is seen rarely. Increased sensitivity to neuroleptic medication may occur. Recurrent falls and syncope may be seen in up to 33%. Neuropsychological testing shows prominent attention deficits, visuospatial impairment, and fronto-subcortical dysfunction.

DIFFUSE LEWY BODY DISEASE—FACT SHEET

Definition
▶ Dementia characterized pathologically by the presence of cortical and brain stem Lewy bodies
▶ Also known as dementia with Lewy bodies and the Lewy body variant of AD
▶ May have concomitant AD

Incidence and Prevalence
▶ No incidence data available
▶ Reported to be the most common cause of dementia after AD
▶ Prevalence in tertiary care centers is estimated at 26% of all dementia cases

Gender and Age Distribution
▶ Age at onset ranges from 68 to 92 years
▶ Slight predilection in men

Clinical Features
▶ Fluctuations in cognitive impairment and level of consciousness
▶ Visual hallucinations
▶ Parkinsonism: bradykinesia, limb rigidity, gait disorder

Radiologic Features
▶ MRI may show generalized atrophy in 60%

Prognosis and Treatment
▶ Duration of disease is 6 to 9 years
▶ Cholinesterase inhibitors decrease psychiatric and behavioral symptoms
▶ Supportive therapy

DIFFUSE LEWY BODY DISEASE—PATHOLOGIC FEATURES

Gross Findings
▶ Diffuse cortical atrophy and ventricular dilatation with concomitant AD
▶ Pallor of the substantia nigra and locus ceruleus

Microscopic Findings
▶ Cortical and brain stem Lewy bodies
▶ Three levels of involvement: brain stem, limbic, and neocortical
▶ Microvacuolation in the temporal cortex
▶ AD changes may be present: diffuse and neuritic plaques, neurofibrillary tangles

Ultrastructural Features
▶ Lewy bodies have radially arranged intermediate filaments associated with granular and vesicular material

Genetics
▶ No genetic abnormalities known

Immunohistochemical Features
▶ Lewy bodies are α-synuclein, ubiquitin, and neurofilament immunoreactive
▶ Lewy neurites are identified with α-synuclein, ubiquitin, or neurofilament antibodies in the CA2/CA3 region of the hippocampus, amygdala, nucleus basalis of Meynert, brain stem, olfactory bulb, intermediolateral column of the spinal cord, and autonomic ganglia
▶ α-Synuclein– and ubiquitin-immunoreactive glial inclusions are also identified in regions where cortical Lewy bodies are found

Pathologic Differential Diagnosis
▶ Parkinson's disease
▶ Alzheimer's disease
▶ Progressive supranuclear palsy
▶ Corticobasal degeneration
▶ Creutzfeldt-Jakob disease
▶ Multiple system atrophy
▶ Frontotemporal lobar degeneration

PATHOLOGIC FEATURES

GROSS FINDINGS

In patients with pure DLBD (i.e., those without associated AD changes), the brain may not show significant atrophy. In DLBD with significant AD changes, diffuse cortical atrophy and ventricular dilatation are seen. Pallor of the substantia nigra and locus ceruleus is usually found in both types.

MICROSCOPIC FINDINGS

The pathologic hallmark of DLBD is the presence of both cortical and brain stem Lewy bodies (see Fig. 6-15). DLBD has been divided into three levels of involvement: brain stem predominant, limbic (transitional), and cortical. Sampling of the brain for evaluation of Lewy

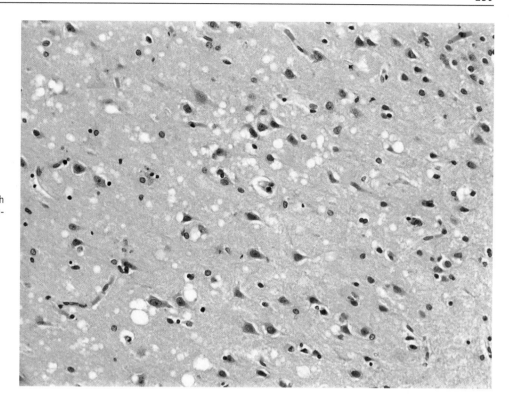

FIGURE 6-17

Diffuse Lewy body disease with spongiform change in the parahippocampal gyrus.

bodies in the brain stem should include the substantia nigra, locus ceruleus, and dorsal nucleus of the vagus. Sampling of the limbic system should include the anterior cingulate cortex, transentorhinal cortex, and middle temporal gyrus. Cortical regions to be evaluated are the middle frontal gyrus and the inferior parietal lobule. Immunohistochemistry with α-synuclein antibody is the best means of identifying cortical Lewy bodies.

Lewy bodies are found in the amygdala in 60% of reported cases of familial AD (including PS1, PS2, and amyloid precursor protein mutations) and occasionally in sporadic AD. Lewy bodies in the amygdala are also found in 50% of individuals with Down syndrome.

Lewy neurites are α-synuclein dystrophic neurites found in DLBD (and PD patients with or without dementia) in the CA2 and CA3 sections of the hippocampus, accessory cortical nuclei of the amygdala, nucleus basalis of Meynert, brain stem (substantia nigra, dorsal vagal nucleus), olfactory bulb, intermediolateral column of the spinal cord, and sympathetic and parasympathetic ganglia (see Fig. 6-16).

Glial cytoplasmic inclusions (α-synuclein and ubiquitin immunoreactive) are found in DLBD. As in PD, they correlate with the distribution of Lewy bodies.

Senile plaques (neuritic plaques and diffuse plaques) are present in most patients with DLBD. However, when present, senile plaques are more frequently of the diffuse subtype than neuritic. In addition, NFTs in the cortex are frequently found only in the mesial temporal lobe structures (hippocampus, entorhinal cortex).

Microvacuolation of the cortex, usually in the parahippocampal gyrus, is frequently seen in association with cortical Lewy bodies and DLBD (Fig. 6-17). The vacuolar pattern is similar to that found in prion disease, but no prion antibody immunoreactivity has been reported in DLBD.

ANCILLARY STUDIES

MRI may show generalized atrophy. However, in contrast to AD, the medial temporal lobe may not be atrophic in about 40% of cases.

DIFFERENTIAL DIAGNOSIS

The clinical differential diagnosis of DLBD includes AD, which may have an atypical clinical course and symptoms, and other diseases with parkinsonism and frequently dementia (multiple system atrophy, progressive supranuclear palsy, and corticobasal degeneration). Pathologically, distinction may be made by identification of cortical and substantia nigra Lewy bodies in DLBD with α-synuclein immunostaining. The presence of abnormal tau deposits in progressive supranuclear palsy and corticobasal degeneration and the absence of Lewy bodies in multiple system atrophy help further clarify the diagnosis. Pathologic distinction of DLBD from PD without dementia or PD with late-onset dementia is often not possible by comparison of the densities of cortical Lewy bodies. However, a recent study has shown that a high density of Lewy bodies in the parahippocampal gyrus may distinguish demented from nondemented patients.

PROGNOSTIC AND THERAPEUTIC CONSIDERATIONS

The duration of disease ranges from 6 to 9 years. Cholinesterase inhibitors have been shown to decrease the behavioral and psychiatric symptoms of DLBD.

MULTIPLE SYSTEM ATROPHY

The term multiple system atrophy (MSA) has recently been redefined as a sporadic progressive adult-onset disease of unknown cause distinguished by the presence of α-synuclein–immunoreactive glial cytoplasmic inclusions. The entities previously called olivopontocerebellar atrophy, Shy-Drager syndrome, and striatonigral degeneration are now encompassed by two groups within MSA: MSA-P (parkinsonian predominant) and MSA-C (cerebellar predominant).

CLINICAL FEATURES

The onset of symptoms is usually in the sixth decade with a range of 33 to 78 years. A male preponderance

has been reported. Familial clustering has not been reported.

The cardinal features of MSA are orthostatic hypotension, parkinsonism, and cerebellar signs and symptoms. MSA-P accounts for 80% of all cases of MSA. Typically, it is manifested as progressive akinesia and rigidity, orofacial dystonia, and dysesthesia. Postural stability is compromised, but falls are not prominent and tremor may be seen. MSA-C is characterized by gait ataxia, limb ataxia, scanning dysarthria, and cerebellar oculomotor disturbances. Dysautonomia occurs in both types. In addition to orthostatic hypotension, symptoms of urogenital dysfunction (impotence and urinary incontinence or retention) and constipation occur.

PATHOLOGIC FEATURES

GROSS FINDINGS

Atrophy and grayish discoloration of the putamen may be seen in MSA-P (Fig. 6-18), whereas in MSA-C, cerebellar, middle cerebellar peduncular, and pontine atrophy are evident. In both types of MSA, the substantia nigra is pale. Slight cortical atrophy may be present.

MULTIPLE SYSTEM ATROPHY—FACT SHEET

Definition
▶ Sporadic progressive adult-onset disease distinguished by the presence of α-synuclein–immunoreactive glial cytoplasmic inclusions
▶ Subdivided into two types: multiple system atrophy, parkinsonian predominant (MSA-P), and multiple system atrophy, cerebellar predominant (MSA-C)

Incidence and Prevalence
▶ Incidence is 3 per 100,000 per year
▶ Prevalence varies from 4 to 16 per 100,000

Gender and Age Distribution
▶ Male sex preponderance
▶ Age at onset ranges from 33 to 78 years
▶ Most often in the sixth decade

Clinical Features
▶ MSA-P: akinesia, rigidity, dystonia, dysesthesia
▶ MSA-C: gait and limb ataxia, dysarthria, oculomotor disturbances
▶ Dysautonomia occurs in both

Radiologic Features
▶ MRI shows atrophy of the caudate nucleus, putamen, cerebellum, and brain stem

Prognosis and Treatment
▶ Duration ranges from 6 to 9 years
▶ MSA-P transiently responds to levodopa

MULTIPLE SYSTEM ATROPHY—PATHOLOGIC FEATURES

Gross Findings
▶ MSA-P: atrophy and discoloration of the putamen, atrophy of the caudate nucleus
▶ MSA-C: atrophy of the cerebellum, middle cerebellar peduncle, and pons
▶ In both types, pallor of the substantia nigra

Microscopic Findings
▶ MSA-P: neuronal loss and astrocytosis in the striatonigral system
▶ MSA-C: cerebellar degeneration with Purkinje cell loss

Ultrastructural Features
▶ Glial cytoplasmic inclusions are composed of both twisted and straight filaments

Genetics
▶ No familial clustering or genetic abnormalities known

Immunohistochemical Features
▶ α-Synuclein–, ubiquitin–, and tau-immunoreactive glial cytoplasmic inclusions are present in the pyramidal, extrapyramidal, limbic, corticocerebellar, and supraspinal autonomic systems

Pathologic Differential Diagnosis
▶ Corticobasal degeneration
▶ Progressive supranuclear palsy

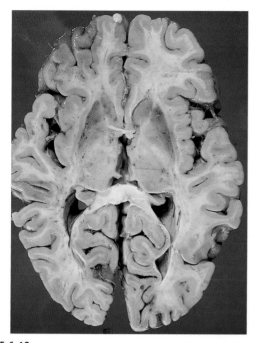

FIGURE 6-18

Multiple system atrophy—parkinsonian predominant. A horizontal slice of brain shows brown discoloration of the putamen bilaterally.

MICROSCOPIC FINDINGS

In MSA-P, neuronal loss with astrocytosis is marked in the striatonigral system (Fig. 6-19). It is most severe in the dorsolateral zone of the caudal putamen and lateral portion of the substantia nigra. In MSA-C, cere-bellar degeneration is most prominent with Purkinje cell loss evident, and the vermis is more affected than the hemispheres.

In each type, neuronal loss and astrocytosis of the basis pontis, accessory and inferior olivary nuclei, intermediolateral cell column, and locus ceruleus are also seen. The cerebellopontine fibers are degenerated. Neuronal loss in the hypothalamus, ventrolateral medulla, and arcuate nucleus is evident. Recent studies have also shown loss of unmyelinated fibers in the sural nerve and abnormalities of respiratory chain complexes in skeletal muscle.

Essential to the diagnosis of each MSA type are glial cytoplasmic inclusions. These inclusions are found in oligodendrocytes of the pyramidal, extrapyramidal, limbic, corticocerebellar, and supraspinal autonomic systems in both types of MSA. Glial cytoplasmic inclusions are argyrophilic (evident on Gallyas and Bielschowsky stains) structures that are ubiquitin and α-synuclein immunoreactive (Fig. 6-20). Immunoreactivity with tau antibodies has been variable. At present it does appear that glial cytoplasmic inclusions are tau immunoreactive, but the immunoreactivity profile differs from that found in AD, corticobasal degeneration, and progressive supranuclear palsy. The inclusions vary in shape and may be conical, oval, triangular, half-moon, sickle, or flame shaped. Ultrastructurally, glial cytoplasmic inclusions are composed of twisted filaments 5 to 18 nm in diameter with a periodicity of 70 to 90 nm. Also present are straight filaments 10 nm in diameter.

Other α-synuclein–immunoreactive inclusions discovered in MSA are in the neuronal cytoplasm, neuronal nucleus, axons, and oligodendrocyte nucleus. These inclusions occur at a much lower density than glial cytoplasmic inclusions do.

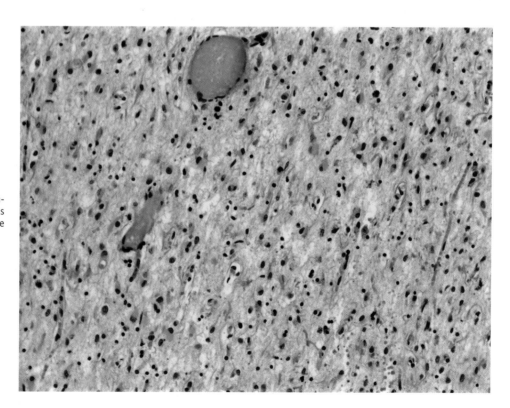

FIGURE 6-19

Multiple system atrophy—parkinsonian predominant. Neuronal loss and astrocytosis of the putamen are present.

ANCILLARY STUDIES

MRI shows atrophy of the caudate nucleus, putamen, cerebellum, and brain stem, regardless of the subtype of MSA. More severe atrophy of the cerebellum is found in MSA-C.

DIFFERENTIAL DIAGNOSIS

Clinically, MSA overlaps with other Parkinson's-plus entities, such as progressive supranuclear palsy and corticobasal degeneration. Pathologically, although oligodendrocyte inclusions have been described in other

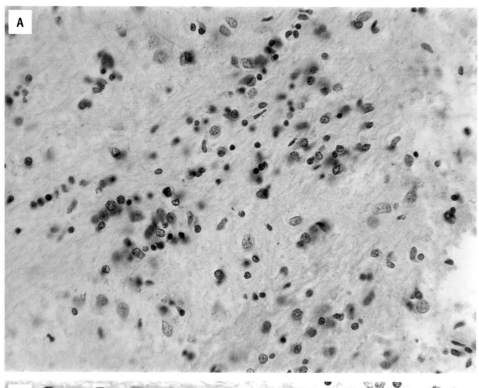

FIGURE 6-20

Multiple system atrophy: α-synuclein–immunoreactive glial cytoplasmic inclusions. **A**, putamen; **B**, base of the pons;

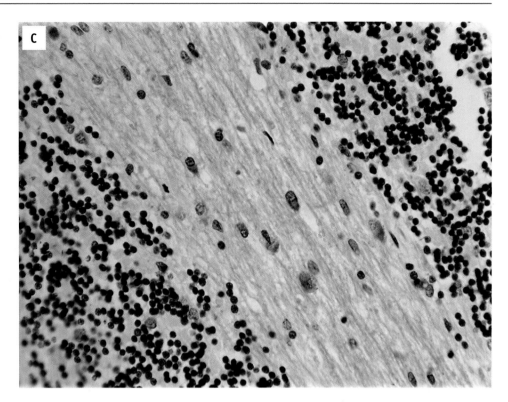

FIGURE 6-20, cont'd
C, cerebellar white matter.

neurodegenerative diseases, the distribution, antigenicity, morphology, and density distinguish glial cytoplasmic inclusions in MSA from other described inclusions. Coiled bodies are oligodendroglial inclusions found primarily in corticobasal degeneration; they are less substantial and voluminous than glial cytoplasmic inclusions. Other glial inclusions prominent in corticobasal degeneration and progressive supranuclear palsy are of astrocytic origin and differ in morphology from glial cytoplasmic inclusions.

PROGNOSTIC AND THERAPEUTIC CONSIDERATIONS

The mean duration varies from 6 to 9 years among studies. Survival is similar in each group. In MSA-P, 30% of patients may respond to levodopa treatment transiently. Otherwise, therapy is supportive.

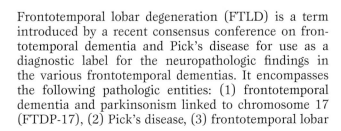

FRONTOTEMPORAL LOBAR DEGENERATION

Frontotemporal lobar degeneration (FTLD) is a term introduced by a recent consensus conference on frontotemporal dementia and Pick's disease for use as a diagnostic label for the neuropathologic findings in the various frontotemporal dementias. It encompasses the following pathologic entities: (1) frontotemporal dementia and parkinsonism linked to chromosome 17 (FTDP-17), (2) Pick's disease, (3) frontotemporal lobar degeneration with ubiquitin-positive and tau-negative deposits without motor neuron disease (FTLD-U) and with motor neuron disease (FTLD-MND), and (4) frontotemporal lobar degeneration without ubiquitin or tau deposits (also known as dementia lacking distinctive histology [DLDH]). FTLD accounts for between 7% and 15% of all dementia in patients younger than 65 years. In addition to the pathologic variability within this category, marked clinical and genetic heterogeneity is found. The clinical findings are variable and not always associated with the same pathologic findings or genetic mutation.

CLINICAL FEATURES

The clinical signs and symptoms associated with FTLD generally fall into one of two categories: changes in behavior or changes in language. In the latter, the impairment is usually classified as semantic dementia or progressive nonfluent aphasia.

Frontotemporal dementia is the label attached to FTLD with behavioral changes and is the most common manifestation of FTLD. It is characterized by significant alterations in personality and social conduct. The patient is usually apathetic and impaired in judgment, abstraction, problem solving, and planning. Repetitive, stereotypic, and compulsive behavior is common. Memory is preserved early in the course; if impairment is evident, it may be secondary to the marked deficits in frontal executive functions. No motor deficits may be evident until late in the disease course, when akinesia and rigidity are present.

FRONTOTEMPORAL LOBAR ATROPHY—FACT SHEET

Definition

▶ Degeneration of the frontal and temporal lobes often in association with abnormal tau or ubiquitin deposits; clinically characterized by dementia with behavioral or language abnormalities and sometimes parkinsonism and motor neuron disease symptoms

▶ Includes the following entities:
  ▶ Frontotemporal dementia and parkinsonism linked to chromosome 17 (FTDP-17)
  ▶ Pick's disease
  ▶ Frontotemporal lobar degeneration with ubiquitin inclusions, with (FTLD-MND) or without (FTLD-U) motor neuron disease
  ▶ Frontotemporal lobar degeneration without tau or ubiquitin deposits (also known as dementia lacking distinctive histology [DLDH])

Incidence and Prevalence

▶ Incidence:
  ▶ 40 to 49 years—2.2 per 100,000 per year
  ▶ 50 to 59 years—3.3 per 100,000 per year
  ▶ 60 to 69 years—8.9 per 100,000 per year
▶ No prevalence data available

Gender and Age Distribution

▶ No gender predilection known
▶ Age distribution:
  ▶ FTDP-17: onset at a mean of 49 years with a range of 25 to 76 years
  ▶ Pick's disease: peak occurrence in the sixth decade with a range of 45 to 65 years
  ▶ FTLD-MND: Range of 39 to 77 years
  ▶ FTLD-U: mean age 65 years; range of 53 to 83 years
  ▶ FTLD without tau/ubiquitin inclusions (DLDH): no data

Clinical Features

▶ Behavioral changes and language abnormalities
▶ Language abnormalities usually fall into one of two categories:
  ▶ Semantic dementia: fluent speech, lack of comprehension
  ▶ Nonfluent aphasia: expressive speech deterioration
▶ No consistent correlations between specific clinical and pathologic findings
▶ FTLD-MND patients may have signs and symptoms of motor neuron disease

Radiologic Features

▶ MRI shows atrophy of the frontal and temporal lobes
▶ Semantic dementia: may show bitemporal atrophy
▶ Nonfluent aphasia: may show atrophy of the left perisylvian region

Prognosis and Treatment

▶ Disease duration ranges from 2 to 17 years
▶ No treatments currently available

Semantic dementia is defined by fluent speech output, lack of comprehension of both the written and spoken word, and impaired face and object recognition. Repetition, visuospatial skills, and memory are preserved. With disease progression, speech output diminishes until late in the course, when the patient is mute.

Primary nonfluent aphasia is a deterioration in expressive language characterized by word retrieval difficulty, effortful, stuttering speech with phonetic and grammatical errors, and a progressive reduction in speech production. Nonverbal abilities, comprehension, and activities of daily living are preserved. Late in the disease course, behavioral changes may also appear.

FTDP-17 has a mean age at onset of 49 years (range, 25 to 76). The disease is autosomal dominant, and at least 80 kindreds have been described with 31 unique tau gene mutations. Extrapyramidal symptoms are seen late in the course and include bradykinesia, rigidity, postural instability, paucity of resting tremor, and poor or no response to dopamine. Clinical phenotypic heterogeneity is seen with different mutations. There is also intrafamilial and interfamilial heterogeneity with the same mutation.

Pick's disease usually occurs in patients between 45 and 65 years of age, is less common in those older than 70, and has a peak incidence in the sixth decade. Most cases of Pick's disease are sporadic. However, mutations in the tau gene and pathologic findings very similar to Pick's disease, including Pick-like bodies, have been reported in patients with frontotemporal dementia. Most of these conditions differ in the type of tau accumulation (3R and 4R instead of 3R only; see later).

FTLD-U and FTLD-MND have been reported to account for more than 50% of all cases of FTLD. In FTLD associated with motor neuron disease, the age at onset ranges from 39 to 77 years. The typical course is 1 to 6 years. In FTLD without clinical or pathologic findings of motor neuron disease, onset is at an older age, the mean being 65 years with a range of 53 to 83 years. The typical course is 4 to 12 years. Motor neuron disease has been described both preceding and following symptoms and signs of cognitive impairment. In motor neuron disease, symptoms usually reflect involvement of the anterior horn cells more than the pyramidal tract. No separate data on the typical age at onset or the course of FTLD without either tau or ubiquitin immunoreactivity (DLDH) are available. In FTLD without tau deposits (not further specified), loci on three chromosomes (3, 9, and 17) associated with the occurrence of familial disease have been identified.

PATHOLOGIC FEATURES

FTDP-17

Gross Findings

Reported brain weights vary from 825 to 1290 g. Atrophy typically involves the frontal and temporal

---

FRONTOTEMPORAL LOBAR ATROPHY—PATHOLOGIC FEATURES

Gross Findings

► In FTDP-17, FTLD-U, FTLD-MND, and DLDH: decreased brain weight and frontotemporal atrophy, most severe in the mesial temporal area; atrophy of the basal ganglia may be present

► Patients with semantic dementia may have bitemporal atrophy, and those with nonfluent aphasia may have left perisylvian atrophy

► Pick's disease: decreased brain weight and severe atrophy of the frontal and temporal lobes with sparing of the posterior superior temporal gyrus

Microscopic Findings

► Each subtype:
  ► Varying degrees of neuronal loss and astrocytosis in the frontotemporal lobes
  ► The basal ganglia and substantia nigra may also show neuronal loss
  ► Typically superficial spongy change in the cortex (second layer)
► In addition:
  ► Pick's disease: Pick bodies (argyrophilic intracytoplasmic inclusions) are most frequently found in the mesial temporal lobe structures, especially dentate granular cell neurons. Pick cells (ballooned or chromatolytic-appearing neurons) found scattered throughout the cortex
  ► FTLD-MND: pathologic findings of motor neuron disease

Ultrastructural Features

► Neuronal and glial tau deposits have been found to be composed of straight and twisted filaments

► Pick bodies: filamentous accumulation (straight or paired/twisted), non–membrane-bound and granular and vesicular material

► Pick cells: accumulation of neurofilament in neuronal cytoplasm

► Ubiquitin-immunoreactive cytoplasmic inclusions in the cortex are randomly arranged, 10- to 15-nm relatively straight filaments

Genetics

► Family history is positive in 50% of all FTLD

► FTDP-17 patients have mutations in the tau gene; the most common is p301L

Immunohistochemical Features

► FTDP-17: tau-immunoreactive deposits:
  ► Neurons: tangles, diffuse stain, dot-like, perinuclear, Pick body–like
  ► Glia (astrocytic or oligodendroglial): tangles, coiled bodies, tufted astrocytes, astrocytic plaques
► Pick's disease: tau-immunoreactive deposits
  ► Pick bodies
  ► Neurites
  ► Glial inclusions
► Pick's disease: neurofilament (phosphorylated)-immunoreactive Pick cells
► FTLD-U and FTLD-MND: ubiquitin-immunoreactive intranuclear inclusions (rod shaped) and cytoplasmic inclusions (dot-like) in the dentate granular cell layer and superficial cortical layer
► DLDH: no tau- or ubiquitin-immunoreactive inclusions

Pathologic Differential Diagnosis

► Corticobasal degeneration
► Progressive supranuclear palsy
► Multiple system atrophy
► Alzheimer's disease

---

cortices, putamen, globus pallidus, amygdala, hippocampus, and hypothalamus. Atrophy of the orbital and cingulate cortices may be present. Asymmetric atrophy may be evident, with the left hemisphere often more severely involved. Pallor of the substantia nigra and locus ceruleus is usually apparent.

Microscopic Findings

Neuronal loss and astrocytosis are seen in the frontal and temporal lobes, including the hippocampus, amygdala, and subiculum. The anterior temporal lobe is often severely involved. Spongy change in superficial layers of the degenerated neocortex is often prominent (Fig. 6-21). Neuronal loss with astrocytosis is also seen in the basal ganglia and substantia nigra. Tau deposits are found in neurons, astrocytes, and oligodendrocytes. Their morphology, cellular and regional location, and density vary with the specific mutation (Fig. 6-22). They may be found in the cerebral cortex, white matter, cerebellum, and brain stem. The neuronal tau deposits include NFTs and diffuse, dot-like, perinuclear, or Pick body–like cytoplasmic immunoreactivity. Tau-positive glial inclusions may be astrocytic or oligodendroglial and appear as tangles, coiled bodies, tufted astrocytes, or astrocytic plaques. Ballooned chromatolytic-like neurons are also frequently present. The presence of these changes illustrates the morphologic overlap of FTLD with the pathologic changes of corticobasal degeneration, progressive supranuclear palsy, and Pick's disease.

PICK'S DISEASE

Gross Findings

Pick's disease is typically associated with focal atrophy involving the frontal and temporal lobes and sparing of the posterior, usually superior, temporal gyrus (Fig. 6-23). The atrophy is often severe and has prompted the terms "knife-edge" or "walnut." The precentral and postcentral gyri are also usually spared. Corresponding enlargement of the frontal and temporal horns of the lateral ventricles also occurs. There may be asymmetric involvement of the cerebral hemispheres, with the dominant hemisphere being more severely involved. Atrophy of the anterior caudate and putamen may also be present.

Microscopic Findings

The essential finding in Pick's disease is the Pick body. This spherical cytoplasmic inclusion is found in neurons in the frontal and temporal cortices, usually layers II and IV. It is also frequent in the mesial temporal lobe structures and limbic cortex. Especially involved are neurons of the dentate granule cell layer of the hippocampus (Fig. 6-24A). They are less frequently found in the anterior frontal, dorsal temporal, or parietal and occipital lobes. The Pick body is argyrophilic and PHF-tau, ubiquitin, and phosphorylated neurofilament immunoreactive (see Fig. 6-24B-D). Electron microscopic examination of a Pick body shows an accumulation of

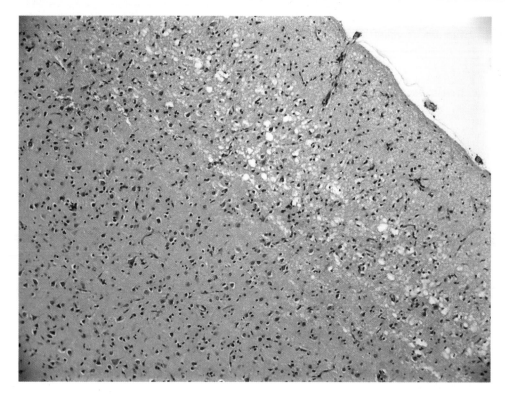

FIGURE 6-21

Frontotemporal lobar degeneration. The superficial temporal cortex shows spongy change of the neuropil in the second cortical layer.

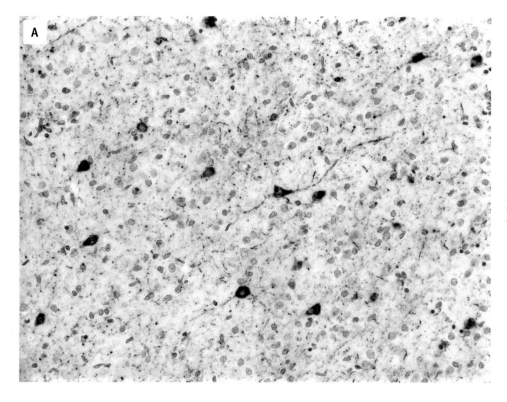

FIGURE 6-22

Frontotemporal lobar atrophy with tau deposition. **A**, Neocortical neuronal and neuritic tau immunoreactivity.

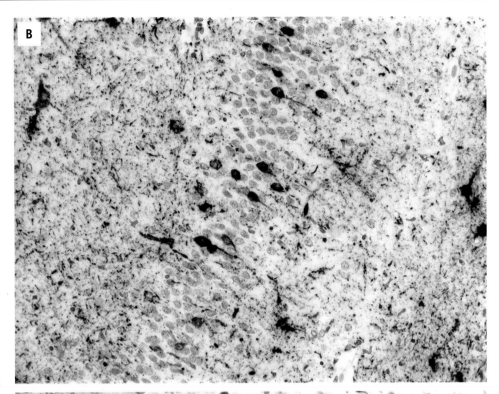

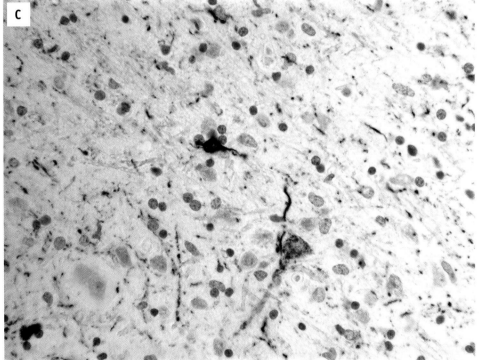

FIGURE 6-22, cont'd

B, Dentate gyrus neuronal and neuritic immunoreactivity. **C**, Tau-immunoreactive glial tangle and neuronal cytoplasm in the temporal cortex.

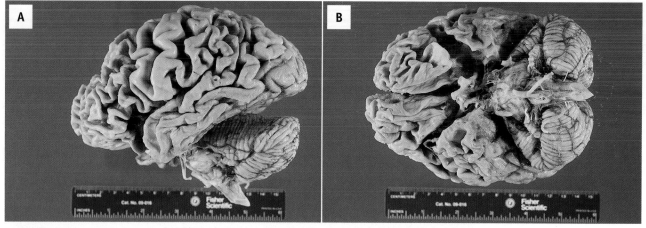

FIGURE 6-23

Pick's disease. Whole-brain lateral (**A**) and ventral (**B**) views show diffuse atrophy affecting the frontal, temporal, and parietal lobes but most severely involving the frontal and temporal lobes and relative sparing of the superior posterior temporal gyrus.

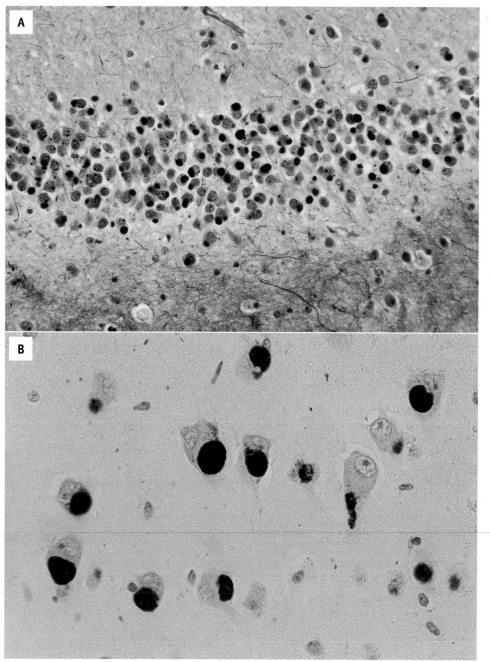

FIGURE 6-24

Pick bodies. **A**, Modified Bielschowsky–stained section of the dentate granular cell layer of the hippocampus showing numerous Pick bodies in the cytoplasm of the dentate neurons. **B**, Immunostaining of a section of the temporal lobe cortex with PHF antibody showing positive staining of intracytoplasmic spherical Pick bodies.

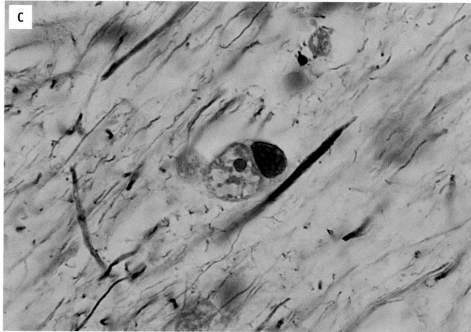

FIGURE 6-24, cont'd
C, Modified Bielschowsky–stained section of the orbital frontal cortex showing a positively stained Pick body. **D**, PHF-immunostained Pick body in the temporal cortex.

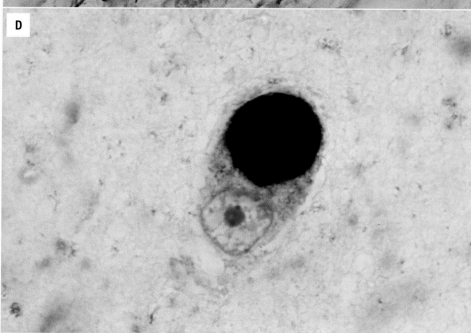

filaments, both straight and paired or twisted. They range in size from 14 to 16 nm to 22 to 24 nm, respectively. Intermixed with the filaments is osmiophilic granular and vesicular material. Neuronal loss, often severe, is associated with Pick bodies (Fig. 6-25A). The astrocytosis is correspondingly severe, mostly in the upper cortical layers and at the gray-white junctions (see Fig. 6-25B). Also found in Pick's disease are Pick cells. These cells are ballooned chromatolytic-like neurons that are immunoreactive with phosphorylated neurofilament antibody and usually located in the middle and lower cortical layers (Fig. 6-26).

The substantia nigra variably shows neuronal loss, and the anterior caudate and putamen frequently show

neuronal loss. White matter is usually pale with loss of myelinated fibers in severely affected cortical regions.

In addition to the Pick bodies and Pick cells, tau-immunoreactive neurites and glial (astrocytic and oligo-dendroglial) inclusions are also found in both the cortex and white matter.

FTLD-U, FTLD-MND, AND DLDH

Gross Findings

FTLD-U, FTLD-MND, and DLDH are usually associated with decreased brain weight and cortical atrophy, most severe in the frontotemporal lobes. Atrophy may be very severe in the mesial temporal lobe structures,

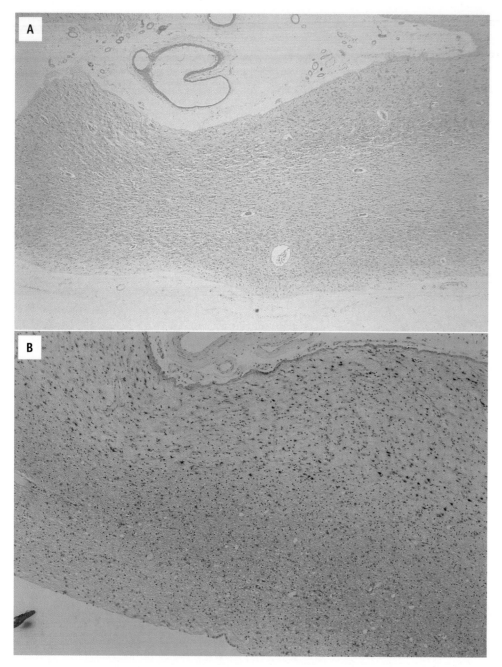

FIGURE 6-25

Pick's disease. **A**, Severe neuronal loss and astrocytosis in the middle temporal gyrus. **B**, Glial fibrillary acidic protein–immunostained section of the temporal gyrus highlighting severe diffuse astrocytosis involving the cortex and white matter.

and compensatory ventricular dilatation occurs. The substantia nigra is usually pale. Atrophy of the basal ganglia may be present. Asymmetry may be evident, especially in patients with primary nonfluent aphasia, and bitemporal atrophy may develop in those with semantic dementia.

Microscopic Findings

Variable neuronal loss and astrocytosis in the frontotemporal lobes are evident. As seen in FTDP-17, laminar spongiosis in layers I to III is present and may be severe (see Fig. 6-21). Both the basal ganglia and substantia nigra generally show neuronal loss and astrocy-

tosis. Ballooned neurons may be seen. In FTLD-U and FTLD-MND, ubiquitin-immunoreactive cytoplasmic dot-like inclusions are present. They are found in the dentate granule cells of the hippocampus and in the superficial cortical layers (Fig. 6-27A and B). Ubiquitin-reactive inclusions may also be seen in the nuclei (often rod shaped) of the dentate granule cells or the superficial cortical layers as well (see Fig. 6-27C and D). These inclusions are nonreactive with tau and α-synuclein antibodies. At present in DLDH, no immunoreactive inclusions have been found, and pathologically, DLDH differs from FTLD-U and FTLD-MND only in the absence of ubiquitin-immunoreactive inclusions. DLDH shows neuronal loss, astrocytosis, and spongy change of

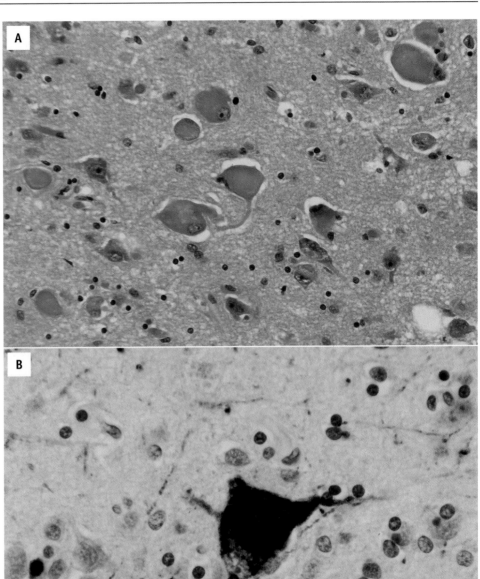

FIGURE 6-26

Pick cells. **A**, Multiple ballooned chromatolytic-like neurons in the amygdala of a patient with Pick's disease. **B**, High-power view of a ballooned neuron in the amygdala in same case showing positive immunostaining with antibody to phosphorylated neurofilament.

the superficial cortex. When the pathologic features of MND are present in a case of FTLD, even in the absence of clinical signs and symptoms of MND it is appropriate to classify the patient as having the FTLD-MND type. It remains to be determined whether FTLD-U and FTLD-MND represent variants of the same disease entity.

ANCILLARY STUDIES

In FTDP-17, assay for mutation of the tau gene may be performed. The most frequently reported mutation is p301L.

Six isoforms of tau are generated by alternative splicing of exons 2, 3, and 10 of the tau gene. These isoforms may be divided into two groups (3R and 4R) that are differentiated by the presence of three or four repeated microtubule-binding domains in exon 10. Western blot analysis of brain tissue from the various FTLDs has shown that some have a predominance of three microtubule-binding repeats (3R tau), others have a predominance of four microtubule-binding repeats (4R tau), and some have both. FTDP-17 brain tissue may contain predominantly 3R, 4R, or both 3R and 4R tau. Pick's disease usually has 3R tau. FTLD-U and DLDH do not contain either 3R or 4R tau.

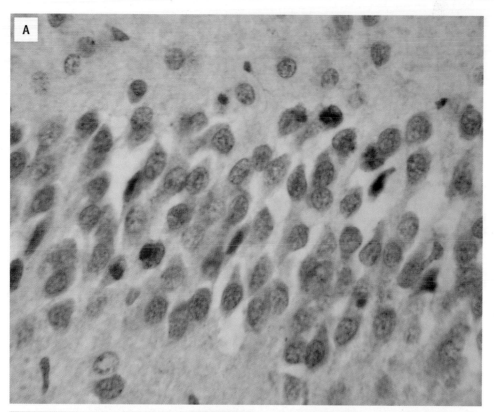

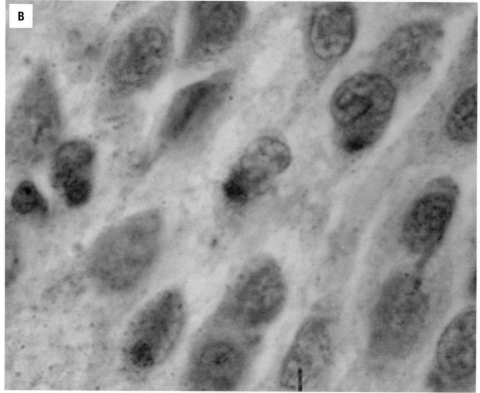

FIGURE 6-27

Frontotemporal lobar degeneration with ubiquitin-immunoreactive deposits. **A**, Immunostaining of dentate gyrus neurons in the hippocampus with ubiquitin antibody. Note the ubiquitin-positive cytoplasmic dot-like inclusions. **B**, High-power image of ubiquitin-positive cytoplasmic dot-like inclusions in the dentate granule cell layer.

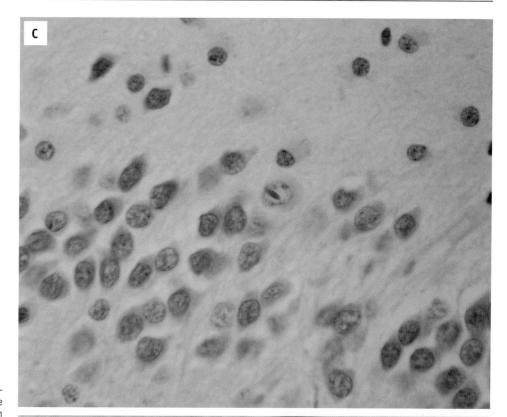

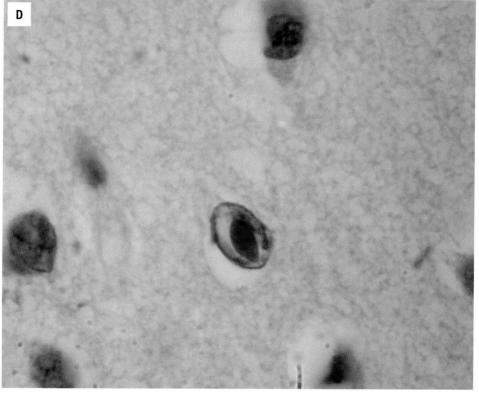

FIGURE 6-27, cont'd

C, Intranuclear ubiquitin-immunore-active inclusion in a dentate granule neuron. **D**, High-power image of an intranuclear ubiquitin-immunoreac-tive inclusion in a second-layer neuron of the frontal cortex.

In FTLD, the electroencephalogram may be normal or show diffuse slowing. MRI reveals atrophy of the frontal and temporal lobes with ventricular dilatation. In patients with semantic dementia, bitemporal atrophy is seen, and in progressive nonfluent aphasia, left perisylvian region atrophy is present.

DIFFERENTIAL DIAGNOSIS

Given the variable clinical and pathologic phenotypes associated with tau mutations, distinction of FTDP-17 from other FTLDs or corticobasal degeneration and progressive supranuclear palsy may be difficult. Genetic testing is able to exclude FTDP-17 readily but is not helpful in distinguishing among other FTLDs, progressive supranuclear palsy, and corticobasal degeneration. Pick's disease may be diagnosed by the presence of characteristic Pick bodies. FTLD-U and FTLD-MND are defined by the presence of ubiquitin-immunoreactive and tau-negative inclusions, as well as the pathologic changes of MND in FTLD-MND. Progressive supranuclear palsy is defined by the presence of globose NFTs in the subcortical nuclei in addition to tufted astrocytes. Corticobasal degeneration has abundant neuropil threads, astrocytic plaques, and ballooned neurons. DLDH is distinguished by frontotemporal degeneration in the absence of tau- or ubiquitin-immunoreactive deposits.

PROGNOSTIC AND THERAPEUTIC CONSIDERATIONS

The average reported duration for all FTLDs varies from 2 to 17 years. No treatments are currently available.

CORTICOBASAL DEGENERATION

Corticobasal degeneration (CBD) has been known by a variety of names since its initial description, including corticodentatonigral degeneration with neuronal achromasia, corticonigral degeneration, and corticobasal ganglionic degeneration.

CLINICAL FEATURES

CBD has a mean age at onset of 63 to 66 years and a range from 47 to 77 years. No sex or ethnic predisposition has yet been described. It is considered a sporadic disease because no definitive familial cases have been identified. Previously reported cases believed to be familial CBD were subsequently reclassified as FTDP-17.

Initial descriptions of CBD focused on findings of progressive asymmetric rigidity, apraxia, and parkin-

---

CORTICOBASAL DEGENERATION—FACT SHEET

Definition

▶ Sporadic disease with progressive rigidity, apraxia, parkinsonism, and occasionally dementia associated with tau deposits in the substantia nigra and perirolandic cortex

Incidence and Prevalence

▶ Incidence is <1 per 100,000 per year
▶ No prevalence data available

Gender and Age Distribution

▶ Mean age at onset, 63 to 66 years (range, 47 to 77)
▶ No gender predilection

Clinical Features

▶ Classically with progressive asymmetric rigidity and apraxia and parkinsonism
▶ May also be manifested as frontal lobe dementia or with progressive aphasia (usually nonfluent)

Radiologic Features

▶ MRI shows asymmetric atrophy of the superior parasagittal perirolandic cortices

Prognosis and Treatment

▶ Average duration, 8 years (range, 5 to 11)
▶ Nonresponsive to levodopa
▶ No therapy currently available

---

sonism, but more recent reports have documented the presence of progressive aphasia and frontal lobe dementia (personality change, disorders of conduct, impaired attention).

PATHOLOGIC FEATURES

GROSS FINDINGS

Atrophy of cortical gyri is most marked in a perirolandic distribution, generally the parasagittal regions. The superior frontal and parietal gyri are usually more involved than the middle and inferior frontal gyri and the temporal or occipital lobes. The atrophy may be asymmetric. In patients with dementia, the cortical atrophy may be more generalized, and those with aphasia are likely to have asymmetric perisylvian atrophy. Pallor of the substantia nigra is usually evident.

MICROSCOPIC FINDINGS

Areas of atrophic cortex show neuronal loss and astrocytosis. Spongiosis of the superficial cortex may be evident. Astrocytosis is also present at the gray-white matter junction, and myelin pallor is seen underlying affected cortical areas. Ballooned chromatolytic-like neurons are seen

---

CORTICOBASAL DEGENERATION—PATHOLOGIC FEATURES

Gross Findings
▶ Perirolandic cortical atrophy
▶ Pallor of the substantia nigra

Microscopic Findings
▶ Neuronal loss and astrocytosis affecting the cortex (preferentially the primary motor and sensory cortices), substantia nigra, and basal ganglia
▶ Argyrophilic and tau-immunoreactive deposits (see below)
▶ Balloon (chromatolytic-like) neurons

Ultrastructural Features
▶ Neuronal and glial inclusions are filaments with a diameter of 20 to 24 nm and paired twisted tubules

Genetics
▶ Sporadic disease
▶ Overexpression of the H1 haplotype
▶ Familial cases previously reported have been reclassified as FTDP-17

Immunohistochemical Features
▶ Tau-immunoreactive deposits:
  ▶ Neuronal cytoplasm
  ▶ Astrocytic plaques
  ▶ Thread-like processes (particularly prominent)
  ▶ Oligodendroglial coiled bodies
▶ Neurofilament-immunoreactive balloon neurons

Pathologic Differential Diagnosis
▶ Alzheimer's disease
▶ Pick's disease
▶ Progressive supranuclear palsy
▶ Frontotemporal lobar degeneration, particularly FTDP-17
▶ Multiple system atrophy

---

in the affected cortex, usually in layers III, V, and VI (Fig. 6-28). These neurons have enlarged eosinophilic to amphophilic cell bodies and are occasionally vacuolated. The cytoplasm is immunoreactive with phosphorylated neurofilament and αB-crystallin and inconsistently with ubiquitin. The periphery of the cytoplasm may immunoreact with tau antibodies. These swollen neurons are also seen in less affected areas of the brain such as the cingulate gyrus, amygdala, insula, and claustrum.

Tau immunostaining of CBD brain tissue reveals a variety of immunoreactive profiles. Diffuse or granular staining of neuronal cytoplasm is seen in cortical neurons (Fig. 6-29A). Occasionally, this staining identifies tangle or skein-like structures. These structures are also prominent in the substantia nigra, locus ceruleus, raphe, and tegmental gray matter. Tau-immunoreactive thread-like processes are very prominent in many areas of the brain (see Fig. 6-29B). They are believed to be predominantly glial in origin, not neuronal. They are found in affected gray and white matter. Also present in white matter are oligodendroglial coiled bodies. These bodies consist of bundles of fibrils coiling around the nucleus. They are tau immunoreactive, α-synuclein negative, and usually ubiquitin negative. Astrocytic plaques are found in the cortex and deep gray matter and consist of a circular collection of tau-immunoreactive processes of astrocytes that resemble senile plaques (Fig. 6-30). Other affected areas of the brain include the caudate and putamen, and the striatal fiber bundles often show neuronal staining with tau antibodies and astrocytic plaques. The ventrolateral nucleus of the thalamus may be affected. The hippocampus and parahippocampal gyrus are usually normal. The substantia nigra shows moderate to severe neuronal loss and astrocytosis and tau-immunoreactive neuronal skein-like inclusions.

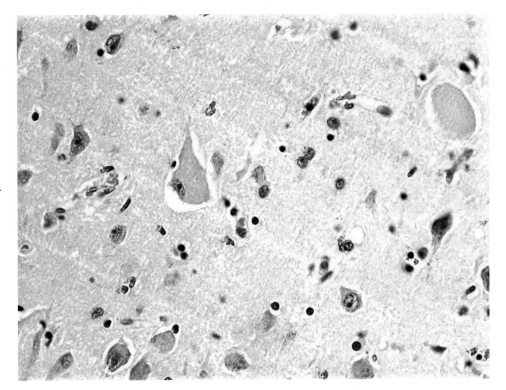

FIGURE 6-28

Corticobasal degeneration: neocortical ballooned neuron.

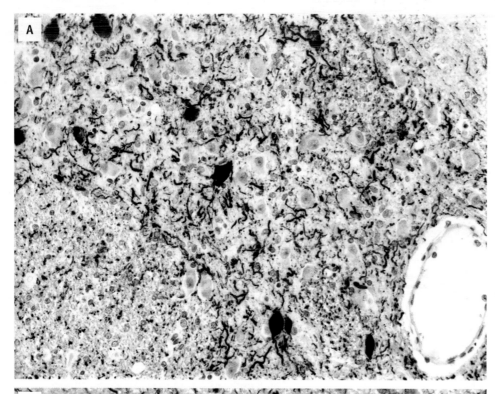

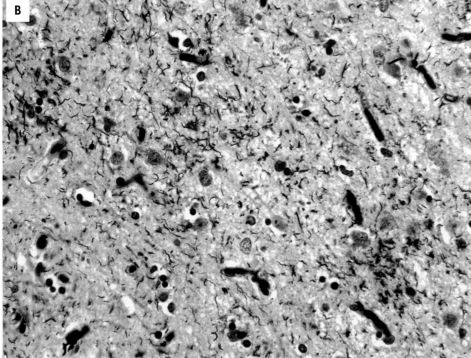

FIGURE 6-29

Corticobasal degeneration. **A**, Tau-immunoreactive neurons and threads in the base of the pons. **B**, Numerous thread-like processes in the lateral putamen (Gallyas stain).

ANCILLARY STUDIES

MRI studies reflect the pattern of cortical atrophy present. Asymmetry and atrophy of the superior parasagittal frontal and parietal lobes have been described. Western blot analysis of CBD brain tissue has shown an accumulation of the four–microtubule-binding repeat form of tau (4R tau). Recently, neuropathologically confirmed cases of CBD have been shown to overexpress the dinucleotide polymorphism, H1 haplotype, as described in progressive supranuclear palsy (see the section "Progressive Supranuclear Palsy"). H1 and H2 are extended haplotypes that cover the entire tau gene.

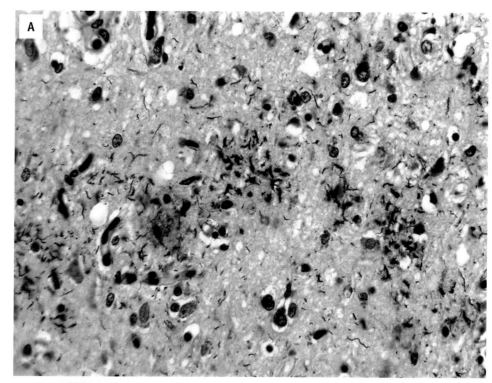

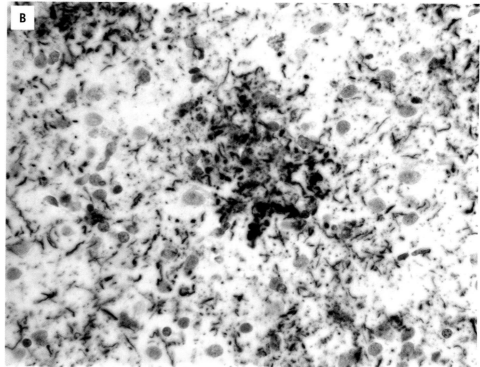

FIGURE 6-30

Corticobasal degeneration. **A,** Three astrocytic plaques (Gallyas stain). **B,** Astrocytic plaque and threads immunostained with tau antibody.

DIFFERENTIAL DIAGNOSIS

CBD may be very difficult to distinguish from FTDP-17 solely on brain examination. Review of the clinical findings and family history may be necessary to separate the two entities. Heterogeneity of both clinical and pathologic findings in CBD has been reported. Patients with typical clinical pictures of CBD have been found to have Alzheimer's or Pick's disease. Conversely, patients found to have CBD pathologically may have frontotemporal dementia. Overlap of CBD with other neurodegenerative pathology has also been reported, specifically, Alzheimer's disease, progressive supranuclear palsy, and frontotemporal lobar degeneration. Distinction may be aided by the presence of tau immunoreactivity and study of the specific morphology of the tau deposits (i.e., tufted astrocytes versus astrocytic plaques, the presence of abundant neuropil threads). Distinction may be further aided by finding 4R tau on Western blot analysis rather than a mixture of 3R and 4R (FTDP-17 may contain either or both) or a predominance of 3R tau (as in Pick's disease).

PROGNOSTIC AND THERAPEUTIC CONSIDERATIONS

CBD has an average duration of 8 years (range, 5 to 11 years). It is not responsive to levodopa therapy. No other treatment is currently available.

PROGRESSIVE SUPRANUCLEAR PALSY

CLINICAL FEATURES

The usual age at onset is between 60 and 65 years. There is a tendency for the disease to occur in men more often than in women. Progressive supranuclear palsy (PSP) is characterized by the presence of gait instability and backward falls early in the clinical course. Also present is vertical supranuclear gaze palsy and parkinsonism (rigidity, slowed movements, and tremor). Frequently accompanying these features is frontal lobe dysfunction (concrete thoughts, perseveration, behavioral disturbances, apathy, disinhibition, depression, anxiety). PSP may be manifested primarily as cognitive impairment, but less commonly than corticobasal degeneration is. The disease is gradually progressive.

PATHOLOGIC FEATURES

GROSS FINDINGS

Mild atrophy of the midbrain with increased size of the aqueduct is seen. In addition, the subthalamic nucleus and superior cerebellar peduncle may be atrophic, and mild cortical atrophy is typically present. Decreased pigmentation of the substantia nigra is evident.

PROGRESSIVE SUPRANUCLEAR PALSY—FACT SHEET

Definition
- Sporadic degenerative disease consisting of parkinsonism, usually gaze palsies and gait abnormalities, and occasionally dementia, with tau deposits in the form of neurofibrillary tangles and glial inclusions in the subcortical gray matter

Incidence and Prevalence
- Incidence is 5.3 per 100,000 per year
- Prevalence is 5 to 6 per 100,000

Gender and Age Distribution
- Usual age at onset is between 60 and 65 years
- Slight predilection for men

Clinical Features
- Gait instability and backward falls
- Vertical supranuclear gaze palsy
- Parkinsonism
- May have cognitive impairment

Radiologic Features
- MRI shows decreased diameter of the midbrain and increased signal within the midbrain and globus pallidus

Prognosis and Treatment
- Median survival is 5 to 6 years
- Generally unresponsive to levodopa

PROGRESSIVE SUPRANUCLEAR PALSY—PATHOLOGIC FEATURES

Gross Findings
- Atrophy of the midbrain and pallor of the substantia nigra
- May see atrophy of the subthalamic nucleus and superior cerebellar peduncle

Microscopic Findings
- Globose neurofibrillary tangles in the subcortical gray matter (globus pallidus, subthalamus, substantia nigra, reticular formation of the midbrain and pons) with neuronal loss and astrocytosis
- Argyrophilic and tau-immunoreactive profiles (see further on)

Ultrastructural Features
- Neurofibrillary tangles are composed of 15- to 18-nm straight filaments

Genetics
- Usually sporadic disease, but familial clustering reported
- Associated with increased presence of the H1 haplotype

Immunohistochemical Features
- A variety of tau-immunoreactive structures are present:
  - Globose neurofibrillary tangles
  - Tufted astrocytes
  - Coiled bodies in oligodendrocytes
  - Neuropil threads

Pathologic Differential Diagnosis
- Parkinson's disease
- Postencephalitic Parkinson's disease
- Parkinsonian-dementia complex of Guam
- Corticobasal degeneration
- Multiple system atrophy
- Frontotemporal lobar degeneration
- Alzheimer's disease

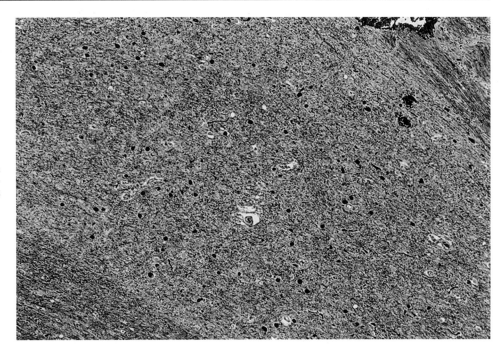

FIGURE 6-31

Progressive supranuclear palsy. A Gallyas-stained section of the subthalamic nucleus shows numerous globose neurofibrillary tangles.

MICROSCOPIC FINDINGS

The key feature of PSP is the presence of globose NFTs in subcortical gray matter. These tangles are predominantly found in the globus pallidus, subthalamic nucleus, substantia nigra, and reticular formations of the midbrain and pons (Figs. 6-31 and 6-32). The striatum, superior colliculus, periaqueductal gray matter, oculomotor complex, locus ceruleus, basis pontis neurons, inferior olivary nuclei, dentate nucleus, and vestibular nucleus are also affected, but usually less severely. The lower layers of the cerebral cortex, especially the frontal cortex and including the precentral gyrus, are also frequently affected. The dentate granule cell neurons of the hippocampus may also contain NFTs. Neuronal loss and astrocytosis parallel the density of NFTs in location and severity. In addition to NFTs, neuropil threads, tufted astrocytes, and coiled bodies (oligodendrocytes) are seen (Fig. 6-33A). All are identified with antibodies to tau protein. Tufted astrocytes have densely packed processes of varying size and length surrounding the nucleus (which is often paired) and are seen mostly in the frontal cortex and striatum (see Fig. 6-33B and C). The coiled bodies of oligodendrocytes are found predominantly in white matter. Electron microscopic examination of NFTs shows that they are composed of 15- to 18-nm straight filaments.

ANCILLARY STUDIES

The type of tau deposited in the brain is primarily 4R. The disease is predominantly a sporadic disease, but familial clustering has been reported. In PSP, haplo-type H1, a dinucleotide polymorphism, confers a slight genetic predisposition to the development of disease. The H1 haplotype appears to be present in all pathologically confirmed cases and is found in 70% of controls. The H1 haplotype has no effect on amount of tau in PSP, age at the onset of disease, or disease severity or survival. MRI scans of PSP patients show a decrease in the diameter of the midbrain (less than 17 mm), increased signal in the midbrain, and increased signal in the globus pallidus.

DIFFERENTIAL DIAGNOSIS

Pathologically, PSP may be confused with corticobasal degeneration or a frontotemporal lobar degenerative condition such as FTDP-17, postencephalitic Parkinson's disease, and the parkinsonian-dementia complex of Guam. Distinction is aided by the absence of globose NFTs and tufted astrocytes in corticobasal degeneration and the presence of a tau gene mutation in FTDP-17. Both postencephalitic Parkinson's disease and the parkinsonian-dementia complex of Guam are distinguished from PSP primarily by clinical features. Clinical overlap with multiple system atrophy occurs, but pathologically it differs by the presence of α-synuclein–immunoreactive glial inclusions and the absence of tau-positive NFTs in multiple system atrophy. Manifestations of PSP with cognitive impairment may lead to a clinical diagnosis of Alzheimer's disease or diffuse Lewy body disease; these conditions are distinguished by the presence of neuritic plaques, NFTs, and/or Lewy bodies.

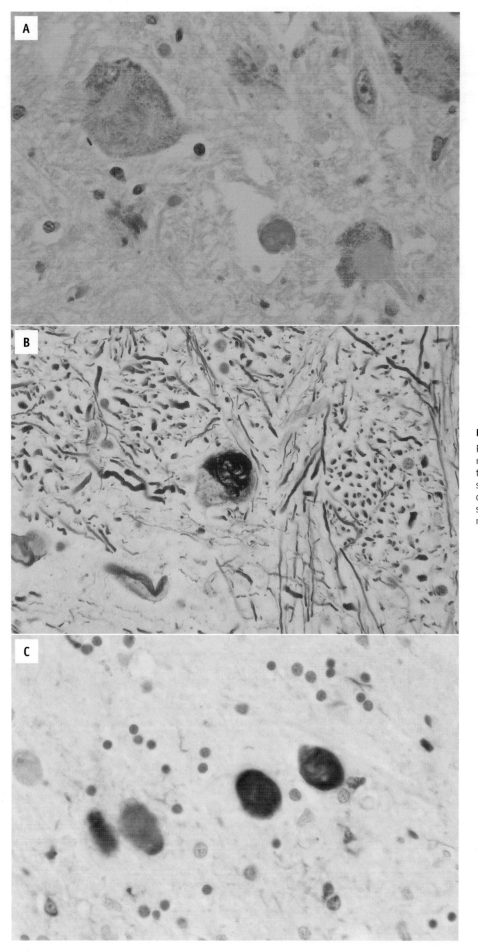

FIGURE 6-32

Progressive supranuclear palsy. **A**, Globose neurofibrillary tangle (NFT) in a neuron of the locus ceruleus. **B**, Bielschowsky-stained globose NFT in a neuron of the dorsal raphe nucleus. **C**, Tau-immuno-stained globose NFT in the subthalamic nucleus.

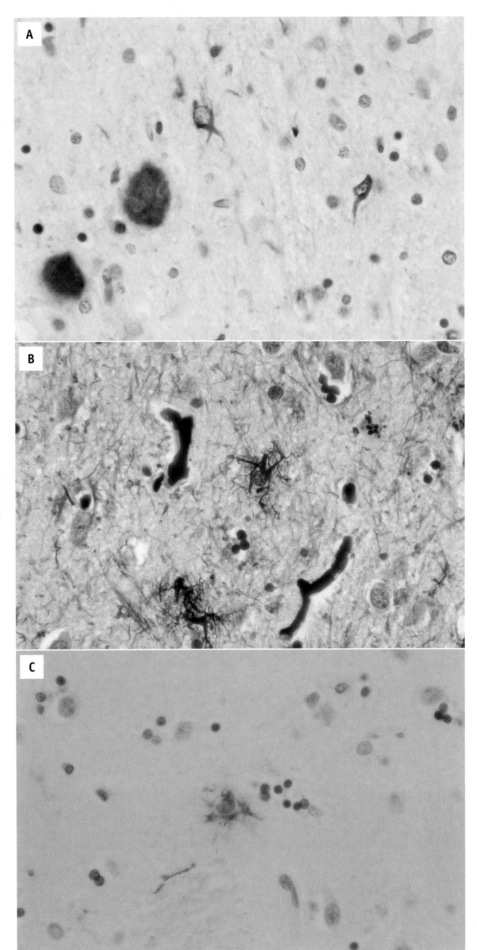

FIGURE 6-33

Progressive supranuclear palsy. **A**, Tau-immunoreactive glial tangles adjacent to two globose neurofibrillary tangles. **B**, Gallyas-stained tufted astrocyte in the putamen. **C**, Tau-immunostained tufted astrocyte also in the putamen.

PROGNOSTIC AND THERAPEUTIC CONSIDERATIONS

PSP is generally unresponsive to levodopa. Median survival is 5 to 6 years from the onset of symptoms.

MOTOR NEURON DISEASES

The term motor neuron disease encompasses a wide variety of diseases with upper motor neuron (UMN) degeneration, lower motor neuron (LMN) degeneration, or both. This chapter discusses two motor neuron diseases: amyotrophic lateral sclerosis (ALS) and spinal muscular atrophy (SMA). ALS most commonly includes degeneration of both UMNs and LMNs or, less commonly, LMNs only (progressive muscular atrophy) or UMNs only (primary lateral sclerosis). SMA exhibits exclusively LMN degeneration.

AMYOTROPHIC LATERAL SCLEROSIS

CLINICAL FEATURES

The mean age at onset is 60 years, and the mean age at death is 64 years. In patients with predominant LMN involvement (approximately 10%), the age at onset is later (mean of 68 years), and the mean age at death is 71. Males younger than 50 years of age are twice as likely to contract the disease as women; after the age of 50 years, the incidence curves are the same.

El Escorial clinical diagnostic criteria for ALS were created in 1994 and revised in 1998. Clinical disease categories of definite, probable, and possible ALS were based on the presence of UMN or LMN signs, or both, in any of four possible regions: bulbar, cervical, thoracic, and lumbosacral.

Signs of UMN degeneration are hyperreflexia, spasticity, loss of dexterity, slowed movements, and pathologic reflexes. LMN signs are weakness, hyporeflexia, muscle atrophy, fasciculations, muscle hypotonicity/flaccidity, and muscle cramps. Classic ALS is manifested as a combination of both UMN and LMN signs. Less commonly, solely progressive muscular atrophy with signs of LMN degeneration only may develop. Similarly but even less frequently, when solely UMN signs occur, the syndrome is called primary lateral sclerosis.

Approximately 10% of ALS patients have an autosomal dominant form of the disease. The clinical and pathologic findings for the most part in this subgroup are the same as in sporadic disease. However, disease onset is more frequently in the legs than in sporadic cases. In 20% of familial ALS cases, disease is due to a mutation in the Cu/Zn superoxide dismutase 1 gene (*SOD1*) located on chromosome 21. This type of ALS has now been designated ALS1. More than 100 muta-

---

AMYOTROPHIC LATERAL SCLEROSIS—FACT SHEET

Definition
▶ Neuromuscular disorder, predominantly sporadic, classically with degeneration of upper and lower motor neurons

Incidence and Prevalence
▶ Incidence is 1 to 3 per 100, 000 per year
▶ Prevalence is 4 to 7 per 100,000

Gender and Age Distribution
▶ Mean age at onset, overall, is 60 years
▶ With predominant lower motor neuron symptoms, mean age at onset is 68 years
▶ Males younger than 50 years are twice as likely to contract the disease as women
▶ Older than 50 years, equal occurrence in the sexes

Clinical Features
▶ ALS typically shows a combination of upper and lower motor neuron signs
▶ Upper motor neuron signs: hyperreflexia, spasticity, pathologic reflexes
▶ Lower motor neuron signs: hyporeflexia, weakness, muscle atrophy and fasciculations
▶ Primary lateral sclerosis: subtype of ALS with predominantly UMN signs
▶ Progressive muscular atrophy: subtype of ALS with predominantly LMN signs

Radiologic Features
▶ Not consistently helpful

Prognosis and Treatment
▶ The mean duration of ALS is 33 months
▶ With predominantly LMN involvement, the mean duration is 21 months

---

tions of the gene have been identified. Disease is due in most cases to point mutations in exons 1, 2, 4, or 5. The mutation results in abnormal protein folding or protein-protein interactions that are hypothesized to result in a toxic gain-of-function effect. Specific mutations do not appear to be associated with specific clinical phenotypes of disease, except for the duration of disease.

Several other types of familial ALS have been associated with specific chromosomes. In a subset of these types, gene products have been identified. ALS2, an autosomal recessive juvenile-onset disease, has been mapped to chromosome 2q33, and the gene product, GTPase regulator, has been identified.

PATHOLOGIC FEATURES

GROSS FINDINGS

Patients have diffuse muscle wasting of the limbs, diaphragm, and intercostal muscles. The cervical and

AMYOTROPHIC LATERAL SCLEROSIS—PATHOLOGIC FEATURES

Gross Findings

▶ Wasting of limbs, diaphragm, and intercostal muscles
▶ The cervical and lumbosacral enlargements of the spinal cord and the anterior motor roots are atrophic and shrunken, respectively
▶ Atrophy of the precentral gyrus may be present in cases of long duration

Microscopic Findings

▶ Loss of anterior horn cells and brain stem motor nuclei neurons
▶ Loss of Betz cells in the primary motor cortex
▶ Loss of myelinated axons of the anterior and lateral corticospinal tracts
▶ Bunina bodies—small round eosinophilic neuronal cytoplasmic inclusions in the anterior horn cells

Ultrastructural Features

▶ Bunina bodies are electron dense and composed of tubules, vesicular structures, and neurofilaments
▶ Ubiquitin-immunoreactive skein-like or spherical structures are bundles of filaments with granules

Genetics

▶ 10% of ALS patients have autosomal dominant familial disease
▶ 20% of familial cases are due to a mutation in the Cu/Zn superoxide dismutase 1 gene on chromosome 21

Immunohistochemical Features

▶ Bunina bodies are cystatin C immunoreactive and ubiquitin negative
▶ Skein-like or spherical inclusions in the anterior horn cells are ubiquitin immunoreactive

Pathologic Differential Diagnosis

▶ Spinal muscular atrophy
▶ Spinal muscular bulbar atrophy (Kennedy's syndrome)
▶ Hereditary spastic paraplegia

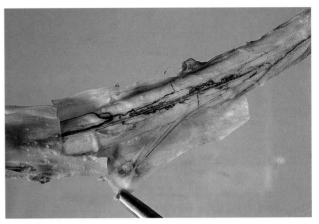

FIGURE 6-34
Amyotrophic lateral sclerosis. An anterior view of the spinal cord shows thinned and translucent anterior spinal roots in comparison to the posterior spinal roots.

are not unique to ALS, but are also seen in spinocerebellar atrophy. Occasionally, ubiquitin-immunoreactive cytoplasmic and nuclear intraneuronal inclusions, as seen in FTLD-U and FTLD-MND, are also present in small neurons of the cerebrum in ALS patients without a history of dementia.

Bunina bodies are small (2 to 4 nm) round eosinophilic neuronal cytoplasmic inclusions characteristically found in the anterior horn cells of the spinal cord in more than 80% of ALS patients (Fig. 6-37). There are greater numbers of Bunina bodies in cases of shorter duration. They are ubiquitin negative and cystatin C immunoreactive. Their nature and origin are unclear, but an association with rough endoplasmic reticulum has been suggested. Ultrastructurally, Bunina bodies are electron dense and contain tubules or vesicular structures and neurofilaments.

Patients with familial ALS associated with a *SOD1* mutation frequently have degeneration of the posterior columns, preferentially the fasciculus cuneatus, Clarke's column, and the spinocerebellar tracts. In addition, distinctive Lewy body–like hyaline inclusions are present in motor neurons, the reticular formation of the brain stem, and Clarke's column. These inclusions are SOD1, ubiquitin, and neurofilament immunoreactive and α-synuclein negative. They have an eosinophilic core with pale peripheral haloes. In addition, astrocytic hyaline inclusions have also been described in two families with ALS caused by a *SOD1* mutation.

lumbosacral enlargements of the spinal cord may be atrophic, and the anterior motor roots are shrunken and gray relative to the sensory roots (Fig. 6-34). Cases of long duration may show atrophy of the precentral gyrus.

MICROSCOPIC FINDINGS

Loss of anterior horn cells and brain stem motor nuclei is evident. Betz cells in the motor cortex also degenerate. Large myelinated axons of the anterior and lateral corticospinal tracts degenerate; myelin loss, macrophages, and variable severity of astrocytosis are evident (Fig. 6-35). Axonal spheroids are also frequently present in the anterior horn (Fig. 6-36A and B). Skeletal muscles show neurogenic atrophy.

Ubiquitin-immunoreactive skein-like or spherical structures in the neuronal cytoplasm of anterior horn cells are found in essentially all patients with ALS (see Fig. 6-36C). These inclusions consist of bundles of filaments, larger than neurofilaments, with granules. They

ANCILLARY STUDIES

Electrophysiologic study of skeletal muscle shows increased spontaneous activity of skeletal muscle and motor unit remodeling and decreased recruitment in chronic disease. No diagnostically useful or consistent MRI scan abnormalities have been found in the brain.

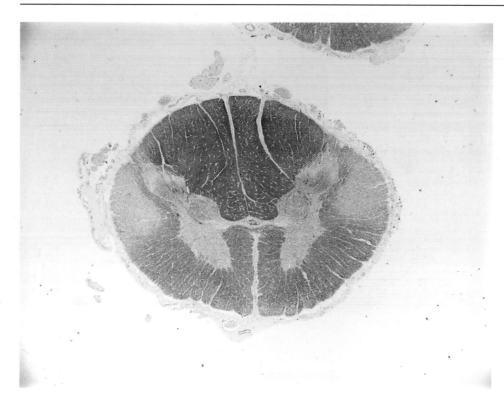

FIGURE 6-35

Amyotrophic lateral sclerosis. A Klüver-Barrera–stained section of the thoracic spinal cord shows degeneration of the lateral corticospinal tracts.

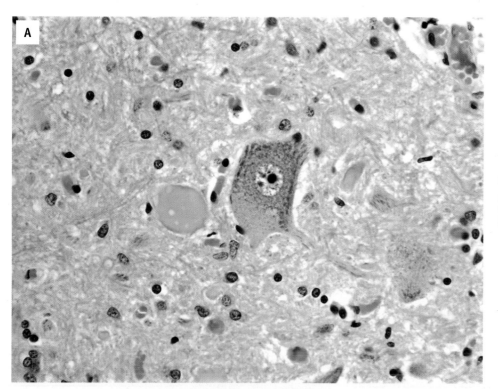

FIGURE 6-36

Amyotrophic lateral sclerosis. **A**, Dystrophic axon adjacent to an anterior horn motor neuron of the spinal cord.

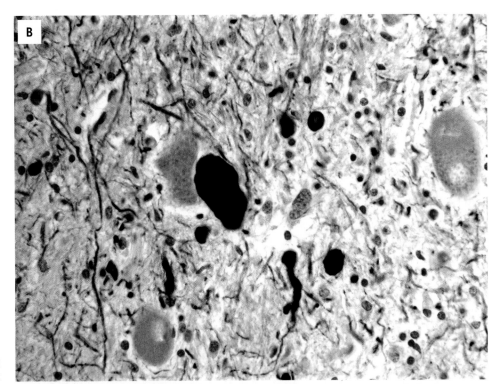

FIGURE 6-36, cont'd
B, Dystrophic axons immunostained with phosphorylated neurofilament antibody in the anterior horn. **C**, Ubiquitin-immunostained spherical cytoplasmic inclusion in an anterior horn motor neuron.

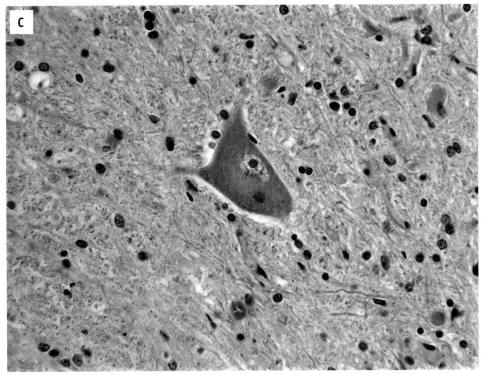

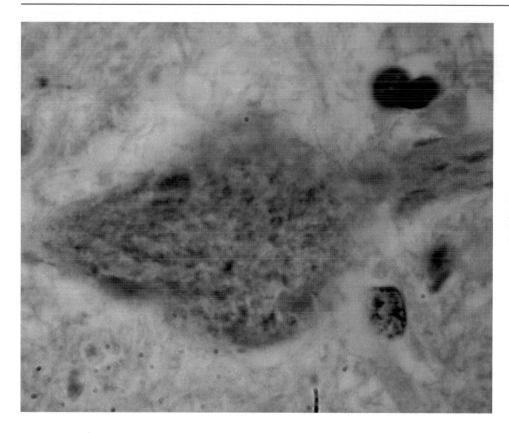

FIGURE 6-37

Amyotrophic lateral sclerosis: anterior horn cell with an eosinophilic beaded cytoplasmic Bunina body.

DIFFERENTIAL DIAGNOSIS

The differential diagnosis clinically includes adult-onset GM_2 gangliosidosis (hexosaminidase deficiency), myasthenia gravis, cervical spondylotic myelopathy, and skull base, foramen magnum, or conus lesions. Distinction of these entities from ALS at autopsy does not usually pose a diagnostic difficulty. SMA, spinal muscular bulbar atrophy (SMBA), and hereditary spastic paraplegia (HSP) may be confused pathologically with ALS. Distinction is aided by lack of corticospinal tract involvement in SMBA and SMA and the presence of posterior column degeneration in HSP. In addition, SMBA is X-linked recessive and associated with sensory neuropathy. SMA patients have mutations in the survival motor neuron gene.

PROGNOSTIC AND THERAPEUTIC CONSIDERATIONS

The mean duration of ALS is 33 months; the mean duration in patients with predominantly LMN findings is 21 months. Survival may be prolonged by mechanical ventilation. Aggressive treatment with noninvasive positive pressure ventilation has been shown to improve the quality of life and survival, but it has no impact on the rate of decline of respiratory function. Riluzole, an antiglutamate agent, has been shown to prolong survival by a mean of 2 months. Aggressive nutritional intervention has also been shown to prolong survival.

SPINAL MUSCULAR ATROPHY

SMA is a hereditary neuromuscular condition consisting of three types, each linked to a deletion or a mutation in the survival motor neuron gene (*SMN1*) on chromosome 5. The three forms are SMA1 (Werdnig-Hoffmann disease), SMA2, and SMA3 (Kugelberg-Welander disease). Each results from a homozygous deletion in the *SMN1* gene. Because asymptomatic members of families with individuals affected by SMA occasionally have the same haplotype as affected family members, it has been suggested that genes adjacent to *SMN1* (specifically *NAIP* and *SMN2*) may be variably affected and modify the disease phenotype.

CLINICAL FEATURES

SMA1 typically has an onset at birth with proximal weakness of limbs and areflexia. In 33%, weakness is detectable prenatally. Weakness progresses over a period of weeks and eventually includes the axial skeleton and diaphragm. SMA2 patients have normal early motor development, but they usually experience the onset of weakness and developmental regression by 3 months. Fasciculations and loss of reflexes are evident; contractures and kyphoscoliosis are usually present. SMA3 is characterized by symptoms of weakness of limbs and absent knee jerk reflexes anywhere from infancy to early childhood. SMA3 onset and progression are gradual in comparison to SMA1, and the disease occasionally occurs sporadically.

SPINAL MUSCULAR ATROPHY—FACT SHEET

Definition

▶ Hereditary neuromuscular disease characterized by motor neuron degeneration and muscle atrophy
▶ Occurs in three forms: SMA1 (Werdnig-Hoffmann disease), SMA2, and SMA3 (Kugelberg-Welander disease)

Incidence and Prevalence

▶ Incidence is 1 in 10,000 to 20,000 live births
▶ Gene carrier frequency is 1 in 50 to 80
▶ No prevalence data available

Gender and Age Distribution

▶ SMA1: onset in infancy, may be manifested in utero (33%)
▶ SMA2: onset at approximately 3 months
▶ SMA3: onset in infancy to early childhood
▶ No gender predilection

Clinical Features

▶ SMA1: proximal weakness of the limbs progressing to include the axial musculature, areflexia, cannot sit unaided
▶ SMA2: learns to sit but not walk, areflexia, fasciculations, contractures, kyphoscoliosis
▶ SMA3: learns to walk but delayed, slow progression of limb weakness, absent knee reflexes

Radiologic Features

▶ Not applicable

Prognosis and Treatment

▶ SMA1: 80% of patients die within 1 year
▶ SMA2: 69% dead by 25 years old
▶ SMA3: statistically normal life span

SPINAL MUSCULAR ATROPHY—PATHOLOGIC FEATURES

Gross Findings

▶ SMA1: atrophic anterior spinal roots

Microscopic Findings

▶ SMA1: characteristic pattern of large groups or fascicles of small rounded atrophic fibers of both types 1 and 2 in skeletal muscle, with scattered single or small groups of markedly hypertrophic type 1 fibers
▶ SMA2: skeletal muscle with a similar pattern as in SMA1
▶ SMA3: adult pattern of denervation
▶ The spinal cord in each subtype of SMA shows loss of anterior horn cells and astrocytosis
▶ Early stages may have chromatolysis and neuronophagia
▶ Chromatolytic cells may be present in the thalamus

Ultrastructural Features

▶ Reflective of denervation of muscle, loss of anterior horn cells, and astrocytosis

Genetics

▶ Autosomal recessive disease caused by homozygous deletions or mutations in the *SMN1* gene on chromosome 5 (q13)
▶ Close association between the extent of the deletion and disease severity
▶ Prenatal diagnosis is possible

Immunohistochemical Features

▶ Not applicable

Pathologic Differential Diagnosis

▶ Myotonic dystrophy
▶ Nemaline myopathy
▶ Congenital fiber-type disproportion
▶ Muscular dystrophy
▶ Amyotrophic lateral sclerosis

PATHOLOGIC FEATURES

Most pathologic descriptions involve SMA1.

GROSS FINDINGS

In SMA1, the anterior spinal roots are thin and atrophic.

MICROSCOPIC FINDINGS

Skeletal muscle in SMA1 shows large groups or fascicles of small rounded atrophic fibers, both types 1 and 2. Scattered single or small groups of markedly hypertrophic type 1 fibers are also evident (Fig. 6-38). At end stage, fibrosis and fatty infiltration may be present. Skeletal muscle in SMA2 shows a pattern similar to SMA1. However, in SMA3, an adult pattern of skeletal muscle denervation is seen.

The spinal cord in each subtype of SMA shows anterior horn cell loss and astrocytosis. In the early stages, chromatolysis and neuronophagia may be evident. In addition, chromatolytic cells are frequently seen in the thalamus. They may have ubiquitin immunoreactivity in their cytoplasm. Ballooned cells filled with neurofilaments may also be noted. No involvement of the corticospinal tracts has been reported.

ANCILLARY STUDIES

Electromyography in each of the SMA types shows denervation.

DIFFERENTIAL DIAGNOSIS

In SMA1 disease, the muscle biopsy changes may suggest myotonic dystrophy, nemaline myopathy, or congenital fiber-type disproportion because of the involvement of type 1 fibers. At end stage, the muscle may suggest a dystrophic process that may be eliminated

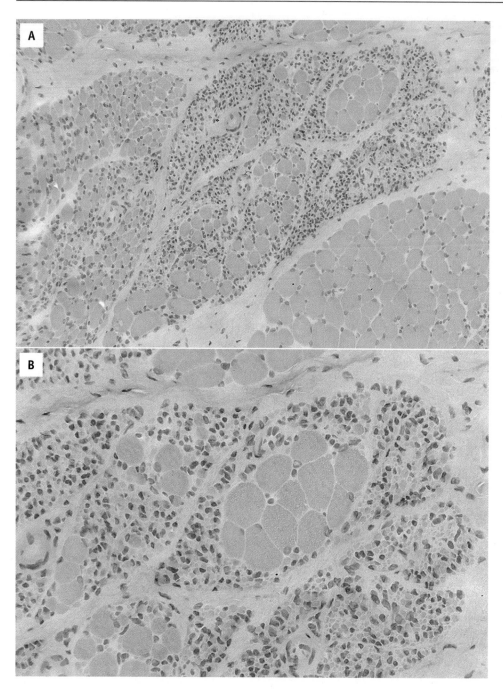

FIGURE 6-38

Werdnig-Hoffman disease. Cross sections (**A** and **B**) of skeletal muscle show severe fascicular atrophy and clusters of markedly hypertrophic fibers.

by immunostaining for dystrophin and dystrophin-associated glycoproteins.

Distinction of SMA from ALS is likely to be facilitated by the presence of corticospinal tract degeneration, Bunina bodies, and ubiquitin skein-like/spherical inclusions in ALS.

PROGNOSTIC AND THERAPEUTIC CONSIDERATIONS

In SMA1, 80% of patients die within 1 year. Patients with SMA2 have a much wider range of survival, with 69% alive at 25 years. SMA3 individuals have a statistically normal life span. Only supportive therapy is available.

TRINUCLEOTIDE REPEAT DISORDERS

The category of trinucleotide repeat disorders is defined by the presence of expansion of triplet repeats of nucleotides. Most of these entities have CAG triplet expansions (Huntington's disease, spinocerebellar ataxias); also expanded is GAA in Friedreich's ataxia. Most data support a toxic gain-of-function pathogenesis. Inheritance may be autosomal dominant, autosomal recessive, or X-linked. These diseases affect the nervous system prominently, but systemic findings are present in several of the disorders (i.e., Friedreich's ataxia).

HUNTINGTON'S DISEASE

Huntington's disease (HD) is a predominantly adult-onset, autosomal dominant chorea caused by a mutation in the HD gene on chromosome 4p16.3. The most common mutation is an expansion of the trinucleotide repeat CAG. The expanded CAG repeat results in an expanded polyglutamine segment near the amino terminus of the huntingtin protein. The CAG repeat size correlates inversely with age at onset and directly with disease severity. The usual repeat length in normal individuals is up to 26; HD is associated with repeat lengths of 36 or greater. Earlier age of onset and an increased number of repeats in the next generation (anticipation) are more likely associated with paternal inheritance. Both mutated and normal forms of huntingtin are expressed in the brain perikarya, axons, synaptosomes, and synaptic terminals of patients with HD.

CLINICAL FEATURES

Adult-onset disease is characterized by chorea. Hypokinesia and bradykinesia are also present to varying degrees in individual patients. Terminally, the patient becomes akinetic and rigid. Psychiatric manifestations are also usually present and range from behavioral abnormalities and depression to paranoia and schizophrenia. The rate of suicide in HD patients is increased. On physical examination, the chorea affects eye movement, facial muscles, tongue, speech, swallowing, and gait. The mean age of adult-onset disease is 40 years.

Juvenile-onset (younger than 20 years) HD accounts for only 1% to 2% of all HD. In juvenile-onset disease, bradykinesia and hypokinesia are prominent, with eventual development of rigidity. Seizures may also occur.

PATHOLOGIC FEATURES

GROSS FINDINGS

Brain weight ranges from 800 to 1000 g. Progressive atrophy of the neostriatum is observed. The pathologic

---

HUNTINGTON'S DISEASE—FACT SHEET

Definition
- Autosomal dominant disease caused by a mutation in the *huntingtin* gene on chromosome 4 and characterized by chorea and psychiatric abnormalities and degeneration of the basal ganglia

Incidence and Prevalence
- No incidence data available
- Prevalence is 5 to 10 per 100,000 in Western countries

Gender and Age Distribution
- No gender predilection
- Mean adult disease onset is 40 years
- Juvenile onset is classified as younger than 20 years

Clinical Features
- Adult onset is characterized by chorea and psychiatric manifestations. Terminally, all patients are akinetic and rigid
- Juvenile-onset disease is manifested as bradykinesia and hypokinesia with eventual rigidity. Seizures may also occur

Radiologic Features
- CT and MRI show caudate atrophy

Prognosis and Treatment
- The mean duration of disease (adult and juvenile) is 17 years
- Supportive therapy to treat movement disorders is available

---

HUNTINGTON'S DISEASE—PATHOLOGIC FEATURES

Gross Findings
- Decreased brain weight
- Progressive atrophy of the caudate and putamen (Vonsattel grades 0 to 4)

Microscopic Findings
- Neuronal loss and astrocytosis of the caudate and putamen developing in a dorsomedial-to-ventrolateral, caudal-to-rostral pattern
- Neuronal loss and minimal astrocytosis in the cerebral cortex (layers III, V, and VI) and mesial temporal lobe structures

Ultrastructural Features
- Nuclear inclusions are composed of a mixture of non–membrane-bound granules and straight and tortuous filaments and fibrils
- Dystrophic neurites are composed of filaments and granules

Genetics
- Autosomal dominant disease caused by a mutation in the *huntingtin* gene on chromosome 4
- Disease caused by expansion of CAG nucleotide repeats
- Size of the CAG repeat correlates inversely with age at onset and directly with the severity of disease
- Normal repeat length is up to 26; HD is associated with lengths of 36 or greater

Immunohistochemical Features
- Intraneuronal nuclear inclusions and dystrophic neurites immunoreactive for ubiquitin and huntingtin proteins in the neostriatum, cortex, and hippocampus

Pathologic Differential Diagnosis
- Pick's disease
- Frontotemporal lobar degeneration
- Corticobasal degeneration
- Multiple system atrophy

changes have been graded by Vonsattel on the basis of both gross and microscopic examination. Grades have been shown to correlate with the degree of clinical impairment determined at the last examination before death. Grade 0 indicates no gross or microscopic changes and is defined by clinical and family histories and DNA analysis. Grade 1 still does not show gross atrophy of the neostriatum, but microscopic changes are evident (see later). Grade 2 indicates gross atrophy of the neostriatum at the level of the nucleus accumbens, but the caudate nucleus still has a slight convex outline. Grade 3 is defined by marked atrophy of the neostriatum, with the caudate nucleus forming a flat line. Grade 4 shows more severe atrophy of the involved areas; the caudate nucleus is shrunken and concave.

In addition to neostriatal atrophy, the parietal and occipital cortices (temporal cortex less involved) also show atrophy. At end stage, atrophy of the globus pallidus, thalamus, brain stem, and cerebellum is also evident. The substantia nigra is usually normally pigmented, but the locus ceruleus has decreased pigmentation.

MICROSCOPIC FINDINGS

Neostriatal involvement progresses in a dorsomedial-to-ventrolateral and caudal-to-rostral direction. GABAergic medium spiny neurons are most susceptible; other neuronal types are unaffected until later-stage disease (Fig. 6-39). It is hypothesized that preferential loss of striatal projections to the lateral pallidum causes chorea. Neuronal loss and astrocytosis are less severe in the globus pallidus and may be partially secondary to wallerian degeneration from loss of input from the striatum.

Nuclear inclusions that are immunoreactive for ubiquitin and huntingtin are present in medium-sized neurons of the neostriatum and all layers of the cortex (Fig. 6-40). Also present in these areas are ubiquitin- and huntingtin-immunoreactive dystrophic neurites.

Microscopic examination to determine the histologic component of the Vonsattel grades is based on examination at three levels: level of the caudate, accumbens, and putamen; level of the globus pallidus; and level of the tail of the caudate (at the lateral geniculate body). These grades are as follows: grade 0—no neuronal loss is discernible on qualitative examination; however, neuronal counts show loss and intranuclear inclusions are present. Grade 1 HD does show neuronal loss and astrocytosis in the dorsomedial caudate, tail of the caudate, and dorsal putamen. The changes are still slight at this stage. Of help in determining their significance is the presence of intranuclear huntingtin- and ubiquitin-immunoreactive inclusions. Grade 2 HD shows extension of the neuronal loss and astrocytosis of the caudate and putamen in a ventrolateral direction. Grade 3 is defined by neuronal loss and astrocytosis involving most of the caudate and putamen. The nucleus accumbens is still relatively unaffected. Grade 4 HD shows severe neuronal loss and astrocytosis involving all of the caudate and putamen, with extension into the nucleus accumbens.

Cerebral involvement primarily affects cortical layers III, V, and VI. In the hippocampus, amygdala, and entorhinal cortex, neuronal loss is evident, but astrocytosis is minimal.

Variable degrees of neuronal loss and astrocytosis are seen in the substantia nigra, thalamus, hypothalamus, subthalamus, claustrum, pons, olivary complex, and Purkinje cells.

The juvenile form of HD has the same pattern of involvement as just detailed, but with more severe changes and extension into the cerebellum. Many cases have cerebellar atrophy with loss of Purkinje and granular cells. In addition, varying degrees of neuronal loss and astrocytosis of the dentate nucleus, thalamus, hippocampus, and neocortex may be seen. Axonal spheroids in the nucleus gracilis have also been described.

ANCILLARY STUDIES

Computed tomographic and MRI scans show caudate atrophy. Genetic testing for the HD mutation is needed for definitive diagnosis.

DIFFERENTIAL DIAGNOSIS

HD may overlap clinically with other causes of chorea, such as senile chorea, benign familial chorea, drug-related chorea, choreoacanthocytosis, Sydenham's chorea, and dentatorubral-pallidoluysian atrophy. Distinction is made easy by the availability of a definitive test for HD, in addition to the absence of HD-associated pathologic changes. Pathologic overlap with HD and other diseases that may show involvement of the anterior caudate and putamen occurs with Pick's disease, frontotemporal lobar degeneration, multiple system atrophy, and corticobasal degeneration. Distinction of HD from these conditions can be achieved by noting the preferential involvement of the dorsal neostriatum and the ubiquitin- and huntingtin-positive nuclear inclusions in HD in contrast to the presence of Pick bodies or other tau-immunoreactive neuronal and glial inclusions in frontotemporal lobar degeneration and corticobasal degeneration and by α-synuclein–immunoreactive inclusions in multiple system atrophy.

PROGNOSTIC AND THERAPEUTIC CONSIDERATIONS

Supportive therapy with medications to treat the movement disorder and psychiatric symptoms is provided. Implantation of fetal cells or stem cells to restore lost function is still at an experimental stage. The mean duration of adult-onset disease is 17 years. The mean duration of juvenile-onset HD is approximately the same; it is of shorter duration when inheritance is from the father and in those with the youngest ages at onset.

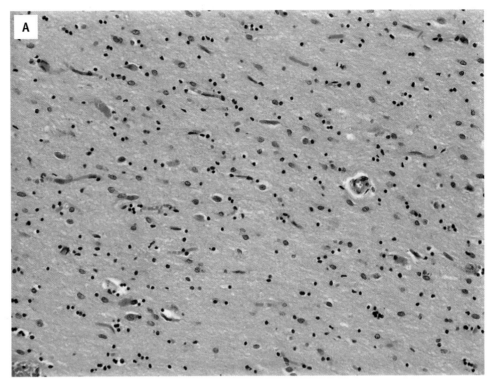

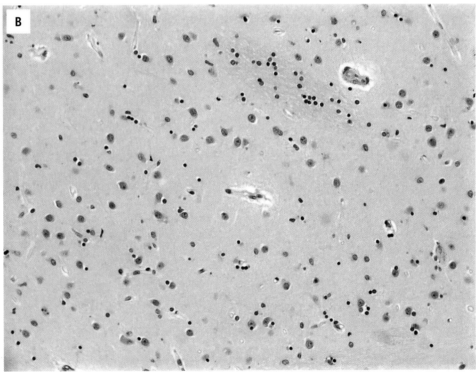

FIGURE 6-39

Huntington's disease. **A**, Anterior caudate nucleus showing neuronal loss and astrocytosis. **B**, Age-matched control anterior caudate nucleus.   *Continued*

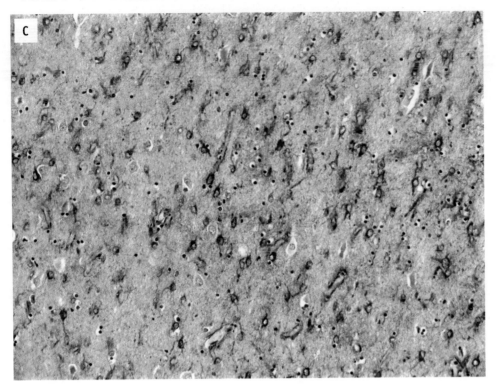

FIGURE 6-39, cont'd

C, Glial fibrillary acidic protein–immunostained anterior caudate nucleus showing severe astrocytosis in a patient with Huntington's disease.

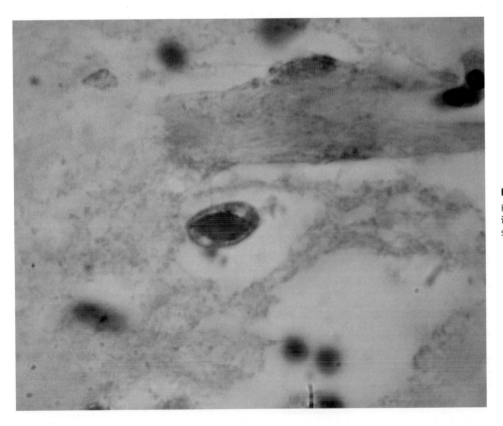

FIGURE 6-40

Huntington's disease: ubiquitin-immunoreactive intranuclear inclusion in a caudate neuron.

SPINOCEREBELLAR ATAXIAS

Spinocerebellar ataxias (SCAs) are dominantly inherited ataxias whose classification is currently based on genetic abnormalities. SCAs are attributed to expansions of triplet nucleotides secondary to mutation. The expansion results in aggregates of polyglutamines, which are hypothesized to result in a toxic gain-of-function effect. At least 21 different SCAs have been reported. Three basic groups have been described: those caused by CAG nucleotide repeats, which account for the majority of SCAs; those caused by noncoding microsatellite expansions; and those classified as episodic ataxias. The most commonly described are SCA2 (olivopontocerebellar atrophy of Menzel) and SCA3 (Machado-Joseph disease). For many SCAs, linkage studies have identified an associated chromosome, but no specific gene or protein product has been described. SCA2 and SCA3 will be described in detail in this review.

SCA2 has a CAG repeat expansion mutation in a gene on chromosome 12. The gene product is a cytoplasmic protein called ataxin-2. The normal repeat length is 14 to 31, whereas expanded repeat lengths range from 32 to 77. SCA3 has a CAG repeat expansion ranging from 53 to 200 (the normal number of repeats is between 12 and 40) that is caused by a mutation on chromosome 14 in the gene for ataxin-3 protein.

CLINICAL FEATURES

In SCA2, the age at onset is usually between 15 and 40 years, but it may occur earlier. Symptoms are gait and limb ataxia, dysarthria, intention tremor, titubation, sensorimotor neuropathy, and abnormal eye movements (slow saccades). Occasionally seen are chorea or dystonia and dementia, and anticipation has been reported in SCA2. Several large kindreds have been reported in Cuba.

SCA3 was originally described in Portuguese families but has since been reported in families of diverse ethnicities. In SCA3, the clinical features are divided into multiple subtypes: type 1 is manifested as dystonia and spasticity, usually in the first 2 decades. Type 2 is the most common form and is characterized by the onset of ataxia, nystagmus, and dysarthria in the second to fourth decades. Type 3 develops between 40 and 60 years of age and is characterized by ataxia and peripheral sensory and motor neuropathy.

PATHOLOGIC FEATURES

GROSS FINDINGS

Severe atrophy of the basis pontis (decreased anterior-posterior diameter), cerebellum, and cervical spinal cord is found in SCA2, with brain weight usually less

---

---

than 1000 g. The pontine tegmentum remains normal in size. In SCA3, the degree of atrophy is most often slight, and brain weight is within normal limits.

MICROSCOPIC FINDINGS

SCA2 • The inferior olivary nucleus, basis pontis gray matter, and cerebellar cortex (both Purkinje cells and internal granular cells) show neuronal loss and astrocytosis (Fig. 6-41). "Torpedoes," or argyrophilic focal swellings of proximal Purkinje cell axons, are present in the granular cell layer. The middle and inferior cerebellar peduncles and the white matter of the cerebellum show axonal loss and astrocytosis. The dentate nucleus is better preserved than the cerebellar parenchyma. Degeneration of the substantia nigra is evident, but the locus ceruleus is intact. Most reports do not describe degeneration of the striatum and pallidum. The exception is an autopsy study of 11 Cuban patients with SCA2 who showed striatal and pallidal involvement. Motor neurons in the brain stem and spinal cord

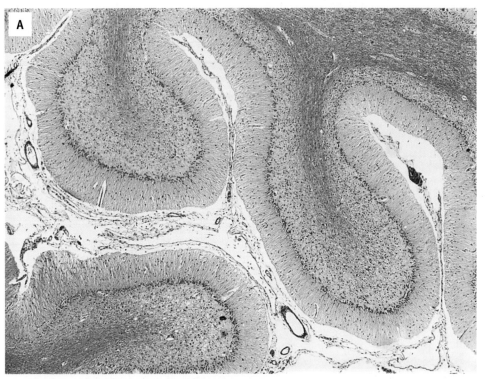

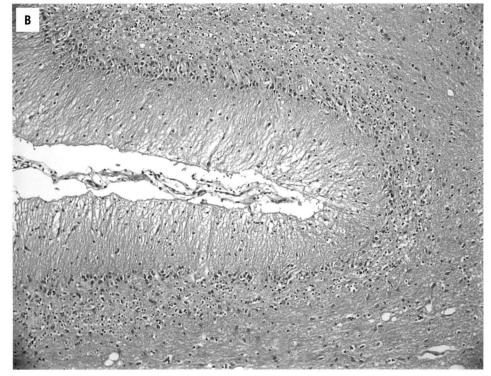

FIGURE 6-41

Spinocerebellar ataxia: severe Purkinje and internal granule cell loss with Bergmann's astrocytosis. **A**, Klüver-Barrera stain. **B**, Hematoxylin-eosin stain.

degenerate, as do the spinocerebellar tracts and posterior columns (tractus gracilis more than the cuneatus). Clarke's column is also affected. Sural nerve biopsy shows axonal loss. Cerebral cortical atrophy may be seen in patients with dementia.

SCA3 • Severe neuronal loss with grumose degeneration is found in the dentate nucleus. Grumose degeneration consists of preterminal axons filled with

mitochondria, vesicles, filaments, and vacuoles. At a light microscopic level, it appears as clumps of eosinophilic granular material adjacent to or overlying the dentate neuron cell bodies. The cerebellar cortex and inferior olivary nuclei are preserved. Degeneration of the superior cerebellar peduncle, spinocerebellar tracts, neurons of Clarke's column, and anterior horn cells is evident. Loss of neurons in the substantia nigra

SPINOCEREBELLAR ATAXIAS—PATHOLOGIC FEATURES

Gross Findings

▶ SCA2: severe atrophy of the basis pontis, cerebellum, and cervical spinal cord. Brain weight is decreased
▶ SCA3: slight degree of atrophy of the posterior fossa structures and spinal cord, with normal brain weight

Microscopic Findings

▶ SCA2:
  ▶ Severe neuronal loss is seen in the inferior olivary nucleus, basis pontis gray matter, cerebellar cortex, and substantia nigra
  ▶ The middle and inferior cerebellar peduncles and cerebellar white matter show axonal loss and astrocytosis
  ▶ Spinocerebellar and posterior columns degenerate
  ▶ Motor neurons and neurons of Clarke's column are lost
▶ SCA3:
  ▶ Severe neuronal loss in the cerebellar dentate nucleus with grumose degeneration
  ▶ The cerebellar cortex and inferior olivary nuclei are preserved
  ▶ Degeneration of the basis pontis gray matter, neurons of Clarke's column, lower motor neurons, and substantia nigra
  ▶ Degeneration of the superior cerebellar peduncle and spinocerebellar tracts
  ▶ Cranial nerve nuclei often affected

Ultrastructural Features

▶ No data available

Genetics

▶ SCA2: CAG repeat expansion secondary to a mutation in the ataxin-2 gene
  ▶ Normal number of repeats is 14 to 31; disease has been reported with 32 to 77 repeats
▶ SCA3: CAG repeat expansion secondary to mutation in the ataxin-3 gene on chromosome 14
  ▶ Normal number of repeats is 12 to 40; disease is found with 53 to 200 repeats

Immunohistochemical Features

▶ IC2, an antibody that recognizes polyglutamine repeats, identifies intranuclear inclusions in many SCAs, including SCA2
▶ SCA3: Ubiquitin and ataxin-3 antibodies identify intranuclear inclusions

Pathologic Differential Diagnosis

▶ Other spinocerebellar ataxias
▶ Friedreich's ataxia

is apparent, and sometimes the globus pallidus (internal segment), putamen, subthalamic nucleus, and basis pontis are also affected. Cranial nerve nuclei may likewise be affected.

Immunocytochemistry with antibodies to ubiquitin and ataxin-3 identifies nuclei in affected areas in SCA3. An antibody (IC2) that recognizes polyglutamine repeats may be used to identify intranuclear inclusions in a variety of SCAs, including SCA2.

ANCILLARY STUDIES

MRI scans in both SCA2 and SCA3 show atrophy of the brain stem, middle cerebellar peduncle, cerebellum, and cervical spinal cord volume. SCA2 is associated with more severe degeneration.

DIFFERENTIAL DIAGNOSIS

Despite clinical and pathologic overlap among the various SCAs, many may be distinguished from each other by detailed clinical, pathologic, and immunocytochemical examination. Confirmation of the classification may be achieved by specific gene analysis.

PROGNOSTIC AND THERAPEUTIC CONSIDERATIONS

The average disease duration of SCA2 is approximately 10 years, and for SCA3 the range is 5 to 12 years. At this time, supportive therapy is all that is available.

FRIEDREICH'S ATAXIA

Friedreich's ataxia (FA), the most common hereditary ataxia, is an autosomal recessive disease caused by a mutation in the *frataxin* gene on chromosome 9. Frataxin, a protein of 210 amino acids, localizes to mitochondria and is hypothesized to bind iron. The most common mutation of the *frataxin* gene causes an expansion of GAA nucleotide repeats and reduced production of the frataxin protein. The normal number of GAA repeats is 6 to 27; in affected individuals the number of expanded alleles ranges from 90 to greater than 100. Genetic studies of FA have shown that 95% of affected individuals are homozygotes with a GAA repeat expansion in the first intron of the gene on chromosome 9. Compound heterozygotes make up the remaining 5%, with one allele containing repeat expansion and the other allele containing a missense, nonsense, or point mutation.

CLINICAL FEATURES

Disease onset is usually near puberty, but it may vary from 2 to 3 years old to later than 25 years. The principal feature is limb and gait ataxia. Also present are sensory loss, muscle weakness, scoliosis, foot deformity, sensorineural hearing loss, diabetes mellitus, and hypertrophic cardiomyopathy. Physical examination shows sensory and cerebellar ataxia, loss of sensation, absent tendon reflexes in the lower extremities, and axonal sensory neuropathy. Eventually, areflexia of all four limbs, up-going toes, pyramidal weakness, and dysarthria are present. Several clinical variants exist: late-onset FA (onset greater than 20 years), FA with

FRIEDREICH'S ATAXIA—FACT SHEET

Definition
► Most common hereditary ataxia caused by GAA triplet nucleotide expansion

Incidence and Prevalence
► No incidence data available
► Prevalence is 2 to 5 per 100,000

Gender and Age Distribution
► Onset is usually during puberty
► Range is from 2 to 3 years to older than 25 years

Clinical Features
► Limb and gait ataxia
► Sensory loss, weakness, sensorineural hearing loss
► Scoliosis, foot deformity, diabetes mellitus, hypertrophic cardiomyopathy

Radiologic Features
► MRI shows spinal cord atrophy with a normal brain stem, cerebellum, and cerebrum

Prognosis and Treatment
► Life expectancy is 35 to 40 years
► Treatment with coenzyme Q and vitamin E has been associated with stabilization and improvement of symptoms

FRIEDREICH'S ATAXIA—PATHOLOGIC FEATURES

Gross Findings
► The spinal cord is atrophic, and the lateral and posterior columns may appear gray
► The posterior roots are thin
► The dentate nucleus may be atrophic

Microscopic Findings
► Severe neuronal loss and astrocytosis in the dentate nucleus
► Atrophy of the superior cerebellar peduncle
► Neuronal loss of the vestibular and cochlear nuclei
► Neuronal loss of the dorsal root ganglia and degeneration of the large myelinated sensory peripheral nerves
► Degeneration of the posterior columns, spinocerebellar tracts, and corticospinal tracts
► Degeneration of the nucleus dorsalis of Clarke

Ultrastructural Features
► Axonal swellings filled with neurofilaments may be present in the dorsal root ganglia
► Occasional descriptions of onion bulbs in peripheral nerve biopsy specimens

Genetics
► Autosomal recessive
► Mutation in the *frataxin* gene on chromosome 9
► Mutation results in expansion of the GAA nucleotide triplet
► Normal number of repeats is 6 to 27; disease is associated with 90 to more than 100.

Immunohistochemical Features
► No specific immunohistochemical features at present

Pathologic Differential Diagnosis
► Spinocerebellar ataxias
► Charcot-Marie-Tooth disease (hypertrophic form)
► Hereditary spastic paraplegia

retained reflexes, and the Acadian type (Louisiana form). There is an inverse correlation between the number of GAA repeats and the frequency of certain clinical characteristics (cardiomyopathy, loss of reflexes in the upper extremities, up-going toes, and scoliosis) and the age at onset.

PATHOLOGIC FEATURES

GROSS FINDINGS

Brain weight is usually normal. The spinal cord is atrophic, and the lateral and posterior columns of the spinal cord may appear gray. The posterior roots are thin in comparison to the anterior spinal roots The dentate nucleus may appear atrophic.

MICROSCOPIC FINDINGS

The dentate nucleus is severely affected, and the superior cerebellar peduncle is atrophic; the cerebellar parenchyma is preserved. Purkinje cells may be lost late in the disease course. In some cases, degeneration of the globus pallidus and subthalamic nucleus is seen. The degree of Betz cell loss is slight. The vestibular and cochlear nuclei show neuronal loss. Dorsal root ganglia show loss of neurons early in the disease course, and loss of the large myelinated sensory axons in peripheral nerves is evident. Degeneration of the posterior

columns, spinocerebellar tracts, and corticospinal tracts is apparent on examination of the spinal cord (Fig. 6-42). The nucleus dorsalis of Clarke shows neuronal loss. Anterior horn cells are preserved.

ANCILLARY STUDIES

Electrophysiologic studies show axonal sensory neuropathy with small or absent sensory action potentials. Motor conduction velocities are slightly decreased or normal.

MRI shows spinal cord atrophy and a normal brain stem, cerebellum, and cerebrum.

DIFFERENTIAL DIAGNOSIS

The differential diagnosis of FA includes other spinocerebellar ataxias, Charcot-Marie-Tooth disease

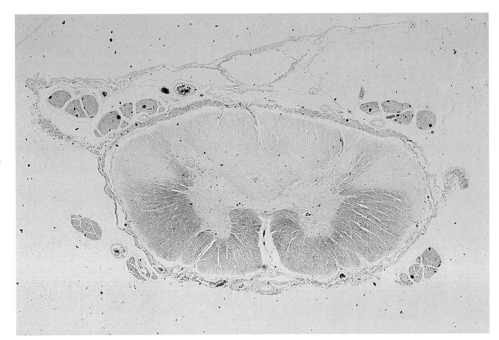

FIGURE 6-42
Friedreich's ataxia. Degeneration of posterior columns, spinocerebellar tracts, and corticospinal tracts are apparent.

(hypertrophic form), and hereditary spastic paraparesis. Differentiation based only on clinical findings may not be possible, but the availability of molecular genetic testing permits specific diagnosis.

PROGNOSTIC AND THERAPEUTIC CONSIDERATIONS

Clinical trials with antioxidants have shown some improvement in the cardiomyopathy. Administration of coenzyme Q and vitamin E has been associated with lack of progression of neurologic signs and echocardiographic abnormalities and also improvement in cardiac and skeletal muscle function. Cardiomyopathy is the most common cause of death. Life expectancy averages 35 to 40 years.

DENTATORUBRAL-PALLIDOLUYSIAN ATROPHY

Dentatorubral-pallidoluysian atrophy (DRPLA), an autosomal dominant spinocerebellar ataxia with high penetrance, occurs most frequently in Japan, but it has also been identified in several North American and European families. The cause of DRPLA is an unstable expansion of CAG expansion repeats found in the *DRPLA* gene on chromosome 12. The number of repeats in DRPLA patients ranges from 54 to 79. The normal number of CAG repeats is 6 to 35. The protein made by the *DRPLA* gene is atrophin-1; its function is unknown, but it is found in neuronal cytoplasm.

CLINICAL FEATURES

DRPLA shows marked clinical heterogeneity between juvenile- and adult-onset disease, but common symptoms are ataxia and dementia. Juvenile-onset (younger than 20 years) DRPLA is manifested as progressive myoclonic epilepsy and consists of ataxia, seizures, myoclonus, and progressive cognitive decline. Adult involvement may occur early (20 to 30 years) or late, and each is usually characterized by choreoathetosis, ataxia, dementia, and psychiatric disturbances. The frequency of seizures decreases with onset after 20 years. In DRPLA there is an inverse correlation between the size of expanded CAG repeats and age at onset. In addition, anticipation is prominent, the effect being greater with paternal transmission.

PATHOLOGIC FEATURES

GROSS FINDINGS

The brain appears small and diffusely atrophic. In juvenile-onset disease, the atrophy is equal in all parts of the brain; in adult-onset disease, the pons and cerebellum are most affected. The cut surface of the brain shows atrophy and discoloration of the globus pallidus, subthalamus, dentate nucleus, and pontine tegmentum.

MICROSCOPIC FINDINGS

Degeneration of both the dentate nucleus and the globus pallidus and disruption of the dentatofugal and pallidofugal systems are essential pathologic

DENTATORUBRAL-PALLIDOLUYSIAN ATROPHY—FACT SHEET

Definition

▶ Type of spinocerebellar ataxia found most commonly in Japan, but reported in North American and European individuals; caused by expansion of CAG trinucleotide repeats

Incidence and Prevalence

▶ No incidence data available
▶ Prevalence is 0.2 to 0.7 per 100,000

Gender and Age Distribution

▶ Juvenile form of disease: age at onset, younger than 20 years
▶ Adult form of disease: age at onset, 20 to 30 years or older

Clinical Features

▶ Common to both adult and juvenile forms: ataxia and dementia
▶ Juvenile form: progressive myoclonic epilepsy, ataxia, and progressive cognitive decline
▶ Adult form: choreoathetosis and psychiatric disturbances

Radiologic Features

▶ MRI shows atrophy of the brain stem and cerebellum

Prognosis and Treatment

▶ No therapy currently available
▶ Duration: adult-onset disease—progressive over a period of 10 to 20 years; juvenile-onset disease is more rapidly progressive

DENTATORUBRAL-PALLIDOLUYSIAN ATROPHY— PATHOLOGIC FEATURES

Gross Findings

▶ Thickened skull bone
▶ Brain weight is decreased and diffuse proportional atrophy is present in both adult and juvenile forms
▶ In the adult form, the pons and cerebellum are most atrophic, and severe atrophy and discoloration may be also be evident in the globus pallidus, subthalamus, dentate nucleus, and pontine tegmentum

Microscopic Findings

▶ The cerebellar dentate nucleus shows severe neuronal loss and grumose degeneration
▶ The external segment of the globus pallidus also has severe neuronal loss and astrocytosis
▶ The red nucleus, caudate, putamen, substantia nigra, and subthalamus show variable degrees of neuronal loss
▶ White matter of the cerebellar/olivary complex, superior cerebellar peduncle is degenerated
▶ The posterior columns, spinocerebellar tracts, corticospinal tracts, and anterior horn cells of the spinal cord are also each degenerated
▶ Eosinophilic round intranuclear inclusions are present in the neurons and glia of affected areas
▶ Cytoplasmic filamentous inclusions are found in the neurons of the dentate nucleus

Ultrastructural Features

▶ Intranuclear inclusions are composed of granular and filamentous non–membrane-bound material

Genetics

▶ Autosomal dominant disease
▶ Mutation in the DRPLA gene on chromosome 12 causes expansion of CAG repeats in the atrophin-1 protein
▶ Normal number of repeats is 6 to 35; in disease, 54 to 79 repeats are found

Immunohistochemical Features

▶ Intranuclear inclusions are ubiquitin and atrophin-1 immunoreactive
▶ Cytoplasmic filamentous inclusions of the dentate neurons are ubiquitin immunoreactive

Pathologic Differential Diagnosis

▶ Other spinocerebellar ataxias
▶ Huntington's disease

---

features of both the adult and juvenile forms of DRPLA. Severe neuronal loss in the dentate nucleus with grumose degeneration and astrocytosis is seen. Some reports have emphasized preferential involvement of the external segment of the globus pallidus, especially in juvenile cases. Variable neuronal loss in the red nucleus, caudate, putamen, substantia nigra, and subthalamic nucleus is also evident. Degeneration of the white matter of the cerebellum, olivary complex, posterior columns, spinocerebellar tracts, corticospinal tracts, and anterior horn cells is likewise apparent.

Eosinophilic round intranuclear inclusions are present; these inclusions are ubiquitin and atrophin-1 immunoreactive. They may also be found in glia. In addition, cytoplasmic filamentous inclusions, also ubiquitin and atrophin-1 immunoreactive, may be found in the dentate nucleus. Electron microscopic examination shows granular and filamentous non–membrane-bound material in the nuclei.

ANCILLARY STUDIES

MRI scans show atrophy of the brain stem and cerebellum.

DIFFERENTIAL DIAGNOSIS

The differential diagnosis in adults includes other spinocerebellar ataxias and Huntington's chorea. Distinction of DRPLA from Huntington's chorea is aided by identification of ataxia and atrophy of the cerebellum and pontine tegmentum on MRI and absence of the huntingtin gene mutation seen in Huntington's disease. SCA3, or Machado-Joseph disease, may be mistaken for

DRPLA. SCA3 shows preferential degeneration of the medial (not lateral) segment of the globus pallidus. In addition, the cerebellar cortex and substantia nigra are affected in SCA3.

PROGNOSTIC AND THERAPEUTIC CONSIDERATIONS

At this time no therapy other than supportive measures is available. Adult-onset disease progresses more slowly (over a period of 10 to 20 years) than the more rapidly progressive juvenile disease.

NEUROAXONAL DYSTROPHIES

Neuroaxonal dystrophies are a group of diseases defined by the presence of axonal swellings or spheroids that occur in the central, peripheral, and autonomic nervous systems. Dystrophic axons occur in a wide variety of conditions: physiologic (attributed to aging), secondary to other diseases or deficiencies (vitamin E deficiency, cystic fibrosis, primary biliary atresia), and in primary degenerations. This section reviews the last category and describes the two diseases in which dystrophic axons form a central feature of the nervous system pathology: neuroaxonal dystrophy and neurodegeneration with brain iron accumulation type 1 (Hallervorden-Spatz disease).

NEUROAXONAL DYSTROPHY (INFANTILE, LATE INFANTILE, JUVENILE, AND ADULT)

CLINICAL FEATURES

Neuroaxonal dystrophy is a rare disease for which no incidence or prevalence data are known. Both sporadic and hereditary (autosomal recessive) forms occur. No mutation or linkage to a specific chromosome has yet been determined. Symptom onset in the infantile form (Seitelberger's disease) is between 6 months and 2 years (mean, 1.3 years). Initial symptoms consist of psychomotor developmental delay or regression, ocular abnormalities (strabismus, nystagmus, uncoordinated eye movements, optic atrophy, and decreased vision), and truncal and gait ataxia. With disease progression, tetraparesis, rigidity, dementia, vision failure, and involvement of the peripheral nervous system are seen.

The late infantile (onset between 2 and 6 years), juvenile (onset between 9 and 21 years), and adult forms of neuroaxonal dystrophy are each very rare. A distinguishing feature of the late infantile form is seizures, in addition to psychomotor regression, spasticity, rigidity, ataxia, and visual disturbances. Abnormalities in gait, speech, and vision and ataxia, spasticity,

athetoid hyperkinesias, psychosis, cranial nerve abnormalities, and dementia develop in patients with the juvenile form. Adult-onset neuroaxonal dystrophy is characterized by changes in personality and by dementia, rigidity, apraxia, and dysarthria.

PATHOLOGIC FEATURES

GROSS FINDINGS

The cerebrum and cerebellum are symmetrically atrophic, and the ventricles are enlarged. The globus pallidus may be enlarged and pale, except in children dying after 4 years, by which time it is rusty brown.

MICROSCOPIC FINDINGS

Dystrophic axons are present in the central, peripheral, and autonomic nervous systems (Fig. 6-43A). These eosinophilic and argyrophilic structures range in size from 20 to 120 μm and are immunoreactive for ubiquitin, amyloid precursor protein, neurofilament, and α-synuclein (see Fig. 6-43B and C). Ultrastructurally, they contain mitochondria, dense multilamellated bodies, vesicles, tubulovesicular profiles, neurofilaments, and amorphous material and frequently also exhibit clefts. Astrocytosis and neuronal loss are evident in affected areas. The areas typically most severely affected are the brain stem, cerebellar cortex, thalamus, globus pallidus, substantia nigra, and spinal cord. Involvement of the autonomic and peripheral nervous systems allows the diagnosis to be made by identification of axonal spheroids on electron microscopic examination of skin or conjunctiva biopsy speci-

mens. In skin biopsy samples, the spheroids are most numerous adjacent to blood vessels, epithelial cells, and eccrine sweat glands. Neuropathologic findings in the late infantile and juvenile forms of neuroaxonal dystrophy are widespread axonal spheroids. Adult-onset disease exhibits involvement of white matter, as well as cortical areas with axonal spheroids. A variant, neuroaxonal leukodystrophy, is characterized by involvement of primarily white matter by axonal spheroids.

ANCILLARY STUDIES

On electroencephalography, most patients show slow background activity and fast rhythms (14 to 22 Hz). Denervation is seen on electromyography. Neuroradiologic examination reveals cerebral and cerebellar atrophy (especially severe in the inferior vermis) on computed tomography (CT) and MRI; some patients show hyperintensity in the cerebellar cortex on T2-weighted images.

DIFFERENTIAL DIAGNOSIS

The clinical manifestations of neuroaxonal dystrophy may also suggest metachromatic leukodystrophy, a gangliosidosis, neuronal ceroid lipofuscinosis, Leigh's disease, Schindler's disease, perinatal brain damage, and neurodegeneration with brain iron accumulation type 1 (Hallervorden-Spatz disease). Neurodegeneration with brain iron accumulation type 1 may show clinical and pathologic overlap with neuroaxonal dystrophy, but it has a mutation in the *PANK2* gene on chromosome 20p and lacks the involvement of the peripheral nervous system seen in infantile neuroaxonal dystrophy. Other diseases with diffuse axonal spheroids occurring secondary to the underlying abnormality are vitamin E deficiency, primary biliary atresia, and cystic fibrosis.

PROGNOSTIC AND THERAPEUTIC CONSIDERATIONS

In the infantile form, death usually occurs between 6 and 12 years. In the late infantile form of neuroaxonal dystrophy, death occurs between 6 and 23 years. At present, no therapy other than supportive care is available.

NEURODEGENERATION WITH BRAIN IRON ACCUMULATION TYPE 1 (HALLERVORDEN-SPATZ DISEASE)

Neurodegeneration with brain iron accumulation type 1 (NBIA) is a rare disease without known incidence or prevalence at this time. It occurs in both autosomal

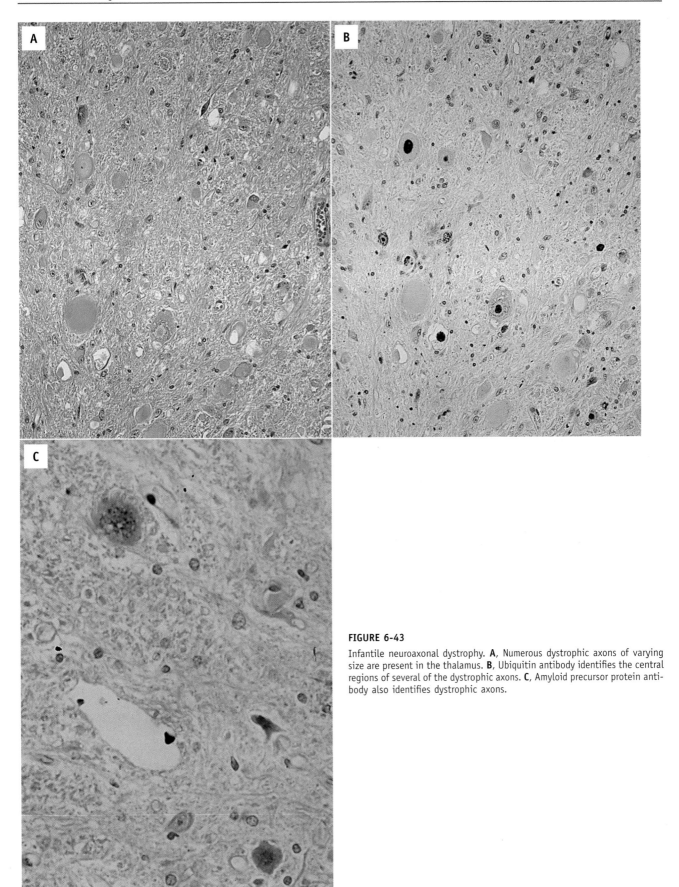

FIGURE 6-43

Infantile neuroaxonal dystrophy. **A**, Numerous dystrophic axons of varying size are present in the thalamus. **B**, Ubiquitin antibody identifies the central regions of several of the dystrophic axons. **C**, Amyloid precursor protein antibody also identifies dystrophic axons.

recessive and sporadic forms and has no known ethnic or gender predisposition. The autosomal recessive form has been linked to chromosome 20p13 and associated with mutations (missense or null) in the *PANK2* gene. The *PANK2* gene codes for pantothenate kinase, which is a rate-determining enzyme in coenzyme A biosynthesis.

CLINICAL FEATURES

NBIA is classified by age at onset and rate of progression. It occurs in childhood (infantile, late infantile, and juvenile) and adulthood. With onset before 10 years, the disease may progress slowly or rapidly; disease in patients who are older at onset usually progresses slowly. Juvenile onset (7 to 15 years) is considered the classic form of NBIA. Symptoms and signs of early-onset disease are gait impairment, spasticity, hyperkinesias (50%), retinitis pigmentosa, optic atrophy, delay in psychomotor and language development, and eventual dystonic rigidity. Hyperkinesias are rare in the infantile and late-infantile types. Later-onset forms may involve dystonia (athetosis, chorea, myoclonus) accompanied by optic atrophy, retinitis pigmentosa, and cognitive impairment.

PATHOLOGIC FEATURES

GROSS FINDINGS

Cerebral and cerebellar atrophy is present. Rust-brown pigmentation is evident in the medial globus pallidus and substantia nigra, pars reticularis.

MICROSCOPIC FINDINGS

Neuronal loss, astrocytosis, and spheroid bodies are evident in the medial globus pallidus and substantia nigra, pars reticularis (Fig. 6-44A). Spheroids may

---

NEURODEGENERATION WITH BRAIN IRON ACCUMULATION TYPE 1 (HALLERVORDEN-SPATZ DISEASE)—FACT SHEET

Definition
► Degenerative disease occurring in both childhood and adulthood and characterized by hyperkinesia and dystonia and accumulation of iron and axonal spheroids in the globus pallidus

Incidence and Prevalence
► No incidence or prevalence data available

Gender and Age Distribution
► No gender predilection
► Occurs in infantile, late infantile, juvenile, and adult forms

Clinical Features
► Early-onset disease (<10 years)—gait impairment, spasticity, hyperkinesias (primarily in the juvenile form), retinitis pigmentosa, optic atrophy, delay in psychomotor and language development, eventual dystonic rigidity
► Late onset forms—dystonia (athetosis, chorea, myoclonus), optic atrophy, retinitis pigmentosa, cognitive impairment

Radiologic Features
► MRI shows bilateral hypointense regions containing an area of increased signal on T2 in the medial globus pallidus, known as the "eye of the tiger" sign
► Atrophy of the cerebrum, cerebellum, and brain stem is also seen along with dilated ventricles

Prognosis and Treatment
► The disease course ranges from 6 to 30 years
► Supportive therapy only

NEURODEGENERATION WITH BRAIN IRON ACCUMULATION TYPE 1 (HALLERVORDEN-SPATZ DISEASE)—PATHOLOGIC FEATURES

Gross Findings
► Rust-brown pigmentation in the medial globus pallidus and substantia nigra
► Atrophy of the cerebrum, cerebellum, and brain stem

Microscopic Findings
► Axonal spheroids, neuronal loss, and astrocytosis are seen primarily in the medial globus pallidus and substantia nigra
► Spheroids are also seen in the thalamus, subthalamus, striatum, brain stem, cerebral cortex, and spinal cord
► Iron is found in spheroids, microglia, and neurons and around vessels
► Lewy bodies and neurofibrillary tangles have been found in affected areas

Ultrastructural Features
► Axonal spheroids contain amorphous granular multilamellated and dense bodies, mitochondria, and tubulovesicular structures

Genetics
► Both sporadic and autosomal recessive disease occurs
► Autosomal recessive disease is associated with missense or null mutations in the *PANK2* gene on chromosome 20, position p13

Immunohistochemical Features
► Axonal spheroids are immunoreactive for amyloid precursor protein, ubiquitin, neurofilament, α-synuclein, and ferritin
► Glial cytoplasmic inclusions are tau and α-synuclein immunoreactive and have been found in affected areas

Pathologic Differential Diagnosis
► Neuroaxonal dystrophy
► Vitamin E deficiency
► Primary biliary atresia
► Cystic fibrosis

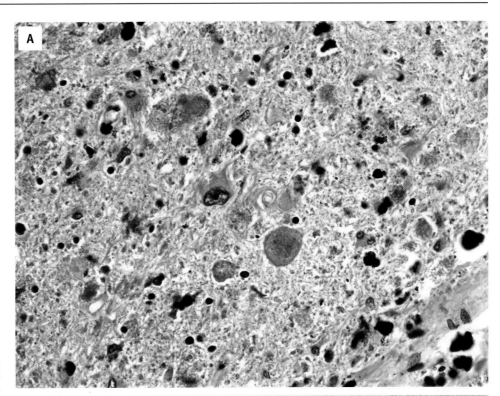

FIGURE 6-44

Neurodegeneration with brain iron accumulation type 1. **A**, Dystrophic axons, pigment, and reactive astrocytes in the substantia nigra. **B**, Iron accumulation in the basal forebrain (iron stain). (Courtesy of Dr. E. Bigio, Northwestern University, Chicago, Illinois.)

also be found in the thalamus, subthalamus, striatum, brain stem, cerebral cortex, and spinal cord. Spheroids are immunoreactive for amyloid precursor protein, ubiquitin, neurofilament, α-synuclein, and ferritin. Electron microscopic examination of the spheroids shows amorphous granular multilamellated and dense bodies, mitochondria, and tubulovesicular structures. Iron is found in the spheroids, as well as in microglia and neurons and around blood vessels (see Fig. 6-44B). Lewy bodies and NFTs have been described in multiple cases of juvenile- and adult-onset disease. In addition, glial cytoplasmic inclusions and dystrophic neurites (each tau and α-synuclein immunoreactive) have been described in NBIA. The peripheral nervous system is not usually affected (as it is in infantile neuroaxonal dystrophy).

ANCILLARY STUDIES

MRI of the brain shows bilateral hypointense regions containing an area of increased signal on T2-weighted images in the medial globus pallidus ("eye of the tiger" sign). Atrophy of the cerebrum, cerebellum, and brain stem and dilated ventricles are also seen. Peripheral blood examination may show acanthocytes and abnormal plasma lipoproteins.

DIFFERENTIAL DIAGNOSIS

Other clinical considerations include juvenile neuronal ceroid lipofuscinosis, juvenile Huntington's disease (rigid form), juvenile Parkinson's disease, GM_1 or GM_2 gangliosidosis, Wilson's disease, subacute sclerosing panencephalitis, perinatal and postnatal disorders, and hereditary ataxias. Distinction from neuroaxonal dystrophy may be difficult, and other entities with secondary accumulation of axonal spheroids should be considered: vitamin E deficiency, primary biliary atresia, and cystic fibrosis.

PROGNOSTIC AND THERAPEUTIC CONSIDERATIONS

Therapy at present is supportive and symptomatic only. The disease is slowly progressive, and typically, the disease course ranges from 6 to 30 years.

SUGGESTED READINGS

Alzheimer's Disease

Arnold SE, Hyman BT, Flory J, et al: The topographical and neuroanatomical distribution of neurofibrillary tangles and neuritic plaques in the cerebral cortex of patients with Alzheimer's disease. Cereb Cortex 1991;1:103-116.

Braak H, Braak E: Neuropathological stageing of Alzheimer-related changes. Acta Neuropathol 1991;82:239-259.

Consensus recommendations for the postmortem diagnosis of Alzheimer disease. The National Institute on Aging and the Reagan Institute Working Group on diagnostic criteria for the neuropathological assessment of Alzheimer disease. Neurobiol Aging 1997;18:S1-S2.

Cummings JL, Cole G: Alzheimer disease. JAMA 2002;287:2335-2338.

Duyckaerts C, Dickson DW: Neuropathology of Alzheimer's disease. In Dickson DW (ed): Neurodegeneration: The Molecular Pathology of Dementia and Movement Disorders. Basel, ISN Neuropath Press, 2003, pp 47-65.

Evans DA, Funkenstein HH, Albert MS, et al: Prevalence of Alzheimer's disease in a community population of older persons: Higher than previously reported. JAMA 1989;262:2551-2556.

Knopman D: Alzheimer type dementia. In Dickson DW (ed): Neurodegeneration: The Molecular Pathology of Dementia and Movement Disorders. Basel, ISN Neuropath Press, 2003, pp 24-39.

Mirra SS, Gearing M, Heyman A: A CERAD Guide to the Neuropathological Assessment of Alzheimer's Disease and Other Dementias. Durham, NC, CERAD, 1994.

Nussbaum RL, Ellis CE: Alzheimer's disease and Parkinson's disease. N Engl J Med 2003;348:1356-1364.

Rogers J, Morrison JH: Quantitative morphology and regional and laminar distributions of senile plaques in Alzheimer's disease. J Neurosci 1985;5:2801-2808.

Zabar Y, Kawas CH: Epidemiology and clinical genetics of Alzheimer's disease. In Clark CM, Trojanowski JQ (eds): Neurodegenerative Dementias: Clinical Features and Pathological Mechanisms. New York, McGraw-Hill, 2000, pp 79-94.

Synucleinopathies

Apaydin H, Ahlskog E, Parisi JE, et al: Parkinson disease neuropathology. Later-developing dementia and loss of the levodopa response. Arch Neurol 2002;59:102-112.

Dale GE, Probst A, Luthert P, et al: Relationships between Lewy bodies and pale bodies in Parkinson's disease. Acta Neuropathol 1992;83:525-529.

Forno LS: Neuropathology of Parkinson's disease. J Neuropathol Exp Neurol 1996;55:259-272.

Harding AJ, Halliday GM: Cortical Lewy body pathology in the diagnosis of dementia. Acta Neuropathol 2001;102:355-363.

Hishikawa N, Hashizume Y, Yoshida M, Sobue G: Clinical and neuropathological correlates of Lewy body disease. Acta Neuropathol 2003;105:341-350.

Hurtig HI, Trojanowski JQ, Galvin J, et al: Alpha-synuclein cortical Lewy bodies correlate with dementia in Parkinson's disease. Neurology 2000;54:1916-1921.

Ince P, McKeith IG: Dementia with Lewy bodies. In Dickson DW (ed): Neurodegeneration: The Molecular Pathology of Dementia and Movement Disorders. Basel, ISN Neuropath Press, 2003, pp 188-199.

Jellinger KA, Mizuno Y: Parkinson's disease. In Dickson DW (ed): Neurodegeneration: The Molecular Pathology of Dementia and Movement Disorders. Basel, ISN Neuropath Press, 2003, pp 159-187.

Kosaka K, Iseki E: Clinicopathological studies on diffuse Lewy body disease. Neuropathology 2000;1:1-7.

McKeith IG, Galasko D, Kosaka K, et al: Consensus guidelines for the clinical and pathologic diagnosis of dementia with Lewy bodies (DLB): Report of the consortium on DLB international workshop. Neurology 1996;47:1113-1124.

Polymeropoulos MH, Lavedan C, Leroy E, et al: Mutation in the α synuclein gene identified in families with Parkinson's disease. Science 1997;276:2045-2047.

Rosenberg CK, Cummings TJ, Saunders AM, et al: Dementia with Lewy bodies and Alzheimer's disease. Acta Neuropathol 2001;102:621-626.

Spillantini MG, Schmidt ML, Lee VM, et al: α Synuclein in Lewy bodies. Nature 1997;388:839-840.

Multiple System Atrophy

Burn DJ, Jaros E: Multiple system atrophy: Cellular and molecular pathology. Mol Pathol 2001;54:419-426

Lantos PL: The definition of multiple system atrophy: A review of recent developments. J Neuropathol Exp Neurol 1998;57:1099-1111.

Lantos P, Quinn N: Multiple system atrophy. In Dickson DW (ed): Neurodegeneration: The Molecular Pathology of Dementia and Movement Disorders. Basel, ISN Neuropath Press, 2003, pp 203-214.

Papp MI, Kahn JE, Lantos PL: Glial cytoplasmic inclusions in the CNS of patients with multiple system atrophy (striatonigral degeneration, olivopontocerebellar atrophy and Shy-Drager syndrome). J Neurol Sci 1989;94:79-100.

Wenning GK, Geser F, Stampfer-Kountchev M, Tison F: Multiple system atrophy: An update. Move Disord 2003;18(Suppl 6):S34-S43.

Frontotemporal Lobar Degeneration

Bergeron C, Morris HR, Rossor M: Pick's disease. In Dickson DW (ed): Neurodegeneration: The Molecular Pathology of Dementia and Movement Disorders. Basel, ISN Neuropath Press, 2003, pp 124-131.

Dickson DW: Pick's disease: A modern approach. Brain Pathol 1998;8:339-354.

Ghetti B, Hutton ML, Wszolek ZK: Frontotemporal dementia and parkinsonism linked to chromosome 17 associated with Tau gene mutations (FTDP-17T). In Dickson DW (ed): Neurodegeneration: The Molecular Pathology of Dementia and Movement Disorders. Basel, ISN Neuropath Press, 2003, pp 86-102.

Houlden H, Baker M, Adamson J, et al: Frequency of *tau* mutations in 3 series of non-AD degenerative dementias. Ann Neurol 1999;46:243-248.

Kertesz A, Kawarai T, Rogaeva E, et al: Familial frontotemporal dementia with ubiquitin-positive, tau-negative inclusions. Neurology 2000;54:818-827.

Kinoshita A, Tomimoto H, Suenaga T, et al: Ubiquitin-related cytoskeletal abnormality in frontotemporal dementia: Immunohistochemical and immunoelectron microscope studies. Acta Neuropathol 1997;94:67-72.

Knopman DS, Petersen RC, Edland SD, et al: The incidence of frontotemporal lobar degeneration in Rochester, Minnesota, 1990 through 1994. Neurology 2004;62:506-508.

Lowe J, Rossor M: Frontotemporal lobar degeneration. In Dickson DW (ed): Neurodegeneration: The Molecular Pathology of Dementia and Movement Disorders. Basel, ISN Neuropath Press, 2003, pp 342-348.

Mann DMA, McDonagh AN, Snowden J, et al: Molecular classification of the dementias. Lancet 2000;355:626.

Neary D, Snowden JS, Mann DMA: Classification and description of frontotemporal dementias. Ann N Y Acad Sci 2000;920:46-51.

Rossor MN. Pick's disease: A clinical overview. Neurology 2001;56(Suppl 4):S3-S5.

Tolnay M, Probst A: Frontotemporal lobar degeneration—tau as a pied piper? Neurogenetics 2002;4:63-75.

Trojanowski JQ, Dickson D: Update on the neuropathological diagnosis of frontotemporal dementias. J Neuropathol Exp Neurol 2001;60:1123-1126.

Zhukareva V, Mann D, Pickering-Brown S, et al: Sporadic Pick's disease: A tauopathy characterized by a spectrum of pathological tau isoforms in gray and white matter. Ann Neurol 2002;51:730-739

Corticobasal Degeneration

Dickson DW: Neuropathologic differentiation of progressive supranuclear palsy and corticobasal degeneration. J Neurol 1999;246(Suppl 2):II/6-II/15.

Dickson DW, Bergeron C, Chin SS, et al: Office of Rare Diseases neuropathologic criteria for corticobasal degeneration. J Neuropathol Exp Neurol 2002;61:935-946.

Dickson D, Litvan I: Corticobasal degeneration. In Dickson DW (ed): Neurodegeneration: The Molecular Pathology of Dementia and Movement Disorders. Basel, ISN Neuropath Press, 2003, pp 115-123.

Doran M, du Plessis DG, Enevoldson TP, et al: Pathological heterogeneity of clinically diagnosed corticobasal degeneration. J Neurol Sci 2003;216:127-134.

Forman MS, Zhukareva V, Bergeron C, et al: Signature tau neuropathology in gray and white matter of corticobasal degeneration. Am J Pathol 2002;160:2045-2053.

Houlden H, Baker M, Morris HR, et al: Corticobasal degeneration and progressive supranuclear palsy share a common tau haplotype. Neurology 2001;56:1702-1706.

Schneider JA, Watts RL, Gearing M, et al: Corticobasal degeneration. Neuropathologic and clinical heterogeneity. Neurology 1997;48:959-969.

Progressive Supranuclear Palsy

Albers DS, Augood SJ: New insights into progressive supranuclear palsy. Trends Neurosci 2001;24:347-352.

Baker M , Litvan I, Houlden H, et al: Association of an extended haplotype in the tau gene with progressive supranuclear palsy. Hum Mol Genet 1999;8:711-715.

Burn DJ, Lees AJ: Progressive supranuclear palsy: Where are we now? Lancet Neurol 2002;1:359-360.

Komori T: Tau-positive glial inclusions in progressive supranuclear palsy, corticobasal degeneration and Pick's disease. Brain Pathol 1999;9:663-679.

Litvan I, Hauw JJ, Bartko JJ, et al: Validity and reliability of the preliminary NINDS neuropathologic criteria for progressive supranuclear palsy and related disorders. J Neuropathol Exp Neurol 1996;55:97-105.

Morris HR, Gibb G, Katzenschlager R, et al: Pathological, clinical and genetic heterogeneity in progressive supranuclear palsy. Brain 2002;125:969-975.

Steele JC, Richardson JC, Olszewski J: Progressive supranuclear palsy. Arch Neurol 1964;10:333-359.

Amyotrophic Lateral Sclerosis

Ikemoto A, Hirano A, Akiguchi I: Neuropathology of amyotrophic lateral sclerosis with extra-motor system degeneration: Characteristics and differences in the molecular pathology between ALS with dementia and Guamanian ALS. Amyotroph Lateral Scler Other Motor Neuron Disord 2000;1:97-104.

Ince PG, Tomkins J, Slade JY, et al: Amyotrophic lateral sclerosis associated with genetic abnormalities in the gene encoding Cu/Zn superoxide dismutase: Molecular pathology of five new cases, and comparison with previous reports and 73 sporadic cases of ALS. J Neuropathol Exp Neurol 1998;57:895-904.

Kato S, Shaw P, Wood-Allum C, et al: Amyotrophic lateral sclerosis. In Dickson DW (ed): Neurodegeneration: The Molecular Pathology of Dementia and Movement Disorders. Basel, ISN Neuropath Press, 2003, pp 350-368.

Majoor-Krakauer D, Willms PJ, Hofman A: Genetic epidemiology of amyotrophic lateral sclerosis. Clin Genet 2003;63:83-101.

Orrell RW, Figlewicz DA: Clinical implications of the genetics of ALS and other motor neuron diseases. Neurology 2001;57:9-17.

Piao Y-S, Wakabayashi K, Kakita A, et al: Neuropathology with clinical correlations of sporadic amyotrophic lateral sclerosis: 102 autopsy cases examined between 1962 and 2000. Brain Pathol 2003;12:10-22.

Przedborski S, Mitsumoto H, Rowland LP: Recent advances in amyotrophic lateral sclerosis research. Curr Neurol Neurosci Rep 2003;3:70-77.

Strong M, Rosenfeld J: Amyotrophic lateral sclerosis: A review of current concepts. ALS and other motor neuron disorders Amyotroph Lateral Scler Other Motor Disord 2003;4:136-143.

Van den Berg-Vos RM, Visser J, Franssen H, et al: Sporadic lower motor neuron disease with adult onset: Classification of subtypes. Brain 2003;126:1036-1047.

Spinal Muscular Atrophy

Harding BN: Spinal muscular atrophy. In Dickson DW (ed): Neurodegeneration: The Molecular Pathology of Dementia and Movement Disorders. Basel, ISN Neuropath Press, 2003, pp 372-375.

Ogino S, Wilson RB: Genetic testing and risk assessment for spinal muscular atrophy (SMA). Hum Genet 2002;111:477-500.

Orrell RW, Figlewicz DA: Clinical implications of the genetics of ALS and other motor neuron diseases. Neurology 2001;57:9-17.

Schmalbruch H, Haase G:. Spinal muscular atrophy: Present state. Brain Pathol 2001;11:231-247.

Huntington's Disease

DiFiglia M, Sapp E, Chase KO, et al: Aggregation of huntingtin in neuronal intranuclear inclusions and dystrophic neurites in brain. Science 1997;277:1990-1993.

Hedreen JC, Roos RAC: Huntington's disease. In Dickson DW (ed): Neurodegeneration: The Molecular Pathology of Dementia and Movement Disorders. Basel, ISN Neuropath Press, 2003, pp 229-241.

Robataille Y, Lopes-Cendes I, Becher M, et al: The neuropathology of CAG repeat diseases: Review and update of genetic and molecular features. Brain Pathol 1997;7:901-926.

Ross CA, Becher MW, Colomer V, et al: Huntington's disease and dentatorubral-pallidoluysian atrophy: Proteins, pathogenesis and pathology. Brain Pathol 1997;7:1003-1016.

Vonsattel JP, Myers RH, Stevens TJ, et al: Neuropathological classification of Huntington's disease. J Neuropathol Exp Neurol 1985;44:559-577.

Spinocerebellar Ataxias

Albin RL: Dominant ataxias and Friedreich ataxia: An update. Curr Opin Neurol 2003;16:507-514.

Estrada R, Galarraga J, Orozco G, et al: Spinocerebellar ataxia 2 (SCA2): Morphometric analyses in 11 autopsies. Acta Neuropathol 1999;97:306-310.

Koeppen AH: The hereditary ataxias. J Neuropathol Exp Neurol 1998;57:531-543.

Margolis RL: The spinocerebellar ataxias: Order emerges from chaos. Curr Neurol Neurosci Rep 2002;2:447-456.

Mizusawa H, Clark HB, Koeppen AH: Spinocerebellar ataxias. In Dickson DW (ed): Neurodegeneration: The Molecular Pathology of Dementia and Movement Disorders. Basel, ISN Neuropath Press, 2003, pp 242-256.

Yagishita S, Inoue M: Clinicopathology of spinocerebellar degeneration; its correlation to the unstable CAG repeat of the affected gene. Pathol Int 1997;47:1-15.

Friedreich's Ataxia

Albin RL: Dominant ataxias and Friedreich ataxia: An update. Curr Opin Neurol 2003;16:507-514.

Alper G, Narayanan V: Friedreich's ataxia. Pedriatr Neurol 2003;28:335-341.

Koeppen AH: The hereditary ataxias. J Neuropathol Exp Neurol 1998;57:531-543.

Robaitaille Y, Klockgether T, Lamarche JB: Friedreich's ataxia. In Dickson DW (ed): Neurodegeneration: The Molecular Pathology of Dementia and Movement Disorders. Basel, ISN Neuropath Press, 2003, pp 257-268.

Wilson RB: Frataxin and frataxin deficiency in Friedreich's ataxia. J Neurol Sci 2003;207:103-105.

Dentatorubral-Pallidoluysian Atrophy

Nanco MA: Clinical aspects of CAG repeat diseases. Brain Pathol 1997;7:881-900.

Oyanagi S: Hereditary dentatorubral-pallidoluysian atrophy. Neuropathology 2000;20:S42-S46.

Robataille Y, Lopes-Cendes I, Becher M, et al: The neuropathology of CAG repeat diseases: Review and update of genetic and molecular features. Brain Pathol 1997;7:901-926.

Ross CA, Becher MW, Colomer V, et al: Huntington's disease and dentatorubral-pallidoluysian atrophy: Proteins, pathogenesis and pathology. Brain Pathol 1997;7:1003-1016.

Takahashi H, Yamada M, Tsuji S: Dentatorubral-pallidoluysian atrophy. In Dickson DW (ed): Neurodegeneration: The Molecular Pathology of Dementia and Movement Disorders. Basel, ISN Neuropath Press, 2003, pp 269-274.

Tsuji S: Dentatorubral-pallidoluysian atrophy: Clinical aspects and molecular genetics. Adv Neurol 2002;89:231-239.

Yagishita S, Inoue M: Clinicopathology of spinocerebellar degeneration: Its correlation to the unstable CAG repeat of the affected gene. Pathol Int 1997;47:1-15.

Neuroaxonal Dystrophies

Aicardi J, Castelein P: Infantile neuroaxonal dystrophy. Brain 1979;102:727-748.

Ceuterick C, Martin JJ: Skin biopsy is useful for diagnosis of infantile neuroaxonal dystrophy. Ann Neurol 1990;28:109-110.

Gordon N: Infantile neuroaxonal dystrophy (Seitelberger's disease). Dev Med Child Neurol 2002;44:849-851.

Jellinger KA, Duda J: Infantile neuroaxonal dystrophy (Seitelberger disease). In Dickson DW (ed): Neurodegeneration: The Molecular Pathology of Dementia and Movement Disorders. Basel, ISN Neuropath Press, 2003, pp 390-393.

Nardocci N, Zorzi G, Farina L, et al: Infantile neuroaxonal dystrophy. Clinical spectrum and diagnostic criteria. Neurology 1999;52:1472-1478.

Ramaekers VT, Lake BD, Harding B, et al: Diagnostic difficulties in infantile neuroaxonal dystrophy. A clinicopathological study of eight cases. Neuropediatrics 1987;18:170-175.

Neurodegeneration with Brain Iron Accumulation Type 1 (Hallervorden-Spatz Disease)

Galvin JE, Giasson B, Hurtig HI, et al: Neurodegeneration with brain iron accumulation, type 1 is characterized by α, β, and γ-synuclein neuropathology. Am J Pathol 2000;157:361-368.

Hayflick SJ, Westaway SK, Levinson B, et al: Genetic, clinical, and radiographic delineation of Hallervorden-Spatz syndrome. N Engl J Med 2003;348:33-40.

Jellinger KA, Duda J: Neurodegeneration with brain iron accumulation, type 1 (Hallervorden-Spatz disease). In Dickson DW (ed): Neurodegeneration: The Molecular Pathology of Dementia and Movement Disorders. Basel, ISN Neuropath Press, 2003, pp 394-399.

Neumann M, Adler S, Schluter O, et al: α-Synuclein accumulation in a case of neurodegeneration with brain iron accumulation type 1 (NBIA-1, formerly Hallervorden-Spatz syndrome) with widespread cortical and brain stem–type Lewy bodies. Acta Neuropathol 2000;100:568-574.

Infections
Kymberly A. Gyure

BACTERIAL INFECTIONS

MENINGITIS

Meningitis is defined as an inflammatory process affecting the leptomeninges and cerebrospinal fluid (CSF) within the subarachnoid space. Acute bacterial (pyogenic) meningitis is a significant cause of death and disability despite major efforts dedicated to the prevention and treatment of this disease. Although meningitis may complicate trauma or surgery, the overwhelming majority of cases are secondary to hematogenous dissemination of bacteria.

CLINICAL FEATURES

In the United States, the incidence of bacterial meningitis is approximately 3 to 5 cases per 100,000 population per year. The etiologic agents causing bacterial meningitis vary with the age of the affected patient; accordingly, knowledge of common pathogens in various age groups is crucial in determining appropriate antibiotic therapy. Neonatal meningitis is due mainly to group B streptococci (*Streptococcus agalactiae*), *Escherichia coli*, and *Listeria monocytogenes*. Before the introduction of effective vaccines, *Haemophilus influenzae* type B was the main cause of meningitis in children between 4 months and 3 years of age. This organism still causes infections in those who have not yet been vaccinated. In children older than 2 years and in young adults, *Neisseria meningitidis* is the primary pathogen; this organism is the agent most commonly responsible for epidemics of meningitis. In older adults, *Streptococcus pneumoniae* is the organism most often responsible for bacterial meningitis. It may be associated with alcoholism, sickle cell disease, and hyposplenism. *L. monocytogenes* is also a cause of meningitis in adults older than 40 years.

Clinical features of meningitis include fever, headache, nausea, vomiting, confusion, and lethargy of acute onset often associated with nuchal rigidity. Kernig's sign, or reflex contraction of the hamstring muscles when extending the leg after flexing the thigh on the body, and Brudzinski's sign, or flexion of both the knees and hips in response to passive flexion of the

---

MENINGITIS—FACT SHEET

Definition
▶ Inflammation of the leptomeninges and CSF within the subarachnoid space

Incidence and Location
▶ Incidence of 3 to 5 cases per 100,000 population per year in the United States

Gender and Age Distribution
▶ Neonates: group B streptococci, *Escherichia coli*, and *Listeria monocytogenes*
▶ Children and young adults: *Neisseria meningitidis*
▶ Older adults: *Streptococcus pneumoniae* and *L. monocytogenes*

Clinical Features
▶ Fever, headache, nausea, vomiting, confusion, and lethargy of acute onset often associated with nuchal rigidity
▶ Kernig's and Brudzinski's signs
▶ CSF findings: cloudiness, increased pressure, neutrophilic leukocytosis, increased protein, markedly decreased glucose

Prognosis and Treatment
▶ 25% fatality rate
▶ Empirical antibiotic therapy based on age and immune status
▶ Vaccination of susceptible individuals

---

neck toward the chest, are common signs of meningeal irritation. CSF changes are often diagnostic and include cloudiness of the CSF, increased pressure, neutrophilic pleocytosis, a raised protein level, and a markedly reduced or absent glucose level. Gram stain is useful in demonstrating the causative organism. Neuroimaging is of little help in diagnosis but may show contrast enhancement of the subarachnoid space.

PATHOLOGIC FEATURES

GROSS FINDINGS

In patients who die of meningitis, the brain is surrounded by creamy yellow or green pus (Fig. 7-1). Pus is first visible at the base of the brain and as thin creamy lines alongside meningeal vessels. These vessels are

---

MENINGITIS—PATHOLOGIC FINDINGS

Gross Findings
▶ The brain is surrounded by creamy yellow or green pus that is often basal and follows the distribution of meningeal blood vessels

Microscopic Findings
▶ Neutrophils in the subarachnoid space
▶ Leptomeningeal veins may be infiltrated

Differential Diagnosis
▶ Leptomeningeal fibrosis

engorged and stand out prominently. In fulminant cases, pus may also be noted within the ventricles (ventriculitis). In those who survive, leptomeningeal fibrosis and consequent hydrocephalus may be evident.

MICROSCOPIC FINDINGS

Microscopically, neutrophils fill the subarachnoid space and are characteristically easiest to find around blood vessels (Fig. 7-2). They may infiltrate the walls of leptomeningeal veins and thereby lead to venous occlusion and hemorrhagic infarction of the underlying brain, which is often edematous. Gram stain may reveal the causative organism, although organisms are frequently not demonstrable in treated cases.

DIFFERENTIAL DIAGNOSIS

The diagnosis of bacterial meningitis is pathologically straightforward. At autopsy, pus in the leptomeninges should be distinguished from the much more commonly encountered age-related leptomeningeal fibrosis. Fibrosis is typically parasagittal rather than basilar in location, does not follow a vascular distribution, and is not movable within the subarachnoid space.

PROGNOSIS AND THERAPY

Untreated bacterial meningitis is uniformly fatal. Even with appropriate antibiotic therapy, the overall case fatality rate is approximately 25%. Empirical antibiotic therapy is based largely on the age and immune status of the patient. Agents effective against most of the commonly

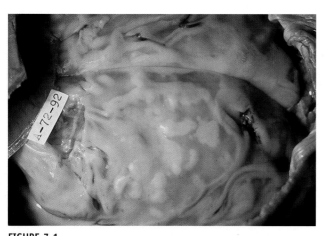

FIGURE 7-1
Meningitis. A thick layer of suppurative exudate surrounds the brain.

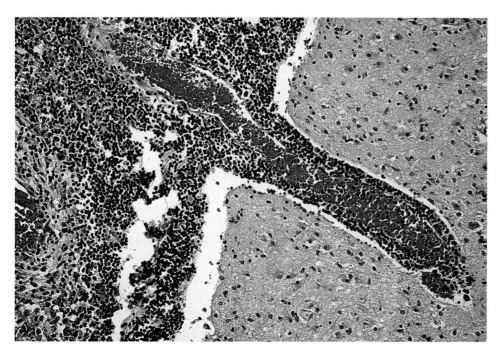

FIGURE 7-2
Meningitis. Neutrophils are present within the subarachnoid space and surrounding blood vessels in the Virchow-Robin spaces.

encountered pathogens include ampicillin and broad-spectrum cephalosporins. Vaccination of susceptible individuals is important in the prevention of meningitis.

BRAIN ABSCESS

An abscess is a localized focus of suppurative inflammation. Most cases are bacterial in origin, with streptococci, staphylococci, and aerobic gram-negative rods being the primary offending agents. Polymicrobial infections are not uncommon. Brain abscesses may arise by direct implantation of organisms, local extension from adjacent foci (especially the paranasal sinuses), or hematogenous spread.

CLINICAL FEATURES

Brain abscesses may occur in any age group. Predisposing conditions include acute bacterial endocarditis, congenital heart disease with a right-to-left shunt, and chronic pulmonary disease. At initial evaluation, patients with cerebral abscesses are found to have progressive focal deficits and signs of increased intracranial pressure. Fever and evidence of a systemic or local source of infection may or may not be apparent.

RADIOGRAPHIC FEATURES

The radiographic appearance of brain abscesses is variable and evolves with time. Early cerebritis may be detected as an area of low attenuation on computed tomography (CT) or as an area of high signal intensity on T2-weighted magnetic resonance imaging (MRI). With time, a collagenous capsule that is dense on CT and of low signal on MRI becomes evident and is classically

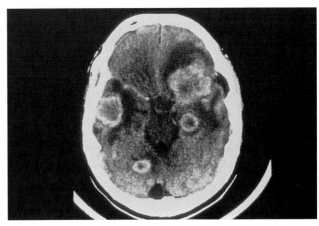

FIGURE 7-3
Brain abscess. A ring-like pattern of enhancement is evident in contrast-enhanced studies (computed tomographic scan).

thinnest on the side nearest the lateral ventricle. A well-defined ring-like pattern of enhancement appears after the administration of contrast material (Fig. 7-3).

PATHOLOGIC FINDINGS

GROSS FINDINGS

Early abscesses are irregular areas of suppuration. With time, a capsule develops. Encapsulation begins as a rim of granulation tissue that ultimately evolves into a firm, fibrous capsule (Fig. 7-4). Satellite lesions, or "daughter" abscesses, may develop, usually inwardly, and may rupture into the ventricular system.

MICROSCOPIC FINDINGS

Microscopically, the center of an abscess consists of necrosis and an inflammatory infiltrate composed of neutrophils and, later, macrophages and lymphocytes. Granulation tissue surrounds the area of inflammation

---

BRAIN ABSCESS—FACT SHEET

Definition
▶ A localized focus of suppurative inflammation

Clinical Features
▶ Predisposing factors: bacterial endocarditis, cyanotic congenital heart disease, chronic pulmonary infection
▶ Progressive focal deficits, signs of increased intracranial pressure
▶ Signs of a systemic infection may be present

Radiographic Features
▶ Fibrous capsule that is thinner nearest the lateral ventricle
▶ Ring enhancing with the administration of contrast material

Prognosis and Treatment
▶ Good prognosis if diagnosed in a timely fashion
▶ Treatment includes antibiotics and occasionally surgery

BRAIN ABSCESS—PATHOLOGIC FINDINGS

Gross Findings
▶ Suppuration surrounded by a fibrous capsule
▶ Satellite lesions

Microscopic Findings
▶ Necrotic center with associated inflammation
▶ Rim consists of granulation tissue that evolves into a fibrous capsule
▶ Entire lesion is surrounded by gliosis and edema

Differential Diagnosis
▶ High-grade glial neoplasm

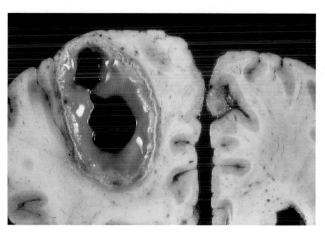

FIGURE 7-4

Brain abscess. Well-developed abscesses are characterized by suppurative necrosis surrounded by a dense, fibrous capsule.

(Fig. 7-5) and eventually develops into a fibrous capsule. This capsule in turn is surrounded by gliotic, edematous brain tissue.

DIFFERENTIAL DIAGNOSIS

Both radiographically and pathologically, brain abscesses are most often confused with high-grade glial tumors. This error in diagnosis is most common at the time of frozen section, when the pathologist is confronted with a highly cellular lesion containing astrocytic cells in the clinical setting of a ring-enhancing lesion thought to be a tumor by the surgeon. The presence of inflammatory cells, including neutrophils and macrophages, should prompt consideration of a nonneoplastic process inasmuch as primary central nervous system (CNS) tumors rarely contain a significant associated inflammatory infiltrate.

PROGNOSIS AND THERAPY

Survival from a brain abscess is the rule in appropriately diagnosed and treated cases; the single most important contributing factor to mortality and permanent neurologic deficit is delay in diagnosis. Most cases are treated with antibiotics. Surgery to drain or remove the abscess is necessary in some instances.

MYCOBACTERIAL INFECTIONS OF THE NERVOUS SYSTEM

Tuberculosis (TB) is the most common mycobacterial infection involving the CNS. TB, which is caused by *Mycobacterium tuberculosis*, a gram-positive, acid-fast rod, remains a major world health problem and is responsible for 3 million deaths per year. CNS involvement is secondary to disease elsewhere in the body, most frequently the lungs. The advent of acquired immunodeficiency syndrome (AIDS) has modified the epidemiology of TB; the immunosuppression characteristic of AIDS has increased the number of people susceptible to TB.

Nontuberculous (atypical) mycobacteria may also infect the CNS. These organisms, including those of the *M. avium* complex, *M. kansasii*, *M. scrofulaceum*, *M. xenopi*, *M. genavense*, and *M. malmoense*, typically produce disease in immunocompromised patients, particularly those with AIDS.

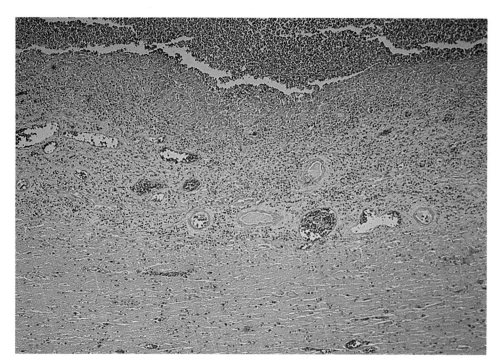

FIGURE 7-5

Brain abscess. A region of central necrosis and inflammation is surrounded by granulation tissue and gliosis.

Leprosy is due to infection by *Mycobacterium leprae*. This organism involves predominantly the peripheral nervous system.

CLINICAL FEATURES

TB meningitis is the most common form of tuberculosis of the CNS. It is manifested as generalized complaints of headache, malaise, mental confusion, and vomiting. CSF findings include increased pressure, a pleocytosis made up of mononuclear cells or a combination of polymorphonuclear and mononuclear cells, elevated protein levels, and a reduced or normal glucose content.

Tuberculomas produce signs and symptoms of a mass lesion. These lesions, which remain a common cause of intracranial masses in tropical countries, occur most often in the first 3 decades of life. There is often a history of exposure to the organism or recognized extracranial disease. The most common signs and symptoms include headache, seizures, papilledema, hemiplegia, and cerebellar dysfunction.

Nontuberculous mycobacteria commonly cause disseminated disease in immunocompromised individuals. The CNS may be affected, but this involvement is usually asymptomatic. When symptomatic CNS involvement does occur, the signs and symptoms are non-specific and include a diffuse encephalopathy, seizures, headache, altered mentation or impaired cognition, nuchal rigidity, lethargy, cranial nerve palsies, and progressive neurologic deterioration.

RADIOGRAPHIC FEATURES

In tuberculous meningitis, there may be radiologic enhancement at the base of the brain. A tuberculoma is a single or multilocular lesion with a peripheral rim of contrast enhancement and a hypodense, necrotic center. Spindle cell pseudotumors may rarely be seen in those with infections caused by atypical mycobacteria; these lesions produce hyperdense masses with surrounding edema on imaging studies.

PATHOLOGIC FEATURES

GROSS FINDINGS

TB meningitis is characterized by a thick, gray exudate that typically involves the base of the brain but subsequently extends to the sylvian fissures and envelopes the spinal cord (Fig. 7-6A). Small nodules or tubercles may be identified in this exudate.

Tuberculomas are round or oval masses. They have necrotic, firm centers and are creamy in color (see Fig. 7-6B). The surrounding rim is gray and gelatinous, and there is much less swelling than around cerebral abscesses.

MYCOBACTERIAL INFECTIONS—FACT SHEET

Definition
- Infections caused by *Mycobacterium tuberculosis* or one of a variety of nontuberculous mycobacteria

Incidence and Location
- Occurs worldwide
- Increased incidence in immunocompromised individuals

Clinical Features
- TB meningitis: headache, malaise, mental confusion, and vomiting
- Tuberculoma: symptoms of a mass lesion
- CSF findings: increased pressure, a pleocytosis made up of mononuclear cells, elevated protein levels, and reduced or normal glucose content
- Nontuberculous mycobacteria: asymptomatic or nonspecific symptoms

Radiographic Features
- Enhancement at the base of the brain in TB meningitis
- Multilocular lesion with a peripheral rim of contrast enhancement and a hypodense, necrotic center (tuberculoma)
- Mycobacterial pseudotumor: hyperdense lesion with surrounding edema

Prognosis and Treatment
- Often fatal without early treatment
- Combination of antimycobacterial agents
- Prophylactic therapy in asymptomatic patients
- BCG (bacille Calmette-Guérin) vaccine

MYCOBACTERIAL INFECTIONS—PATHOLOGIC FEATURES

Gross Findings
- TB meningitis: thick, gray exudate that typically involves the base of the brain
- Tuberculoma: round or oval mass with a necrotic, firm center; creamy in color
- Abscesses may also occur

Microscopic Findings
- TB meningitis: lymphocytes, plasma cells, and tubercles with necrotic centers surrounded by epithelioid histiocytes and lymphocytes; obliterative endarteritis
- Tuberculoma: necrotizing granulomatous inflammation surrounded by gliotic brain tissue
- Acid-fast organisms difficult to identify
- Nontuberculous mycobacteria: poorly formed granulomas; perivascular lymphocytes and macrophages with acid-fast organisms; spindle cell pseudotumors

Ancillary Studies
- Polymerase chain reaction (PCR) to identify mycobacterial DNA

Differential Diagnosis
- Fungal infections
- Sarcoidosis

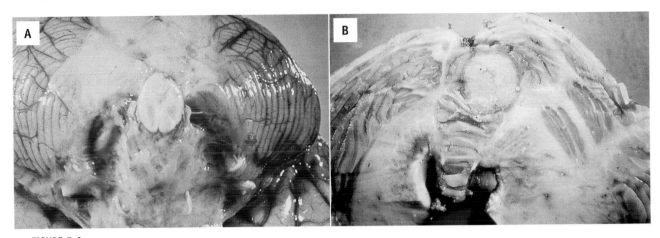

FIGURE 7-6

Tuberculosis. **A**, Tuberculous meningitis typically involves the base of the brain. Small nodules or tubercles may be identified within the exudate. **B**, Tuberculous infection of the CNS may also take the form of mass lesions or tuberculomas.

TB may also produce abscesses, particularly in patients with AIDS. Epidural spinal abscesses are usually a complication of TB of the spine (Pott's disease).

MICROSCOPIC FINDINGS

In TB meningitis, one sees lymphocytes, other mononuclear inflammatory cells, and tubercles composed of a central area of necrosis surrounded by epithelioid cells and lymphocytes. Langhans giant cells may also be seen but are typically sparse. Meningeal blood vessels may be involved with resulting fibrinoid necrosis and thrombosis. So-called endarteritis obliterans, characterized by thickening of the vascular intima by collagenous fibrosis, may be present. The diagnosis is definitively established by identifying acid-fast organisms with either a Ziehl-Neelsen stain (Fig. 7-7) or an auramine-rhodamine fluorescent technique. Organisms are often difficult to identify, especially if treatment has been initiated; therefore, a negative acid-fast stain does not completely exclude the diagnosis.

Tuberculomas are also characterized by necrotizing granulomatous inflammation. Typically, they consist of a caseous center surrounded by epithelioid histiocytes, giant cells, and lymphocytes (Fig. 7-8). The surrounding brain tissue is gliotic. Again, organisms may be difficult to identify.

Nontuberculous mycobacteria may also produce granulomatous inflammation, but the granulomas are typically poorly formed. Perivascular infiltrates composed of lymphocytes and macrophages, some of which contain acid-fast organisms (Fig. 7-9), may be seen in symptomatic patients. Rarely, spindle cell pseudotumors, which are identical to those seen in other organ systems in immuno-

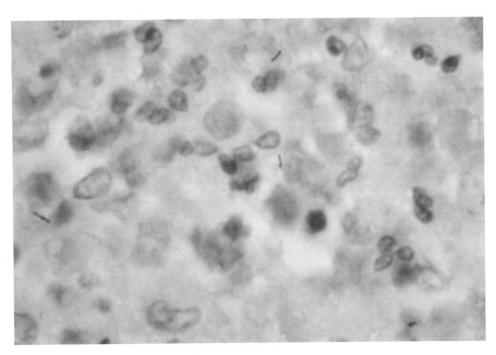

FIGURE 7-7

Tuberculosis. Acid-fast organisms, seen with a Ziehl-Neelsen stain, are often difficult to identify and should be searched for carefully in suspected cases of tuberculosis.

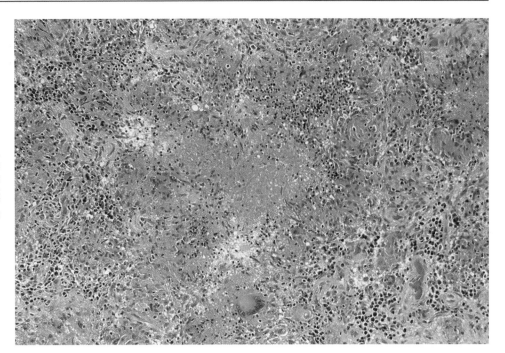

FIGURE 7-8

Tuberculosis. Necrotizing granulomatous inflammation is typical of this infection. Areas of central caseous necrosis are surrounded by an inflammatory infiltrate composed of epithelioid histiocytes, Langhans giant cells, and lymphocytes.

compromised patients, may be present. They are composed of spindle cells arranged in fascicles associated with lymphocytes, plasma cells, and occasional neutrophils. Acid-fast bacilli may be seen within the spindled cells.

ANCILLARY STUDIES

Detection of mycobacterial DNA sequences with the polymerase chain reaction (PCR) method is a useful diagnostic procedure when organisms cannot be identified by conventional means.

DIFFERENTIAL DIAGNOSIS

Necrotizing granulomatous inflammation is characteristic of TB. However, other infectious processes, particularly those caused by fungi, can produce a similar pattern of inflammation and need to be considered in the differential diagnosis. A combination of acid-fast and methenamine silver or periodic acid–Schiff (PAS) stains is useful in establishing a diagnosis when granulomas are encountered. The granulomas of sarcoidosis are typically non-necrotizing; however, necrosis can occur in this disorder. The diagnosis of sarcoidosis is

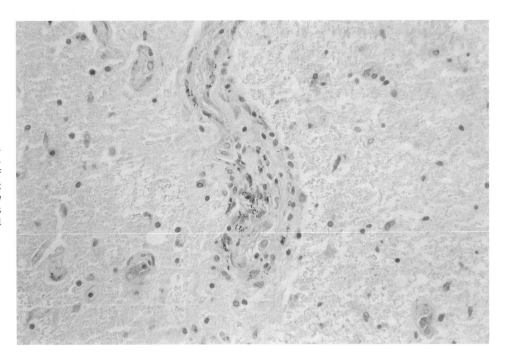

FIGURE 7-9

Nontuberculous mycobacterial infection. Perivascular infiltrates of lymphocytes and macrophages, some of which contain filamentous, acid-fast organisms (Ziehl-Neelsen stain), may be seen in symptomatic patients with disseminated mycobacterial infections.

one of exclusion and should be considered only after infectious causes have been ruled out.

PROGNOSIS AND THERAPY

Disseminated TB is often fatal unless treated early. A combination of antimycobacterial agents, including isoniazid, rifampin, pyrazinamide, ethambutol, and streptomycin, is used to minimize the possibility of antibiotic resistance, which has become an increasingly common problem. Prophylactic treatment of those infected with *M. tuberculosis* but free of disease is useful in preventing CNS disease. An attenuated vaccine developed from a strain of *M. bovis* by Calmette and Guérin (the BCG vaccine) is used in some groups but may cause infection, particularly in immunosuppressed patients.

NEUROSYPHILIS

Syphilis is caused by the spirochete *Treponema pallidum*. This organism is transmitted in adults by venereal contact or in children transplacentally from mother to fetus. Neurosyphilis occurs predominantly in patients with tertiary syphilis, although meningitis or cranial nerve palsies can occur during the acute disseminated phase of infection.

CLINICAL FEATURES

Although the incidence of syphilis is decreasing in industrialized countries, there is a rise in the number of cases in developing countries, as well as in certain patient populations, including those with AIDS. In patients in whom tertiary syphilis develops, asymptomatic neurosyphilis is common. The clinical findings in symptomatic patients are extremely variable, and neurosyphilis has been termed "the great imitator" of other diseases because the clinical presentation is often atypical and misleading. Those with human immunodeficiency virus (HIV) infection are more likely to progress to symptomatic neurosyphilis and to have an accelerated course.

Patients with meningovascular neurosyphilis present with signs of chronic meningitis. If the vascular component of the disease is severe, infarcts may develop. Extension of the inflammatory process into cranial and spinal nerves and blood vessels may produce optic atrophy or cranial nerve palsies. If the meningeal exudate organizes, symptoms of obstructive hydrocephalus may develop.

Paretic neurosyphilis occurs when brain tissue is invaded by the treponemal organisms. In this form of the disease, which has been termed "general paresis of the insane," an insidious, progressive loss of mental and physical functions develops, with mood alterations terminating in severe dementia. Argyll Robertson pupils, which show accommodation but do not react to light, are seen in this form of tertiary neurosyphilis.

Tabes dorsalis results from damage to the sensory nerves in the dorsal roots of the spinal cord. Sensory disturbances, including "lightning pains," and loss of deep tendon reflexes are typical findings. Impaired joint position sense with ataxia and loss of pain sensation leading to skin and joint damage (Charcot joints) are also observed.

Stigmata of congenital syphilis include interstitial keratitis, chorioretinitis, and deafness. In congenitally infected children, all the aforementioned neurosyphilitic syndromes may eventually develop.

PATHOLOGIC FEATURES

GROSS FINDINGS

Thickened, fibrotic meninges are characteristic of meningovascular neurosyphilis. When the infection is confined to the cervical region, the term "pachymeningitis cervicalis hypertrophica" has been applied. Syphilitic gummas, which vary from 0.1 to 4 cm in diameter, may occur in the meninges, where they are usually attached to the dura and the underlying brain, in which they become embedded. Gummas are generally round, reddish tan to gray, and firm and rubbery with a central area of necrosis.

The brains of patients suffering from paretic neurosyphilis are shrunken and firm and covered by thick, opaque leptomeninges. The atrophy is most marked frontally (Fig. 7-10), and the ventricles are typically greatly enlarged. The ependyma may have a fine ground-

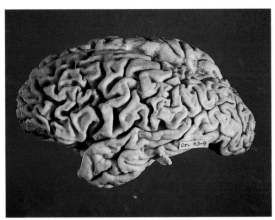

FIGURE 7-10

Neurosyphilis. In paretic neurosyphilis, there is prominent frontal atrophy.

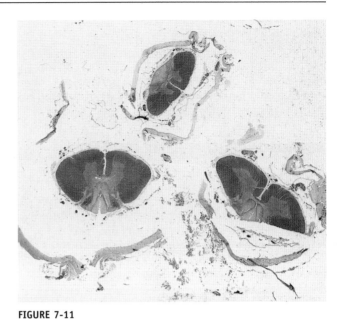

FIGURE 7-11

Neurosyphilis. In tabes dorsalis, there is myelin loss affecting the posterior columns of the spinal cord (Luxol fast blue myelin stain).

glass appearance because of extensive granular ependymitis.

In long-standing tabes dorsalis, degeneration of the posterior columns leads to an excavated dorsal surface of the spinal cord. The posterior nerve roots are gray and shrunken.

Microscopic Findings

In meningovascular neurosyphilis, an admixture of lymphocytes and plasma cells is present in association with fibrosis. The vascular component, termed "Heubner's arteritis," is a form of endarteritis obliterans with crescentic, collagenous thickening of the vascular intima. Lymphocytes and plasma cells are present in the adventitia, cuffing the vasa vasorum, and may penetrate the media. Gummas, if present, consist of a central area of necrosis surrounded by epithelioid histiocytes, multinucleated foreign body–type giant cells, lymphocytes, plasma cells, and focal fibrosis.

The cerebral cortex in paretic neurosyphilis is atrophic and lacks a normal laminar architectural pattern. There is loss of neurons with proliferation of astrocytes and microglial cells. The microglial cells are hypertrophied and elongated and often contain abundant iron, which may be highlighted with a Perls stain. The cerebral cortex has been described as having a "wind-swept" or "bush fire" appearance. There may be perivascular lymphocytes and plasma cells, and treponemal organisms may occasionally be demonstrated with special stains (modified Steiner or Warthin-Starry silver stains).

Tabes dorsalis is characterized by a loss of myelinated axons in the dorsal nerve roots and pallor and atrophy in the dorsal columns (Fig. 7-11). Typically, no significant inflammatory infiltrate is found, and organisms are not identifiable.

NEUROSYPHILIS—PATHOLOGIC FEATURES

Gross Findings

▶ Meningovascular neurosyphilis: thick, opaque meninges and gummas
▶ Paretic neurosyphilis: atrophy, meningeal fibrosis, large ventricles, granular ependymitis
▶ Tabes dorsalis: excavated dorsal spinal cord, atrophic and gray dorsal nerve roots

Microscopic Findings

▶ Meningovascular neurosyphilis: lymphocytes and plasma cells, obliterative endarteritis, necrotizing granulomatous inflammation in gummas
▶ Paretic neurosyphilis: loss of cerebral laminar architecture with neuronal loss and proliferation of astrocytes and microglial cells; organisms may be identified
▶ Tabes dorsalis: loss of myelinated axons in nerve roots with pallor and atrophy of the dorsal columns; no organisms

Differential Diagnosis

▶ Tuberculosis and other causes of granulomatous inflammation
▶ Tabes dorsalis: subacute combined degeneration, vacuolar myelopathy, tropical spastic paraparesis

---

Differential Diagnosis

The obliterative endarteritis seen in meningovascular syphilis is similar to and should be distinguished from that seen in tuberculosis. Similarly, syphilitic gummas must be distinguished from other forms of granulomatous inflammation. The differential diagnosis of tabes dorsalis includes subacute combined degeneration of the spinal cord as a result of vitamin B_{12} deficiency, the vacuolar myelopathy of AIDS, and tropical spastic paraparesis.

PROGNOSIS AND THERAPY

Treatment of neurosyphilis is largely preventive; the disease should be treated in its primary stage. Undetected cases often respond to large doses of penicillin.

NEUROBORRELIOSIS (LYME DISEASE)

Lyme disease is a multisystem infectious disease caused by the tick-borne spirochete *Borrelia burgdorferi*. It occurs primarily in certain areas of North America, Europe, and Asia, locations reflecting the distribution of *Ixodes* ticks, which are required for disease transmission. Involvement of the central and peripheral nervous systems is a common manifestation of this disease.

CLINICAL FEATURES

Lyme disease has three clinical stages. In the first stage, one sees the characteristic skin lesion, erythema chronicum migrans. In the second stage, which occurs weeks to months later, neurologic or cardiac problems develop. Nervous system manifestations include lymphocytic meningitis, cranial neuropathy, or radiculoneuritis. Less commonly, a mild encephalopathy characterized by cognitive and memory impairment develops. Neurologic symptoms may also be a feature of the third stage, which typically occurs several years later. Arthritis is the main clinical problem in this stage of the disease.

PATHOLOGIC FEATURES

Only a few documented reports of the pathologic findings in Lyme disease of the CNS have been published. These reports have demonstrated perivascular inflammation or vasculitis and multifocal areas of demyelina-

---

NEUROBORRELIOSIS (LYME DISEASE)—PATHOLOGIC FEATURES

► Perivascular inflammation or vasculitis
► Periventricular demyelination

---

tion involving the periventricular white matter. Diagnosis relies on clinical judgment and the demonstration of a specific immune response.

PROGNOSIS AND THERAPY

Oral treatment with doxycycline or parenteral treatment with cephalosporins is effective in the majority of patients.

WHIPPLE'S DISEASE

Whipple's disease is a rare multisystem disorder caused by *Tropheryma whippelii*, a gram-positive actinomycete.

CLINICAL FEATURES

Whipple's disease is typically systemic in nature, although isolated CNS involvement has been reported. Men are affected much more frequently than women, and most cases occur between the fourth and seventh decades of life. Common symptoms include arthralgias, weight loss, steatorrhea, lymphadenopathy, and hyperpigmentation. CNS findings include dementia, gaze palsies, and myoclonus. Focal enhancing and nonenhancing lesions may be present radiologically.

NEUROBORRELIOSIS (LYME DISEASE)—FACT SHEET

Definition
► A multisystem disease caused by the spirochete *Borrelia burgdorferi*

Incidence and Location
► Parts of North America, Europe, and Asia

Clinical Features
► 1st stage: erythema chronicum migrans
► 2nd stage: nervous system disease and cardiac involvement
► 3rd stage: arthritis
► Lymphocytic meningitis, cranial neuropathy, radiculoneuritis

Prognosis and Treatment
► Treated successfully with doxycycline or cephalosporins

WHIPPLE'S DISEASE—FACT SHEET

Definition
► A rare systemic disease caused by *Tropheryma whippelii*

Gender and Age Distribution
► Much more common in men
► Fourth through seventh decades

Clinical Features
► Systemic findings: arthralgias, weight loss, steatorrhea, lymphadenopathy, hyperpigmentation
► CNS findings: dementia, gaze palsies, myoclonus

Radiographic Features
► Multiple focal lesions

Prognosis and Treatment
► Fatal if untreated
► Responds dramatically to antibiotic therapy

PATHOLOGIC FEATURES

Histologic findings include small collections of macrophages that are often perivascular in location (Fig. 7-12). A lymphoplasmacytic infiltrate and gliosis are also present. The macrophages are lipid laden and filled with sickle-shaped organisms that are PAS, gram, and methenamine silver positive.

ANCILLARY STUDIES

ULTRASTRUCTURAL FEATURES

The bacillary nature of the organisms may be confirmed with electron microscopy. Lamellar, partially degraded bacterial cell walls may also be identified with this method.

WHIPPLE'S DISEASE—PATHOLOGIC FEATURES

Histologic Findings
▶ Collections of perivascular lipid-laden macrophages
▶ PAS-, gram-, and methenamine silver–positive organisms

Ultrastructural Features
▶ Bacillary organisms and lamellar bacterial cell walls

Differential Diagnosis
▶ *Mycobacterium avium* complex infection

DIFFERENTIAL DIAGNOSIS

The diagnosis of Whipple's disease is not usually difficult if the entity is considered. The differential diagnosis includes infection with organisms of the *M. avium* complex, which are also present within macrophages in a perivascular location and are PAS and gram positive.

PROGNOSIS AND THERAPY

Untreated cerebral Whipple's disease may progress to death in 6 to 12 months. However, this infection responds dramatically to appropriate antibiotic therapy, thus highlighting the need for accurate diagnosis.

ACTINOMYCOSIS

Actinomyces species are rare, but treatable, causes of CNS infection. They are anaerobic, gram-positive organisms with a worldwide distribution. *A. israelii* and *A. bovis* produce most infections in humans.

CLINICAL FEATURES

Lesions in the CNS are usually secondary to a focus elsewhere in the body and spread to the brain hematogenously or by direct extension. Risk factors include dental infections or recent tooth extraction, head trauma, gastrointestinal tract surgery, chronic otitis or sinusitis, chronic osteomyelitis, tetralogy of Fallot, or infection of an intrauterine device. Patients have symptoms of either a space-occupying lesion or meningitis.

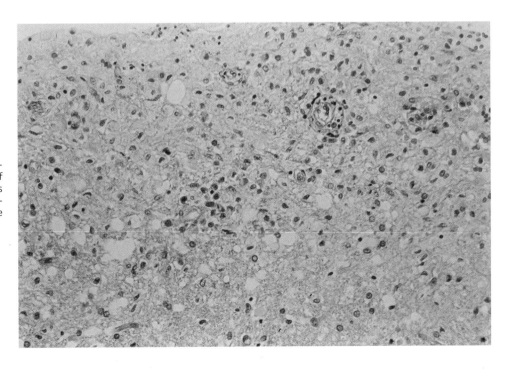

FIGURE 7-12
Whipple's disease. Microscopic findings in Whipple's disease consist of an inflammatory infiltrate that is composed predominantly of macrophages and associated with reactive astrocytosis.

PATHOLOGIC FEATURES

Actinomycosis of the CNS typically results in abscess formation. The lesions show central necrosis with an inflammatory infiltrate composed predominantly of neutrophils. Colonies of branching organisms form the characteristic sulfur granules (Fig. 7-13). These granules in turn are surrounded by chronic inflammation and granulation tissue.

DIFFERENTIAL DIAGNOSIS

The branching organisms should be distinguished from *Nocardia* species. The latter organisms are acid-fast.

PROGNOSIS AND THERAPY

Even with appropriate treatment, CNS actinomycosis has a significant mortality rate, and approximately half the survivors have neurologic sequelae. Optimal management consists of combined adequate surgical drainage and prolonged antibiotic therapy.

NOCARDIOSIS

CNS involvement is a well-described complication of nocardial infection; CNS disease accounts for approximately 5% to 35% of reported nocardial infections. Most cases are caused by *Nocardia asteroides*, a gram-positive, acid-fast, aerobic, and filamentous bacterium.

CLINICAL FEATURES

CNS disease caused by *Nocardia* is generally thought to occur via hematogenous dissemination from an infection in the lungs. Most patients are men, and the mean

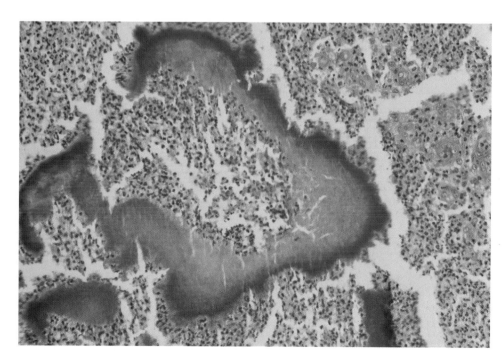

FIGURE 7-13

Actinomycosis. The sulfur granule, which is characteristic of actinomycosis, is a purplish mass of filamentous organisms.

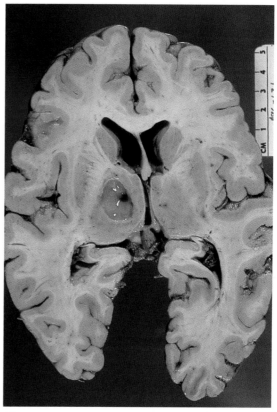

FIGURE 7-14

Nocardiosis. *Nocardia* may produce abscesses, meningitis, or both.

age of patients is 40 years. Predisposing factors include immunosuppression, especially organ transplantation, and CNS trauma or invasive CNS procedures. Patients typically present with a subacute onset of signs and symptoms, including head or neck pain, nausea and vomiting, or altered mental status. CSF findings include a neutrophilic pleocytosis with decreased glucose levels.

PATHOLOGIC FEATURES

Nocardia may produce either abscesses (Fig. 7-14), meningitis, or both. The abscesses are typically similar to those found in other bacterial infections, although a granulomatous reaction can sometimes be seen. The organisms appear as thin, branching filaments and may be identified with a tissue Gram stain, silver stains, or modified acid-fast stains (Fig. 7-15).

DIFFERENTIAL DIAGNOSIS

Nocardial abscesses are similar to those produced by other bacterial organisms, and a high index of suspicion

is necessary to make the correct diagnosis. The organisms should be distinguished from those causing actinomycosis. The latter fail to stain with acid-fast stains.

PROGNOSIS AND THERAPY

The diagnosis of nocardiosis is often delayed, which results in suboptimal treatment in some cases. Mortality with this infection ranges from 25% to 75%. A variety of antibacterial agents, including the sulfonamides, are effective in the treatment of this organism.

OTHER BACTERIAL INFECTIONS

Subdural empyema and extradural (epidural) abscesses may develop as a result of spread from an infection in the adjacent skull bones or paranasal sinuses. When this process occurs in the spinal epidural space, there may be compression of the underlying spinal cord, which constitutes a neurosurgical emergency (and leads to a possible after-hours frozen section).

Sarcoidosis is a granulomatous, multisystem disorder of unknown etiology. It is thought to be a disorder of immune complex deposition that triggers a granulomatous response. As of yet, no specific organism has been

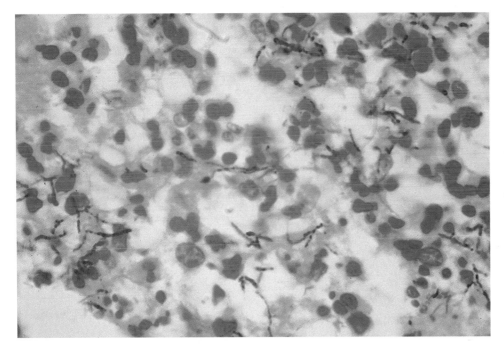

FIGURE 7-15

Nocardiosis. The organisms are thin, branching filaments (tissue Gram stain).

unequivocally associated with this disease. Neurosarcoidosis typically affects the base of the brain, especially the hypothalamus and optic region, and produces a variety of neurologic manifestations, including cranial nerve deficits, long tract signs, autonomic dysfunction, and endocrine abnormalities. Its pathologic features are similar to those in other organs systems. Typically, one sees non-necrotizing granulomatous inflammation (Fig. 7-16).

Leptospirosis is caused by the spirochete *Leptospira interrogans*. Clinical meningitis is frequent in this disease, and encephalitis or myelitis can occur in some cases. A form of the disease referred to as severe icteric leptospirosis, or Weil's disease, is characterized by liver and renal dysfunction, decreased level of consciousness, and widespread vasculitis with hemorrhage, including subarachnoid and intracerebral bleeding.

Brucellosis (Malta fever) is a zoonosis transmitted to humans by raw dairy products or by direct contact with animal products such as the placenta. Manifestations of neurobrucellosis include meningitis, encephalitis, myelitis, radiculoneuritis, and vascular syndromes.

Cat-scratch disease, caused by *Bartonella henselae*, may rarely affect the CNS. An acute encephalopathy with diffuse cerebral dysfunction is most commonly observed. Most infections resolve without treatment, and infection may be confirmed serologically.

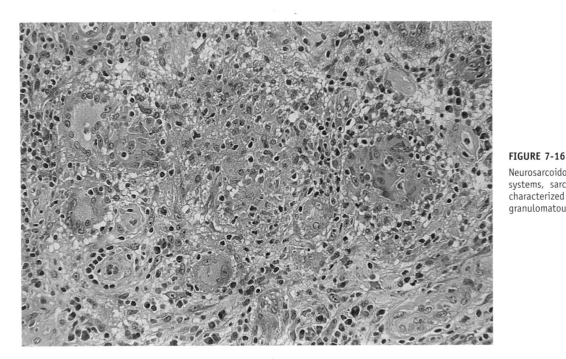

FIGURE 7-16

Neurosarcoidosis. As in other organ systems, sarcoidosis of the CNS is characterized by non-necrotizing granulomatous inflammation.

Finally, bacteria may cause neurologic damage indirectly by the production of toxins. Bacteria producing CNS toxins include those causing diphtheria, tetanus, botulism, and shigellosis.

FUNGAL INFECTIONS

Fungal infections (mycoses) of the CNS are most commonly seen in immunocompromised patients. Most CNS infections occur secondarily via hematogenous dissemination from a primary focus, usually in the lung. Infection by fungal organisms may result in meningitis, parenchymal infections, or a combination of these patterns. In general, organisms that appear as yeasts in tissue cause meningitis, whereas those that form hyphae in tissue cause parenchymal lesions. In many instances the organisms can be visualized in tissue sections stained with routine hematoxylin-eosin; however, special stains such as methenamine silver and PAS are often used to highlight fungi.

CRYPTOCOCCOSIS

Cryptococcosis is caused by *Cryptococcus neoformans*, an encapsulated, spherical budding yeast found in soil and wood that have been contaminated with bird excreta.

CLINICAL FEATURES

Cryptococcosis occurs in all races and is more common in men. It sometimes develops spontaneously in previously healthy individuals; however, in up to 85% of cases it is associated with debilitating illnesses. Predisposing conditions include lymphoproliferative disorders, alcoholism, advanced age, generalized malnutrition, corticosteroid therapy, organ transplantation, collagen vascular diseases, and AIDS. Patients present with signs and symptoms of subacute or chronic meningitis. Other findings include cranial nerve disturbances, papilledema, amblyopia, strabismus, diplopia, ptosis, and deafness.

PATHOLOGIC FEATURES

GROSS FINDINGS

In most cases, the leptomeninges are thickened and opaque, particularly over the base of the brain and cerebellum. Hydrocephalus may be present in chronic cases. Parenchymal lesions resemble soap bubbles (Fig. 7-17); this appearance is related to exuberant capsular material produced by the proliferating organisms. Lesions are most commonly seen in the basal ganglia and thalamus. Rarely, masses of fungi aggregate in an inflammatory lesion, a finding referred to as a cryptococcoma.

MICROSCOPIC FINDINGS

The inflammatory infiltrate in cryptococcosis is typically scant. Granulomatous inflammation may be seen in some cases. The organisms may form small colonies,

---

CRYPTOCOCCOSIS—FACT SHEET

Definition
▶ An infection caused by the budding yeast *Cryptococcus neoformans*

Incidence and Location
▶ Occurs worldwide

Gender and Age Distribution
▶ More common in men

Clinical Features
▶ 85% of patients have other debilitating conditions
▶ Subacute or chronic meningitis

Prognosis and Treatment
▶ Steadily progressive course in most cases
▶ Fluconazole is the drug of choice

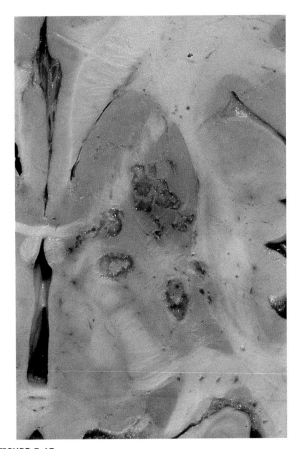

FIGURE 7-17

Cryptococcosis. Lesions with a soap bubble appearance are characteristic and are typically found in the basal ganglia.

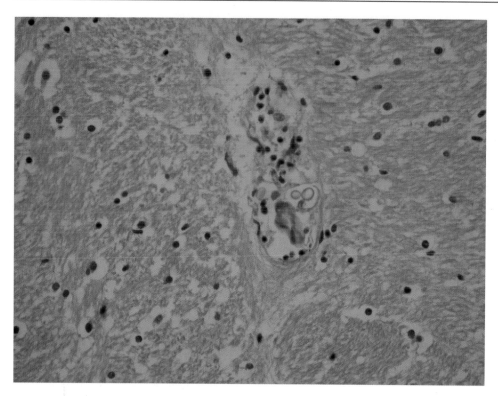

FIGURE 7-18
Cryptococcosis. The yeasts causing cryptococcosis are faintly staining and tend to cluster about blood vessels. Budding forms may be present.

CRYPTOCOCCOSIS—PATHOLOGIC FEATURES

Gross Findings
▶ Thickening and opacification of the leptomeninges
▶ Soap bubble lesions in the basal ganglia
▶ Cryptococcoma

Microscopic Findings
▶ Scant inflammatory infiltrate
▶ Narrow-based budding yeasts

Differential Diagnosis
▶ Blastomycosis
▶ Corpora amylacea

---

usually around blood vessels. They stain faintly with hematoxylin-eosin but can be highlighted with PAS, mucicarmine, alcian blue, or methenamine silver stains (Fig. 7-18). Small buds may be attached to the main body by a short neck.

DIFFERENTIAL DIAGNOSIS

The yeast forms of *C. neoformans* must be distinguished from those of *Blastomycosis dermatitidis*, which are slightly larger and exhibit broad-based budding. These organisms may also be confused with corpora amylacea, which exhibit a similar staining pattern.

PROGNOSIS AND THERAPY

Cryptococcosis typically runs a steadily progressive course ranging from a few weeks to 6 months. Periods of relapse and remission are common in untreated individuals. Fluconazole is the drug of choice in the treatment of this organism.

CANDIDIASIS

Candidiasis is thought to be the most common fungal infection involving the CNS. *Candida* has a worldwide distribution and is a saprophyte that is part of the normal digestive, genital, and cutaneous flora.

CLINICAL FEATURES

Candida species involve the CNS by hematogenous dissemination from a primary focus elsewhere in the body. The portal of entry of the fungus may also be intravenous when therapeutic or recreational drugs are administered by this route. Hematogenous dissemination is promoted by a variety of conditions, including long-term antibiotic or corticosteroid therapy, indwelling catheters, hyperalimentation lines, abdominal surgery, diabetes, burns, malignancies, intravenous drug abuse, and AIDS. The clinical signs and symptoms of CNS candidiasis are those of a low-grade meningitis.

CANDIDIASIS—FACT SHEET

Definition
▶ An infection caused by saprophytic *Candida* species

Clinical Features
▶ Occurs in patients with a wide variety of other conditions
▶ Low-grade meningitis

Prognosis and Treatment
▶ May be treated with amphotericin B and 5-fluorocytosine

CANDIDIASIS—PATHOLOGIC FEATURES

Gross Findings
▶ Microabscesses in the distribution of the anterior and middle cerebral arteries

Microscopic Findings
▶ Small foci of cerebritis
▶ Yeast forms and pseudohyphae

Differential Diagnosis
▶ Other yeasts
▶ Hyphal organisms

PATHOLOGIC FEATURES

GROSS FINDINGS

The brain is often grossly normal. Microabscesses may be present and are most commonly seen in the distribution of the anterior and middle cerebral arteries.

MICROSCOPIC FINDINGS

Histologically, candidiasis is characterized by small foci of cerebritis (Fig. 7-19). Granulomatous inflammation may be seen in some cases. Both yeast forms and pseudohyphae may be present and are faintly basophilic in hematoxylin-eosin–stained sections. The organisms stain intensely with both PAS and methenamine silver (Fig. 7-20).

DIFFERENTIAL DIAGNOSIS

Candida species may be confused with both other yeasts and hyphal organisms. The pseudohyphae are con-stricted at the point of septation and therefore differ from true hyphae.

PROGNOSIS AND THERAPY

Candidiasis usually occurs in patients with other serious diseases, and the prognosis of patients with this disorder depends on the course of these other conditions. Treatment of CNS candidiasis is with amphotericin B and 5-fluorocytosine.

ASPERGILLOSIS

Aspergillosis is caused by several different fungal species, but most cases are due to *Aspergillus fumigatus* or *flavus*. These organisms are found in soil, plants, and decaying matter. CNS infection occurs via hematogenous

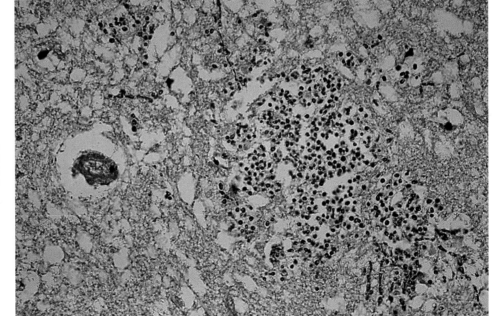

FIGURE 7-19

Candidiasis. CNS candidiasis is characterized by multiple microscopic abscesses. The organisms are faintly basophilic in hematoxylin-eosin–stained sections.

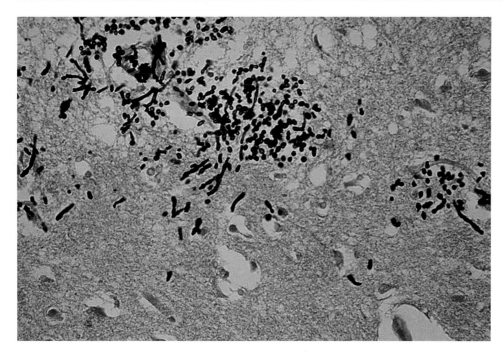

FIGURE 7-20
Candidiasis. The organisms are highlighted by a methenamine silver stain. Both yeast forms and pseudohyphae are present.

dissemination; the usual portal of entry is the respiratory tract. Some cases are the result of direct extension from the paranasal sinuses or from head trauma.

CLINICAL FEATURES

Aspergillosis typically occurs in the settings of corticosteroid and immunosuppressive therapy, prolonged antibiotic use, neoplastic disorders, collagen vascular diseases, diabetes mellitus, organ transplantation, neutropenia, chronic lung disease (especially cavitary tuberculosis), hepatic failure, cardiovascular surgery, alcoholism, intravenous drug or marijuana abuse, and generalized malnutrition. Interestingly, it is uncommon in AIDS patients. Focal neurologic deficits are common. Other frequently encountered signs and symptoms include headache, hemiparesis, seizures, fever, paralysis of cranial nerves, and abnormal plantar reflexes.

PATHOLOGIC FEATURES

GROSS FINDINGS

Multiple lesions are usually present and most often involve areas supplied by the anterior and middle cerebral arteries. Because the fungus is highly angiotropic, foci of hemorrhagic necrosis are common (Fig. 7-21).

MICROSCOPIC FINDINGS

The inflammatory response depends in part on the immune status of the patient, and both neutrophilic and granulomatous inflammatory infiltrates may be seen. Blood vessels are typically involved and show thrombosis and invasion of their walls by fungi. The organisms are septate hyphae that branch at acute angles (Fig. 7-22).

ASPERGILLOSIS—FACT SHEET

Definition
▶ An infection caused by various *Aspergillus* species

Clinical Features
▶ Occurs in immunocompromised patients
▶ Focal neurologic deficits
▶ Common symptoms include headache, hemiparesis, and seizures

Prognosis and Treatment
▶ Poor prognosis
▶ Amphotericin B and flucytosine are the drugs of choice

ASPERGILLOSIS—PATHOLOGIC FEATURES

Gross Findings
▶ Multiple lesions
▶ Foci of hemorrhagic necrosis

Microscopic Findings
▶ Neutrophilic and/or granulomatous inflammation
▶ Vascular invasion and thrombosis
▶ Septate hyphae that branch at acute angles

Differential Diagnosis
▶ Mucormycosis
▶ Other mycoses caused by septate hyphal organisms
▶ Large myelinated axons or cortical blood vessels

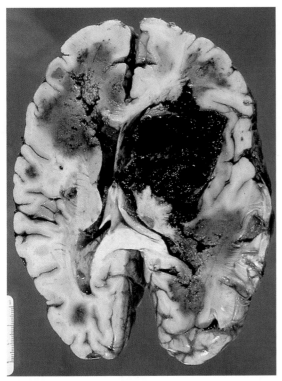

FIGURE 7-21

Aspergillosis. Hemorrhagic abscesses are typical of aspergillosis and are characteristically found in the distribution of the anterior and middle cerebral arteries.

DIFFERENTIAL DIAGNOSIS

These organisms must be distinguished from the Zygomycetes (see the next section), which are typically more irregular and broader. Large myelinated axons in swollen brain tissue and delicate, branching cerebral cortical blood vessels can also be confused with these organisms. Because of the similarity of *Aspergillus* species to other hyphal organisms, one cannot make a definitive diagnosis of aspergillosis by histopathology alone; culture of the organisms is required to confirm the diagnosis. A diagnosis of "fungal organisms consistent with aspergillosis" is appropriate in most cases.

PROGNOSIS AND THERAPY

Disseminated aspergillosis has a poor prognosis, and the diagnosis of CNS involvement is made mostly after death at postmortem examination. Treatment options include amphotericin B and flucytosine.

MUCORMYCOSIS (ZYGOMYCOSIS)

Mucormycosis, also known as zygomycosis, is caused by members of the Zygomycetes, most commonly *Absidia*, *Mucor*, and *Rhizopus*. These organisms are ubiquitous and are found in soil, manure, and decaying vegetation. Unlike most other fungal infections involving the CNS, CNS mucormycosis (rhinocerebral mucormycosis) results from direct venous invasion through the orbital plate from a primary site of infec-

FIGURE 7-22

Aspergillosis. *Aspergillus* species appear in tissue as septate hyphae that branch at acute angles and typically invade blood vessel walls.

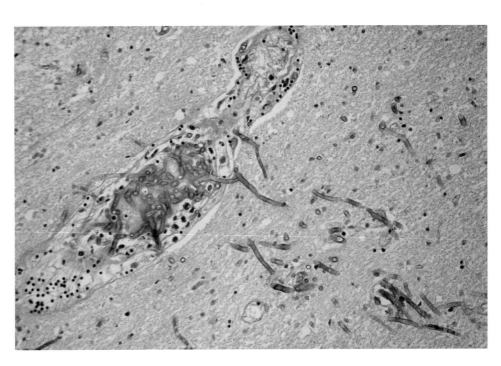

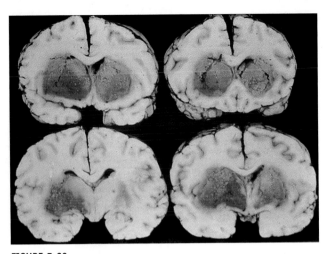

FIGURE 7-23
Mucormycosis. Hemorrhagic lesions are typical and most often involve the basal frontal lobes or the deep gray nuclei.

tion on the skin of the face or in the mucosa of the nose and nasopharynx. Hematogenous dissemination may also occur.

CLINICAL FEATURES

Rhinocerebral mucormycosis is classically seen in the setting of diabetic ketoacidosis. Signs and symptoms often result from involvement of the orbit and include unilateral ophthalmoplegia, proptosis, edema of the eyelid, corneal edema, and blindness. Hematogenous dissemination to the CNS occurs in patients who are intravenous drug abusers and those who are immunosuppressed.

PATHOLOGIC FEATURES

GROSS FINDINGS

Rhinocerebral mucormycosis is characterized grossly by necrotic, hemorrhagic lesions that most commonly involve the base of the frontal lobes. When CNS involvement results from hematogenous dissemination, hemorrhagic lesions are often present in the deep gray nuclei (Fig. 7-23).

MICROSCOPIC FINDINGS

The Zygomycetes typically elicit a minimal inflammatory response that is predominantly neutrophilic. These fungi, like *Aspergillus* species, are highly angiotropic and are often identified within the walls of blood vessels. They appear as broad, nonseptate, irregular (ribbon-like) hyphae that branch at right angles (Fig. 7-24).

DIFFERENTIAL DIAGNOSIS

Aspergillus species, particularly when treated, can resemble the Zygomycetes. Special stains (PAS and methenamine silver) are useful in demonstrating septations in the former.

PROGNOSIS AND THERAPY

Rhinocerebral mucormycosis has a poor prognosis. The illness often runs a fulminating course, with death within a few days. Improvement can occur after treatment of the diabetic ketoacidosis, and surgical extirpation combined with antifungal agents (amphotericin B, trimethoprim-sulfamethoxazole) is effective in some cases.

COCCIDIOIDOMYCOSIS

Coccidioidomycosis, caused by *Coccidioides immitis*, is a geographically restricted mycosis. It is endemic in the southwestern United States. The organism exists in soil, and infection occurs when spores are inhaled through infected dust.

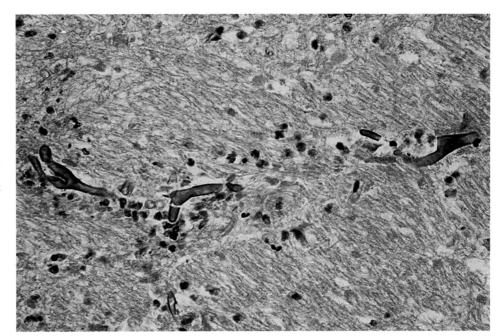

FIGURE 7-24
Mucormycosis. These organisms appear in tissue as nonseptate, ribbon-like hyphae that branch at right angles.

CLINICAL FEATURES

Infection with *C. immitis* initially produces a mild febrile illness. Infection of the lungs follows in many cases. Coccidioidomycosis of the CNS occurs when the disease disseminates; disseminated disease develops most commonly in the nonwhite population and in patients who are pregnant, diabetic, or immunosuppressed, including those with AIDS. Common clinical symptoms include aphasia, hemiparesis, confusion, restlessness, and mental depression. Symptoms of acute hydrocephalus may also occur.

PATHOLOGIC FEATURES

GROSS FINDINGS

CNS coccidioidomycosis is typically manifested as a subacute or chronic meningitis. One sees thickened, cloudy, opacified leptomeninges associated with small nodules. These findings are most prominent at the base of the brain. Gross parenchymal lesions may occur but are unusual.

MICROSCOPIC FINDINGS

C. immitis typically elicits a necrotizing granulomatous inflammatory response. Vascular involvement may be prominent. In tissue sections, the distinctive spherules of coccidioidomycosis are easily identified with hematoxylin-eosin staining (Fig. 7-25). When the spherules rupture, they release endospores that may

---

COCCIDIOIDOMYCOSIS—FACT SHEET

Definition
▶ An infection caused by the dimorphic fungus *Coccidioides immitis*

Incidence and Location
▶ Endemic in the southwestern United States

Clinical Features
▶ Occurs most commonly in nonwhites and those who are pregnant, diabetic, or immunosuppressed
▶ Focal symptoms or generalized complaints
▶ Acute hydrocephalus may occur

Prognosis and Treatment
▶ Often terminal in immunocompromised patients
▶ Intravenous amphotericin B is the drug of choice

COCCIDIOIDOMYCOSIS—PATHOLOGIC FEATURES

Gross Findings
▶ Basal meningitis with the formation of small nodules

Microscopic Findings
▶ Granulomatous inflammation with spherules
▶ Endospores may elicit an acute inflammatory response

Differential Diagnosis
▶ Other causes of granulomatous inflammation (tuberculosis, other fungi)
▶ Blastomycosis

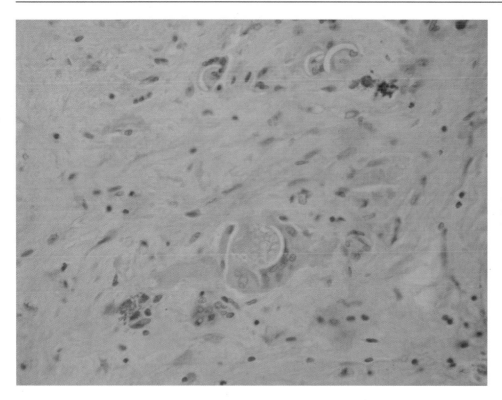

FIGURE 7-25
Coccidioidomycosis. This infection is characterized by spherules that typically elicit a granulomatous response.

provoke an acute inflammatory response and are best identified with a methenamine silver stain.

DIFFERENTIAL DIAGNOSIS

Differential diagnostic considerations include other causes of necrotizing granulomatous inflammation, including tuberculosis and other fungal infections. The endospores may be confused with other yeasts, especially *Blastomyces dermatitidis*. Identification of the classic spherules allows a correct diagnosis in most cases.

PROGNOSIS AND THERAPY

The prognosis of coccidioidomycosis depends in part on the immune status of the patient. Disseminated disease in immunosuppressed patients is often a terminal event. Treatment of this disease is with intravenous amphotericin B.

BLASTOMYCOSIS

Blastomycosis (North American blastomycosis) is caused by *B. dermatitidis*, an organism found in soil and decaying wood. This infection is endemic in the southeastern United States. CNS infection with this organism is rare.

CLINICAL FEATURES

B. dermatitidis gains access to the body via the respiratory tract and commonly infects the lungs and the skin. Infection occurs most commonly in adult men, especially agricultural workers. Predisposing conditions are not necessary for CNS disease to develop, although cerebral blastomycosis does occur in the setting of AIDS. The most common symptoms in cases with CNS involvement are headaches and neck stiffness. Eventually, convulsions, mental deterioration, confusion, and lethargy develop.

BLASTOMYCOSIS—FACT SHEET

Definition
▶ An infection caused by the dimorphic fungus *Blastomyces dermatitidis*

Incidence and Location
▶ Endemic in the southeastern United States

Gender and Age Distribution
▶ Most common in adult males

Clinical Features
▶ Lung and skin lesions are typical
▶ CNS symptoms include headaches and neck stiffness

Prognosis and Treatment
▶ Amphotericin B is used in those with CNS involvement

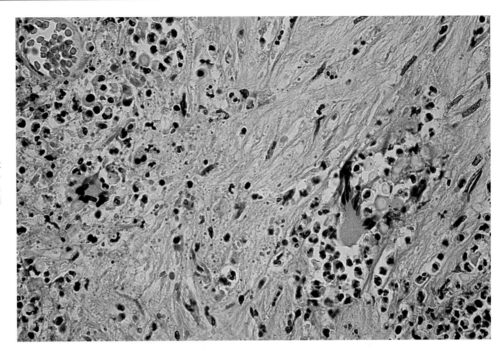

FIGURE 7-26
Blastomycosis. Yeasts that exhibit broad-based budding are characteristic of blastomycosis. This organism elicits a mixed granulomatous and suppurative inflammatory reaction.

PATHOLOGIC FEATURES

GROSS FINDINGS

Cerebral blastomycosis typically produces leptomeningitis with adjacent granulomas. Brain or dural abscesses may also occur.

MICROSCOPIC FINDINGS

B. dermatitidis characteristically elicits a mixed granulomatous and suppurative reaction. The fungi, which are basophilic in hematoxylin-eosin–stained material, are best visualized with PAS or methenamine silver stains and appear as broad-based budding yeasts (Fig. 7-26).

DIFFERENTIAL DIAGNOSIS

The differential diagnosis of blastomycosis includes other fungal infections such as coccidioidomycosis,

cryptococcosis, and paracoccidioidomycosis. Identification of fungal forms with broad-based buds allows a correct diagnosis.

PROGNOSIS AND THERAPY

Individuals with a normal immune system can often mount a successful defense against this organism. When CNS involvement occurs, amphotericin B is the drug of choice.

HISTOPLASMOSIS

Histoplasmosis occurs throughout the world. In the United States it occurs most commonly in the Ohio, Mississippi, and St. Lawrence River Valleys. The causative organism, *Histoplasma capsulatum*, is present in soil and dust contaminated with chicken, bird, or bat excreta.

CLINICAL FEATURES

CNS involvement in histoplasmosis is uncommon and occurs in those with disseminated disease. Risk factors for dissemination, usually from a focus in the lung, include immunosuppression as a result of burns, antibiotics, steroids, or AIDS. Histoplasmosis is characterized by splenomegaly, emaciation, irregular pyrexia, leukopenia, and anemia. Symptoms of meningitis may occur in those with CNS involvement.

BLASTOMYCOSIS—PATHOLOGIC FEATURES

Gross Findings
▶ Leptomeningitis with adjacent granulomas

Microscopic Findings
▶ Mixed granulomatous and suppurative reaction
▶ Broad-based budding yeasts

Differential Diagnosis
▶ Other yeast infections

PATHOLOGIC FEATURES

GROSS FINDINGS

Histoplasmosis causes diffuse or basilar meningitis with thickening of the leptomeninges, particularly around the base of the brain. Intraparenchymal lesions also occur and may mimic neoplasms (Fig. 7-27).

MICROSCOPIC FINDINGS

Histoplasmosis is characterized microscopically by necrotizing granulomatous inflammation. Nodular collections of histiocytes may also be seen. Organisms are found within the cytoplasm of macrophages. In hematoxylin-eosin–stained sections, they appear to be surrounded by a halo (Fig. 7-28). Methenamine silver staining is useful in demonstrating the organisms and differentiating them from other intracytoplasmic microbes.

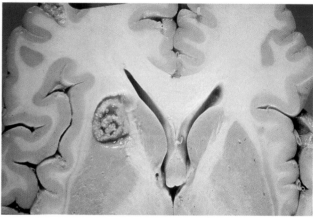

FIGURE 7-27

Histoplasmosis. CNS histoplasmosis is characteristically manifested as meningitis; however, parenchymal lesions that may resemble a neoplastic process can sometimes occur.

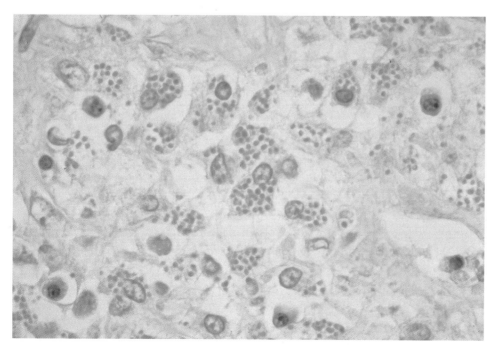

FIGURE 7-28

Histoplasmosis. Intracellular yeast forms are present within macrophages.

DIFFERENTIAL DIAGNOSIS

Histoplasmosis needs to be distinguished from other causes of granulomatous inflammation, including tuberculosis and other fungal infections. The intracytoplasmic organisms may resemble those of toxoplasmosis or leishmaniasis; special stains are often helpful in this differential diagnosis. *Candida* species may also be confused with *H. capsulatum* but are typically somewhat larger and extracellular in location.

PROGNOSIS AND THERAPY

Treatment options for disseminated histoplasmosis remain problematic. Amphotericin B is typically used with other agents, including azoles, sulfonamides, and arsenical and antimony compounds.

OTHER FUNGAL INFECTIONS

Other fungal infections that may involve the CNS include paracoccidioidomycosis (South American blastomycosis), chromoblastomycosis, sporotrichosis, and pseudallescheriasis.

VIRAL INFECTIONS

Viral infections of the CNS may result in a so-called aseptic meningitis or meningoencephalitis. Viral meningitis is typically less severe than its bacterial counterpart, and most patients recover without complications. Members of the enterovirus family are a common cause. Viral encephalitis is characterized by the histologic triad of perivascular chronic inflammation, microglial nodules, and neuronophagia (Fig. 7-29). CNS viral infections may be diagnosed by examination of CSF, PCR of CSF or tissue, culture of the causative virus, or brain biopsy.

HERPES ENCEPHALITIS

Herpes simplex virus (HSV) encephalitis is the most common sporadic, nonseasonal encephalitis and is usually caused by HSV-1 (herpes labialis). HSV-2 (herpes genitalis) may also affect the CNS. It is a cause of aseptic meningitis in immunocompetent individuals, a cause of generalized encephalitis in neonates born by vaginal delivery to women with active primary HSV infection, and a cause of acute, necrotizing encephalitis in immunosuppressed patients.

HERPES ENCEPHALITIS—FACT SHEET

Definition
▶ An infection caused by herpes simplex viruses (HSV-1 and HSV-2)

Gender and Age Distribution
▶ HSV-1 encephalitis: adolescents and young adults
▶ HSV-2 encephalitis: neonates

Clinical Features
▶ HSV-1: fever, headache, seizures, personality and mood changes, mental status changes
▶ HSV-2: vesicular skin lesions and keratoconjunctivitis, poor feeding, irritability, lethargy, seizures

Radiographic Features
▶ Increased T2 signal in the temporal lobes, insular cortex, and inferior frontal lobes

Prognosis and Treatment
▶ HSV-1: significant morbidity and mortality despite acyclovir therapy
▶ HSV-2: long-term neurologic sequelae

CLINICAL FEATURES

HSV encephalitis may occur at any age but has its highest incidence in adolescence and young adulthood. Patients present with fever, headache, seizures, and mental status changes and may rapidly progress to coma and death. Alterations in mood, memory, and behavior are characteristic. Only about 10% of patients have a history of previous labial infection.

Neonates with disseminated HSV-2 infection typically have vesicular skin lesions and signs of keratoconjunctivitis. CNS involvement is usually manifested nonspecifically and includes poor feeding, irritability, lethargy, and seizures.

RADIOGRAPHIC FEATURES

The radiologic features of HSV encephalitis often suggest the diagnosis. One sees lesions in the temporal lobes (often bilateral), the insular cortex, and the inferior frontal lobes. These lesions are often hemorrhagic and are characterized by increased signal on T2-weighted MRI. A cortical or gyriform pattern of enhancement may be present.

PATHOLOGIC FEATURES

GROSS FINDINGS

Grossly, HSV encephalitis is characterized by bilateral, typically asymmetric, hemorrhagic necrosis affecting the temporal lobes, the insulae, the cingulate gyri, and the posterior orbitofrontal cortices (Fig. 7-30). The

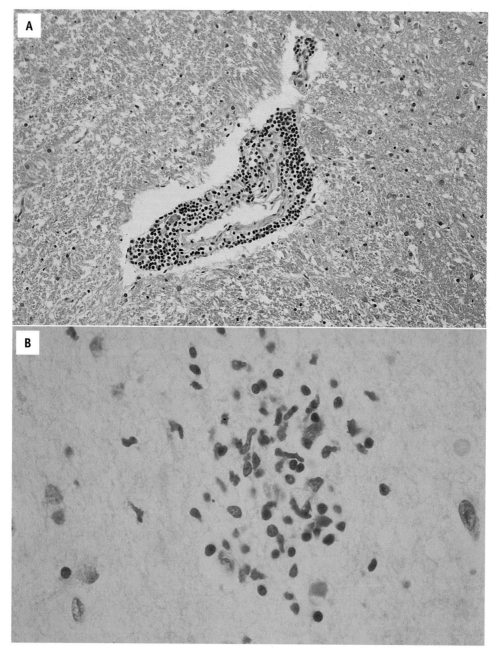

FIGURE 7-29
Viral encephalitis. Viral infections of the CNS are characterized by perivascular chronic inflammation (**A**), microglial nodules (**B**), and neuronophagia.

brain is usually swollen, and lateral transtentorial herniation is a common finding.

MICROSCOPIC FINDINGS

Microscopically, one sees necrosis associated with a macrophage-rich inflammatory infiltrate. Neurons with eosinophilic cytoplasm resembling the "red and dead" neurons seen in infarcts are present. Features suggestive of a viral infection, including perivascular chronic inflammation and microglial nodules, are present but often sparse. Even more difficult to identify are the characteristic Cowdry A intranuclear inclusions, which are

eosinophilic and surrounded by a halo (Fig. 7-31). These inclusions are present in both neurons and glial cells. One may also see neurons with homogeneous, wine-red nuclei with a stained-glass appearance.

ANCILLARY STUDIES

ULTRASTRUCTURAL FEATURES

The diagnosis of HSV encephalitis may be confirmed by electron microscopy. Viral particles may be found in

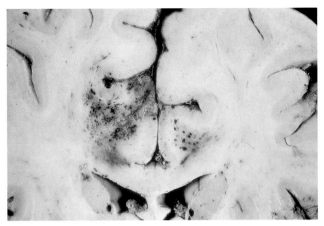

FIGURE 7-30

Herpes encephalitis. Necrotizing, hemorrhagic lesions affecting the limbic structures are characteristic of HSV encephalitis.

HERPES ENCEPHALITIS—PATHOLOGIC FEATURES

Gross Findings

▶ Hemorrhagic necrosis of limbic structures with brain swelling and herniation

Microscopic Findings

▶ Necrosis, macrophages, and eosinophilic neurons
▶ Sparse perivascular inflammation and microglial nodules
▶ Cowdry A intranuclear inclusions

Ultrastructural Features

▶ Hexagonal capsids surrounding a central nucleoid

Immunohistochemistry

▶ Useful in many cases

Differential Diagnosis

▶ Infarct

---

the nucleus and are hexagonal with a central nucleoid (Fig. 7-32).

IMMUNOHISTOCHEMISTRY

Because the characteristic inclusions are often difficult to identify, particularly in treated patients, immunostaining for viral antigens is often used to confirm the diagnosis.

OTHER

PCR amplification of viral DNA in the CSF has now largely supplanted brain biopsy as the main diagnostic procedure in HSV encephalitis. Confirmation of the diagnosis by culture is also useful.

DIFFERENTIAL DIAGNOSIS

The microscopic pathologic features of HSV encephalitis often mimic an infarct. Attention to the presence of perivascular chronic inflammation, microglial nodules, and viral inclusions, if present, is necessary to render the correct diagnosis.

PROGNOSIS AND THERAPY

Without treatment, HSV encephalitis is usually a fatal disease. Even with treatment with acyclovir, approxi-

FIGURE 7-31

Herpes encephalitis. Intranuclear Cowdry A inclusions are diagnostic but often difficult to identify, particularly in patients receiving antiviral therapy.

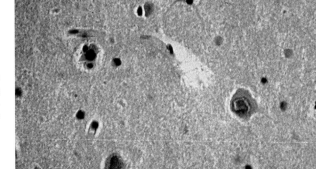

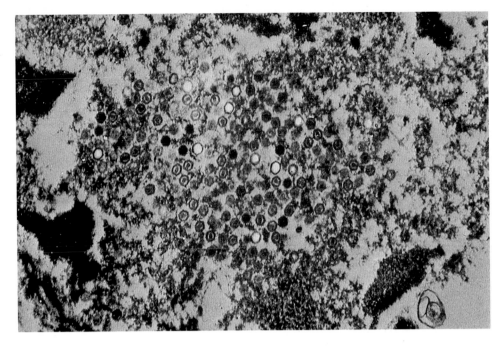

FIGURE 7-32
Herpes encephalitis: ultrastructural findings. The viral particles are hexagonal with a central nucleoid.

mately 20% of patients die, and many survivors have persistent neurologic dysfunction, including impairment of memory. Morbidity and mortality are greatest in the very young and the elderly.

Neonatal HSV infection is also associated with significant morbidity and mortality. Long-term neurologic complications include microcephaly, seizure disorders, ophthalmologic defects, cerebral palsy, and mental retardation.

VARICELLA-ZOSTER VIRUS INFECTION

Varicella-zoster virus (VZV) is a herpesvirus that exclusively affects humans. It is the cause of chickenpox (varicella), an acute febrile exanthematous illness. After resolution of the chickenpox, the virus becomes latent in neurons of the cranial and spinal ganglia. Reactivation of VZV usually leads to disorders of the peripheral nervous system, including shingles (zoster) and postherpetic neuralgia. However, in immunocompetent elderly persons or immunocompromised patients, VZV may produce disease of the CNS.

CLINICAL FEATURES

The clinical features of VZV infection of the CNS depend in part on the immune status of the affected patient. CNS complications of VZV infection may develop in immunocompetent persons after either varicella or zoster, and an accompanying rash may or may not be present. Myelitis occurs when the virus spreads centrally along peripheral nerves toward the spinal cord and is characterized clinically by paraparesis, a sensory level, and sphincter impairment. The virus may also

VARICELLA-ZOSTER VIRUS INFECTION—FACT SHEET
Definition
▶ A group of disorders resulting from infection by varicella-zoster virus
Clinical Features
▶ A rash in the distribution of a dermatome may be present
▶ Immunocompetent patients: myelitis, stroke
▶ Immunocompromised patients: diffuse encephalitis
Prognosis and Treatment
▶ Immunocompetent patients may survive and recover
▶ Progressive disease in immunocompromised individuals
▶ Antiviral agents

spread to the large blood vessels at the base of the brain. In some affected patients, zoster develops in the ophthalmic division of the trigeminal nerve (herpes zoster ophthalmicus), and days to weeks later, stroke develops with hemiplegia contralateral to the zoster.

Immunocompromised patients tend to have disseminated disease. Common clinical findings include headache, fever, vomiting, mental status changes, and focal neurologic deficits, including focal weakness. A progressive and sometimes fatal myelitis may also develop in this patient population.

RADIOGRAPHIC FEATURES

MRI often shows abnormalities in patients with CNS manifestations of VZV infection. Focal areas of enhancement are observed in patients with myelitis. In the setting of disseminated VZV encephalitis, large and small infarcts are present in the cortical and subcortical gray and white matter.

PATHOLOGIC FEATURES

Neuropathologic findings in patients with myelitis include inflammation of the meninges, necrosis, demyelination, and microglial cell proliferation. The brains of patients in whom stroke develops show inflammation of the walls of large vessels, including the internal carotid artery and its branches, a process that has been termed granulomatous angiitis. Immunocompromised patients have evidence of small vessel vasculopathy. Ependymitis as well as demyelinating lesions may also develop. Intranuclear Cowdry A inclusion bodies may be seen in multiple cell types.

ANCILLARY STUDIES

Antibodies directed against VZV antigens are available to confirm the tissue diagnosis of VZV infection. VZV DNA may be detected in both CSF and tissue by PCR.

DIFFERENTIAL DIAGNOSIS

The differential diagnosis of VZV infection is broad and depends on the immune status of the patient and the initial clinical syndrome. The presence of a rash in the distribution of a single dermatome is a useful diagnostic clue. Identification of viral antigens or viral DNA allows a specific diagnosis to be made.

PROGNOSIS AND THERAPY

The prognosis of CNS involvement by VZV depends on the immune status of the patient. Most immunocompetent patients survive and improve substantially, whereas immunocompromised patients typically have a progres-

sive course. Antiviral agents are useful in the treatment of VZV infections.

CYTOMEGALOVIRUS ENCEPHALITIS

Cytomegalovirus (CMV) is the largest member of the herpesvirus family and gets its name from the unique morphologic changes that it induces in infected cells. It is distributed worldwide, and in the United States, more than 80% of the population is seropositive for this virus by the age of 35 years.

CLINICAL FEATURES

CMV infection of the brain in adults usually occurs in AIDS patients. Other immunosuppressed patients, including transplant patients, may be affected, and rarely this virus causes disease in immunocompetent individuals. Patients often have minimal neurologic deficits or may be asymptomatic. In the setting of advanced HIV infection, patients with CMV encephalitis present with confusion, gait disturbances, cranial nerve palsies, hyperreflexia, abnormal serum electrolytes, and retinitis.

Symptomatic disease of the CNS also occurs in neonates who are infected in utero. Most of these cases are due to a primary maternal infection in pregnancy, and the risk of fetal complications is highest when the infection is acquired during the first trimester. Disseminated cytomegalic inclusion disease is manifested shortly after birth with petechiae, hepatosplenomegaly, jaundice, microcephaly, and chorioretinitis.

RADIOGRAPHIC FEATURES

In severe cases, usually seen in the setting of advanced AIDS, there may be evidence of hydrocephalus with associated periventricular enhancement. Neonates with CMV infection may have foci of intracranial mineralization that may be detected by ultrasound.

PATHOLOGIC FEATURES

GROSS FINDINGS

The neuropathologic appearance of the brain in CMV infection is variable; there may be no gross evidence of this infection. Ependymal necrosis may be present in those with CMV ventriculitis, and rarely, large necrotic lesions resembling infarcts may be identified.

The brain in neonatal CMV infection is usually small and may show porencephaly or polymicrogyria. Less frequent findings include hydrocephalus and cerebellar hypoplasia. Foci of calcification and cystic spaces may be noted on sectioning.

MICROSCOPIC FINDINGS

Diffuse microglial nodules characterize most cases of CMV encephalitis. Scattered cytomegalic cells that contain both intranuclear and intracytoplasmic viral inclusions (Fig. 7-33) are usually associated with these nodules. Any cell type within the CNS may be infected, but the virus is often identified within ependymal cells, and cytomegalic cells may largely replace the normal ependyma. There is often little or no associated inflammatory infiltrate in this setting.

CYTOMEGALOVIRUS—PATHOLOGIC FEATURES

Gross Findings
▶ The brain is often grossly normal
▶ Necrosis of the ependyma or other necrotizing lesions may be seen
▶ Neonates: microcephaly, porencephaly or polymicrogyria, calcifications, and cystic spaces

Microscopic Findings
▶ Diffuse microglial nodules
▶ Cytomegalic cells with intranuclear and intracytoplasmic inclusions

Ancillary Studies
▶ Immunohistochemistry

Differential Diagnosis
▶ HIV encephalitis
▶ Other opportunistic infections

ANCILLARY STUDIES

IMMUNOHISTOCHEMISTRY

The characteristic viral inclusions are evident in most cases of CMV encephalitis. Immunohistochemistry for viral antigens may be used to confirm the diagnosis in difficult cases.

DIFFERENTIAL DIAGNOSIS

The CNS manifestations of CMV infection are difficult to distinguish from those of HIV encephalitis or other opportunistic infections. Identification of the

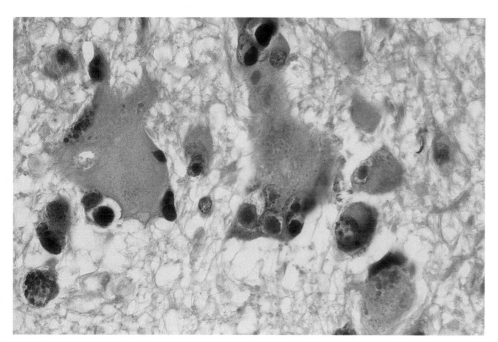

FIGURE 7-33

Cytomegalovirus encephalitis. Cytomegalic cells, which are enlarged and contain both intranuclear and intracytoplasmic inclusions, are typical of this infection.

characteristic viral inclusions in the setting of subacute encephalitis allows a correct diagnosis.

PROGNOSIS AND THERAPY

The prognosis of adult patients with CMV encephalitis is related to their underlying condition. Antiviral agents have improved the outcome of CMV infection. Neonatal infections often run a fatal course, and surviving infants may have severe mental retardation, seizures, spasticity, hearing loss, and optic atrophy.

POLIOMYELITIS

Poliovirus is a member of the enterovirus group. Infection with this virus has largely been controlled by effective immunization; however, poliomyelitis still occurs in less developed countries. In Western countries, cases occur as a result of infection by other enteroviruses or are due to reversion of vaccine-associated poliovirus to a virulent form.

CLINICAL FEATURES

Infection with poliovirus occurs by the fecal-oral route, and before widespread immunization, it most commonly occurred in young children. A nonspecific gastroenteritis develops in most infected patients. Paralytic disease occurs in 1% to 2% of infected patients and is characterized by flaccid paralysis with muscle wasting and hyporeflexia. Bulbar involvement is noted in some cases and may lead to respiratory compromise.

PATHOLOGIC FEATURES

GROSS FINDINGS

In the acute phase of poliomyelitis, the brain and spinal cord are usually macroscopically normal. In severe cases, vascular congestion, petechial hemorrhages, and

---

POLIOMYELITIS—FACT SHEET

Definition
▶ A paralytic illness caused by poliovirus

Clinical Features
▶ Prodrome of gastroenteritis
▶ Flaccid paralysis with muscle wasting and hyporeflexia

Prognosis and Treatment
▶ Largely controlled by immunization
▶ Postpolio syndrome

POLIOMYELITIS—PATHOLOGIC FEATURES

Gross Findings
▶ Acute: normal brain and spinal cord in most cases
▶ Chronic: atrophy of the anterior spinal nerve roots

Microscopic Findings
▶ Acute: perivascular chronic inflammation and neuronophagia
▶ Chronic: neuronal loss and gliosis of the anterior horns of the spinal cord, neurogenic atrophy of skeletal muscle

Differential Diagnosis
▶ West Nile virus encephalomyelitis

---

foci of necrosis may be seen. Chronically, there is atrophy of the anterior nerve roots of the spinal cord.

MICROSCOPIC FINDINGS

Acutely, poliomyelitis is characterized by inflammation affecting predominantly the anterior horns of the spinal cord. Perivascular chronic inflammation and neuronophagia are prominent. A neutrophilic infiltrate may also be seen in some cases. Clusters of microglial cells are evident in sites of neuronal destruction (Fig. 7-34). In patients who survive the acute illness, one sees neuronal loss and gliosis of the anterior horns. There is a loss of axons with fibrosis in the anterior nerve roots. Affected skeletal muscles show neurogenic atrophy.

DIFFERENTIAL DIAGNOSIS

The differential diagnosis of poliomyelitis includes other disorders affecting predominantly the anterior horn cells of the spinal cord. A form of West Nile virus encephalomyelitis causes a syndrome that is clinically and pathologically similar to poliomyelitis.

PROGNOSIS AND THERAPY

A late complication of poliovirus termed postpolio syndrome is seen in a significant percentage of survivors of paralytic polio. This disorder, which occurs 30 to 40 years after the acute illness, is characterized by progressive weakness associated with decreased muscle bulk and pain.

PROGRESSIVE MULTIFOCAL LEUKOENCEPHALOPATHY

Progressive multifocal leukoencephalopathy (PML) is a demyelinating disease of the CNS that results from infection of oligodendroglial cells by JC virus (a

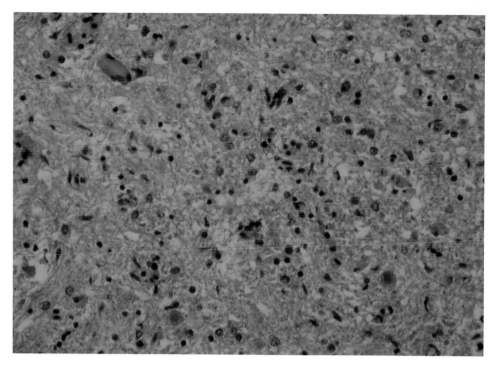

FIGURE 7-34
Poliomyelitis. Destruction of the anterior horn cells of the spinal cord is evident. Clusters of microglial cells remain where neurons once were.

papovavirus). It occurs almost exclusively in immuno-compromised patients. Before the AIDS epidemic, most patients with PML had lymphoproliferative disorders as the underlying cause of their immunosuppression. It is now a disease of the young and middle-aged populations affected by AIDS.

CLINICAL FEATURES

Patients with PML typically present with focal neurologic deficits, including weakness, visual deficits, and

---

PROGRESSIVE MULTIFOCAL LEUKOENCEPHALOPATHY—FACT SHEET

Definition
▶ A demyelinating disease caused by JC virus infection of oligodendroglial cells

Clinical Features
▶ Occurs in immunocompromised patients
▶ Patients present with focal neurologic deficits
▶ JC virus DNA may be detected in CSF by PCR

Radiologic Features
▶ Hyperintense signal on T2-weighted MRI
▶ Minimal enhancement

Prognosis and Treatment
▶ Mean survival of 4 to 6 months
▶ Reduction of immunosuppression is helpful in some cases

---

cognitive abnormalities. The clinical differential diagnosis is broad and encompasses other AIDS-related illnesses, including toxoplasmosis, CNS lymphoma, and HIV encephalitis. Demonstration of JC virus DNA in CSF by PCR is useful in establishing the diagnosis clinically.

RADIOGRAPHIC FEATURES

The diagnosis of PML is strongly supported by radiographic imaging. Hyperintense signal abnormalities of white matter on T2-weighted MRI are highly suggestive of the diagnosis in an appropriate clinical setting. Contrast enhancement, when present, is faint and peripheral.

PATHOLOGIC FEATURES

GROSS FINDINGS

Macroscopically, one sees multiple foci of demyelination. Lesions are typically subcortical in the cerebral hemispheres and have a predilection for the parieto-occipital regions (Fig. 7-35). The cerebellum and brain stem may also be affected.

MICROSCOPIC FINDINGS

As in other demyelinating diseases, one sees myelin loss with an associated macrophage-rich infiltrate. The infected oligodendroglial nuclei are enlarged and hyperchromatic; some have a ground-glass appearance typical of viral infection (Fig. 7-36). Bizarre astrocytes with lobulated, hyperchromatic nuclei are also present.

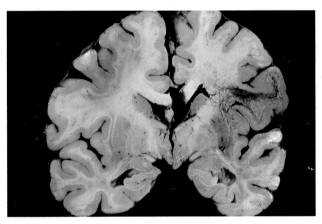

FIGURE 7-35

Progressive multifocal leukoencephalopathy. Areas of subcortical demyelination, which in some cases appear grossly necrotic, are characteristic of this disorder.

**PROGRESSIVE MULTIFOCAL LEUKOENCEPHALOPATHY—
PATHOLOGIC FEATURES**

Gross Findings

▶ Demyelinating lesions in subcortical white matter
▶ Predilection for the parieto-occipital regions

Microscopic Findings

▶ Myelin loss with a macrophage-rich background
▶ Enlarged oligodendrocyte nuclei with a ground-glass appearance
▶ Bizarre astrocytes

Ultrastructural Findings

▶ Filamentous and spherical viral particles ("spaghetti and meatballs")

Differential Diagnosis

▶ Other demyelinating diseases (multiple sclerosis, leukodystrophies)
▶ Astrocytoma

ANCILLARY STUDIES

ULTRASTRUCTURAL FEATURES

The virions of JC virus may be identified in the nuclei of oligodendroglial cells by electron microscopic examination. These virions measure approximately 30 to 45 nm in diameter and appear as both filamentous and spherical forms (so-called spaghetti-and-meatball appearance) (Fig. 7-37).

IMMUNOHISTOCHEMISTRY

The presence of viral inclusions within oligodendrocyte nuclei may be confirmed by immunohistochemical staining for JC or SV40 (a related papovavirus) virus.

DIFFERENTIAL DIAGNOSIS

In addition to other demyelinating disorders, because of the presence of bizarre astrocytes, the differential diagnosis of PML includes astrocytic neoplasms. Attention to the clinical history and the presence of macrophages in the background should alert the pathologist to suspect a reactive/inflammatory process.

PROGNOSIS AND THERAPY

The prognosis of PML in the setting of immunosuppression is poor; the median survival in this patient

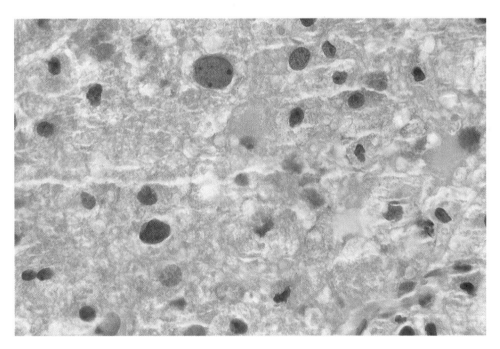

FIGURE 7-36

Progressive multifocal leukoencephalopathy. Enlarged oligodendroglial nuclei with a ground-glass appearance are characteristic of this viral infection.

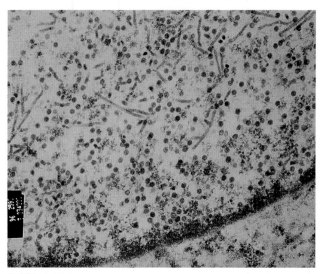

FIGURE 7-37
Progressive multifocal leukoencephalopathy: ultrastructural findings. Viral particles are seen within an oligodendrocyte nucleus and are both filamentous and spherical in appearance.

population is 4 to 6 months. Highly active antiretroviral therapy (HAART) may have a salutary effect on survival, and when immunosuppression can be reduced (i.e., in the setting of organ transplantation), some patients experience partial recovery and prolonged survival.

SUBACUTE SCLEROSING PANENCEPHALITIS

CLINICAL FEATURES

Subacute sclerosing panencephalitis (SSPE) is a rare disease caused by a defective form of the measles virus.

SUBACUTE SCLEROSING PANENCEPHALITIS—FACT SHEET

Definition
▶ A rare disorder caused by a defective measles virus

Gender and Age Distribution
▶ Occurs in children
▶ Boys affected more commonly than girls

Clinical Features
▶ Occurs years after measles infection
▶ Symptoms include personality changes, intellectual deterioration, seizures, myoclonus, and clumsiness

Radiologic Features
▶ Increased signal in white matter on T2-weighted MRI

Prognosis and Treatment
▶ Progressive disorder resulting in death

It develops in approximately one per million measles cases and typically affects children. The disease occurs several years after the initial measles infection, and boys are affected approximately twice as often as girls. SSPE is a chronic disorder characterized by personality changes, intellectual deterioration, seizures, myoclonus, and clumsiness.

RADIOGRAPHIC FEATURES

MRI shows diffuse signal abnormalities affecting predominantly the white matter.

PATHOLOGIC FEATURES

GROSS FINDINGS

The brain is grossly atrophic in most cases of SSPE. The white matter is abnormally firm and may have a mottled gray appearance.

MICROSCOPIC FINDINGS

The microscopic findings are those of chronic encephalitis and include perivascular chronic inflammation, microglial cell proliferation, and neuronophagia. Affected white matter is gliotic. Intranuclear eosinophilic inclusions surrounded by a halo may be seen within neurons, and subtle intracytoplasmic inclusions may also be identified. Oligodendroglial nuclei exhibit a ground-glass appearance similar to that seen in progressive multifocal leukoencephalopathy (Fig. 7-38). Neurofibrillary tangles may be identified in some cases.

DIFFERENTIAL DIAGNOSIS

The histologic findings of SSPE are similar to those seen in most viral encephalitides. Identification of both intranuclear and intracytoplasmic inclusions in an appropriate clinical setting allows a correct diagnosis to be made.

SUBACUTE SCLEROSING PANENCEPHALITIS—PATHOLOGIC FEATURES

Gross Findings
▶ Atrophy and mottled gray matter

Microscopic Findings
▶ Chronic encephalitis
▶ Intranuclear and intracytoplasmic inclusions
▶ Neurofibrillary tangles

Differential Diagnosis
▶ Other viral encephalitides

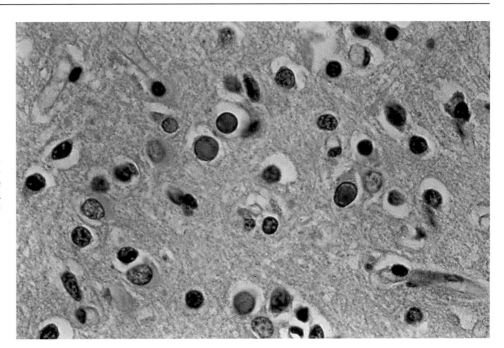

FIGURE 7-38
Subacute sclerosing panencephalitis. Intranuclear inclusions within oligo-dendroglial cells, similar to those present in progressive multifocal leukoencephalopathy, may be seen in this disorder.

PROGNOSIS AND THERAPY

SSPE is a progressive disease that results in death within 2 years in most cases. There is no effective treatment; however, vaccination for measles has resulted in a decreased incidence of this fatal disease.

RABIES

CLINICAL FEATURES

Rabies encephalitis is typically caused by the introduction of rabies virions into deep soft tissue by an animal bite, although aerosol transmission with infection of exposed neuroepithelial cells in the olfactory epithelium may also occur. The virus, an RNA member of the rhabdovirus family, reaches the CNS via intra-axonal transport.

Clinical illness begins with a nonspecific flu-like syndrome, and some patients experience pain or paresthesia at the original exposure site. These symptoms are followed by an acute neurologic syndrome characterized by hyperactivity, disorientation, bizarre behavior, and hallucinations. Hydrophobia, or pharyngeal and laryngeal spasm when attempting to drink, is characteristic but seen in only 30% to 50% of patients. These symptoms are often episodic and alternate with periods of calm. A paralytic variant characterized by seizures and constant high fever is less common.

PATHOLOGIC FEATURES

The brain and spinal cord typically are grossly normal in cases of rabies encephalitis. Microscopically, one sees

---

RABIES—FACT SHEET

Definition
▶ A fatal infection caused by rabies virus (rhabdovirus)

Clinical Features
▶ Nonspecific, flu-like prodrome
▶ Acute neurologic illness characterized by hyperactivity, disorientation, bizarre behavior, and hallucinations
▶ Uncommon paralytic variant—seizures and high fever

Prognosis and Treatment
▶ Fatal in nonimmunized patients
▶ Postexposure prophylaxis prevents clinical illness

RABIES—PATHOLOGIC FEATURES

Microscopic Findings
▶ Intracytoplasmic inclusions in the hippocampus and cerebellum—Negri and lyssa bodies
▶ Perivascular chronic inflammation, microglial nodules, and neuronophagia

Ultrastructural Findings
▶ Filamentous core surrounded by viral nucleocapsids

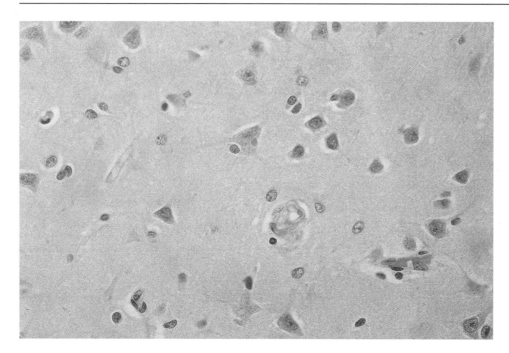

FIGURE 7-39

Rabies. Negri bodies, which are diagnostic of rabies infection, are intracytoplasmic, well-demarcated eosinophilic inclusions typically seen in the hippocampus and cerebellum.

a variable distribution of perivascular chronic inflammation, microglial nodules, and neuronophagia. Intracytoplasmic viral inclusions, termed Negri bodies, are diagnostic and are most abundant in the pyramidal neurons of the hippocampus and in cerebellar Purkinje cells. Classic Negri bodies are round to oval, sharply demarcated, and eosinophilic with fine basophilic stippling (Fig. 7-39). In addition, one may see more irregular, less sharply demarcated inclusions termed lyssa bodies.

ANCILLARY STUDIES

ULTRASTRUCTURAL FEATURES

Both Negri and lyssa bodies are composed of a central or granular filamentous core surrounded by viral nucleocapsids budding into dilated cisternae of the endoplasmic reticulum.

IMMUNOHISTOCHEMISTRY

Demonstration of viral nucleocapsid antigens by immunohistochemistry or immunofluorescence is necessary to confirm a diagnosis of rabies encephalitis.

DIFFERENTIAL DIAGNOSIS

The diagnosis of rabies encephalitis is straightforward once it is suspected and the characteristic viral inclusions are sought.

PROGNOSIS AND THERAPY

Clinical rabies infection is virtually always fatal in non-immunized humans. Current strategies focus on prevention and timely prophylactic treatment of rabies exposure. When performed properly, thorough wound cleansing, postexposure vaccination, and administration of human rabies hyperimmune globulin prevent the development of clinical illness.

ARTHROPOD-BORNE VIRUSES (ARBOVIRUSES)

The arboviruses are responsible for most outbreaks of epidemic viral encephalitis. The most common viruses causing these epidemics belong to four main groups: the alphavirus subgroup of togaviruses (Eastern equine encephalitis, Western equine encephalitis, and Venezuelan equine encephalitis), the flaviviruses (St. Louis encephalitis, Japanese B encephalitis, Murray Valley encephalitis, and West Nile virus encephalitis), the bunyaviruses (California encephalitis and La Crosse encephalitis), and the reoviruses (Colorado tick fever encephalitis). These viruses have animal (horses and small mammals) or bird hosts and mosquito or tick vectors.

CLINICAL FEATURES

Most patients with arbovirus encephalitis have nonspecific, flu-like symptoms lasting a few days. These symptoms are followed by seizures, confusion, drowsiness, and meningism. West Nile virus may cause a paralytic syndrome similar to poliomyelitis.

PATHOLOGIC FEATURES

The arboviruses produce findings typical of any viral encephalitis, including perivascular chronic inflammation, microglial nodules, and neuronophagia. There is also evidence of leptomeningitis. Most lesions are found in gray matter, and some viruses, including West Nile virus, have a predilection for the brain stem and spinal cord (Fig. 7-40). Small foci of necrosis may be present, and some viruses (Eastern equine encephalitis virus, California encephalitis virus, and Colorado tick fever virus) may cause a vasculitis. In fulminating cases of Japanese B encephalitis and Murray Valley encephalitis, a neutrophilic inflammatory infiltrate may be seen. Viral inclusions are typically not identified in the arbovirus encephalitides.

ANCILLARY STUDIES

PCR analysis of serum, CSF, or brain tissue allows identification of the specific arbovirus causing disease in some cases.

DIFFERENTIAL DIAGNOSIS

The differential diagnosis of arbovirus encephalitis includes other causes of viral encephalitis.

PROGNOSIS AND THERAPY

Most arbovirus infections are subclinical. The age of the host and strain of the virus are important determinants of disease severity.

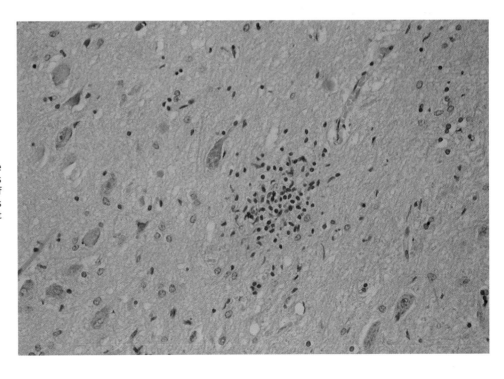

FIGURE 7-40

Arboviruses (West Nile virus). The histologic features of the arbovirus encephalitides are similar to those of viral encephalitis in general. In this case, microglial nodules are evident in a section from the brain stem.

HUMAN IMMUNODEFICIENCY VIRUS INFECTION

Neurologic dysfunction develops in up to 60% of patients with AIDS during the course of their illness, and neuropathologic changes may be demonstrated in as many as 90% of brains from this patient population. These findings include opportunistic infections involving the CNS, discussed in other sections of this chapter; primary CNS lymphomas; a variety of disorders affecting peripheral nerves and skeletal muscle; and lesions thought to be directly related to the HIV virus, including aseptic meningitis, HIV encephalitis, and vacuolar myelopathy, which are discussed in this section.

CLINICAL FEATURES

Primary HIV infection is usually accompanied by constitutional symptoms similar to those of mononucleosis or influenza. Aseptic meningitis is a common manifestation of primary infection, and virus can be isolated from CSF in this patient population. Most patients recover from this acute disorder and remain asymptomatic for a variable, but usually long, time.

In a subset of patients with late-stage AIDS, a diffuse encephalopathy termed the AIDS dementia complex or HIV-1–associated cognitive/motor complex develops that is not attributable to an opportunistic infection. The symptoms of this disorder are those of subcortical dementia and include forgetfulness, inability to concentrate, irritability, apathy, mild confusion, ataxia, leg weakness, and tremor.

A myelopathy termed vacuolar myelopathy may also develop in AIDS sufferers. Symptoms of this illness include leg weakness, spastic paraparesis, sensory ataxia, and incontinence.

Finally, in infants of HIV-infected mothers, neurologic problems may develop and include microcephaly with mental retardation and motor developmental delay.

RADIOGRAPHIC FEATURES

Imaging of the brain in patients with HIV-1–associated cognitive/motor complex shows diffuse cortical atrophy, abnormalities of the cerebral white matter, and ventricular dilatation.

PATHOLOGIC FEATURES

GROSS FINDINGS

The brains of HIV-infected individuals are often grossly normal or may exhibit diffuse atrophy with hydrocephalus ex vacuo. Subtle, ill-defined regions of grayish discoloration of the white matter may be observed in some cases.

MICROSCOPIC FINDINGS

The precise pathologic substrate for the clinical findings in patients with AIDS is unclear. Many individuals with cognitive and motor abnormalities exhibit a pathologic picture that has been termed HIV-1 encephalitis. This encephalitis is characterized by a diffuse or multifocal accumulation of microglia, including ill-defined microglial nodules. Perivascular chronic inflammatory cells may also be seen, but because

---

HUMAN IMMUNODEFICIENCY VIRUS INFECTION—FACT SHEET

Definition
▶ Infection by the retrovirus causing AIDS
▶ Neurologic manifestations may be due to direct effects of the virus, opportunistic infections, or primary CNS lymphomas

Clinical Features
▶ Aseptic meningitis at the time of seroconversion
▶ AIDS dementia complex or HIV-1–associated cognitive/motor complex: subcortical dementia
▶ Vacuolar myelopathy: leg weakness, spastic paraparesis, sensory ataxia, and incontinence

Radiologic Features
▶ Diffuse atrophy with ventricular enlargement
▶ Abnormalities in white matter

Prognosis and Treatment
▶ Highly active antiretroviral therapy (HAART) has improved the outcome
▶ Patients with HIV-associated cognitive disorders have a poor prognosis

---

HUMAN IMMUNODEFICIENCY VIRUS INFECTION— PATHOLOGIC FEATURES

Gross Findings
▶ Atrophy with hydrocephalus ex vacuo
▶ Subtle white matter changes

Microscopic Findings
▶ HIV encephalitis: increase in microglia with ill-defined microglial nodules, multinucleated giant cells
▶ Vacuolar myelopathy: vacuolation of white matter tracts in the lateral and posterior columns
▶ Infants and children: mineralization of blood vessels in the basal ganglia

Differential Diagnosis
▶ Opportunistic infections
▶ Primary CNS lymphoma
▶ Vacuolar myelopathy: subacute combined degeneration of the spinal cord

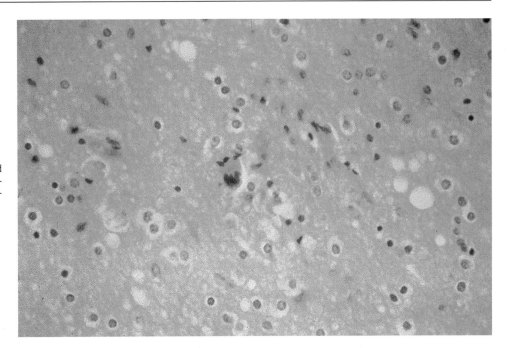

FIGURE 7-41

HIV encephalitis. Multinucleated giant cells, derived from macrophages, are characteristic of HIV-associated encephalitis.

these individuals are immunosuppressed, the degree of inflammation is often minimal. Characteristic macrophage-derived multinucleated cells may be observed and are diagnostic (Fig. 7-41). In most cases, there is also diffuse pallor of the white matter with associated gliosis.

The brains of infants and children affected by AIDS have similar findings and in addition show mineralization of the walls of blood vessels, particularly those of the basal ganglia.

Patients with HIV-associated myelopathy (vacuolar myelopathy) have vacuolar changes and myelin damage in the lateral and posterior columns of the spinal cord (Fig. 7-42). These changes are most prominent at the thoracic levels.

ANCILLARY STUDIES

Viral particles may be ultrastructurally identified within macrophages and free in the extracellular space.

Immunohistochemistry for the p24 viral antigen highlights the multinucleated cells in cases of HIV-1 encephalitis.

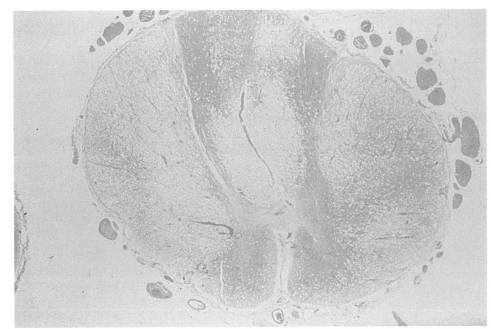

FIGURE 7-42

Vacuolar myelopathy of AIDS. Myelin loss is evident in the posterior and lateral columns of the spinal cord.

DIFFERENTIAL DIAGNOSIS

The differential diagnosis of neurologic symptoms in HIV-infected individuals is extensive. A variety of opportunistic infections and primary CNS lymphomas must be considered. The pathology of vacuolar myelopathy is similar, if not identical to that seen in subacute combined degeneration secondary to vitamin B_{12} deficiency, and although serum vitamin B_{12} levels are normal in patients with vacuolar myelopathy, there is some evidence to suggest that alterations in metabolic pathways involving this vitamin may play a role in the pathogenesis of vacuolar myelopathy.

PROGNOSIS AND THERAPY

HAART has changed the course of neurologic complications in HIV-infected patients. The most dramatic benefit of HAART is a restored immune system, and opportunistic infections are now decreasing in incidence. This therapy has had less of an effect on HIV-associated cognitive disorders, which remain an important source of morbidity in this patient population. The prognosis for these patients remains poor, and most survive for less than 1 year after diagnosis.

TROPICAL SPASTIC PARAPARESIS

CLINICAL FEATURES

Tropical spastic paraparesis, also known as HTLV-1–associated myelopathy, is a rare disorder caused by the human retrovirus HTLV-1. This virus is endemic in southern Japan, the Caribbean, Africa, and South America, where as many as 30% of the population may harbor the virus. HTLV-1 is best known for causing an aggressive T-cell leukemia, but a paralytic disease develops in about 0.25% of those infected. This disorder, which develops months to years after infection, is

---

TROPICAL SPASTIC PARAPARESIS—FACT SHEET

Definition
▶ A paralytic infection caused by the retrovirus HTLV-1

Clinical Features
▶ Endemic in parts of Japan, the Caribbean, Africa, and South America
▶ Slowly progressive spastic weakness, sensory disturbances, and difficulties with bladder control

Prognosis and Treatment
▶ Immunosuppressive therapy is helpful in some cases
▶ Progressive impairment in most patients

TROPICAL SPASTIC PARAPARESIS—PATHOLOGIC FEATURES

Gross Findings
▶ Thickened spinal meninges
▶ Atrophy of the spinal cord

Microscopic Findings
▶ Perivascular lymphocytic inflammation and microglial nodules affecting the gray and white matter

Differential Diagnosis
▶ Other viral infections

---

characterized clinically by slowly progressive spastic weakness of the lower limbs, sensory disturbances, and difficulties with bladder control. HTLV-1 may also cause an inflammatory myopathy similar to polymyositis.

PATHOLOGIC FEATURES

GROSS FINDINGS

Grossly, the spinal meninges may be thickened, and atrophy of the spinal cord may be seen. These changes are generally most prominent at the thoracic and lumbar levels.

MICROSCOPIC FINDINGS

Both gray and white matter are affected in tropical spastic paraparesis. Perivascular chronic inflammation and microglial nodules are typical. The inflammatory infiltrate consists predominantly of T cells and may involve the meninges and proximal nerve roots.

DIFFERENTIAL DIAGNOSIS

The pathologic features of tropical spastic paraparesis are nonspecific and similar to those seen in other viral infections of the CNS.

PROGNOSIS AND THERAPY

Some patients with this disease improve with immunosuppressive therapy; however, tropical spastic paraparesis is a progressive disease, and most patients are wheelchair bound within 10 years.

OTHER VIRAL INFECTIONS

Other members of the herpesvirus family that may affect the CNS include Epstein-Barr virus (EBV) and human herpes virus type 6 (HHV-6). EBV may rarely cause meningitis, encephalitis, or cranial neuritis, but it is better known as a pathogenic factor in the development of primary CNS lymphomas in immunosuppressed patients. HHV-6 causes exanthem subitum (roseola or sixth disease) in immunocompetent children and may rarely cause meningoencephalitis with gray and white matter necrosis or demyelination in immunosuppressed patients.

Encephalitis is a rare complication of adenovirus infection and occurs predominantly in immunosuppressed patients. There are few reports of the neuropathologic findings in this condition; however, basophilic intranuclear inclusions similar to those seen in other organ systems have been described.

In addition to causing subacute sclerosing panencephalitis, the measles virus is also responsible for a rare form of encephalitis termed measles inclusion body encephalitis, in which many neurons and some glial cells contain nuclear and cytoplasmic eosinophilic inclusions. Other paramyxoviruses that may have rare CNS manifestations include the mumps virus, which may cause aseptic meningitis or transverse myelitis, and the Hendra and Nipah viruses.

Congenital rubella infection has largely been eliminated by effective vaccination programs, but it does occur rarely. The most common neurologic abnormalities are sensorineural deafness and encephalitis. Mineralization of vessels in the deep gray nuclei and white matter has been described. A panencephalitis (progressive rubella panencephalitis) similar to subacute sclerosing panencephalitis may also occur.

PARASITIC INFECTIONS

TOXOPLASMOSIS

Toxoplasmosis is a worldwide infection caused by the intracellular protozoan *Toxoplasma gondii*. The definitive host for this parasite is the cat; humans become infected by ingesting mature oocysts passed by cats in their feces or cysts in the meat of infected animals, by receiving blood from a person with active infection, or in the womb by passage of organisms from an acutely infected mother. Infection of the CNS usually develops by reactivation of a previously acquired primary infection.

CLINICAL FEATURES

In immunocompetent hosts, *T. gondii* typically produces subclinical infection. Some patients may have nonspecific symptoms, including lymphadenitis, fever, malaise, and weight loss. In immunocompromised individuals, particularly those with AIDS, the usual findings are those of encephalitis. Commonly encountered symp-

---

TOXOPLASMOSIS—FACT SHEET

Definition
▶ An infection caused by the protozoan *Toxoplasma gondii*

Clinical Features
▶ Occurs most commonly in immunocompromised patients and as a congenital infection
▶ Symptoms are nonspecific

Radiologic Features
▶ Contrast-enhancing lesions surrounded by edema

Prognosis and Treatment
▶ Treated with a combination of pyrimethamine and sulfonamide

---

toms include headache, disorientation, and drowsiness. Large lesions may produce symptoms due to mass effect.

The manifestations of in utero infection depend on the time at which the parasite is acquired during gestation. Infection early in pregnancy leads to abortion of the fetus. Infections acquired later in the gestational period produce stigmata of chronic infection in the fetus. Most infants are born prematurely and frequently die within 1 or 2 years.

RADIOLOGIC FEATURES

The lesions of toxoplasmosis are typically contrast enhancing and surrounded by a variable amount of edema. In affected neonates, paraventricular calcification is typical.

PATHOLOGIC FEATURES

GROSS FINDINGS

The brain lesions in toxoplasmosis are typically necrotic and may have areas of hemorrhage (Fig. 7-43).

TOXOPLASMOSIS—PATHOLOGIC FEATURES

Gross Findings
▶ Necrotic, focally hemorrhagic lesions

Microscopic Findings
▶ Coagulative necrosis with variable inflammation
▶ Encysted bradyzoites and free tachyzoites at the periphery of the lesion

Differential Diagnosis
▶ CNS lymphoma
▶ Other causes of brain abscesses

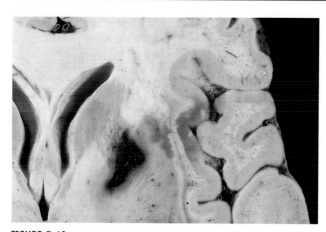

FIGURE 7-43

Toxoplasmosis. In immunosuppressed patients, toxoplasmosis produces mass lesions with necrotic centers.

MICROSCOPIC FINDINGS

Histologically, CNS lesions are composed of discrete areas of coagulative necrosis with prominent necrotic blood vessels. The inflammatory response is variable and may consist of both acute and chronic inflammatory cells. The degree of inflammation depends in part on the degree of immunosuppression. Organisms are characteristically located at the periphery of the lesion. The parasites may be free in tissue (tachyzoites) or may be present as collections of encysted, basophilic organisms (bradyzoites) (Fig. 7-44).

ANCILLARY STUDIES

Both bradyzoites and tachyzoites may be identified by electron microscopy. The tachyzoite forms have an apical complex of organelles. Immunohistochemistry is useful in identifying the tachyzoite forms of the organism. The encysted bradyzoites also stain with antibodies directed against *T. gondii* antigens.

DIFFERENTIAL DIAGNOSIS

The differential diagnosis of cerebral toxoplasmosis includes other causes of focal or mass lesions in immunocompromised patients. Most commonly, toxoplasmosis is confused clinically with primary CNS lymphomas. Other infections causing brain abscesses should also be included in the differential diagnosis.

PROGNOSIS AND THERAPY

Toxoplasmosis is a treatable infection, and prophylactic therapy with a combination of pyrimethamine and sulfonamide is often used in immunocompromised patients. Clindamycin is an alternative choice. Lifelong therapy is needed.

CEREBRAL AMEBIASIS

CLINICAL FEATURES

Despite rare examples of cerebral involvement in *Entamoeba histolytica* infections, most cases of CNS amebiasis result from infection by the free-living amebas *Naegleria*, *Acanthamoeba*, and *Balamuthia*.

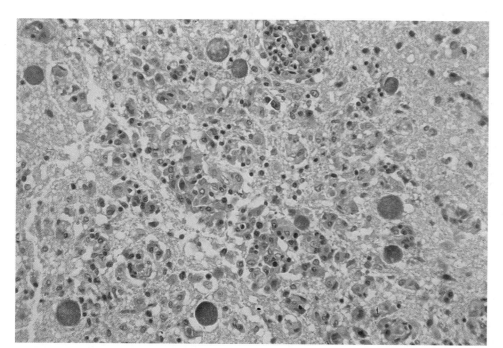

FIGURE 7-44

Toxoplasmosis. The encysted forms of the organism (bradyzoites) are easily identifiable in tissue sections and are typically found at the periphery of the lesion.

Infection by *Naegleria fowleri* is the cause of primary amebic meningoencephalitis (PAM). The infection is acquired by exposure to polluted water in ponds, swimming pools, and man-made lakes, and the typical victims are children and young adults who have been swimming and diving during the hot summer months. The clinical course of PAM is rapid, and the disease is characterized by severe frontal headaches, nausea, vomiting, and a stiff neck followed by coma.

Acanthamoeba species and *Balamuthia mandrillaris* produce an opportunistic infection referred to as granulomatous amebic encephalitis (GAE). This disorder is typically seen in the setting of chronic alcoholism, pregnancy, HIV/AIDS, systemic lupus erythematosus, or bone marrow suppression secondary to chemotherapy. GAE is a chronic, clinically protracted illness characterized by headache, personality changes, slight fever, seizures, hemiparesis, cranial nerve palsies, and depressed levels of consciousness and coma. Species of *Acanthamoeba* may also produce a vision-threatening keratitis in contact lens wearers using homemade cleaning solutions.

PATHOLOGIC FEATURES

GROSS FINDINGS

Brains from patients with PAM are edematous and congested. The olfactory bulbs and orbitofrontal cortices are hemorrhagic and necrotic. The cerebral hemispheres are also edematous in GAE, and the leptomeninges contain a purulent exudate. Multiple foci of softening and necrosis are present throughout the cerebrum, cerebellum, and brain stem.

MICROSCOPIC FINDINGS

In PAM there is a scant fibrinopurulent exudate, and amebic trophozoites are found around blood vessels within the Virchow-Robin spaces. No cyst forms are present. In GAE, both trophozoites and cysts may be seen within necrotic cerebral tissue (Fig. 7-45). Chronic inflammation, which may or may not be granulomatous, is characteristic.

ANCILLARY STUDIES

In PAM, motile amebic trophozoites can be observed moving in CSF when one or two drops of unstained CSF are placed on a glass slide, which is then topped with a coverslip and examined under low magnification with a lowered diaphragm or darkfield illumination.

DIFFERENTIAL DIAGNOSIS

Amebic trophozoites may be easily mistaken for macrophages. They may be recognized as organisms by the presence of a prominent karyosome.

PROGNOSIS AND THERAPY

PAM is a rapidly fatal illness; only a few patients have been reported to survive. Proper disinfection of the water in swimming pools with chlorine is useful in preventing the disease. There is also no effective therapy for GAE at the present time. Amebic keratitis may be prevented by using proper cleaning solutions.

CEREBRAL MALARIA

CLINICAL FEATURES

Malaria remains a major health care problem in many parts of the world. The most important complication

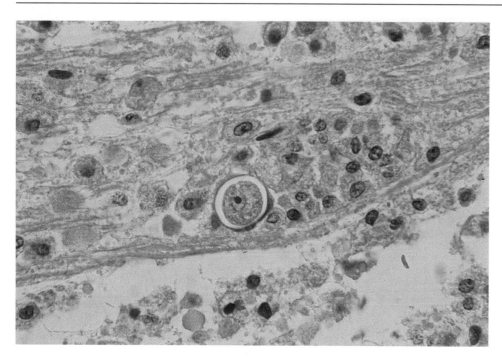

FIGURE 7-45
Granulomatous amebic meningoen-cephalitis. Amebic cysts resembling macrophages are typically perivascular in location.

CEREBRAL MALARIA—FACT SHEET

Definition
▶ Involvement of the CNS in *Plasmodium falciparum* infection

Clinical Features
▶ Diffuse encephalopathy

Prognosis and Treatment
▶ Mortality rate of 30% to 50%
▶ Permanent neurologic impairment in 10%

CEREBRAL MALARIA—PATHOLOGIC FEATURES

Gross Findings
▶ Petechial hemorrhages in white matter

Microscopic Findings
▶ Petechial hemorrhages
▶ Sequestered red blood cells in the microvasculature with deposition of pigment
▶ Dürck's granuloma

Ancillary Studies
▶ Peripheral blood smear examination

---

of severe disease is cerebral malaria, which is seen in infections with *Plasmodium falciparum*. This disorder is a diffuse encephalopathy associated with seizures and loss of consciousness. Few localizing signs are present in most patients.

PATHOLOGIC FEATURES

GROSS FINDINGS

The most consistent gross finding in patients dying of cerebral malaria is the presence of petechial hemorrhages, which are usually most prominent in the white matter. There is generally minimal associated edema.

MICROSCOPIC FINDINGS

In addition to petechial hemorrhages, one typically sees parasitized erythrocytes sequestered within cerebral microvessels (Fig. 7-46). Deposition of pigment, the granules of which are smaller and darker than formalin

pigment, occurs in the lining of blood vessels. A proliferation of microglia, astrocytes, and lymphocytes, termed Dürck's granuloma, may be seen in some cases and is thought to represent a region of healed hemorrhage.

ANCILLARY STUDIES

Most cases of malaria are diagnosed on the basis of examination of peripheral blood smears.

PROGNOSIS AND TREATMENT

Cerebral malaria generally has a poor prognosis, with a mortality rate of 30% to 50% even with appropriate treatment and support. Up to 10% of those who recover suffer some sort of permanent neurologic impairment.

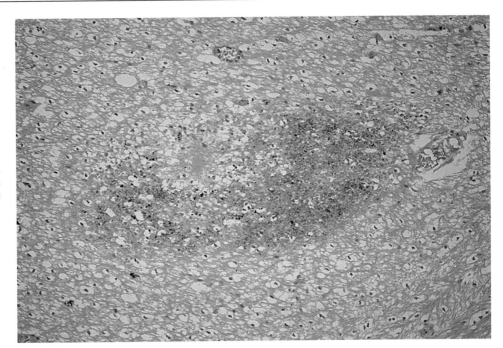

FIGURE 7-46
Cerebral malaria. Petechial hemorrhages associated with the deposition of malarial pigment are seen in this infection.

NEUROCYSTICERCOSIS

CLINICAL FEATURES

Neurocysticercosis is caused by *Taenia solium* larvae, which develop after the ingestion of eggs excreted in human feces and is the most frequent human neuroparasitosis. It is endemic in many parts of the world, and in the United States it is most commonly seen in the southwest. Neurocysticercosis may occur at any age, and it affects males slightly more frequently than females. Seizures are the most common clinical mani-

festation, and in endemic regions, cysticercosis is one of the major causes of late-onset epilepsy.

RADIOLOGIC FEATURES

MRI reveals a wide spectrum of lesions that may affect the meninges, brain tissue, and/or ventricular system. Small lesions with a contrast-enhancing rim and internal point of enhancement are characteristic.

PATHOLOGIC FEATURES

GROSS FINDINGS

The lesions of neurocysticercosis are characteristically cystic and have thin, translucent, membranous walls (Fig. 7-47). The cysts are filled with clear fluid and may contain a pearly white, invaginated scolex. They

---

NEUROCYSTICERCOSIS—FACT SHEET

Definition
► An infection of the CNS caused by the ingestion of *Taenia solium* eggs

Clinical Features
► Most commonly seen in the southwestern United States
► Seizures

Radiographic Features
► Lesions may affect the meninges, brain tissue, or ventricular system
► Rim-enhancing cysts

Prognosis and Treatment
► Drug therapy plus steroids
► Surgery in selected cases

NEUROCYSTICERCOSIS—PATHOLOGIC FEATURES

Gross Findings
► Cysts with thin, translucent, membranous walls

Microscopic Findings
► Cysts have three layers—cuticular, cellular, and reticular
► A scolex may be present
► Variable chronic inflammatory response

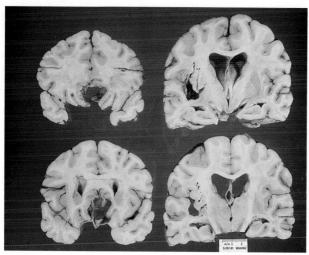

FIGURE 7-47

Neurocysticercosis. In this case, cysts may be identified at the base of the frontal lobe and within the septum pellucidum.

may be seen within brain tissue, in the leptomeninges, or within the ventricular system.

MICROSCOPIC FINDINGS

The cyst wall has three layers: an outer or eosinophilic cuticular layer that has a smooth contour beneath which are bundles of muscle fibers, a middle cellular layer with dark-staining nuclei, and an inner reticular layer containing loosely arranged fibrils, excretory canaliculi, and calcareous corpuscles (Fig. 7-48). In favorable sections one may also see suckers and a rostellum armed with hooklets. Degenerating organisms elicit an acute and chronic inflammatory response.

PROGNOSIS AND THERAPY

The severity of neurocysticercosis depends on the number and location of organisms. Albendazole is an effective agent; however, dead organisms release antigens that may enhance the inflammatory response and produce more symptoms. Therefore, the concomitant use of steroids with drug therapy is recommended. In some cases, surgical intervention is preferable to drug therapy.

NEUROSCHISTOSOMIASIS

CLINICAL FEATURES

Schistosomiasis is an infection caused by trematodes of the genus *Schistosoma*. *S. haematobium*, *S. japonicum*, and *S. mansoni* are the most important to humans and the most widely distributed. Schistosomes may reach the CNS at any time from the moment that the worms have matured and their eggs have been laid; for this reason, neuroschistosomiasis may be observed with any of the clinical forms of schistosomal infection. In situ egg deposition follows the anomalous migration of adult worms in rare cases; in most instances the eggs embolize to the brain and spinal cord from the portal mesenteric system.

Cerebral involvement in schistosomiasis occurs most commonly with *S. japonicum* infection. Most patients are men between 20 and 40 years of age. Signs and symptoms of increased intracranial pressure and focal neurologic deficits, including seizures accompanied by loss of consciousness, headache, visual abnormalities,

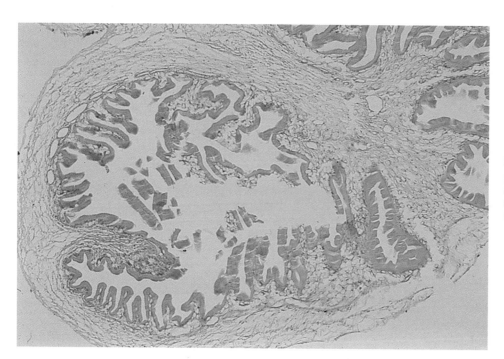

FIGURE 7-48

Neurocysticercosis. Organisms are easy to identify and are composed of an eosinophilic, wavy cyst wall with underlying stroma.

NEUROSCHISTOSOMIASIS—FACT SHEET

Definition
▶ A CNS infection caused by trematodes of the genus *Schistosoma*

Gender and Age Distribution
▶ Males most commonly affected
▶ Adult patients between 20 and 40 years of age

Clinical Features
▶ *S. japonicum*: increased intracranial pressure and focal neurologic deficits
▶ *S. mansoni*: transverse myelitis

Prognosis and Treatment
▶ Most cases are asymptomatic
▶ Oxamniquine and praziquantel

PATHOLOGIC FEATURES

GROSS FINDINGS

The macroscopic changes in neuroschistosomiasis consist of a conglomerate of yellow-white nodules that vary in size and are well defined. Small foci of necrosis are typically seen.

MICROSCOPIC FINDINGS

As in other organs affected by schistosomal infection, the periovular inflammatory response is typically granulomatous (Fig. 7-49). Schistosomal eggs may be seen in inflamed areas or be unassociated with inflammation.

sensory disturbances, papilledema, hemiparesis, and dysphasia, are typical and vary according to the site of the cerebral lesions. Spinal cord involvement in the form of a rapidly progressive transverse myelitis may occur with *S. mansoni* infection and typically affects the lumbosacral segments of the spinal cord. Nonspecific changes of hepatic encephalopathy may also occur in patients with schistosomiasis and are attributable to portal hypertension.

Radiologic findings in neuroschistosomiasis are nonspecific, and laboratory evaluations are of little help in establishing the diagnosis.

NEUROSCHISTOSOMIASIS—PATHOLOGIC FEATURES

Gross Findings
▶ Multiple well-defined, yellow-white nodules

Microscopic Findings
▶ Granulomatous inflammation
▶ Eggs apart from and within inflamed areas

Differential Diagnosis
▶ Other causes of granulomatous inflammation

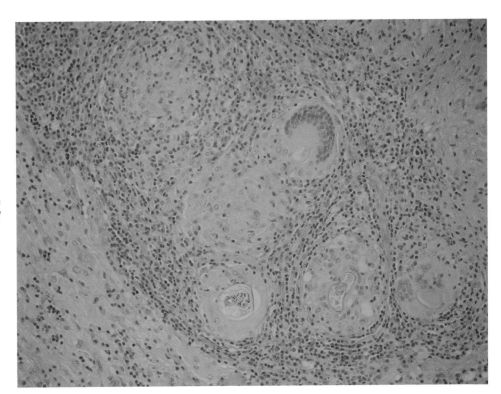

FIGURE 7-49

Neuroschistosomiasis. The eggs in schistosomiasis are surrounded by granulomatous inflammation.

DIFFERENTIAL DIAGNOSIS

The differential diagnosis of neuroschistosomiasis encompasses other causes of granulomatous inflammation, including other infectious processes, sarcoidosis, and vasculitis.

PROGNOSIS AND THERAPY

Most cases of neuroschistosomiasis are probably asymptomatic and overshadowed by systemic symptoms. Treatment is the same as for systemic disease (oxamniquine and praziquantel). Corticosteroids may be added in patients with severe edema and mass effect.

TRYPANOSOMIASIS

CLINICAL FEATURES

African trypanosomiasis (sleeping sickness) is endemic in sub-Saharan Africa. It is transmitted by the bite of the tsetse fly and is caused by *Trypanosoma brucei rhodesiense* and *T. brucei gambiense*. In the more severe *T. brucei rhodesiense* infection, involvement of the CNS follows 3 to 4 weeks after infection with the development of a primary chancre and is characterized by diffuse meningoencephalitis. Common symptoms include indifference, lassitude, and daytime somnolence. Electroencephalographic (EEG) studies show profound abnormalities. *T. brucei gambiense* infections result in subacute or chronic meningoencephalitis.

TRYPANOSOMIASIS—FACT SHEET

Definition
▶ A group of disorders (African and American forms) caused by protozoa of the family Trypanosomatidae

Incidence and Location
▶ African trypanosomiasis: occurs in African countries situated below the Saharan belt
▶ American trypanosomiasis (Chagas' disease): endemic in South America

Gender and Age Distribution
▶ Chagas' disease: usually acquired during childhood

Clinical Features
▶ African trypanosomiasis: indifference, lassitude, and daytime somnolence
▶ Chagas' disease: encephalitis acutely and megaviscera chronically

Prognosis and Treatment
▶ African trypanosomiasis: melarsoprol
▶ Chagas' disease: multiple antiparasitic agents

American trypanosomiasis (Chagas' disease) is endemic in parts of Latin America. It is transmitted by reduviid bugs and caused by *Trypanosoma cruzi*. This form of trypanosomiasis is usually acquired during childhood and has acute and chronic forms. The acute form of the illness is often asymptomatic; however, a severe illness characterized by encephalitis and myocarditis develops in a small percentage of patients. Involvement of the autonomic peripheral nervous system resulting in digestive megaviscera is typical of the chronic form.

PATHOLOGIC FEATURES

GROSS FINDINGS

In African trypanosomiasis, macroscopic changes may be scanty. The leptomeninges may appear opaque, particularly at the base of the brain, and the brain is typically swollen and congested. In the American form, the changes are similar, but with the addition of petechial hemorrhages.

MICROSCOPIC FINDINGS

The histologic features of African trypanosomiasis are those of diffuse meningoencephalitis with a prominent perivascular chronic inflammatory infiltrate. Microglial nodules may also be present. Plasma cells with small peripheral nuclei and cytoplasm filled with Russell bodies, the so-called morular or Mott cells, are characteristic (Fig. 7-50). Trypanosomes are not usually identifiable.

Chagas' disease is characterized by microglial nodules associated with amastigote forms of the parasite, which are often seen within the cytoplasm of glial cells. Macrophages, endothelial cells, and neurons may also contain organisms. Cerebral infarcts may occur secondary to associated cardiac disease with accompanying thromboembolism.

TRYPANOSOMIASIS—PATHOLOGIC FEATURES

Gross Findings
▶ Cerebral edema and congestion

Microscopic Findings
▶ African trypanosomiasis: diffuse meningoencephalitis with morular/Mott cells, no organisms
▶ Chagas' disease: microglial nodules with amastigotes in glial cells

Ancillary Studies
▶ Peripheral blood or CSF examination for trypomastigotes

Differential Diagnosis
▶ Histoplasmosis, toxoplasmosis

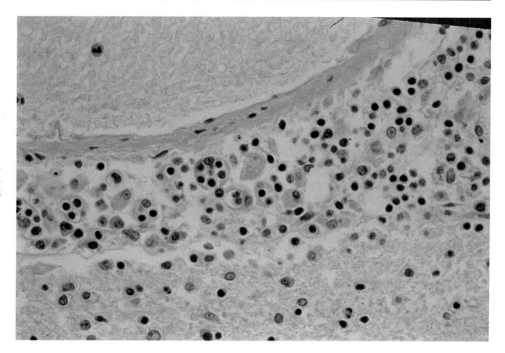

FIGURE 7-50

African trypanosomiasis. A perivascular inflammatory infiltrate composed predominantly of plasma cells is characteristic of this infection.

ANCILLARY STUDIES

Both forms of trypanosomiasis may be diagnosed by identifying the causative organisms (trypomastigotes) in peripheral blood smears. Rarely, trypanosomes may be identified in CSF.

DIFFERENTIAL DIAGNOSIS

The amastigote forms of *T. cruzi* must be distinguished from other intracellular organisms of similar size, including *Histoplasma capsulatum* and *Toxoplasma gondii*.

PROGNOSIS AND THERAPY

CNS involvement by African sleeping sickness is treated with melarsoprol. This drug is very toxic, and corticosteroids are usually given to reduce the likelihood of melarsoprol-induced encephalopathy.

Treatment of *T. cruzi* infection is more problematic, and there is no single effective treatment. Nifurtimox, benznidazole, itraconazole, and fluconazole may be of value in the acute phase of the disease.

OTHER PARASITIC INFECTIONS

Cerebral echinococcosis results from dissemination of the larvae of the tapeworm *Echinococcus granulosus* and produces hydatid cysts similar to those found in the liver (the usual site of infection in echinococcosis). Other parasitic infections in which the CNS may rarely be involved include sparganosis and paragonimiasis.

SPONGIFORM ENCEPHALOPATHIES

The transmissible spongiform encephalopathies, or prion diseases, are a group of neurodegenerative, uniformly fatal disorders of humans and animals. Human forms include Creutzfeldt-Jakob disease (CJD), Gerstmann-Sträussler-Scheinker disease (GSS), fatal familial insomnia (FFI), kuru, and new-variant CJD (vCJD). Common to all is the accumulation of an abnormally aggregated and protease-resistant form of the mammalian prion protein (PrP). Most cases are sporadic, although familial and iatrogenic examples are well recognized.

CLINICAL FEATURES

CJD is the most common of the spongiform encephalopathies and occurs worldwide with an incidence of approximately one case per million population per year. Most cases are sporadic and occur in patients between 50 and 70 years of age. The typical clinical course is that of a rapidly progressive dementia. Other common symptoms include myoclonus, particularly startle myoclonus, visual or cerebellar disturbances, pyramidal dysfunction, and akinetic mutism. Periodic sharp wave complexes on EEG testing are characteristic, and elevated levels of protein 14-3-3 in CSF may be useful in supporting the clinical diagnosis. Approximately 10% to 15% of cases are familial with an autosomal dominant pattern of inheritance; these cases are due to mutations, deletions, or insertions in the PrP gene located on the short arm of chromosome 20. Iatrogenic transmission via contaminated neurosurgical instruments or contaminated dural grafts, corneal trans-

SPONGIFORM ENCEPHALOPATHIES—FACT SHEET

Definition
▶ A group of fatal neurodegenerative disorders caused by the accumulation of protease-resistant prion protein

Incidence and Location
▶ One case per million population per year
▶ New-variant Creutzfeldt-Jakob disease (vCJD) most common in the United Kingdom

Gender and Age Distribution
▶ Sporadic forms in patients between 50 and 70 years of age
▶ Hereditary and iatrogenic forms affect younger patients

Clinical Features
▶ Rapidly progressive dementia with myoclonus, visual/cerebellar disturbances, pyramidal signs, and akinetic mutism
▶ Periodic sharp wave complexes on electroencephalography
▶ Elevated protein 14-3-3 in CSF
▶ Gerstmann-Sträussler-Scheinker (GSS) disease: autosomal dominant inheritance with cerebellar ataxia
▶ Fatal familial insomnia (FFI): autosomal dominant inheritance with progressive insomnia
▶ vCJD: younger patients with early psychiatric symptoms

Prognosis and Treatment
▶ Uniformly fatal
▶ No known therapy

plants, or human pituitary hormone injections has been documented in more than 100 cases.

GSS is an autosomal dominant illness characterized by severe cerebellar ataxia and spastic paraparesis. Dementia develops late in the course of the disease, which is typically more prolonged than that of CJD. FFI also exhibits an autosomal dominant pattern of inheritance. This illness is characterized by progressive insomnia, dysautonomia, and dementia. Kuru is a disorder confined to the Fore tribe of New Guinea and is thought to be transmitted via ritualistic cannibalism. This disease is largely extinct; occasional new cases are thought to be related to the long incubation period for the disease. vCJD, first reported in the United Kingdom, is a recently identified variant of CJD believed to be due to the transmission of an animal prion disease, bovine spongiform encephalopathy, to humans. Patients with vCJD are younger than those with the sporadic form, typically have more prominent early psychiatric and behavioral symptoms, and often fail to demonstrate typical EEG changes.

RADIOGRAPHIC FEATURES

Radiographic studies are of limited value in the diagnosis of prion diseases, although increased signal in the basal ganglia on T2-weighted and proton-density MRI is characteristic. In cases of vCJD, increased signal is seen in the pulvinar.

PATHOLOGIC FEATURES

GROSS FINDINGS

Grossly, there is little to distinguish the spongiform encephalopathies from other neurodegenerative disorders. Brains from these patients are either grossly normal or exhibit mild, diffuse atrophy.

MICROSCOPIC FINDINGS

The spongiform encephalopathies are characterized by the histologic triad of neuronal loss, gliosis, and spongiform change (Fig. 7-51). Amyloid plaques, referred to as kuru plaques (Fig. 7-52), are found in about 10% of cases of sporadic CJD. In GSS, one sees multicentric plaques composed of a dense core of amyloid surrounded by smaller globules of amyloid. They are most numerous in the molecular layer of the cerebellum. In vCJD, the so-called florid plaque, which consists of an amyloid core surrounded by a halo of spongiform change, is a distinguishing finding. FFI is characterized by severe neuronal loss and gliosis in thalamic nuclei; spongiform change and amyloid plaques are not easily identified.

ANCILLARY STUDIES

Monoclonal antibodies directed against PrP have been developed and are useful in confirming the diagnosis of a prion disorder. One characteristically sees a granular staining pattern in areas of spongiform change; kuru plaques, when present, are also positive.

SPONGIFORM ENCEPHALOPATHIES—PATHOLOGIC FEATURES

Gross Findings
▶ Mild, diffuse atrophy

Microscopic Findings
▶ Neuronal loss, gliosis, spongiform change, and amyloid (kuru) plaques
▶ Florid plaques in vCJD

Genetics
▶ Mutations, deletions, or insertions in the PrP gene (chromosome 20)

Differential Diagnosis
▶ Vacuolation as a result of edema or artifact
▶ Status spongiosis

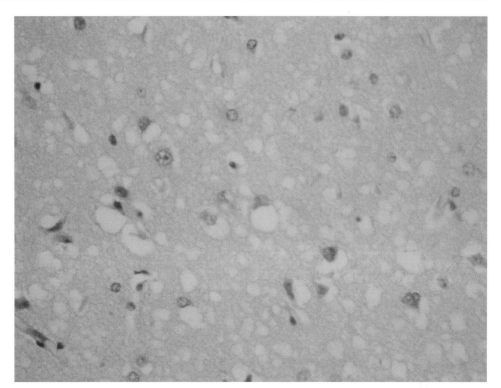

FIGURE 7-51

Spongiform encephalopathies. The spongiform encephalopathies are characterized by the histologic triad of neuronal loss, gliosis, and spongiform change.

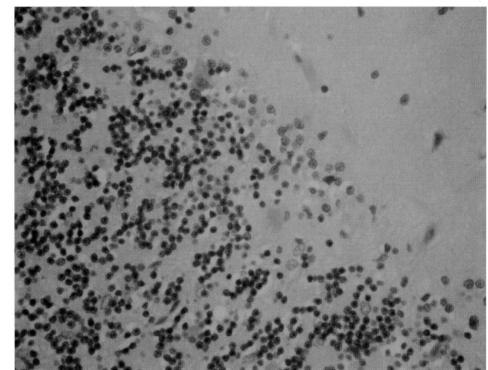

FIGURE 7-52

Creutzfeldt-Jakob disease: kuru plaques. Amyloid plaques are seen in approximately 10% of cases of CJD and are seen here in the cerebellum.

Confirmation of the presence of PrP by Western blotting is at the present time considered to be the gold standard for the pathologic diagnosis of prion disorders. In vCJD, PrP has been identified in tonsillar tissue, and biopsy of the tonsils has been suggested by some as a diagnostic procedure for this variant.

DIFFERENTIAL DIAGNOSIS

From a histologic standpoint, the differential diagnosis of spongiform encephalopathies includes vacuolation of brain tissue as a result of edema or as an artifactual change, as well as "status spongiosis," which is characterized by extensive neuronal loss, gliosis, and pericellular vacuoles secondary to cell shrinkage and is seen as an end-stage process in a number of other neurodegenerative disorders. The vacuoles in true spongiform change are within the neuropil and sometimes within neurons rather than pericellular in location.

PROGNOSIS AND THERAPY

Unfortunately, the spongiform encephalopathies are uniformly fatal. In sporadic CJD, the mean survival time is 5 months. There is currently no useful therapy; studies are under way to identify compounds that may inhibit PrP formation and/or aggregation.

SUGGESTED READINGS

Bacterial Infections

Bross JE, Gordon G: Nocardial meningitis: Case reports and review. Rev Infect Dis 1991;13:160-165.

Calfee DP, Wispelwey B: Brain abscess. Semin Neurol 2000;20:353-360.

Gray F: Bacterial infections. Brain Pathol 1997;7:629-647.

Gyure KA, Prayson RA, Estes ML, Hall GS: Symptomatic *Mycobacterium avium* complex infection of the central nervous system: A case report and review of the literature. Arch Pathol Lab Med 1995;119:836-839.

Morrison A, Gyure KA, Stone J, et al: Mycobacterial spindle cell pseudotumor of the brain: A case report and review of the literature. Am J Surg Pathol 1999;23:1294-1299.

Nachmann SA, Pontrelli L: Central nervous system Lyme disease. Semin Pediatr Infect Dis 2003;14:123-130.

Rosenstein NE, Perkins BA, Stephens DS, et al: Meningococcal disease. N Engl J Med 2001;344:1378-1388.

Scheld WM: Whipple disease of the central nervous system. J Infect Dis 2003;188:797-800.

Smego RA Jr: Actinomycosis of the central nervous system. Rev Infect Dis 1987;9:855-865.

Fungal Infections

Chimelli L, Mahler-Araújo MB: Fungal infections. Brain Pathol 1997;7:613-627.

Gottfredsson M, Perfect JR: Fungal meningitis. Semin Neurol 2000;20:307-322.

Kleinschmidt-Demasters BK: Central nervous system aspergillosis: A 20-year retrospective series. Hum Pathol 2002;33:116-124.

Lee SC, Dickson DW, Casadevall A: Pathology of cryptococcal meningoencephalitis: Analysis of 27 patients with pathogenetic implications. Hum Pathol 1996;27:839-847.

Mischel PS, Vinters HV: Coccidioidomycosis of the central nervous system: Neuropathological and vasculopathic manifestations and clinical correlates. Clin Infect Dis 1995;20:400-405.

Sanchez-Portocarrero J, Perez-Cecilia E, Corral O, et al: The central nervous system and infection by *Candida* species. Diagn Microbiol Infect Dis 2000;37:169-179.

Wheat LJ, Batteiger BE, Sathapatayavongs B: *Histoplasma capsulatum* infections of the central nervous system. A clinical review. Medicine (Baltimore) 1990;69:244-260.

Viral Infections

Arribas JR, Storch GA, Clifford DB, Tselis AC: Cytomegalovirus encephalitis. Ann Intern Med 1996;125:577-587.

Berger JR, Major EO: Progressive multifocal leukoencephalopathy. Semin Neurol 1999;19:193-200.

Esiri MM: Viruses and rickettsiae. Brain Pathol 1997;7:695-709.

Gray F, Keohane C: The neuropathology of HIV infection in the era of highly active antiretroviral therapy (HAART). Brain Pathol 2003;12:79-83.

Kleinschmidt-DeMasters BK, Gilden DH: The expanding spectrum of herpesvirus infections of the nervous system. Brain Pathol 2001;11:440-451.

Kleinschmidt-DeMasters BK, Gilden DH: Varicella-zoster infections of the nervous system: Clinical and pathologic correlates. Arch Pathol Lab Med 2001;125:770-780.

Kling E, Mistler E, Gyure KA: Neuropathologic findings in West Nile virus encephalomyelitis. Pathol Case Rev 2004;9:20-22.

Mrak RE, Young L: Rabies encephalitis in humans: Pathology, pathogenesis and pathophysiology. J Neuropathol Exp Neurol 1994;53:1-10.

Petito CK: Brain pathology in human immunodeficiency virus infection. Pathol Case Rev 2004;9:11-15.

Sharer LR: Pathology of HIV-1 infection of the central nervous system. A review. J Neuropathol Exp Neurol 1992;51:3-11.

Uhlmann EJ, Storch GA: Viral encephalitis. Lab Med 2001;6:317-323.

Parasitic Infections

Chimelli L, Scaravilli F: Trypanosomiasis. Brain Pathol 1997;7:599-611.

Falangola MF, Reichler BS, Petito CK: Histopathology of cerebral toxoplasmosis in human immunodeficiency virus infection: A comparison between patients with early-onset and late-onset acquired immunodeficiency syndrome. Hum Pathol 1994;25:1091-1097.

Martinez AJ, Visvesvara GS: Free-living, amphizoic and opportunistic amebas. Brain Pathol 1997;7:583-598.

Peoc'h MY, Gyure KA, Morrison AL: Postmortem diagnosis of cerebral malaria. Am J Forensic Med Pathol 2000;21:366-369.

Pittella JEH: Neuroschistosomiasis. Brain Pathol 1997;7:649-662.

Pittella JEH: Neurocysticerosis. Brain Pathol 1997;7:681-693.

Turner G: Cerebral malaria. Brain Pathol 1997;7:569-582.

Spongiform Encephalopathies

Castellani RJ: Variant Creutzfeldt-Jakob disease: An overview. Pathol Case Rev 2004;9:16-19.

Kretzschmar HA: Diagnosis of prion diseases. Clin Lab Med 2003;23:109-128.

Johnson RT, Gibbs CJ Jr: Creutzfeldt-Jakob disease and related transmissible spongiform encephalopathies. N Engl J Med 1998;339:1994-2004.

Ward HJT, Head MW, Will RG, Ironside JW: Variant Creutzfeldt-Jakob disease. Clin Lab Med 2003;23:87-108.

Will RG, Ironside JW, Zeidler M, et al: A new variant of Creutzfeldt-Jakob disease in the UK. Lancet 1996;347:921-925.

8 Metabolic and Toxic Disorders
Dimitri P. Agamanolis

LYSOSOMAL STORAGE DISORDERS

Lysosomal storage diseases (LSDs) are rare disorders caused by genetically transmitted lysosomal enzyme deficiencies. The resulting lysosomal accumulation of uncleaved substrates impairs cell function and causes cell death. Although some LSDs have been known for more than 100 years, the concept of lysosomal storage did not crystallize until the 1960s, after lysosomes were discovered by DeDuve and the electron microscope became available. LSDs involve all organ systems but affect the brain and the skeleton most severely. They usually begin early in life and are inexorably progressive, and most are fatal in childhood. For these reasons they are an important problem in genetics, pediatrics, and child neurology.

BIOLOGY OF LYSOSOMES AND LYSOSOMAL ENZYMES

Lysosomes contain enzymes that biodegrade diverse molecules. Lysosomal enzymes are glycoproteins that are active in an acid pH. The enzymes are produced in the endoplasmic reticulum and are brought into lysosomes by means of a specific receptor-mediated mechanism. Most lysosomal enzymes cleave sugar chains that are attached to glycolipids, glycoproteins, and other compounds.

Primary lysosomes are round to oval organelles measuring 0.2 to 0.8 µm. They have a phospholipid bilayer membrane and contain 40 or so enzymes (phosphatases, nucleases, glycosidases, proteases, peptidases, sulfatases, phospholipases) that are active near pH 4.5. The acid environment is maintained by proton pumps in the lysosomal membrane. These enzymes are capable of hydrolyzing most biomolecules (mostly damaged or nonfunctional compounds) produced by cells or brought into cells by endocytosis. They obtain their substrates by merging with endosomes, phagosomes, and autophagosomes.

Lysosomal enzymes are glycoproteins. They are synthesized in the rough endoplasmic reticulum and glycosylated in the smooth endoplasmic reticulum. As they travel through the Golgi, they have a mannose-6-phosphate (M6P) molecule attached to them. By binding to complementary M6P receptors located on the Golgi membrane, the M6P marker enables lysosomal enzymes to home into parts of the Golgi that bud off to form lysosomes. The M6P marker also helps internalize lysosomal enzymes from the extracellular space, including those administered for treatment. Attachment of M6P to the lysosomal enzyme protein is catalyzed by the sequential action of N-acetylglucosamine (GlcNAc) phosphotransferase, which adds N-acetylglucosamine-1-phosphate to the mannose residue on the lysosomal enzyme, and α-N-acetylglucosaminidase, which removes the acetylglucosamine to expose the M6P marker. Two lysosomal enzymes, glucocerebrosidase and acid phosphatase, are located in the lysosomal membrane and do not require the M6P marker. Proteolytic processing and other modifications, which begin in the prelysosomal compartments and end when the enzymes are in the lysosomes, trim and modify the lysosomal enzyme proteins, stabilize their molecules, and protect them from internal proteolytic digestion.

Most enzymes that are involved in LSDs cleave sugar chains that are attached to glycoproteins (glycoproteinoses) and glycolipids (sphingolipidoses), disaccharide chains of glycosaminoglycans (mucopolysaccharidoses), and glycogen (Pompe's disease). Farber's disease and Wolman's disease are the only LSDs in which the catalytic action of the respective enzymes is directed against lipid molecules. Some of the neuronal ceroid lipofuscinoses are thought to be caused by defects involving proteases.

MECHANISMS OF LYSOSOMAL ENZYME DEFICIENCY

The most common cause of lysosomal enzyme deficiency is mutation of the gene coding for the lysosomal enzyme. Less frequent causes include failure of addition of the M6P marker, which targets lysosomal proteins to lysosomes, absence of various cofactors (saposins, "protective" protein, GM_2 activator), errors in post-translational modification of enzyme proteins, defects in lysosomal transport, and drug-induced lysosomal dysfunction.

Lysosomal enzymes are encoded by nuclear genes. Most LSDs are due to mutations of these genes that result in absence of the enzyme protein or in a catalytically inactive or unstable polypeptide. Less frequently, enzyme deficiency and storage arise by other mechanisms described later (Table 8-1).

TABLE 8-1

Mechanisms of Lysosomal Enzyme Deficiency

Mutations of lysosomal enzyme genes

No addition of the mannose-6-phosphate marker

Absence of saposins, "protective" protein, GM_2 activator

Errors of post-translational modification

Drug-induced lysosomal dysfunction

Defects in lysosomal transport

Failure of addition of the M6P marker (because of deficiency of GlcNAc) results in an inability to segregate lysosomal enzymes into lysosomes. The enzymes then leak into the cytosol and are inactivated by the slightly alkaline pH, which leads to deficiency of multiple lysosomal enzymes and accumulation of diverse substrates in many cells and organs. GlcNAc deficiency causes I-cell disease, a severe LSD characterized by psychomotor retardation and a Hurler phenotype (see "Mucopolysaccharidoses" later), and a milder variant, pseudo-Hurler polydystrophy. The name of this condition, I (inclusion)-cell disease, describes the storage vacuoles that develop in cultured fibroblasts and in vivo (Fig. 8-1).

Sphingolipid activator proteins (saposins) bind substrate molecules and link up with lysosomal enzymes. In the absence of these activators, substrate is not presented to the lysosomal enzyme. There are four saposins—A, B, C, and D—all derived from a single precursor by different pathways of proteolytic processing. Mutations of all saposins have been described and cause rare variants of GM_2 gangliosidosis, metachromatic leukodystrophy, and Gaucher's disease. Combined deficiency of β-galactosidase and sialidase (galactosialido-sis) is caused by the absence of a "protective" 32-kd lysosomal protein that assembles these two enzymes into a functional complex.

Multiple sulfatase deficiency is characterized by decreased activity of all sulfatases that are coded by different genes. The cause of this LSD is thought to be an error in post-translational modification of sulfatases.

The products of lysosomal degradation are small molecules that either diffuse freely through the lysosomal membrane or are taken out of lysosomes via carrier-mediated transport. Defects in the lysosomal membrane transport system cause sialic acid storage, its milder variant Salla disease, and cystinosis. In cystinosis, birefringent cystine crystals damage the cornea and glomeruli and accumulate in the histiocytes of bone marrow, lymphoid tissue, and other organs (Fig. 8-2). An error in lysosomal transport of cholesterol also causes Niemann-Pick disease type C.

More than 50 drugs and plant chemicals with a cationic amphophilic structure and diverse pharmacologic activity can induce lysosomal storage of phospholipids (myelinoid bodies) and glycoconjugates. Some of these drugs concentrate in lysosomes and, because they are weak bases, inactivate acid hydrolases by raising the pH. Other drugs form complexes with polar lipids that inhibit their degradation or impair lysosomal function by other mechanisms. In most instances, drug-induced lysosomal storage is reversible when use of the offending agent is discontinued.

LYSOSOMAL STORAGE DISORDERS IN GENERAL

PREVALENCE AND GENETICS

The combined prevalence of all LSDs at birth has been estimated to be between 11.1 and 14 per 100,000,

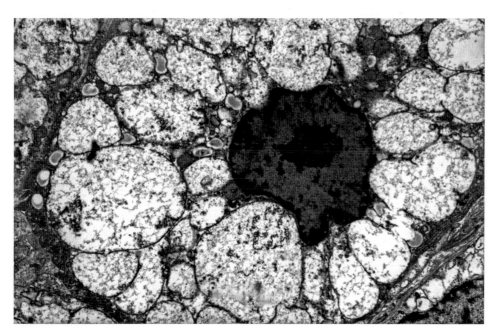

FIGURE 8-1

Vacuoles in fibroblasts in I-cell disease.

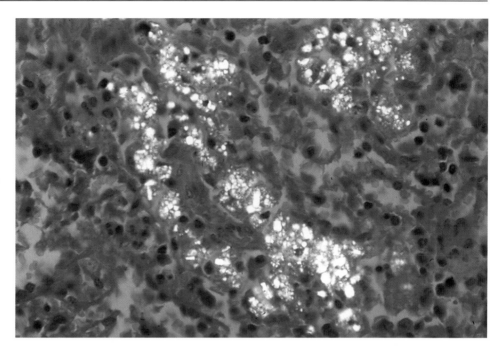

FIGURE 8-2

Cystinosis: birefringent cystine crystals in the kidney.

and that of Gaucher's disease, the single most common LSD, 1.16 to 1.75 per 100,000. The prevalence of the mucopolysaccharidoses, the most common group of LSDs, has been found to be 4.44 per 100,000. There is significant variation in the prevalence of individual LSDs among different ethnic and racial groups (Table 8-2). In the Netherlands, the most common LSD is Pompe's disease (2 per 100,000), and the most frequent group of LSDs is the lipidoses (6.2 per 100,000). Two LSDs, Fabry's disease and Hunter's syndrome, are X-linked recessive. All the rest are autosomal recessive.

CLINICAL PHENOTYPES

Most LSDs cause one of four basic clinical-pathologic phenotypes: neuronal lipidosis, leukodystrophy, storage histiocytosis, and mucopolysaccharidosis (MPS) or the Hurler phenotype. These phenotypes overlap in several LSDs. Some LSDs (Fabry's disease, Niemann-Pick disease type C) exhibit protean manifestations involving many organ systems. Other LSDs (Farber's lipogranulomatosis, Wolman's disease, Pompe's disease) cause distinct clinical and pathologic changes.

The neuronal lipidosis phenotype is caused by lysosomal storage in the neuronal perikaryon. This phenotype is characterized by slowing of psychomotor development, eventual loss of acquired motor and perceptual skills, dementia, myoclonus, epilepsy, visual loss and, ultimately, progression to a vegetative state. The cherry-red spot that is seen in some LSDs with this phenotype is caused by lysosomal storage in the perifoveal ganglion cell layer. Although it is the principal manifestation of GM_1 and GM_2 gangliosidosis and type A and B Niemann-Pick disease, neuronal lipidosis also occurs in type C and D Niemann-Pick disease, the neuronal ceroid lipofuscinoses, the mucopolysacchari-

doses (in which neurons store gangliosides), and most glycoproteinoses.

The leukodystrophy phenotype, seen mainly in metachromatic leukodystrophy and Krabbe's disease, is caused by loss of oligodendrocytes and myelin and is characterized clinically by psychomotor retardation, spasticity, ataxia, visual loss, and demyelinative peripheral neuropathy.

The storage histiocytosis phenotype is caused by lysosomal storage in monocyte-macrophage cells and is characterized by hepatosplenomegaly and occasionally also by hematopoietic and skeletal abnormalities. This phenotype is seen primarily in Gaucher's disease and Niemann-Pick disease.

The MPS phenotype, seen in the mucopolysaccharidoses, glycoproteinoses, and GM_1 gangliosidosis, is due to visceral, soft tissue, and skeletal changes resulting

---

TABLE 8-2

Lysosomal Storage Diseases with a High Incidence in Ethnic Groups

GM_2 gangliosidosis (Tay-Sachs disease): Ashkenazi

Gaucher's disease: Ashkenazi, Sweden (type III neuronopathic)

Aspartylglucosaminuria: Finland

Infantile sialic acid storage and Salla disease: Finland

INCL: Finland

JNCL-INCL: Northern Europe—Scandinavia

Neimann-Pick disease: Nova Scotia

INCL, infantile neuronal ceroid lipofuscinosis; JNCL, juvenile neuronal ceroid lipofuscinosis.

LYSOSOMAL STORAGE DISORDERS IN GENERAL—DISEASE FACTS AND PATHOLOGIC FEATURES

Prevalence and Genetics

▶ Combined prevalence of 11.1 to 14 per 100,000. Two LSDs, Fabry's disease and Hunter's syndrome, are X-linked. All others are autosomal recessive. Certain LSDs such as Gaucher's disease and Tay-Sachs disease are frequent among Ashkenazi Jews and other ethnic groups. Each LSD shows allelic diversity, which accounts for its phenotypic variability

Clinical Phenotypes

▶ Four core clinical-pathologic phenotypes are recognized: neuronal lipidosis, leukodystrophy, storage histiocytosis, and mucopolysaccharidosis

Pathologic Changes

▶ Uncleaved substrate accumulates intracellularly in membrane-bound (lysosomal) compartments. Lamellar products are seen in most sphingolipidoses, and reticulogranular material is observed in the mucopolysaccharidoses. Accumulation of substrate in the extracellular matrix occurs in the mucopolysaccharidoses and other LSDs

Pathogenesis

▶ Cell damage is caused by the mechanical effects of storage. Impaired recycling and toxicity of the stored materials also play a role

Biochemical-Phenotypic Correlation

▶ The phenotype of LSDs depends on which cells and tissues have to function with a defective or absent enzyme

Genotype-Phenotype Correlation

▶ The phenotype of LSDs depends on which cells and tissues use the defective enzyme. Their severity depends on residual enzyme activity, which is determined by the type of mutation. Some mutations abolish all enzymatic activity and therefore result in severe phenotypes. Other mutations leave some residual activity and thus cause milder disease. The multicatalytic function of some lysosomal enzymes causes overlapping phenotypes

Diagnosis

▶ Enzyme assay of leukocytes and other cells is the standard method. Assay of amniocytes and cells obtained by chorionic villus sampling is used for prenatal diagnosis. Urine chromatography can be used as a screening test in some LSDs. Molecular analysis is impractical because of genetic variability. Morphology can contribute to the diagnosis

Therapy

▶ The most promising therapy is enzyme replacement, which has been shown to be effective in Gaucher's disease and is being introduced in Fabry's disease

from lysosomal storage of water-soluble glycoconjugates and consists of coarse facial features, organomegaly, and dysostosis multiplex. The most exaggerated form of these changes is the "Hurler" phenotype (see "Mucopolysaccharidoses" later). Many mucopolysaccharidoses have secondary neuronal lipidosis, which accounts for the central nervous system (CNS) manifestations.

PATHOLOGIC CHANGES

Lysosomal storage distends the cytoplasm. This distention is most impressive when it affects large pyramidal cells (Fig. 8-3). Water-soluble materials are washed out during processing, and a clear or vacuolated cytoplasm is left (Fig. 8-4). Glycolipids have a finely granular or foamy appearance and are sudanophilic and periodic acid–Schiff (PAS) positive. In the sphingolipidoses and other LSDs with neuronal storage, lysosomes also accumulate in axon hillocks and dendrites and cause spherical or torpedo-like swellings (Fig. 8-5). Increased cytoplasmic mass results in organomegaly. Thus, megalencephaly occurs early in the gangliosidoses. However, the end result of the storage is cell death followed by cerebral atrophy and gliosis (Figs. 8-6 and 8-7). These changes are the pathologic substrate of the neuronal lipidosis phenotype. Neuronal lipidosis involves autonomic neurons and retinal ganglion cells. Rectal biopsy with detection of storage in enteric ganglia (Fig. 8-8) was frequently used for the diagnosis of sphingolipidoses before biochemical methods were available. Ganglioside storage in the cellular perifoveal ganglion cell layer creates an opaque yellowish halo that accentuates the red color of the fovea. The fovea appears as a "cherry-red spot" on funduscopic examination.

In metachromatic leukodystrophy and Krabbe's disease, lipid accumulation involves oligodendroglial and Schwann cells. When oligodendroglial cells die, the lipid is picked up by macrophages that accumulate in white matter. Dysfunction and loss of myelin-producing cells causes loss of myelin. These findings are the substrate of the leukodystrophy phenotype. Storage of water-soluble materials in mesenchymal and epithelial cells and in the extracellular matrix correlates with the MPS phenotype, and accumulation in monocyte-macrophage cells is the substrate of the storage histiocytosis phenotype.

The storage material accumulates in membrane-bound (i.e., intralysosomal) particles (Fig. 8-9) that have acid phosphatase activity (Fig. 8-10). Acid phosphatase has been used as a lysosomal marker since the time that lysosomes were discovered by DeDuve. The fine structure of the stored material gives a general idea of its chemical composition but is not specific. In general, sphingolipids assume membranous forms that are arranged concentrically or in parallel stacks (membranous cytoplasmic bodies [MCBs], zebra bodies) (Figs. 8-11 and 8-12). Concentric lamellae are more common in the gangliosidoses and zebra bodies in the mucopolysaccharidoses (in which neurons store gangliosides), but none of these structures are specific for any given type of sphingolipidosis, and they are usually found in various combinations in all of them. Mucopolysaccharides (glycosaminoglycans [GAGs]) are highly soluble in water and are lost in processing, with only clear cells visible by light microscopy and sparse reticulogranular structures by electron microscopy (see Figs. 8-1 and 8-9). Other LSDs with storage of water-soluble compounds have a similar appearance.

Text continued on p. 347

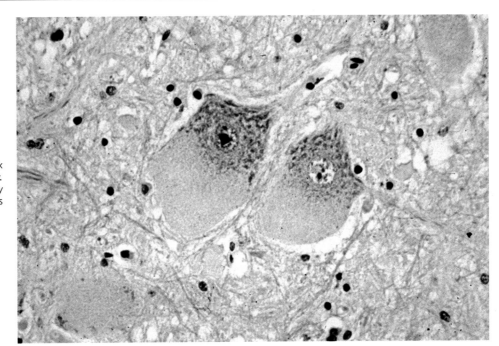

FIGURE 8-3

Neuronal ballooning in Niemann-Pick type C disease. (Reproduced from *www.akronchildrens.org/neuropathology* with permission of Akron Children's Hospital.)

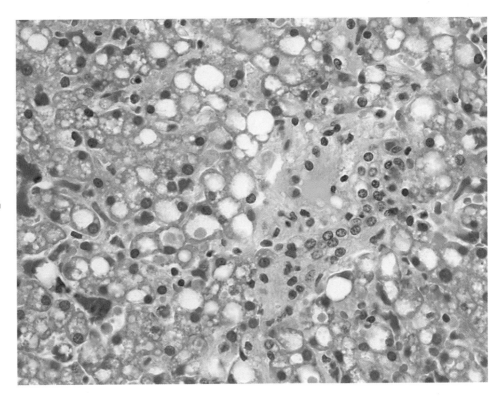

FIGURE 8-4

Distended clear hepatocytes in mucopolysaccharidosis.

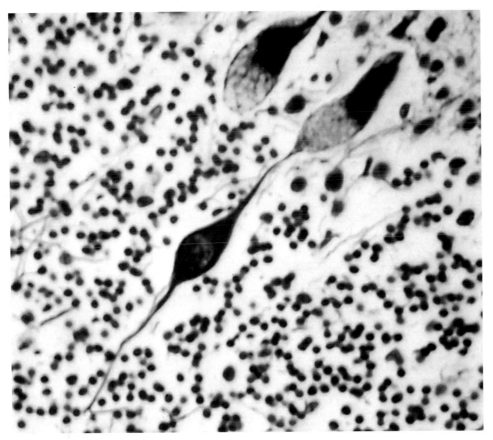

FIGURE 8-5

Torpedo-like swelling of a Purkinje cell dendrite in GM$_1$ gangliosidosis. (Reproduced from *www.akronchildrens. org/neuropathology* with permission of Akron Children's Hospital.)

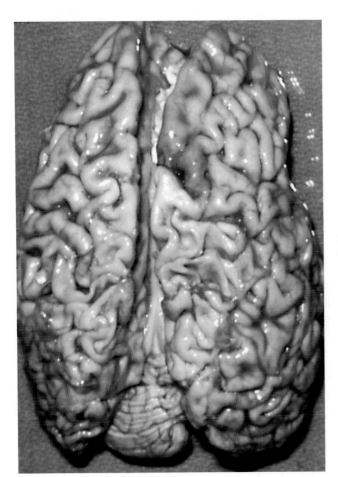

FIGURE 8-6

Cerebral atrophy in GM$_1$ gangliosidosis.

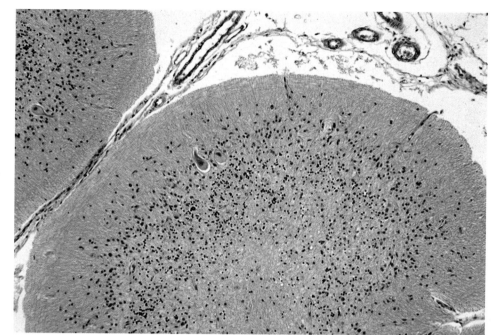

FIGURE 8-7

Cerebellar atrophy in GM$_1$ gangliosidosis.

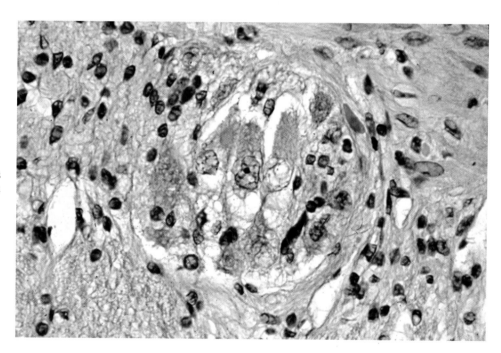

FIGURE 8-8

Distended vacuolated ganglion cells in the Auerbach plexus in GM$_1$ gangliosidosis.

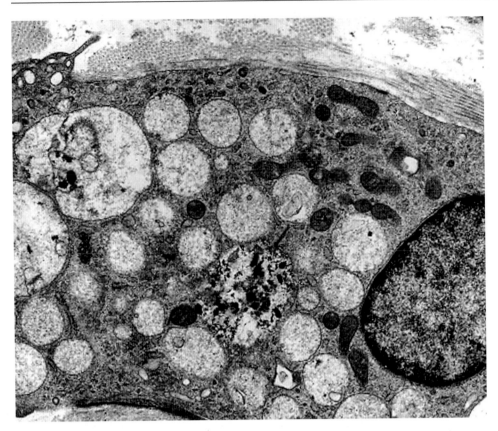

FIGURE 8-9

Membrane-bound reticulogranular material in fibroblasts in mucopolysaccharidosis.

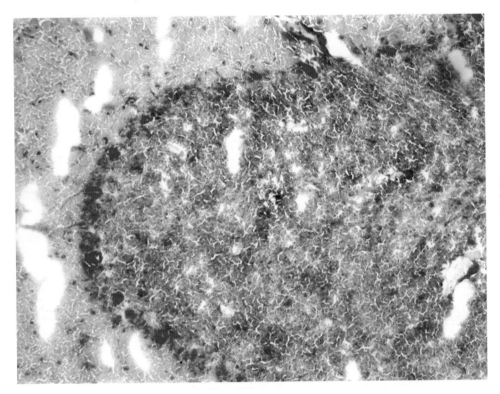

FIGURE 8-10

Intense acid phosphatase activity in Purkinje cells in mucopolysaccharidosis.

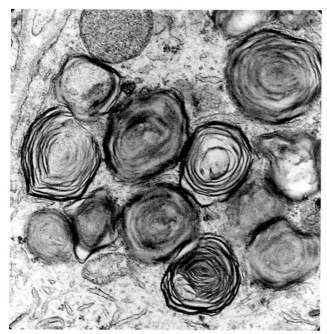

FIGURE 8-11
Concentric lamellar bodies in GM₁ gangliosidosis.

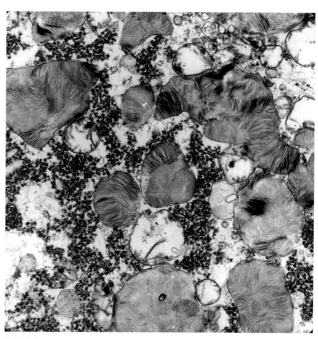

FIGURE 8-12
Zebra bodies in mucopolysaccharidosis.

In some instances, such as Gaucher's disease and globoid cell leukodystrophy, the morphologic appearance is diagnostic. For the most part, however, light and electron microscopy is nonspecific. Thus, at the cellular level, all ganglioside-storing LSDs look the same and the mucopolysaccharidoses are indistinguishable from one another and from the glycoproteinoses.

Special techniques supplement light and electron microscopy. Loss of GAGs can be prevented to some extent by adding the cationic dye toluidine blue to the fixatives and buffers used for electron microscopy. Metachromatic stains are diagnostic in metachromatic leukodystrophy and helpful in the mucopolysaccharidoses. Cystine crystals can be identified under polarized light (see Fig. 8-2), and ceroid-lipofuscin is autofluorescent (Fig. 8-13). Because in most LSDs the stored material is a glycoconjugate, lectin histochemistry and immunoelectron microscopy can be used to characterize the storage products.

FIGURE 8-13
Autofluorescent products in neuronal ceroid lipofuscinosis.

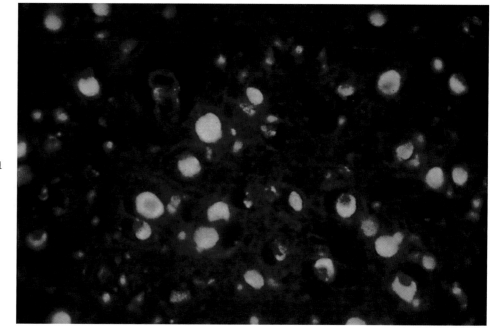

PATHOGENESIS: HOW CELLS AND TISSUES ARE DAMAGED IN THE LYSOSOMAL STORAGE DISORDERS

Cell injury in LSDs is primarily due to the mechanical effects of storage, specifically, displacement of organelles, disruption of cytoplasmic circulation, and in the case of neurons, impaction of axons and dendrites. This process leads to cellular dysfunction and loss, which is most critical for neurons and oligodendrocytes. Storage does not interfere directly with synthetic processes or energy metabolism. In most LSDs, the stored material is chemically inert. In some gangliosidoses, toxic byproducts of the stored gangliosides are also produced and cause additional cell damage. One such example is globoid cell leukodystrophy, in which psychosine, a metabolite of galactocerebroside, is toxic to oligodendrocytes. Impaired recycling and imbalance of membrane lipids in the gangliosidoses cause membrane and synaptic abnormalities that probably account for the early neurologic dysfunction before neurons are lost. In addition, the abnormal chemical composition of myelin lipids may play a role in myelin breakdown in the leukodystrophies, but loss of myelin-producing cells is more important.

Whereas the primary pathology of LSDs is intracellular, in many of them, significant changes also develop in the extracellular matrix. Some of these changes represent scarring from loss of parenchymal elements. In the mucopolysaccharidoses and other LSDs with an MPS phenotype, extracellular accumulation of GAGs and other glycoconjugates causes the severe soft tissue changes that are central to their phenotype.

BIOCHEMICAL-PHENOTYPIC CORRELATION

The type and distribution of substrate in various tissues determines what cells and organ systems are affected in the LSDs. Lysosomal activity also varies between tissues and at different stages of development, depending on substrate turnover. For instance, acid maltase deficiency most severely affects tissues with high glycogen turnover, such as the liver, heart, and skeletal muscle; hexosaminidase A deficiency affects primarily neurons that have the highest GM_2 content and turnover, especially during the phase of dendritic sprouting; and the mucopolysaccharidoses affect connective tissue and the skeleton, which contain a large amount of GAGs. Although LSDs affect all cells and organs, two classes of cells are most vulnerable: (1) neurons, because of their large size, the high ganglioside content of their membranes, and the fact that they do not regenerate and (2) phagocytic cells, which are easily overloaded because of their high burden of substrate turnover.

As lysosomes swell in LSDs, their proton pumps cannot maintain the acid environment. The consequent rise in lysosomal pH leads to generalized loss of enzyme activity. This lysosomal "exhaustion" may also explain the accumulation of diverse products in LSDs (see "Mucopolysaccharidoses" later).

GENOTYPE-PHENOTYPE CORRELATION

The severity of each LSD depends primarily on residual enzyme activity, which correlates with the genotype. Several mutations of each lysosomal enzyme gene can occur. Some of these mutations cause severe enzyme deficiency, whereas others allow some enzyme to be produced. Because of this allelic diversity and because many patients are compound heterozygotes, no two cases of any given LSD are exactly alike. Normally, cells produce about 10 times the amount of lysosomal enzymes that are needed to carry out cellular function. LSD heterozygotes, with about half-normal enzyme activity, are phenotypically normal. In every tissue there is a threshold of lysosomal enzyme activity, usually 10% to 20% of normal, that is required to maintain normal function. Storage develops when enzyme activity falls below this critical level. Some LSDs such as Gaucher's disease show significant clinical variability within the same genotype, thus suggesting that additional genetic and environmental factors contribute to the phenotype.

The molecular defect in LSDs is present from the time of conception, and the biochemical defect is expressed in amniocytes, trophoblasts, and fetal tissues, thereby allowing prenatal diagnosis in the first trimester by enzyme testing. Typical pathologic changes also develop before the second trimester. Fetal and neonatal tissues have the highest regenerative ability, but by the same token, the period of growth and development challenges the capacity of the lysosomal system with the highest substrate turnover. This is especially true in the developing brain, in which large numbers of primitive neurons are eliminated by programmed death. As a consequence, severe enzyme mutations are clinically apparent prenatally or in early childhood. Mutations allowing for higher (but below threshold) residual activity cause symptoms later in life. For instance, in Tay-Sachs disease, severe hexosaminidase deficiency causes diffuse neuronal storage in the first few months of life and is fatal within 1 or 2 years. Mutations resulting in somewhat higher hexosaminidase activity have a later onset, milder symptoms, a more chronic course, and affect neuronal groups selectively.

Lysosomal enzymes are not substrate specific. They are specific for certain residues and linkages and break these linkages in whatever molecules they occur. Thus, hexosaminidases cleave β-hexosamine from glycolipids and glycoproteins, enzymes involved in glycoprotein degradation also degrade glycosphingolipids, and GAG-cleaving enzymes participate in the degradation of several classes of GAGs. Deficiency of a single multicatalytic enzyme causes storage of diverse compounds and thus creates overlapping phenotypes. For example, β-galactosidase deficiency causes GM_1 gangliosidosis and keratan sulfate storage (MPS IV-B—type B Morquio's syndrome). Conversely, several enzymes participate in degradation of the same molecule. Deficiency of any of these enzymes may cause storage of similar compounds and result in a shared phenotype. Thus, the Sanfilippo syndrome can be caused by four different gene mutations, and the Morquio syndrome phenotype can result from deficiency of either β-galactosidase or galactosamine-6-sulfatase.

DIAGNOSIS OF LYSOSOMAL STORAGE DISORDERS

The gold standard in the laboratory diagnosis of LSDs is enzyme assay. Because the enzyme deficiency is expressed in all tissues, albeit not equally, a diagnosis can be made by testing samples obtained by relatively non-invasive methods, such as serum, plasma, white cells, amniocytes, cells obtained by chorionic villus sampling (CVS), and cultured skin fibroblasts. Enzyme assay can also be used to detect carriers. Some LSDs can be diagnosed by assaying a leukocyte pellet. In most instances in which multiple enzymes need to be evaluated, cultured fibroblasts or amniocytes must be used.

Urine chromatography is a useful screening test for many LSDs. The pattern of glycoconjugates secreted in urine can identify several mucopolysaccharidoses and glycoproteinoses, but it is not specific because storage of similar compounds may result from different enzyme defects. Because of the great genotypic diversity that characterizes all LSDs, molecular analysis is impractical for primary diagnosis. However, when the mutation is known, molecular analysis can be used for carrier detection and prenatal diagnosis.

Morphology evaluation combining light microscopy, electron microscopy, and ancillary studies is an important tool in the diagnosis and investigation of LSDs. Anatomic studies reliably reveal the presence of a storage process and can narrow the differential down to a presumptive diagnosis, which is important for guiding biochemical, molecular, and genetic studies. Because small amounts of substrates are asymptomatically stored in many cell types, characteristic pathologic changes can be detected by minimally invasive sampling of a variety of cells and tissues such as amniotic fluid, skin, conjunctiva, bone marrow, and circulating leukocytes (Fig. 8-14). In several LSDs, although enzymatic diagnosis is available, morphology can also provide a specific diagnosis (Table 8-3).

In a few LSDs, morphology is the only diagnostic modality. Morphology is the only means of detecting drug-induced LSDs, helps in understanding the pathogenesis of cell and tissue injury, and is indispensable in evaluating the effects of treatment. The pathology of many LSDs is incompletely described, but systematic anatomic study can still make significant contributions to our understanding.

TREATMENT OF LYSOSOMAL STORAGE DISORDERS

Bone marrow transplantation (BMT) is currently recommended for type 3 Gaucher's disease, Hurler's syndrome, Maroteaux-Lamy syndrome, asymptomatic late infantile metachromatic leukodystrophy, juvenile- and adult-onset metachromatic leukodystrophy, and juvenile- and adult-onset Krabbe's disease. The experience with the rare human cases in which BMT has been attempted is

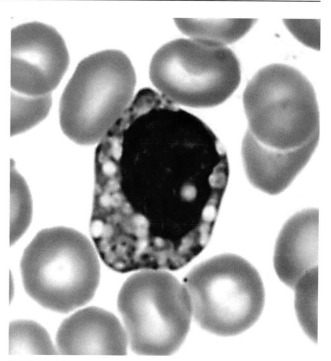

FIGURE 8-14
Vacuolization of a circulating monocyte in I-cell disease.

not encouraging. Although delivery of the missing enzyme to the brain has been demonstrated in experimental animals and progression of the disease has been slowed in some cases, arrest or reversal of the disease has not occurred. BMT has some effect on extraneural pathology, and limited success has been reported in type 1 Gaucher's disease and a few other disorders. BMT does not reverse brain damage that has already occurred and is

TABLE 8-3

Lysosomal Storage Diseases with Diagnostic Morphology

Disease	Diagnostic Finding
Gaucher's disease	Gaucher cells, characteristic fine structure
Globoid cell leukodystrophy	Globoid cells, characteristic fine structure
Metachromatic leukodystrophy	Metachromasia, characteristic fine structure
Farber's lipogranulomatosis	Lipid granulomas, characteristic fine structure
Fabry's disease	Vascular, renal pathology
Pompe's disease	Lysosomal glycogen storage myopathy
Wolman's disease	Adrenal calcification, lipid droplets, cholesterol crystals
Neuronal ceroid lipofuscinoses	Characteristic ultrastructure

most effective if performed early in the course of the disease. Enzyme replacement therapy, although very expensive, has been successful in type 1 Gaucher's disease and seems promising in Fabry's disease. Gene therapy is being explored in experimental models.

Based on the chemical structure of the stored material, LSDs can be divided into four major groups—sphingolipidoses, mucopolysaccharidoses, glycoproteinoses, and ceroid lipofuscinoses—and several other individual entities. An account of the core features of each group and brief descriptions of the most common LSDs follow.

SPHINGOLIPIDOSES

DEFINITION AND CHEMISTRY

The sphingolipidoses are a diverse group of LSDs caused by deficiencies in the lysosomal enzymes responsible for sphingolipid degradation. Sphingolipids consist of a backbone of ceramide (*N*-acylsphingosine) with various attached side chains. They are major constituents of cell membranes, and gangliosides are especially rich in neuronal membranes. Deficiency of sphingolipid degradation enzymes results in the accumulation of undegraded ceramide compounds, especially in the brain. Sphingolipids have a hydrophobic and a hydrophilic side and tend to form bilayers in aqueous moieties. This property is replicated in the storage products of some sphingolipidoses that form MCBs.

GENERAL CLINICAL AND PATHOLOGIC FEATURES

Eight sphingolipidoses are recognized (Table 8-4). Fabry's disease is X-linked; all other sphingolipidoses are autosomal recessive.

GM_1 gangliosidosis, GM_2 gangliosidosis, and type A and B Niemann-Pick disease cause neuronal storage (neuronal lipidosis). GM_2 gangliosidosis and type A and B Niemann-Pick disease also cause visceral storage (storage histiocytosis). Enlarged, lipid-filled lysosomes balloon the neural soma (see Fig. 8-3) and expand axons and dendrites (see Fig. 8-5), thereby blocking axoplasmic flow. The axonal swellings are covered by ectopic dendritic spines. Aberrant dendritogenesis is thought to contribute to the neurologic dysfunction. Two sphingolipidoses, metachromatic leukodystrophy and Krabbe's disease, cause primarily white matter disease (leukodystrophy) and are described elsewhere. Gaucher's, Farber's, and Fabry's diseases cause unique phenotypes and are described separately.

GM_1 GANGLIOSIDOSIS

CLINICAL FINDINGS

GM_1 gangliosidosis is manifested in infancy with severe psychomotor retardation and a full-blown Hurler phe-

---

SPHINGOLIPIDOSES—DISEASE FACTS AND PATHOLOGIC FEATURES

Definition
▶ A group of LSDs caused by deficiencies in enzymes that degrade sphingolipid

Storage Materials
▶ Sphingolipids (ceramide compounds)

Prevalence
▶ Gaucher's disease is the most common LSD (1.16 to 1.75 per 100,000). Gaucher's disease and Tay-Sachs disease are frequent in Ashkenazi Jews

Inheritance
▶ Fabry's disease is X-linked recessive; all other sphingolipidoses are autosomal recessive

Clinical Phenotypes
▶ Neuronal lipidosis, leukodystrophy, storage histiocytosis, mucopolysaccharidosis, and other individual entities

Pathology
▶ Storage of gangliosides in neurons initially causes neuronal ballooning and then neuronal loss
▶ Involvement of oligodendroglia and Schwann cells causes myelin loss
▶ Storage in monocyte-macrophage cells causes hepatosplenomegaly

---

GM_1 GANGLIOSIDOSIS—DISEASE FACTS AND PATHOLOGIC FEATURES

Definition
▶ An autosomal recessive LSD caused by a deficiency of β-galactosidase and characterized by neuronal lipidosis and mucopolysaccharidosis-like somatic changes

Storage Materials
▶ GM_1 ganglioside, keratan sulfate, glycoproteins

Clinical Phenotype
▶ Neuronal lipidosis, mucopolysaccharidosis

Gross Findings
▶ Megalencephaly initially followed by cerebral and cerebellar atrophy

Microscopic Findings
▶ Neuronal ballooning, meganeurites
▶ Clear epithelial and mesenchymal cells similar to the mucopolysaccharidoses

Ultrastructural Features
▶ Membranous cytoplasmic bodies in neurons
▶ Sparse reticulogranular material in epithelial and mesenchymal cells

TABLE 8-4

The Sphingolipidoses

Disease	Enzyme	Locus	Stored Material	Phenotype
GM$_1$ gangliosidosis, Morquio type C	β-Galactosidase	3p21.33	GM$_1$ ganglioside Keratan sulfate Glycoprotein	NL, CRS, MPS
GM$_2$ gangliosidoses			GM$_2$ gangliosides	NL, CRS
Tay-Sachs disease	Hex A	15q23-24		
Sandhoff's disease	Hex A & B	5q13 (Hex B)		
GM$_2$ activator deficiency	Hex A & B	5q31.3-32.1		
Niemann-Pick A & B	Sphingomyelinase	11p15.1-p15.4	Sphingomyelin	NL, CRS, SH
Gaucher's disease	Glucocerebrosidase Glucosylsphingosine	1q21	Glucosylceramide	SH
Krabbe's disease	Galactocerebrosidase Psychosine	14q24.3-32.1	Galactosylceramide	LD
Metachromatic leukodystrophy	Arylsulfatase A Galactosylsphingosine	22q13.31-tes	Galactosylsulfatide	LD, PN
Fabry's disease	α-Galactosidase	Xq22.1	Trihexosylceramide	PN, NL, AK, SA, HD
Farber's granulomatosis	Ceramidase	8p22-p21.3	Ceramide	LD, NL, CRS, HF

AK, angiokeratoma; CRS, cherry-red spot; HD, heart disease; HF, hydrops fetalis; LD, leukodystrophy; MPS, mucopolysaccharidosis; NL, neuronal lipidosis; PN, peripheral neuropathy; SA, storage angiopathy; SH, storage histiocytosis.

notype (see "Mucopolysaccharidoses" later), including coarse facial features (Fig. 8-15), dysostosis multiplex, corneal clouding, and organomegaly. A cherry-red spot is seen in 50% of patients. Patients with infantile onset usually die before 2 years of age. Later-onset variants have a milder neurologic picture (which includes dystonia and ataxia) and milder somatic and skeletal findings. An allelic variant called type B Morquio's syndrome is phenotypically similar to type A Morquio's syndrome (MPS IV-A) and consists primarily of skeletal changes (short-trunk dwarfism) with normal intelligence but without organomegaly or corneal clouding. The neurologic symptoms in type B Morquio's syndrome develop not as a result of CNS storage but rather as a consequence of atlantoaxial dislocation.

PATHOLOGIC FINDINGS

The neuropathologic changes in infantile and late infantile GM$_1$ gangliosidosis consist of lipid storage in the neuronal soma (neuronal ballooning) (see Fig. 8-3) and proximal axon. Storage also occurs in sensory and autonomic ganglionic neurons (see Fig. 8-8). On electron microscopic examination, the storage material consists of MCBs (see Fig. 8-11). In early phases of the disease, the brain is large. GM$_1$ ganglioside, normally accounting for 20% of brain gangliosides, increases to 80% to 90%. As the disease progresses, neuronal loss and gliosis occur and cerebral atrophy develops (see

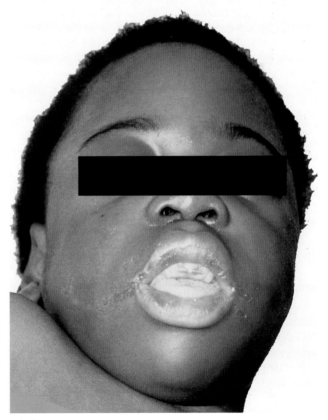

FIGURE 8-15

Coarse facial features in GM$_1$ gangliosidosis.

Figs. 8-6 and 8-7). Storage in retinal ganglion cells results in cherry-red spots. Patients with GM_1 gangliosidosis also have skeletal, soft tissue, and visceral changes similar to Hurler's syndrome.

GM_2 GANGLIOSIDOSES

The GM_2 gangliosidoses (Table 8-5) are a prime example of the genotypic complexity and phenotypic diversity of LSDs. GM_2 accumulation can result from deficiency of hexosaminidase A (Hex A), hexosaminidase B (Hex B), or the GM_2 activator, a polypeptide that forms a complex with GM_2 ganglioside that is important for its degradation. Both Hex A and Hex B are multicatalytic and metabolize oligosaccharides, glycolipids, glycoproteins, and GAGs with terminal GlcNAc or GalNAc. Only Hex A catabolizes GM_2 ganglioside.

Tay-Sachs Disease

CLINICAL FINDINGS

Deficiency of the α subunit (and Hex A) causes Tay-Sachs disease, the prototype of LSDs and the first LSD to be described. Patients with classic infantile Tay-Sachs disease present in the first year of life and die by 5 years of age. They have profound psychomotor retardation, myoclonus, hypotonia, and cherry-red spots. Variants caused by milder mutations begin later and have a subacute or chronic course characterized by seizures, ataxia, spasticity, choreoathetosis, and motor neuron disease with little or no cognitive dysfunction.

GM_2 GANGLIOSIDOSES—DISEASE FACTS AND PATHOLOGIC FEATURES

Definition
- ▶ A group of autosomal recessive LSDs caused by deficiencies in hexosaminidase A (Tay-Sachs disease), hexosaminidase B (Sandhoff's disease), and the GM_2 activator

Storage Material
- ▶ GM_2 ganglioside

Clinical Phenotype
- ▶ Neuronal lipidosis, blindness, cherry-red spots

Gross Findings
- ▶ Megalencephaly initially, followed by cerebral atrophy

Microscopic Findings
- ▶ Neuronal lipidosis early, neuronal loss and gliosis late

Ultrastructural Features
- ▶ Membranous cytoplasmic bodies

TABLE 8-5

The GM_2 Gangliosidoses

Hex A: α and β subunits. Catabolizes GM_2

Hex B: Two β subunits. Catabolizes GM_2, glycoproteins, glycosaminoglycans

Tay-Sachs disease: Hex A deficiency, α-subunit mutation

Sandhoff's disease: Hex A and B deficiency, β-subunit mutation

Activator deficiency: GM_2 activator deficiency

PATHOLOGIC CHANGES

The neuropathology of infantile Tay-Sachs disease is generalized neuronal lipidosis indistinguishable from GM_1 gangliosidosis. The brain is larger than normal initially, but by the end of the clinical course, severe neuronal loss and brain atrophy occur. GM_2 ganglioside, normally a minor component of total brain gangliosides, increases to 90% of brain gangliosides. The few late-onset cases that have been studied show similar, but less severe, changes throughout the brain, more severe storage in spinal cord neurons and dorsal root ganglia, and more diverse and heterogeneous lysosomal contents.

Sandhoff's Disease and GM_2 Activator Deficiency

The clinical profile and pathology of activator deficiency are similar to Tay-Sachs disease. β-Subunit mutations cause Hex A and Hex B deficiency (Sandhoff's disease). The neurologic manifestations and neuropathology of Sandhoff's disease are similar to those of Tay-Sachs disease, but Sandhoff's disease also shows hepatosplenomegaly and visceral storage of oligosaccharides, glycoproteins, and glycolipids. No such visceral storage is seen in Tay-Sachs disease.

NIEMANN-PICK DISEASE TYPES A AND B

Niemann-Pick disease types A and B is caused by mutations in the sphingomyelinase gene and results in lysosomal storage of sphingomyelin. Type C Niemann-Pick disease and its variant type D (see later) are caused by defects in intracellular cholesterol circulation. Niemann-Pick type A has a high incidence among Ashkenazi Jews and becomes clinically apparent in infancy because of progressive neurologic deterioration, cherry-red spots, and massive hepatosplenomegaly; it is usually fatal within 2 to 3 years. Niemann-Pick type B has an onset in infancy or childhood and results in massive hepatosplenomegaly and pulmonary infiltrates. There is little or no neurologic involvement, and patients survive to adulthood. The visceral pathology of type A and B Niemann-Pick disease consists of foamy histiocytes in the bone marrow (Fig. 8-16), spleen, lymph nodes, hepatic sinusoids, and pulmonary

alveoli. The stored sphingomyelin takes the form of small concentric lamellar bodies. Similar material accumulates in the CNS and autonomic neurons, brain macrophages and microglia, retinal ganglion cells, and other non-neuronal cells. Neuronal storage causes ballooning leading to neuronal degeneration and loss and severe cerebral and cerebellar atrophy.

GAUCHER'S DISEASE

GENETICS AND CLINICAL FINDINGS

Gaucher's disease is an LSD characterized by storage of glucocerebroside (glucosylceramide) in monocyte-macrophage cells because of deficiency of glucocerebrosidase (glucosylceramidase). With an estimated birth frequency of 1 per 50,000, it is the most common LSD in white individuals. Gaucher's disease is caused by mutations of the *GBA* gene located on 1q21. Four mutations account for the vast majority of all forms of Gaucher's disease, although more than 200 mutations have been described. The phenotype is predictable in some mutations. In others there is marked phenotypic variability, even among monozygotic twins with Gaucher's disease.

Three clinical phenotypes are recognized. The most common by far is type 1, the prevalence of which in Ashkenazi Jews is 1 per 855 with a carrier frequency of 1 per 18. Type 1 Gaucher's disease develops in childhood to early adulthood and is characterized by hepatosplenomegaly with occasional splenic infarcts,

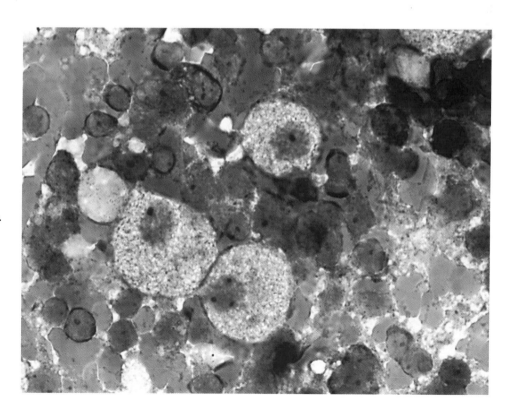

FIGURE 8-16
Niemann-Pick cells in bone marrow.

GAUCHER'S DISEASE—DISEASE FACTS AND PATHOLOGIC FEATURES

Definition

▶ An autosomal recessive LSD caused by a deficiency of glucocerebrosidase and storage of glucocerebroside in monocyte-macrophage cells

Storage Material

▶ Glucocerebroside

Prevalence

▶ 1.16 to 1.75 per 100,000. Type 1 Gaucher's disease is the most common LSD

Clinical Findings

▶ Type 1: storage histiocytosis causing hepatosplenomegaly, bone disease, anemia, thrombocytopenia
▶ Type 2: storage histiocytosis and severe neurologic abnormalities starting in infancy and causing death by 2 to 4 years
▶ Type 3 is similar to type 2 but milder

Radiologic Features

▶ Osteopenia, lytic or sclerotic bone lesions, osteonecrosis, fractures

Gross Findings

▶ Hepatosplenomegaly

Microscopic Findings

▶ Gaucher cells: large monocyte-macrophage cells with a "wrinkled tissue paper" appearance. They are found in lymph nodes, bone marrow, spleen, hepatic sinusoids. In type 2 Gaucher's disease, Gaucher cells are present in perivascular CNS spaces

Ultrastructural Features

▶ Tubular inclusions in lysosomes

bone disease (osteopenia, focal lytic or sclerotic lesions, osteonecrosis, pathologic fractures, chronic bone pain), anemia and thrombocytopenia as a result of hypersplenism, pulmonary interstitial infiltrates, and other manifestations. Neurologic manifestations from spinal cord or root compression secondary to bone disease may develop in patients with type 1 Gaucher's disease, but there is no primary CNS involvement. In type 2 (acute neuronopathic) Gaucher's disease, neurologic manifestations (stridor, strabismus and other oculomotor abnormalities, swallowing difficulty, opisthotonos, spasticity) appear before the age of 2 years, progress rapidly, and lead to death by 2 to 4 years of age. Some patients have non-immune fetal hydrops and ichthyosiform or collodion skin changes. Patients with type 2 Gaucher's disease also have hepatosplenomegaly similar to type 1. There is no special ethnic prevalence for type 2. Type 3 (subacute neuronopathic) Gaucher's disease is frequent in northern Sweden and has clinical manifestations similar to those of type 2, but it is more slowly progressive such that patients may survive into their 20s and 30s.

DIAGNOSIS AND THERAPY

The gold standard in the diagnosis of Gaucher's disease is assay of acid β-glucosylceramidase activity in blood leukocytes. The diagnosis can also be made by finding Gaucher cells in bone marrow aspirates. Enzyme assay of amniocytes and CVS cells can also be performed for prenatal diagnosis but is unreliable for carrier detection. Molecular testing is available on a clinical basis and can be used for carrier detection in at-risk relatives.

Gaucher's disease is the first LSD that was successfully managed by enzyme replacement. Alglucerase, a placental preparation of glucocerebrosidase, has proved effective in more than 1000 patients with Gaucher's disease, and imiglucerase, the recombinant form of the enzyme that recently became available, is equally effective. This success story has opened the door for consideration of similar therapies in other LSDs.

PATHOLOGIC CHANGES

The pathology of Gaucher's disease consists of lysosomal storage of glucocerebroside in cells of the monocyte-macrophage system. Glucocerebroside storage leads to a characteristic cellular alteration in these cells—the Gaucher cells. Gaucher cells have a large cytoplasmic mass with a striated appearance that has been likened to "wrinkled tissue paper" or "crumpled silk" (Fig. 8-17). This change is caused by the storage of twisted bundles of tubules (Fig. 8-18) in large, irregularly branching lysosomal compartments. These inclusions are unique and diagnostic for Gaucher's disease. Biochemically, they consist of glucocerebroside, the main sources of which are thought to be the membranes of blood cells phagocytosed by monocytes-macrophages. A similar cellular alteration (pseudo-Gaucher cells) is sometimes seen in the marrow of patients with chronic myelogenous leukemia.

Gaucher cells are present in the bone marrow, spleen, lymph nodes (see Fig. 8-18), hepatic sinusoids, and other organs and tissues in all forms of Gaucher's disease but account for only a small fraction of the mass of the liver and spleen in Gaucher's disease. Cytokines released by Gaucher cells induce an inflammatory response that plays a significant role in the organomegaly and systemic manifestations of Gaucher's disease. An increased incidence of cancer, including lymphoma, myeloma, and bone tumors, has been reported in patients with Gaucher's disease. Rare Gaucher cells without other pathology also occur in the leptomeninges and Virchow-Robin spaces in type 1 Gaucher's disease. In type 2 and 3 Gaucher's disease, there are numerous Gaucher cells in the perivascular spaces and rare Gaucher cells in brain parenchyma (Fig. 8-19). No part of the CNS is spared, but the brain stem and deep nuclei are more severely affected than the cortex and account for most neurologic deficits.

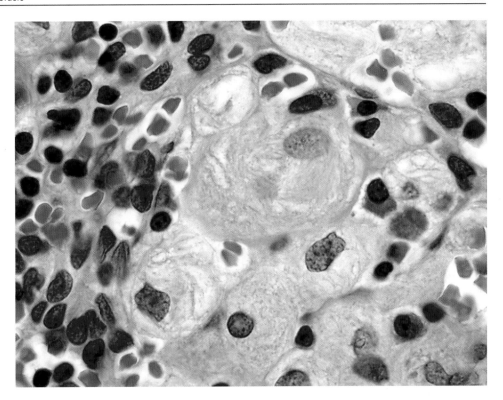

FIGURE 8-17
Gaucher cells in the spleen.

Along with the presence of Gaucher cells there is neuronophagia, neuronal loss, and gliosis. Except for the rare finding of tubular inclusions in neurons, no neuronal storage is seen. Neuronal degeneration and loss have been attributed to the neurotoxic action of glucosylsphingosine, a byproduct of glucocerebroside not normally present in the brain.

FABRY'S DISEASE

GENETICS AND CLINICAL FINDINGS

Fabry's disease (α-galactosidase deficiency) is one of two X-linked LSDs, the other being MPS II (Hunter's syndrome). The gene for α-galactosidase is located on Xq22.

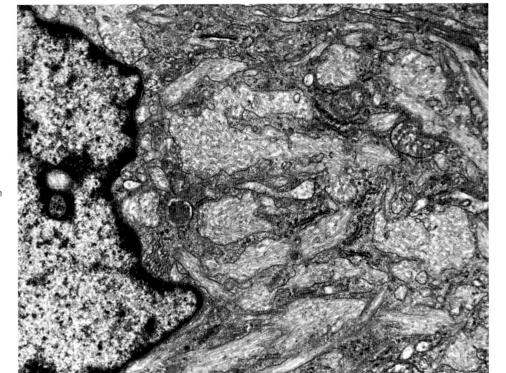

FIGURE 8-18
Tubular lysosomal inclusions in Gaucher's disease.

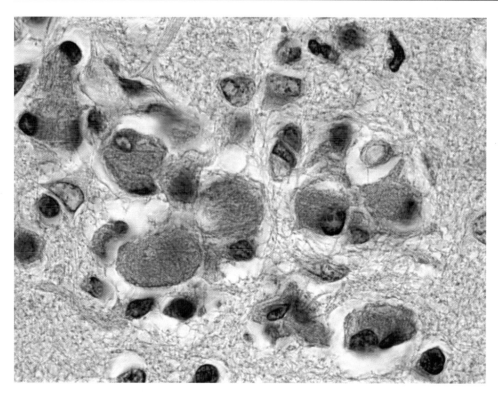

FIGURE 8-19
Gaucher cells in the brain in type 2 Gaucher's disease.

More than 190 mutations have been reported. Fabry's disease becomes clinically apparent in adolescence or young adult life with peripheral neuropathy, cutaneous lesions, renal disease, corneal opacities, and cataracts. The peripheral neuropathy is characterized by intermittent episodes of disabling, burning limb pain that are often precipitated by stress, exercise, and increased temperature. No significant weakness or muscle atrophy occurs. Cutaneous telangiectases (angiokeratoma corporis diffusum) cover the body in a bathing trunk distri-

---

FABRY'S DISEASE—DISEASE FACTS AND PATHOLOGIC FEATURES

Definition
▶ An X-linked LSD with multiorgan pathology caused by a deficiency of α-galactosidase

Storage Material
▶ Trihexosylceramide

Clinical Manifestations
▶ Neuropathy, angiokeratoma, renal failure, hypertension, heart disease, corneal opacities

Pathologic Changes
▶ Lipid storage in vascular cells, Schwann cells, neurons, cardiac myocytes
▶ Ischemic pathology in the brain and heart

Ultrastructural Findings
▶ Membrane-bound lamellar structures

---

bution. Renal dysfunction progresses to renal failure with hypertension and cardiac and cerebrovascular complications. Heart involvement is manifested by mitral insufficiency, cardiac arrhythmias, cardiomyopathy, angina, and myocardial infarction. Four percent to 8% of unselected patients with hypertrophic nonobstructive cardiomyopathy have Fabry's disease. There are renal and cardiac variants of Fabry's disease that lack the classic multisystem manifestations. Males with Fabry's disease generally die in their 30s or 40s from renal failure, heart disease, or cerebrovascular disease. Female carriers are usually asymptomatic, but some may have mild manifestations beginning in their 40s, most commonly corneal opacities. Enzyme replacement therapy with recombinant α-galactosidase A, now in clinical trials, is a major advance in the treatment of Fabry's disease.

PATHOLOGIC CHANGES

The pathology of Fabry's disease consists of widespread lysosomal storage of birefringent lipids in epithelial, mesenchymal, and neural cells (Fig. 8-20). On electron microscopic examination, the membrane-bound deposits have a lamellar configuration (Fig. 8-21). Endothelial and vascular smooth muscle cells are most severely affected. Vascular involvement causes endothelial injury, thrombosis, and ischemic changes and weakens vessel walls, thereby leading to telangiectasia of cutaneous, conjunctival, and retinal vessels. Involvement of glomerular cells (see Fig. 8-20) and renal tubular epithelium explains the renal complications. Heart disease is due to lipid storage in cardiac myocytes (cardiomyopathy)

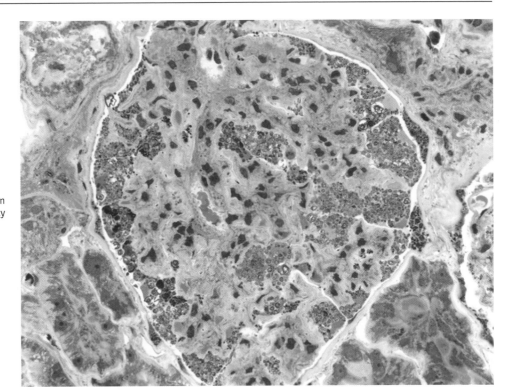

FIGURE 8-20

Lipid deposits in a glomerulus in Fabry's disease (semithin epoxy section, toluidine blue stain).

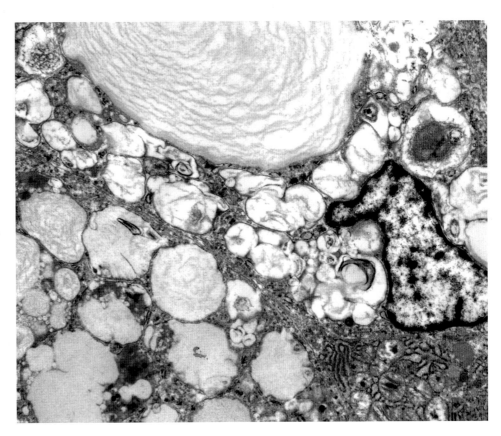

FIGURE 8-21

Lamellar structures in Fabry's disease.

and ischemia. The CNS complications of Fabry's disease are primarily due to ischemia and hypertension, but storage in neurons, glial cells, and the leptomeninges also occurs. Sural nerve biopsy in Fabry's disease shows loss of small myelinated and unmyelinated fibers and lipid deposits in vascular cells, perineurial cells, and Schwann cells. Storage in sensory and autonomic ganglionic neurons also occurs.

FARBER'S LIPOGRANULOMATOSIS

CLINICAL FINDINGS

Farber's lipogranulomatosis, a rare autosomal recessive deficiency of acid ceramidase, has a wide phenotypic spectrum. In its classic infantile form, it is manifested in the first few months of life with a striking characteristic combination of painful, swollen deformed joints, particularly in the hands and feet, subcutaneous nodules, and hoarseness from the development of granulomas in the larynx. As the disease progresses, granulomas cause skeletal deformities and affect the lungs, liver, heart, and other organs. Patients have psychomotor retardation and usually die in 2 to 3 years. Milder forms have a later onset and longer survival with mild neurologic involvement. Cherry-red spots associated with progressive neurologic symptoms are seen in some patients. A severe, rapidly fatal phenotype is manifested as neonatal hydrops and hepatosplenomegaly.

PATHOLOGIC CHANGES

The granulomas of Farber's disease consist of foamy histiocytes that have accumulated ceramide and are associated with lymphoplasmacytic infiltrates and scarring. They deform and destroy soft tissues, bones, and viscera

---

FARBER'S LIPOGRANULOMATOSIS—DISEASE FACTS AND PATHOLOGIC FEATURES

Definition
▶ A rare autosomal recessive LSD caused by a deficiency of ceramidase

Storage Material
▶ Ceramide

Clinical Findings
▶ Arthropathy, multisystem pathology as a result of lipid granulomas, psychomotor retardation

Pathology
▶ Lipid granulomas in joints and viscera, lipid storage in neurons

Ultrastructure
▶ Lamellar (zebra) bodies, "banana" bodies

---

and cause organomegaly by their sheer volume. The stored material is PAS positive and consists of diverse structures, including curved tubular structures, lamellar profiles (zebra bodies), and banana bodies (electron-lucent inclusions with dense rims). Neuronal storage also occurs, especially in large neurons of the spinal cord, brain stem, and cerebellum and to a lesser extent in the cerebral cortex. The white matter shows myelin loss and gliosis.

MUCOPOLYSACCHARIDOSES

DEFINITION AND CHEMISTRY

The mucopolysaccharidoses are inherited metabolic disorders caused by impaired lysosomal degradation of mucopolysaccharides (GAGs). GAGs are long unbranched molecules of repeating disaccharides. They are attached to core proteins and form proteoglycan complexes that consist of 95% carbohydrate and 5% protein. GAGs are produced by most cells, including brain cells, and are found mainly on the surface of cells and in the extracellular matrix. They are primarily structural molecules but perform a variety of other biologic functions. Proteoglycans form a network with collagen fibers that contributes to the structural stability and toughness of connective tissue and cartilage. The large amount of water that GAGs attract cushions tissues from mechanical stress and is important for nutrient circulation. Synthesis of GAGs occurs by the stepwise addition of sugar molecules. Degradation of GAGs begins with their internalization by endocytosis, followed by stepwise removal of sugar molecules by glycosidases and sulfatases, which occurs in lysosomes. Deficiency of these enzymes results in the accumulation of four GAGs in lysosomes and the extracellular matrix: dermatan sulfate, heparan sulfate, keratan sulfate, and chondroitin sulfate.

PREVALENCE AND GENETICS

As a group, the mucopolysaccharidoses are the most common LSDs. They are autosomal recessive with the exception of MPS II (Hunter's syndrome), which is X-linked. As in other LSDs, different enzyme defects can cause the same phenotype (e.g., MPS III—Sanfilippo's syndrome and MPS IV—Morquio's syndrome), and allelic heterogeneity results in a wide phenotypic spectrum (e.g., MPS I—Hurler's syndrome, MPS II—Hunter's syndrome, and MPS VII—Sly's syndrome).

CLINICAL MANIFESTATIONS

The mucopolysaccharidoses share certain core clinical features. They are progressive multisystem disorders characterized by coarse facial features, skeletal and joint abnormalities, organomegaly, corneal clouding, cardiovascular disease, and CNS involvement. MPS I-H

TABLE 8-6
The Mucopolysaccharidoses

MPS Type	Syndrome	Chromosomal Locus	Enzyme	Stored GAG	Clinical Findings
MPS I	Hurler Scheie Hurler-Scheie	4p16.3	α-L-Iduronidase	DS, HS	H, MR, DM, CC, HD
MPS II	Hunter	Xq28	Iduronate sulfatase	DS, HS	H, MR, DM, HD
MPS III-A	Sanfilippo A	17q25.3	Heparan *N*-sulfatase	HS	MR
MPS III-B	Sanfilippo B	17q21	α-*N*-acetyl glucosaminidase	HS	MR
MPS III-C	Sanfilippo C	Chr 14	Acetyl-CoA: α-glucosaminide acetyltransferase	HS	MR
MPS III-D	Sanfilippo D	12q14	*N*-acetylglucosamine-6-sulfatase	HS	MR
MPS IV-A	Morquio A	16q24.3	Galactose-6-sulfatase	KS, CS	DM, CC, HD
MPS IV-B	Morquio B	3p21.33	β-Galactosidase	KS	DM, CC, HD
MPS VI	Maroteaux-Lamy	5q13-q14	Arylsulfatase B	DS	H, DM, CC, HD
MPS VII	Sly	7q21.11	β-Glucuronidase	DS, HS, CS	H, MR, DM, CC, HF
MPS IX		3p21.2-p21.3	Hyaluronidase	Hyaluronan	

CC, corneal clouding; CS, chondroitin sulfate; DM, dysostosis multiplex; DS, dermatan sulfate; H, Hurler phenotype; HD, heart disease; HF, hydrops fetalis; HS, heparan sulfate; KS, keratan sulfate; MR, mental retardation.

(Hurler's syndrome), the most severe MPS phenotype, is described in detail in the next section as a prototype, and the variation among the other mucopolysaccharidoses in the expression of key clinical findings is discussed later and presented in Table 8-6.

MUCOPOLYSACCHARIDOSIS I-H (HURLER'S SYNDROME)

CLINICAL FINDINGS

Patients with MPS I-H are normal at birth, with clinical manifestations beginning to develop in the first year of life. MPS I-H is diagnosed in most patients by 18 months, and they die before they reach 10 years. The first abnormality to appear may be inguinal or umbilical hernia, followed by coarsening of facial features. Corneal clouding occurs in all patients, and open-angle glaucoma and retinal degeneration may cause additional visual impairment. Cardiovascular involvement consists of aortic and mitral insufficiency, hypertrophic cardiomyopathy with arrhythmias, and ischemic heart disease secondary to coronary artery stenosis. The skeletal manifestations of MPS I-H constitute the syndrome of dysostosis multiplex (Fig. 8-22), which consists of an enlarged skull, thick calvaria, J-shaped sella, broad clavicles, oar-shaped ribs, scoliosis, abnormal vertebrae, flared iliac wings, dysplastic acetabula, and shortened long bones with

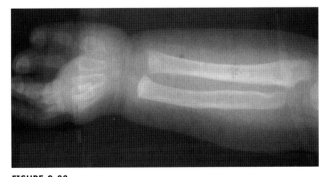

FIGURE 8-22

Mucopolysaccharidosis, dysostosis multiplex: thickened forearm bones.

thickened cortices. Thickening of synovium and soft tissues causes progressive joint stiffening and distortion, clawhand deformity, and carpal tunnel and other nerve entrapment syndromes. Thickening of the tongue, tonsils, adenoids, and other soft tissues of the oropharynx causes upper airway obstruction, noisy breathing, and copious nasal discharge. Eustachian tube obstruction leads to middle ear infections, which are the main cause of the hearing loss seen in patients with severe MPS I-H. The abdomen protrudes because of hepatosplenomegaly. The Hurler phenotype, which has prompted the insensitive term "gargoylism," consists of short stature, protruding abdomen, and coarse facial features (Fig. 8-23). Delay in neurologic development is usually evident by 1 year of age, followed by regression

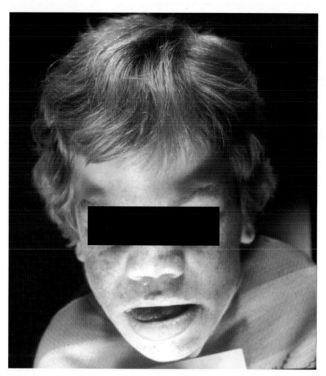

FIGURE 8-23

Coarse facial features in mucopolysaccharidosis. (Reproduced from *www.akronchildrens.org/neuropathology* with permission of Akron Children's Hospital.)

MUCOPOLYSACCHARIDOSIS I-H (HURLER'S SYNDROME)— DISEASE FACTS AND PATHOLOGIC FEATURES

Definition
▶ An LSD with an accumulation of glycosaminoglycans (GAGs) and severe neurologic, skeletal, and visceral abnormalities

Clinical Findings
▶ Psychomotor retardation, coarse facial features, protuberant abdomen, short stature, corneal clouding, heart disease

Radiologic Findings
▶ Dysostosis multiplex, hydrocephalus

Laboratory Findings
▶ GAGs in urine, vacuolated lymphocytes

Diagnosis
▶ Urinary screening for GAGs, enzyme testing (leukocytes, fibroblasts, amniocytes, CVS cells), DNA testing

General Pathology
▶ Hepatosplenomegaly, myocardial fibrosis, thickening of the endocardium and cardiac valves

Neuropathology
▶ Gross: thickening of the arachnoid membrane, hydrocephalus, late cortical atrophy
▶ Microscopic: expansion of perivascular CNS spaces, neuronal lipidosis
▶ Electron microscopic: reticulogranular material in epithelial and mesenchymal cells, lamellar material (zebra bodies and membranous cytoplasmic bodies) in neurons

---

and severe psychomotor retardation. Imaging studies show hydrocephalus and arachnoid cysts. Additional neurologic damage is caused by spinal cord compression secondary to spondylolisthesis or thickening of the dura.

Patients with mild MPS I (Scheie's syndrome) and intermediate MPS I (Hurler-Scheie syndrome) have a later onset of the disease and may survive to adulthood. Corneal clouding and all other somatic manifestations develop at a slower pace but may become severe because of the prolonged survival. Intellectual impairment is mild or absent.

VISCERAL AND SKELETAL PATHOLOGY

In extraneural tissues, the key cellular pathology of MPS is cellular swelling with a clear or vacuolated appearance on light microscopic examination (see Fig. 8-4). GAGs form a loose branching fibrillary network, but are lost in processing because they are highly soluble in water. Electron microscopy shows distended lysosomes that are empty or contain sparse reticulogranular structures (Fig. 8-24; see also Fig. 8-9). Accumulation of GAGs in the extracellular matrix, presumably caused by deficient recycling and probably also by discharge from dying cells, is central to the phenotype of MPS I-H and other mucopolysaccharidoses. Extracellular GAGs are also lost during processing but can be demonstrated in frozen sections with metachromatic stains and in paraffin sections with colloidal iron stains.

The tissue and organ pathology in mucopolysaccharidoses is due to the combined intracellular and extracellular accumulation of GAGs. Cellular swelling is responsible for the organomegaly. GAG storage in connective tissue matrix and fibroblast dysfunction explain the thickening and deformity of connective tissues, the thick swollen skin, coarse facial features, macroglossia, arthropathy, cardiovascular pathology, and corneal opacity. The cardiac pathology of MPS I-H consists of thickening of heart valves and the endocardium leading to mitral and aortic stiffening and regurgitation (Fig. 8-25). This pathology is compounded by myocardial ischemia secondary to intimal thickening of the coronary arteries (Fig. 8-26). The cornea is a fibrous structure consisting of fibroblasts in a collagenous stroma. GAG storage in corneal fibroblasts (Fig. 8-27) causes corneal clouding and loss of vision. The skeletal pathology of dysostosis multiplex has not been described. Despite GAG storage in chondrocytes and cartilage matrix, growth plates appear normal or slightly disorganized. Numerous clear cells are seen in the periosteum, and osteoblasts also store GAGs. Presumably, the dysostosis is due to a disturbance in enchondral and periosteal osteogenesis caused by an excess of GAGs in matrix and osteoblast dysfunction as a result of intracellular GAG storage.

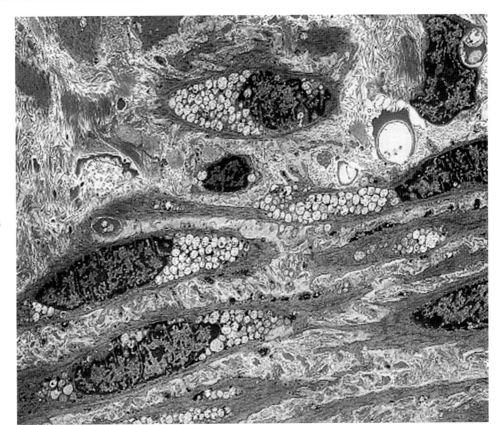

FIGURE 8-24

Mucopolysaccharidosis with vacuoles in fibroblasts.

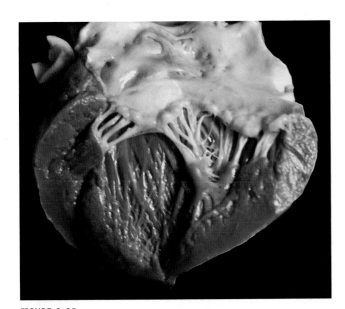

FIGURE 8-25

Myocardial hypertrophy and thickening of the endocardium, cardiac valves, and chordae tendineae in mucopolysaccharidosis.

NEUROPATHOLOGIC CHANGES

The neuropathologic changes in the mucopolysaccharidoses fall under three categories:

1. Entrapment neuropathies, optic nerve compression, and compression myelopathy are secondary to the skeletal and soft tissue changes.

2. GAG deposition causes thickening of the arachnoid membrane and its granulations and resultant impaired circulation of cerebrospinal fluid (CSF) and hydrocephalus (Fig. 8-28). The arachnoid membrane is opaque (Fig. 8-29), and there is cystic expansion of perivascular Virchow-Robin spaces (Fig. 8-30).

3. The most devastating CNS pathology of MPS I-H is a process of neuronal lipidosis, including axonal and dendritic swelling from the accumulation of GM_2 and GM_3 gangliosides, cholesterol, and other lipid materials (Fig. 8-31; see also Fig. 8-3). These products assume the form of concentric or parallel stacks of membranes (zebra bodies) (see Fig. 8-12). This pathology, which is seen in all mucopolysaccharidoses with psychomotor retardation, is indistinguishable from other gangliosidoses. The gangliosides that are deposited in the zebra bodies do not require mucopolysaccharide-cleaving enzymes for their degradation. Ganglioside storage in the mucopolysaccharidoses has been attributed to inhibition of neuraminidase and other ganglioside-cleaving enzymes secondary to GAG accumulation in lysosomes. Although neurons process GAGs and GAGs are present in the CNS interstitial space, lysosomal or interstitial GAG storage is not apparent.

CLINICAL AND PATHOLOGIC FINDINGS IN OTHER MUCOPOLYSACCHARIDOSES

The dysostosis in MPS III and VII is milder than that in MPS I-H and II (see also Table 8-6). The skeletal

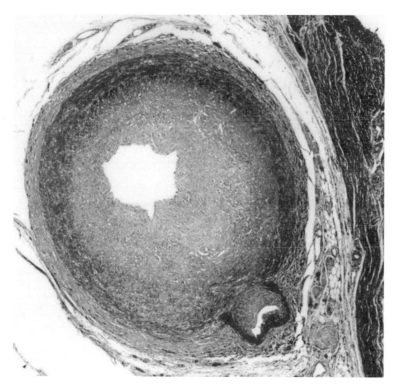

FIGURE 8-26
Intimal thickening of the coronary artery in mucopolysaccharidosis.

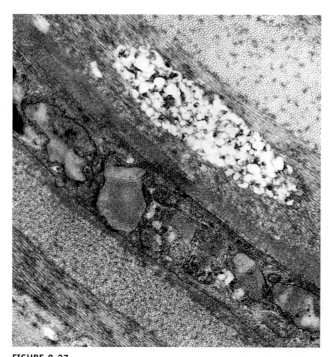

FIGURE 8-27
Glycosaminoglycan storage in corneal fibroblasts in mucopolysaccharidosis.

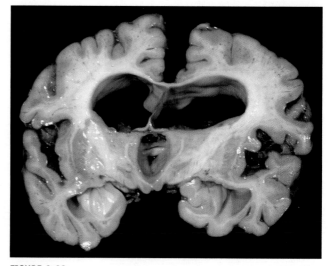

FIGURE 8-28
Hydrocephalus in Hurler's syndrome.

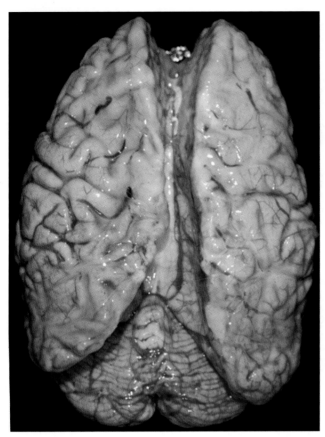

FIGURE 8-29

Meningeal opacity in mucopolysaccharidosis.

dysplasia in MPS IV (Morquio's syndrome) most severely affects the vertebral column and causes a short-trunk dwarfism and atlantoaxial dislocation as a result of odontoid hypoplasia and ligamentous laxity. The only neurologic problem in MPS IV is compression myelopathy. As a rule, heparan sulfate accumulation correlates with psychomotor retardation and dermatan sulfate accumulation with skeletal and mesenchymal abnormalities. In addition to these differences between mucopolysaccharidoses, within each group, especially MPS I, II, and VII, there is molecular heterogeneity leading to phenotypic variability. MPS IV (Morquio's syndrome) and MPS VII cause placental edema and nonimmune hydrops fetalis. The pathogenesis of the hydrops in these cases is poorly understood but may be related to the release of hydrophilic glycoconjugates in the matrix.

DIAGNOSIS OF MUCOPOLYSACCHARIDOSIS

Analysis of urinary GAGs can be used as a preliminary screening test. A definitive diagnosis can be made by enzyme assays of leukocytes, cultured fibroblasts, or serum. Enzyme assay of amniotic fluid or CVS cells is used for prenatal diagnosis. Enzyme analysis does not distinguish carriers from normal individuals who are at the lower range of normal enzyme activity. With the exception of the Sanfilippo type C syndrome, genes causing the mucopolysaccharidoses have been mapped and sequenced, and many mutations have been described. However, the great genetic heterogeneity and frequent compound heterozygosity of the mucopolysaccharidoses make DNA analysis impractical for primary diagnosis. When the mutant alleles are known, mutation analysis can be performed for detection of carriers and prenatal diagnosis (see Table 8-6).

FIGURE 8-30

Expansion of perivascular CNS spaces as a result of mucopolysaccharide deposition in Hurler's syndrome.

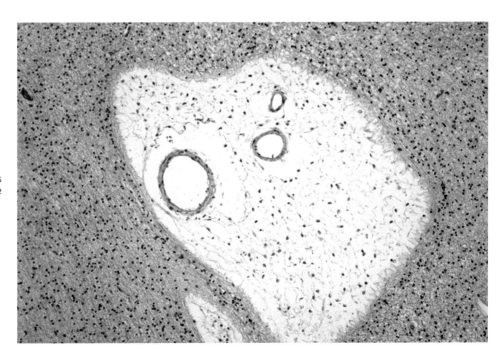

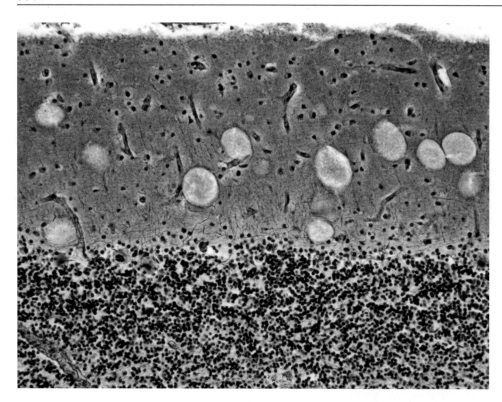

FIGURE 8-31

Expansion of Purkinje cell dendrites as a result of ganglioside storage in the Sanfilippo C syndrome.

GLYCOPROTEINOSES

DEFINITION AND CLASSIFICATION

The glycoproteinoses are a group of LSDs that share features with the mucopolysaccharidoses and sphingolipidoses (Table 8-7).

They are caused by deficiencies of enzymes involved in the degradation of glycoproteins and gangliosides. The stored materials are oligosaccharides, glycopeptides, and glycolipids. All glycoproteinoses are autosomal recessive and panethnic, with the exception of aspartylglycosaminuria, which is largely confined to Finland.

CLINICAL FINDINGS

The multicatalytic action of the deficient lysosomal enzymes in the glycoproteinoses explains the diversity of storage products and their hybrid phenotypes,

TABLE 8-7

Glycoproteinoses

Disease	Enzyme/Protein	Locus	Stored Material	Clinical Findings
Sialidosis	Acid sialidase	6p21.3	Sialyloligosaccharides	H, MR, M, DM, CRS, HF, NS
α-Mannosidosis	α-Mannosidase	19p13.2q12	α-Mannose oligosaccharides	H, MR, DM
β-Mannosidosis	β-Mannosidase	4q22-q25	β-Mannose oligosaccharides	
Fucosidosis	α-Fucosidase	1p34	Fucose oligosaccharides, glycolipids	H, MR, DM, AK
Aspartylglucosaminuria	Aspartylglucosaminidase	4q32-q33	Glycoasparagines Aspartylglucosamine	H, MR, M
Schindler's disease	α-N-acetylgalactosaminidase	22q13	α-N-acetylgalactosamine	MR

CRS, cherry-red spot; DM, dysostosis multiplex; H, Hurler phenotype; HF, hydrops fetalis; M, myoclonus; MPS, mucopolysaccharidosis; MR, mental retardation; NS, nephrotic syndrome.

GLYCOPROTEINOSES—DISEASE FACTS AND PATHOLOGIC FEATURES

Definition

▶ A group of autosomal recessive LSDs caused by deficiencies in enzymes involved in the degradation of glycoproteins and gangliosides. The glycoproteinoses combine phenotypic features of mucopolysaccharidoses and gangliosidoses

Clinical Findings

▶ Psychomotor retardation, coarse facial features, skeletal abnormalities, myoclonus, cherry-red spots, angiokeratoma, nonimmune fetal hydrops

Laboratory Diagnosis

▶ Urine thin-layer chromatography or electrophoresis
▶ Enzyme assay on leukocytes and cultured fibroblasts, amniocytes, and CVS cells

Gross Findings

▶ Hepatosplenomegaly

Microscopic Findings

▶ Clear vacuoles in leukocytes, mesenchymal and epithelial cells, neurons, and glial cells
▶ Neuroaxonal swellings in Schindler's disease

Ultrastructural Features

▶ Reticulogranular material, membranous cytoplasmic bodies, lipofuscin-like products

---

which include elements of glycoproteinoses and sphingolipidoses. In particular, the role of glycoproteins as structural molecules and components of mucinous secretions explains the resemblance of the connective tissue matrix and skeletal pathology to that of the mucopolysaccharidoses.

Like other LSDs, the glycoproteinoses are progressive disorders. They resemble the mucopolysaccharidoses in that most of them have the core clinical components of coarse facial features, skeletal abnormalities, and psychomotor retardation. However, even these core components may be absent or very mild in some glycoproteinoses. For instance, mannosidosis and fucosidosis have mild kyphosis and no true dysostosis multiplex, and Schindler's disease has severe neurologic deterioration without skeletal abnormalities. Other features such as corneal opacity, organomegaly, and heart disease are even more variable. Variations in severity within each group further widen the phenotypic spectrum. Diverse neurologic manifestations, including myoclonus, are seen in sialidosis and Schindler's disease. Moreover, several glycoproteinoses present unique and distinctive clinical features such as cherry-red spots (sialidosis), angiokeratoma (β-mannosidosis and fucosidosis), and nephrotic syndrome (sialidosis).

The most significant phenotypic variation is seen in sialidosis. Three sialidosis phenotypes are distinguished. Sialidosis I is characterized by juvenile to adult onset, cherry-red spots, and myoclonus without

dysostosis or psychomotor retardation; sialidosis II (mucolipidosis I, childhood dysmorphic sialidosis) is characterized by severe neurologic and somatic abnormalities; and severe neonatal sialidosis is characterized by fetal and neonatal hydrops, nephrotic syndrome, and early death.

PATHOLOGIC CHANGES

The core pathology of the glycoproteinoses consists of neurovisceral storage of highly water-soluble oligosaccharides. Such storage results in vacuolization of multiple cell types, including leukocytes, mesenchymal cells, epithelial cells, neurons, and glial cells. By light microscopy, the vacuoles are clear or contain a small amount of metachromatic material. On electron microscopic examination, the vacuoles are membrane bound and contain sparse reticulogranular or floccular material that represents oligosaccharides left over after tissue processing. In fucosidosis, stored glycolipids appear in neurons as reticulogranular material, membranous bodies, and lipofuscin-like products. The pathology of Schindler's disease is unique and consists of neuroaxonal dystrophy in which tubular, vesicular, and lamellar material is stored in axons. No other neurovisceral storage is seen. However, type 2 Schindler's disease, a milder form of this entity reported from Japan (Kanzaki's disease), shows clear cytoplasmic vacuoles in somatic cells and angiokeratoma. In advanced disease, neuronal storage in the glycoproteinoses leads to neuronal loss, gliosis, and cerebral atrophy.

LABORATORY DIAGNOSIS

Urinary screening by thin-layer chromatography or electrophoresis reveals an abnormal pattern of oligosaccharides and glycopeptides. Vacuolated lymphocytes and membrane-bound vacuoles with reticulogranular material in skin, conjunctiva, and other biopsy tissue provide additional evidence of lysosomal storage. A definitive diagnosis can be achieved by enzyme assay of leukocytes or cultured fibroblasts, and prenatal diagnosis can be accomplished by enzyme testing of amniocytes and CVS cells.

NEURONAL CEROID LIPOFUSCINOSES

DEFINITION AND CHEMISTRY

Lipofuscin is an undegradable material that is formed in the free radical–rich environment of lysosomes by peroxidation of membrane phospholipids. It appears in several tissues with advancing age and is an indicator of free radical injury. The neuronal ceroid lipofuscinoses (NCLs) are a group of autosomal recessive disorders characterized clinically by progressive psychomotor retardation, seizures, and blindness and pathologically by lysosomal accumulation in neurons and other cells of PAS-positive, acid-fast, autofluorescent (see Fig. 8-13) lipopigments similar to ceroid and lipofuscin. With an estimated incidence of 1 per 12,500 to 25,000, the NCLs are among the most frequent hereditary neurodegenerative diseases in childhood and one of the most common groups of LSDs. Batten reported the first case of NCL in 1903 and described the clinical and pathologic findings in juvenile NCL in 1914. The name Batten's disease is used for all NCLs but should more specifically apply to juvenile NCL.

Although the NCLs have been known for 100 years, their genetic and molecular basis is still poorly understood. Eight genes causing NCLs have been identified, and seven have been mapped. The two best-known genes, *CLN1* and *CLN2*, code for the lysosomal enzymes palmitoyl protein thioesterase 1 (PPT1) and tripeptidyl peptidase 1 (TPP1), respectively. PPT1 cleaves long-chain fatty acid chains from proteins, and TPP1 cleaves tripeptides from small proteins before further degradation by other proteases. The in vivo substrates of these enzymes are not known with certainty. They are also found in extralysosomal locations such as synapses, and their intracellular location in extraneural cells is not the same as it is in neurons. The products of the other NCL genes are less well characterized. The storage products in the NCLs are of two types. Saposins A and D are stored in infantile NCL, whereas subunit C of mitochondrial adenosine triphosphate (ATP) synthase is stored in all other NCLs.

CLINICAL AND PATHOLOGIC FINDINGS

The uncertainties about their molecular basis notwithstanding, the NCLs are clinically and pathologically indistinguishable from other LSDs that have the neuronal lipidosis phenotype. Four main clinical NCL phenotypes—infantile NCL, late infantile NCL, juvenile NCL, and adult NCL—and several other rarer types are recognized (Table 8-8).

Infantile NCL is most common in Finland. The other NCLs occur worldwide. The light microscopic changes are similar in all NCLs, but the fine structure of the storage material is different and is the basis of their pathologic recognition. Neuronal storage leads to neuronal loss and cerebral and cerebellar atrophy, which may be mild or extreme depending on the type of NCL and the duration of illness. In addition to the retina and CNS, subclinical storage with the same fine structure occurs in a variety of other tissues, including endothelial cells, Schwann cells, smooth and skeletal muscle, sweat glands, and lymphocytes. Examination of these tissues and cells may be used for diagnosis.

Patients with infantile NCL are normal at birth and develop normally for a few months, but within 1 year of age, microcephaly, hypotonia, myoclonus, seizures, ataxia, progressive psychomotor retardation, and blindness develop, and they die between 8 and 13 years of age. Neurons and glial cells in infantile NCL contain membrane-bound granular osmiophilic deposits (Fig. 8-

---

NEURONAL CEROID LIPOFUSCINOSES—DISEASE FACTS AND PATHOLOGIC FEATURES

Definition

▶ A group of autosomal recessive disorders characterized clinically by neurologic deterioration and pathologically by accumulation of lipofuscin-like products in neurons and other cells

Prevalence

▶ 1 per 12,500 to 25,000. Among the most common LSDs

Genetics

▶ Autosomal recessive
▶ Eight genes causing NCLs have been identified

Enzyme Defects

▶ Probably lysosomal proteases in some NCLs

Clinical Findings

▶ Four clinical entities: infantile (INCL), late infantile (LINCL), juvenile (JNCL), and adult (ANCL)
▶ Hypotonia, myoclonus, seizures, ataxia, psychomotor retardation, blindness. Dementia in ANCL

Laboratory Diagnosis

▶ Electron microscopy of lymphocytes and biopsies of skin, conjunctiva, and other tissues
▶ Enzyme testing and molecular analysis are also available for some NCLs

Gross Findings

▶ Cerebral and cerebellar atrophy in advanced stages of NCLs

Microscopic Findings

▶ Neuronal ballooning
▶ Neuronal loss and gliosis in advanced disease

Ultrastructural Features

▶ Granular osmiophilic deposits in INCL, curvilinear bodies in LINCL, fingerprint profiles in JNCL, mixed products in ANCL (see Table 8-8)

TABLE 8-8
Neuronal Ceroid Lipofuscinoses

Type	Gene	Locus	EM	Storage
Infantile	*CLN1*	1p32	GROD	Saposin A & D
Late infantile	*CLN2*	11p15	CLB	SCMAS
Juvenile	*CLN3*	16p12	FP	SCMAS
Adult	*CLN4*	Unknown	Mixed	SCMAS

CLB, curvilinear bodies; EM, electron microscopy; FP, fingerprint profiles; GROD, granular eosinophilic deposits; SCMAS, subunit C of mitochondrial ATP synthase.

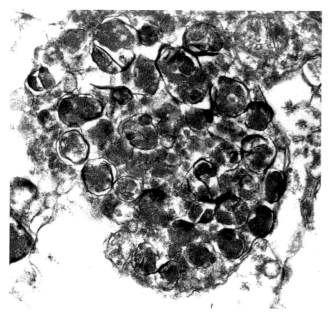

FIGURE 8-32

Granular osmophilic deposits (GRODs) in adult neuronal ceroid lipofuscinosis.

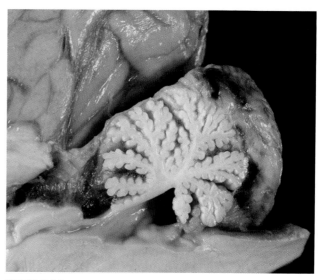

FIGURE 8-34

Cerebellar atrophy in late infantile neuronal ceroid lipofuscinosis.

32). In patients surviving beyond 3 to 4 years of age, virtually all cortical neurons are lost, and there is striking cerebellar atrophy.

Patients with late infantile NCL present between 2 and 4 years of age with seizures, myoclonus, and ataxia.

Psychomotor regression and blindness ensue, and death occurs between 10 and 30 years of age. The storage material in late infantile NCL consists of curvilinear profiles (Fig. 8-33). Patients with advanced disease have severe cerebral and cerebellar atrophy (Fig. 8-34).

Juvenile NCL begins between 4 and 10 years of age with rapidly progressive visual loss that leads to blindness in 2 to 4 years. Seizures and myoclonus appear later, and progressive psychomotor retardation and focal neurologic deficits develop and lead to death by 20 to 30 years of age. The storage material takes the form of fingerprint bodies (Fig. 8-35). The brain shows neuronal

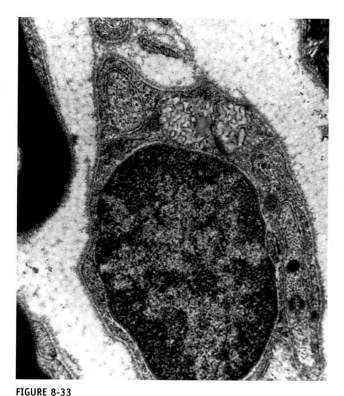

FIGURE 8-33

Curvilinear bodies in a Schwann cell in late infantile neuronal ceroid lipofuscinosis.

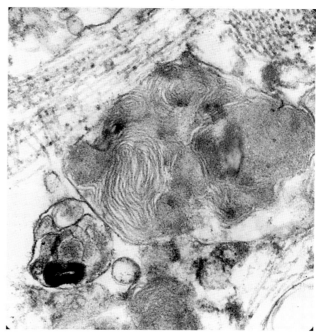

FIGURE 8-35

Fingerprint profiles in juvenile neuronal ceroid lipofuscinosis.

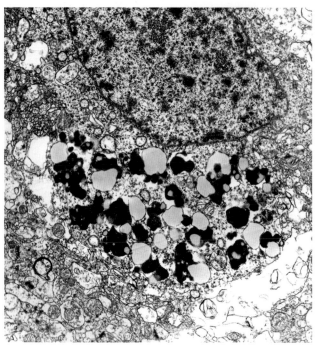

FIGURE 8-36

Lipofuscin-like deposits in adult neuronal ceroid lipofuscinosis.

loss and cortical atrophy, but not of the extreme degree seen in infantile and late infantile NCL.

Adult NCL becomes clinically apparent on average by 30 years of age. Some patients present with myoclonus, ataxia, and dementia and others with behavioral abnormalities and dementia. Progressive neurodegeneration leads to death in 10 years. The storage material in adult NCL is a mixture of fingerprint bodies (Fig. 8-36), granular osmiophilic deposits, and rectilinear profiles. Neuronal loss and cortical atrophy are not as pronounced as in the other NCLs.

DIAGNOSIS

The diagnosis of NCLs is based on clinical findings and electron microscopy of blood lymphocytes or biopsy samples of skin, conjunctiva, and other tissues. The enzyme activity of PPT1 and TPP1 in leukocytes, skin fibroblasts, amniocytes, and CVS cells can be used for diagnosis, prenatal diagnosis, and carrier detection. Molecular genetic testing of *CLN1*, *CLN2*, and *CLN3* gene mutations is also available on a clinical basis.

NIEMANN-PICK DISEASE TYPE C

DEFINITION AND CHEMISTRY

Niemann-Pick disease type C (NPC) and its variant type D are caused by defects in intracellular cholesterol circulation that result in moderate lysosomal storage of phospholipids and glycolipids (including GM_2 ganglioside) and derangement of glycolipid metabolism. Recycled cholesterol from plasma membranes and endocytosed low-density lipoprotein (LDL) cholesterol particles are normally hydrolyzed in endosomes-lysosomes, and cholesterol is then transported back to the plasma membrane. In NPC, uptake and hydrolysis are normal, but subsequent cholesterol transport is arrested and thereby leads to the accumulation of cholesterol in perinuclear lysosomes. This transport also involves other lysosomal contents, which accumulate because they cannot be moved out of lysosomes. NPC is a panethnic disease with protean clinical manifestations that may develop from fetal life to adulthood.

GENETICS AND CLINICAL FINDINGS

NPC is autosomal recessive. Ninety-five percent of cases are caused by mutations of the *NPC1* gene on 18q11-q12. The product of this gene is a membrane protein in the endoplasmic reticulum that is thought to be involved in intracellular sorting of cholesterol and glycosphingolipids. More than 100 mutations of *NPC1* have been reported. Five percent of NPC cases are caused by mutations of the *HE1/NPC2* gene on 14q24.3, which codes for a cholesterol-binding protein. At an estimated prevalence of 1 per 150,000 in Europe, NPC is much more

---

NIEMANN-PICK DISEASE TYPE C—DISEASE FACTS AND PATHOLOGIC FEATURES

Definition
▶ An autosomal recessive disorder of intracellular cholesterol processing

Prevalence
▶ 1 per 150,000 in Europe
▶ Panethnic

Stored Material
▶ Cholesterol, sphingolipids

Clinical Phenotype
▶ Neuronal lipidosis, storage histiocytosis, liver disease, hypotonia, fetal ascites

Laboratory Diagnosis
▶ Filipin test

Gross Findings
▶ Hepatosplenomegaly—normal brain initially, cortical atrophy in advanced cases

Microscopic Findings
▶ Niemann-Pick cells in viscera, ballooned neurons in the brain

Ultrastructural Features
▶ Membranous cytoplasmic bodies

frequent than Niemann-Pick disease types A and B combined. Type D Niemann-Pick disease refers to a genetic cluster of this disease in Nova Scotia.

Infantile-onset NPC may be manifested as fetal ascites, neonatal hepatitis, hypotonia, and delay in psychomotor development. Neurologic symptoms predominate when the onset is in childhood. In addition to psychomotor retardation, neurologic findings include impaired vertical gaze, dystonia, speech abnormality, and seizures. Similar neurologic manifestations developing at a slower pace and psychiatric illness characterize adolescent and adult disease.

PATHOLOGIC CHANGES

The viscera in NPC are infiltrated by foamy histiocytes (Fig. 8-37) that contain membrane-bound lamellar structures and lucent vacuoles (Fig. 8-38). Similar products accumulate in neuronal lysosomes and cause neuronal ballooning (see Fig. 8-3), meganeurites (see Fig. 8-5), and eventually neuronal loss and cerebral and cerebellar atrophy. Additionally, NPC causes axonal swellings, which are especially prominent in early-onset disease, and neurofibrillary tangles indistinguishable from those of Alzheimer's disease, which are seen in adult-onset forms. The viscera in NPC show a moderate accumulation of unesterified cholesterol, sphingolipids, phospholipids, and glycolipids. Cholesterol and sphingolipid concentrations in brain are normal, but there is a moderate reduction of sphingolipids and a change in glycolipid composition.

DIAGNOSIS

The biochemical diagnosis of NPC is made by determining the ability of cultured fibroblasts to esterify cholesterol (Filipin test). In this test, the culture medium is loaded with LDL cholesterol. Normal fibroblasts esterify cholesterol, which is then incorporated into cell membranes. NPC fibroblasts do not. Unesterified cholesterol accumulates in perinuclear lysosomes and is detected by the fluorescent stain Filipin. The Filipin test can also be applied to amniocytes and CVS cells for prenatal diagnosis. Molecular testing for NPC1 is available on a clinical basis and is used for carrier detection and prenatal diagnosis when the mutation is known.

POMPE'S DISEASE (GLYCOGENOSIS TYPE II)

GENETICS AND CLINICAL FINDINGS

This LSD was described by the Dutch physician Pompe in 1932. In 1963, Hers reported that Pompe's disease was caused by the absence of α-glucosidase (acid maltase), the first LSD in which deficiency of a lysosomal hydrolase was proved. This landmark discovery was the foundation of the concept of LSDs and led to the discovery of other lysosomal enzyme deficiencies. The function of acid α-glucosidase is to degrade glycogen particles that enter lysosomes inadvertently. Thus, cells with a high glycogen content such as myocytes and hepatocytes are severely affected. The disease has no effect on energy generation.

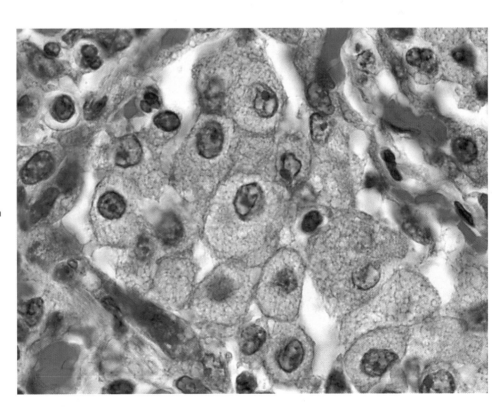

FIGURE 8-37

Niemann-Pick cells in the lungs in type C Niemann-Pick disease.

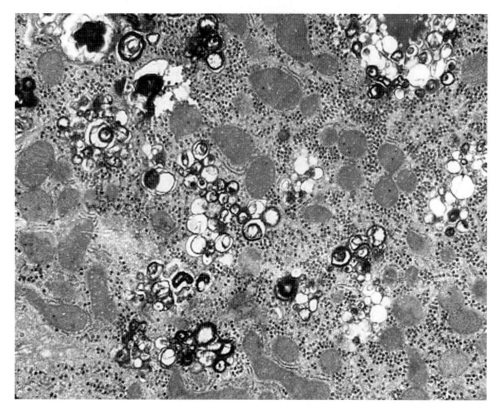

FIGURE 8-38
Lamellar bodies and vacuoles in hepatocyte in type C Niemann-Pick disease.

The gene for acid α-glucosidase is located on 17q25.2-q25.3. More than 40 mutations have been described. Pompe's disease is the most frequent LSD in the Netherlands and the most common form of glycogen storage disease in Taiwan. It is genetically and phenotypically diverse. Patients with the classic infantile form of the disease present early in infancy with severe hypotonia, cardiomegaly (Fig. 8-39), macroglossia, and hepatomegaly and die before they reach their second birthday. Milder variants are manifested later in life (sometimes in the sixth decade), primarily with myopathy, and show great intrafamilial variability in the age of onset and severity of symptoms.

POMPE'S DISEASE (GLYCOGENOSIS TYPE II)— DISEASE FACTS AND PATHOLOGIC FEATURES

Definition
► An autosomal recessive deficiency of acid maltase that causes lysosomal glycogen storage in the heart, skeletal muscle, liver, and other tissues

Storage Material
► Glycogen (lysosomal)

Prevalence
► Rare worldwide but the most common LSD in the Netherlands

Clinical Phenotype
► Hypotonia, cardiomegaly, hepatomegaly, and early death in the infantile form (Pompe's disease)
► Adult-onset myopathy in milder variants

Gross Findings
► Cardiomegaly, macroglossia, hepatomegaly

Microscopic and Ultrastructural Findings
► Membrane-bound (lysosomal) and diffuse monoparticulate glycogen accumulation

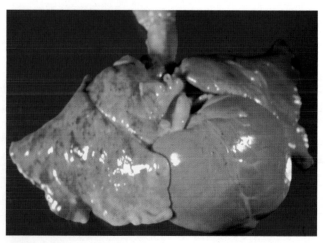

FIGURE 8-39
Cardiomegaly in Pompe's disease.

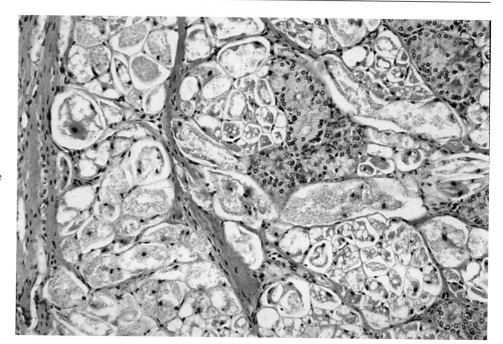

FIGURE 8-40
Glycogen storage in myocytes of the tongue in Pompe's disease.

PATHOLOGIC CHANGES

The pathology of Pompe's disease is characterized by massive lysosomal and extralysosomal accumulation of normal monoparticulate glycogen in skeletal and cardiac muscle (Fig. 8-40), hepatocytes (Fig. 8-41), and many other tissues, including neurons, glial cells, and Schwann cells. Swollen lysosomes impair muscle function initially by crowding out contractile filaments and later by causing myocyte loss. Diffuse (extralysosomal) accumulation is due to saturation of the lysosomal pathway and release of glycogen from lysosomes. The pathology in the late-onset variant is confined to skeletal muscle and consists of a vacuolar myopathy (Fig. 8-42) with membrane-bound and diffuse glycogen.

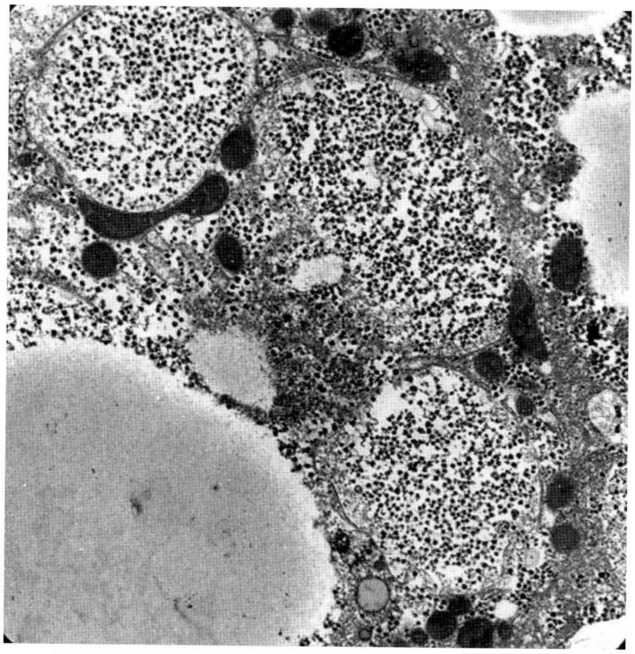

WOLMAN'S DISEASE AND CHOLESTERYL ESTER STORAGE DISEASE

Wolman's disease and cholesteryl ester storage disease are due to a deficiency of acid lipase, which hydrolyzes cholesteryl esters in lipoproteins. Patients present in infancy with hepatosplenomegaly, abdominal distention, steatorrhea, and other gastrointestinal manifestations and usually die before reaching their first birthday. Radi-

FIGURE 8-41
Lysosomal and diffuse storage of monoparticulate glycogen in hepatocytes in Pompe's disease.

WOLMAN'S DISEASE AND CHOLESTERYL ESTER STORAGE DISEASE—DISEASE FACTS AND PATHOLOGIC FEATURES

Definition
▶ A rare autosomal recessive LSD caused by a deficiency of acid lipase

Storage Material
▶ Triglycerides and cholesteryl esters

Clinical Phenotype
▶ Hepatosplenomegaly, steatorrhea

Pathologic Findings
▶ Deposition of sudanophilic lipid material in many tissues and organs
▶ No neuronal storage

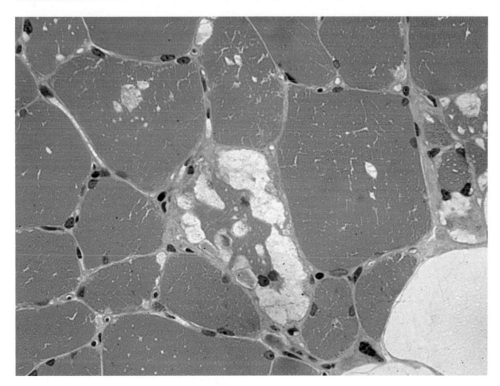

FIGURE 8-42

Vacuolar myopathy in adult-onset acid maltase deficiency.

ologic demonstration of adrenal calcifications is diagnostic. Cholesteryl ester storage disease, an allelic variant, has a milder course. The pathology consists of deposition of cholesteryl esters and triglycerides in all organs and tissues (Fig. 8-43). Sudanophilic droplets accumulate in hepatocytes, Kupffer cells, adrenal cortical cells, smooth muscle and vascular endothelium, histiocytes in the leptomeninges and choroid plexus, Schwann cells, microglial cells, perivascular brain histiocytes, and other cell types. There is no evidence of neuronal storage in the CNS, but sudanophilic droplets have been reported in ganglion cells, histiocytes, and other cell types.

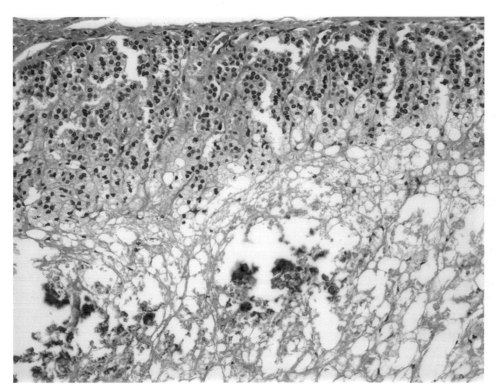

FIGURE 8-43

Lipid storage and calcification in the adrenal cortex in Wolman's disease.

PEROXISOMAL DISORDERS

THE PEROXISOME

ANATOMY OF PEROXISOMES

Peroxisomes (also known as microbodies, microperoxisomes, diaminobenzidine-positive particles, catalosomes, catalase-positive particles) are small, membrane-bound organelles that average 0.5 μm in diameter. They are most abundant in hepatocytes and renal tubular cells but are present in virtually all cells. In the mature brain, peroxisomes are confined to oligodendroglial cells. In the developing CNS, they are found in neuroblasts, immature neurons, and oligodendrocytes. The term peroxisome, coined by DeDuve, refers to the ability of these organelles to generate H_2O_2. Peroxisomes can be identified on light microscopy by their catalase activity using the diaminobenzidine reaction. They can also be localized by immunohistochemistry by using antibodies to catalase and other peroxisomal membrane and matrix proteins. Particulate staining indicates the presence of peroxisomes. Diffuse staining or cytoplasmic localization of catalase indicates the absence of peroxisomes. Peroxisomes in plants (glyoxysomes) are important for photorespiration and for the glyoxylate cycle in which fatty acids are converted to sugars and stored in seeds.

The significance of peroxisomes in human metabolic disease became apparent in 1973 when Goldfischer reported that peroxisomes were absent in Zellweger's syndrome (ZS). Elucidation of the metabolic functions of peroxisomes began with the discovery that patients with ZS had elevated very long chain fatty acids (VLCFAs) in plasma and decreased plasmalogens in tissues and red blood cells (RBCs).

BIOCHEMISTRY AND FUNCTIONS OF PEROXISOMES

The most important functions of peroxisomes are listed in Table 8-9.

TABLE 8-9

Biochemistry and Functions of Peroxisomes

H_2O_2 generation
Oxidation of very long chain fatty acids and phytanic acid
Plasmalogen biosynthesis
Cholesterol biosynthesis
Glyoxylate detoxification
Amino acid metabolism
Purine metabolism
Bile acid metabolism

H_2O_2 Generation • Peroxisomes generate H_2O_2 and use it to oxidize a variety of substances, including phenol, formic acid, and alcohol. This reaction is important for detoxification of toxic molecules. Excess H_2O_2, which is toxic in itself, is converted by catalase to H_2O and O_2.

β-Oxidation and Phytanic Acid Processing • β-Oxidation is a process by which the alkyl chains of fatty acids are shortened by two carbon atoms at a time. The shortened fatty acids are further β-oxidized in mitochondria. The acetyl coenzyme A (CoA) that is generated is exported into the cytosol and used in a variety of biosynthetic reactions. The bulk of β-oxidation is performed in mitochondria, which oxidize short-, medium-, and many long-chain fatty acids. Peroxisomes oxidize mostly VLCFAs, such as C24:0 and especially C26:0, and pristanic acid, a product of phytanic acid. Phytanic acid is derived entirely from dietary sources and can be β-oxidized only after removal of its terminal carboxyl group by the peroxisomal phytanoyl-CoA hydrolase, a reaction that is called α-oxidation. Deficiency of this enzyme causes Refsum's disease. β-Oxidation of phytanic acid and dihydroxycholestanoic and trihydroxycholestanoic acid (DHCA and THCA) also plays a role in bile acid synthesis.

Plasmalogen Synthesis • The ether linkage of ether-linked phospholipids (plasmalogens) is catalyzed by the peroxisomal dihydroacetone-phosphate acyltransferase (DHAPAT) and alkyldihydroacetone-phosphate synthase (alkyl-DHAP synthase). Although plasmalogens are the most abundant (80% to 90%) phospholipids in myelin, they do not appear to be involved in the myelin abnormalities of peroxisomal disorders. Plasmalogen deficiency is seen in rare disorders caused by isolated defects of DHAPAT and alkyl-DHAP synthase and is also a feature of rhizomelic chondrodysplasia punctata and other peroxisomal biogenesis disorders.

Cholesterol Biosynthesis • Many enzymes of cholesterol biosynthesis are localized in peroxisomes, and patients with peroxisomal disorders have defective cholesterol biosynthesis.

Glyoxylate Detoxification • Glyoxylate, a toxic metabolite of alanine, is converted to glycine by the peroxisomal enzyme alanine glyoxylate aminotransferase. Deficiency of this enzyme results in an increase in gly-

---

THE PEROXISOME—DISEASE FACTS AND PATHOLOGIC FEATURES

Anatomy of Peroxisomes
▶ Small membrane-bound organelles with catalase activity, abundant in hepatocytes and renal cells

Main Biochemical Functions
▶ H_2O_2 generation, β-oxidation of very long chain fatty acids, plasmalogen synthesis, cholesterol biosynthesis, bile acid metabolism

Peroxisomal Biogenesis
▶ Peroxisomes contain no RNA or DNA. A vesicle develops first, proteins are embedded in its wall, and peroxisomal enzymes are imported into the matrix

oxylate, which is then converted to oxalate by lactate dehydrogenase.

Amino Acid Metabolism • Peroxisomes are involved in the metabolism of two amino acids: lysine and alanine. Pipecolic acid, a product of lysine, is converted to α-aminoadipate by peroxisomal pipecolic acid oxidase. This pathway is active in the brain. Elevation of pipecolic acid is seen in peroxisomal biogenesis disorders. Pipecolic acid is thought to be an agonist of γ-aminobutyric acid (GABA).

BIOGENESIS OF PEROXISOMES

The peroxisome has a single membrane that encloses the peroxisomal matrix. The peroxisomal membrane is a lipid bilayer with embedded peroxisomal membrane proteins. Peroxisomes have no DNA or ribosomes. All peroxisomal membrane proteins and enzymes of the peroxisomal matrix are encoded by nuclear genes, synthesized on free ribosomes, and imported into the peroxisomes. The biogenesis of peroxisomes probably begins with the formation of a vesicle with a lipid bilayer wall. It is not clear how this first step is accomplished, and there is no evidence that this preperoxisomal vesicle is pinched off of the endoplasmic reticulum. Once the vesicle wall is in place, proteins are inserted into the lipid bilayer. These proteins stabilize the peroxisomal membrane and, together with cytosolic proteins, take part in the importation of enzymes into the peroxisomal matrix. When the mature peroxisome reaches critical volume, it divides into two daughter peroxisomes. The proteins that are involved in peroxisomal

biogenesis are called peroxins. Some of them are embedded in the peroxisomal membrane and others are cytosolic. Peroxins are encoded by *PEX* genes. Fifteen human and 23 yeast *PEX* genes are known. Enzymes targeted for the peroxisomal matrix are tagged with two types of short amino acid sequences called peroxisomal targeting signals, PTS1 and PTS2. PTS1 is attached to the C-terminus of the protein and is the recognition signal for most peroxisomal enzymes. PTS2 is attached to the N-terminus and identifies a few peroxisomal enzymes. In the cytosol, peroxisomal enzymes bind to specific receptor proteins, PEX5 for PTS1 enzymes and PEX7 for PTS2 enzymes. The enzyme-receptor complex docks onto peroxisomal membrane proteins, the enzyme separates from the receptor and is translocated into the peroxisome, and the receptor is then released back into the cytosol.

PEROXISOMAL DISORDERS IN GENERAL

There are two types of peroxisomal disorders: single peroxisomal enzyme deficiencies and peroxisomal biogenesis disorders (Table 8-10).

The former are caused by mutations in genes encoding specific enzymes. Peroxisomal biogenesis disorders are caused by mutations in *PEX* genes that are involved in the biogenesis and function of peroxisomes; these disorders are characterized by deficiencies of multiple peroxisomal enzymes and, in some cases, by absence or reduction of the number of peroxisomes. X-linked adrenoleukodystrophy (XALD) is also classified as a peroxisomal disorder but has a different pathogenesis:

TABLE 8-10
Peroxisomal Disorders

Disease		Transmission	PEX Gene/Enzyme	Loci	Pathology
PBDs	Zellweger spectrum (ZS, NALD, IRD)	AR	Pex1 Matrix protein import	7q21-22 and other	NMD, white matter disease, liver disease
	Rhizomelic chondrodysplasia punctata	AR	Pex7 PTS2 receptor	6q22-q24	Skeletal abnormalities, microcephaly, cerebellar atrophy
Single enzyme defects	D-Bifunctional protein deficiency	AR	17β-Hydroxysteroid dehydrogenase	5q2	NMD, white matter abnormality, liver disease
	Adult Refsum's disease	AR	Phytanoyl-CoA hydroxylase	10pter-p11.2	Hypertrophic neuropathy, long tract degeneration, retinitis pigmentosa
Nonperoxisomal	X-linked adrenoleukodystrophy	X-linked	VLCFA transport (ALDP) ATP-binding cassette, subfamily D	Xq28	Leukodystrophy Adrenal atrophy

ALDP, adrenoleukodystrophy transport protein; AR, autosomal recessive; IRD, infantile Refsum's disease; NALD, neonatal adrenoleukodystrophy; NMD, neuronal migration defect; PBD, peroxisomal biogenesis disorder; ZS, Zellweger's syndrome.

PEROXISOMAL DISORDERS IN GENERAL—DISEASE FACTS AND PATHOLOGIC FEATURES

Peroxisomal Disorders

► There are two types of peroxisomal disorders:
  ► Peroxisomal biogenesis disorders characterized by the absence of multiple peroxisomal enzymes and, in some cases, the absence of peroxisomes
  ► Single peroxisomal enzyme deficiencies with intact peroxisomes

Genetics

► All peroxisomal disorders are autosomal recessive except for X-linked adrenoleukodystrophy

Laboratory Diagnosis

► Elevated very long chain fatty acids, decreased plasmalogens, decreased or absent hepatic peroxisomes in peroxisomal biogenesis disorders

Neuropathologic Abnormalities

► Neuronal migration defects, leukodystrophy or other white matter abnormality, lipid deposition in the CNS, hepatic fibrosis and cirrhosis, adrenocortical ballooned and striated cells

---

it is caused by mutations of ALDP, a transmembrane protein similar to the cystic fibrosis transmembrane regulator that is involved in transporting C26:0-CoA ester across the peroxisomal membrane. XALD is more frequent than all other peroxisomal disorders combined.

COMPLEMENTATION GROUPS

Insight into the etiology of peroxisomal biogenesis disorders was gained by complementation experiments in which fibroblasts from patients with two different disorders were cocultured. Sharing of genes in cells derived from such cultures leads to correction of biochemical abnormalities in the individual cell lines. On the basis of such experiments, peroxisomal biogenesis disorders have been divided into 12 complementation groups

(CGs), each of which is caused by mutation of one *PEX* gene. One of these groups, CG11, is caused by mutations in *PEX7* and correlates with the distinct phenotype of rhizomelic chondrodysplasia punctata, which accounts for 17% of peroxisomal biogenesis disorders studied by complementation. Fifty-seven percent of peroxisomal biogenesis disorders are caused by mutations in *PEX1* and have a wide phenotypic spectrum that encompasses ZS, neonatal adrenoleukodystrophy (NALD), and infantile Refsum's disease (IRD). The rest are caused by mutations in other *PEX* genes and also fall into the ZS-NALD-IRD spectrum.

GENETICS OF PEROXISOMAL DISORDERS

All peroxisomal disorders except one are autosomal recessive. The only exception is XALD. As in other genetic disorders, several mutations in each gene are seen, some of them causing severe and some milder phenotypes. Mutations in different genes can cause a similar phenotype. The unique biogenesis of peroxisomes and the multiple interactions of *PEX* genes explain the genetic and phenotypic complexity of peroxisomal disorders. For instance, defects in genes that are important for the assembly of peroxisomes can result in total absence or a severe decrease in the number of peroxisomes, a situation that does not occur in other organelle disorders. Single gene defects can either impair peroxisomal enzyme import and lead to a deficiency in multiple peroxisomal enzymes or can cause isolated enzyme deficiencies.

LABORATORY DIAGNOSIS OF PEROXISOMAL DISORDERS

The laboratory diagnosis of peroxisomal disorders should start with determination of plasma VLCFAs and RBC plasmalogens (Table 8-11). This screen distinguishes the ZS spectrum of peroxisomal biogenesis disorders and the phenotypically similar single β-oxidation enzymopathies from rhizomelic chondrodysplasia punctata and XALD.

TABLE 8-11
Laboratory Diagnosis of Peroxisomal Disorders

Abnormality	ZS	NALD	IRD	Single β-Oxidation Enzyme Defects	RCDP	XALD
Plasma VLCFAs	Increased	Increased	Increased	Increased	Normal	Increased
RBC plasmalogens	Decreased	Decreased	Decreased	Normal	Decreased	Normal
Hepatic peroxisomes	Absent	Decreased/normal	Normal	Normal	Normal	Normal

IRD, infantile Refsum's disease; NALD, neonatal adrenoleukodystrophy; RCDP, rhizomelic chondrodysplasia punctata; XALD, X-linked adrenoleukodystrophy; ZS, Zellweger's syndrome.

Among the ZS spectrum disorders, the biochemical abnormalities are most severe in ZS, intermediate in NALD, and mildest in IRD. Plasmalogen deficiency is most severe in young patients. If this initial screen is abnormal, further analysis of DHCA, THCA, phytanic, pristanic, and pipecolic acids and measurements of fatty acid β-oxidation and plasmalogen synthesis in fibroblasts distinguish the ZS spectrum peroxisomal biogenesis disorders from single β-oxidative enzyme deficiencies. Phytanic acid levels depend on dietary intake and may be normal in newborns. In the ZS spectrum, peroxisomes are absent or severely reduced, and the catalase in hepatocytes has a diffuse (cytosolic) as opposed to the normal particulate (peroxisomal) distribution. Prenatal diagnosis can be facilitated by study of catalase activity in chorionic villi, determination of enzyme activity and plasmalogen content in uncultured CVS cells and cultured amniocytes, and DNA analysis.

TREATMENT OF PEROXISOMAL DISORDERS

The only peroxisomal disorder that can be effectively treated is adult Refsum's disease. Dietary restriction decreases blood levels and the tissue burden of phytanic acid. Progression of the neuropathy is arrested, nerve conduction velocity improves, and nerve biopsy specimens show myelin regeneration. CNS manifestations do not improve, but further deterioration is arrested and patients live longer. Therapy aiming to improve the biochemical abnormalities of peroxisomal biogenesis disorders (supplementation of plasmalogens, decrease in VLCFAs) has not worked. Supplementation of docosahexaenoic acid, which is deficient in patients with peroxisomal biogenesis disorders, is being evaluated.

The following section describes the ZS spectrum, rhizomelic chondrodysplasia punctata, and the two best-known single peroxisomal enzyme deficiencies, D-bifunctional protein deficiency and adult Refsum's disease. XALD is described elsewhere.

THE ZELLWEGER SPECTRUM

ZS, NALD, and IRD were initially described as separate entities. It is now clear that they represent a phenotypic spectrum, the ZS spectrum, that is caused by mutations in *PEX* genes that result in abnormal peroxisomal biogenesis. ZS is the most severe end of the spectrum and IRD the least severe. The ZS spectrum accounts for about 80% of peroxisomal biogenesis disorders and rhizomelic chondrodysplasia punctata for 17%. Their combined incidence is 1 per 50,000 births. Hyperpipecolic acidemia, once considered a separate entity, is now thought to be part of the ZS spectrum. The ZS spectrum is caused by mutations of 10 *PEX* genes (more than half are due to mutations in PEX1, which is involved in matrix protein import). Mutations of the same gene can cause different phenotypes, either ZS, NALD, or IRD. Conversely, mutations of different genes can cause the

same phenotype. A detailed account of ZS and brief descriptions of NALD and IRD follow.

CLINICAL FINDINGS

ZS, described by Zellweger and named "cerebro-hepatorenal syndrome" by Passarge and "Zellweger syndrome" by Opitz, is characterized clinically by dysmorphic features, congenital abnormalities, calcific

---

THE ZELLWEGER SPECTRUM—DISEASE FACTS AND PATHOLOGIC FEATURES

Definition
▶ A peroxisomal biogenesis disorder characterized by dysmorphic features, calcific stippling of the patellae, liver disease, neuronal migration abnormalities, and white matter changes
▶ The Zellweger syndrome, neonatal adrenoleukodystrophy, and infantile Refsum's disease are parts of the Zellweger spectrum

Inheritance
▶ Autosomal recessive

Gene Loci
▶ 7q21.22 and other

Enzyme/Protein Defects
▶ PEX1 (involved in protein import) and several other peroxins

Clinical Findings
▶ Prominent forehead, flat supraorbital ridges, large fontanelles and other dysmorphic features, liver disease, hypotonia, seizures, absent neurologic development

Radiologic Features
▶ Calcific stippling of the patellae

Laboratory Diagnosis
▶ Elevated VLCFAs, decreased plasmalogens, decreased or absent hepatic peroxisomes

Neuropathologic Findings
▶ Gross: perisylvian pachygyria with surrounding polymicrogyria
▶ Microscopic: abnormal cortical cytoarchitecture; cerebellar microgyria and heterotopia; dysplasia of the inferior olives; reduced white matter mass with deficient myelin; accumulation of sudanophilic lipids in neurons, glial cells, macrophages, and the neuropil

Ultrastructural Features
▶ Cholesterol clefts, membranous bodies, and fiber-like (trilamellar) inclusions in brain cells
▶ Trilamellar inclusions in adrenocortical cells

Pathology in Other Organs
▶ Hepatic fibrosis and cirrhosis, absent peroxisomes in hepatocytes, renal cortical cysts, ballooned striated adrenocortical cells

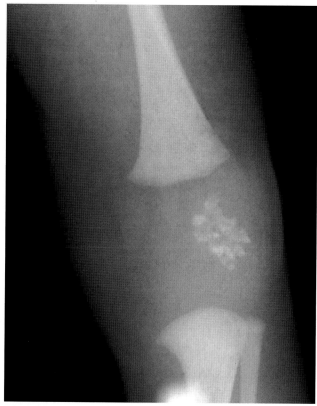

FIGURE 8-44
Calcific stippling of the patella in the Zellweger syndrome.

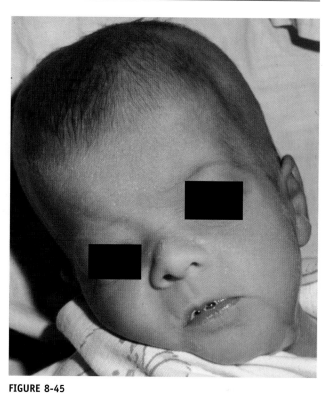

FIGURE 8-45
Dysmorphic features in the Zellweger syndrome: prominent forehead, hypertelorism, broad nasal bridge.

stippling of the patellae (Fig. 8-44), liver disease, and severe neurologic manifestations. The dysmorphic features consist of a prominent forehead, hypertelorism, epicanthal folds, flat supraorbital ridges, a broad nasal bridge, micrognathia, large fontanelles, and a flat occiput (Fig. 8-45). Neurologic manifestations include hypotonia, decreased sucking, absent or decreased tendon reflexes, absent or weak Moro reflex, seizures, abnormal electroencephalogram (EEG), nystagmus, and contractures. Most ZS patients exhibit failure to thrive and die by 6 months of age. Longer survival and some neurologic development have been reported in rare ZS variants.

GENERAL PATHOLOGIC CHANGES

The liver is enlarged in the majority of ZS patients and shows cholestasis, fibrosis in 76%, and micronodular cirrhosis in 37% (Fig. 8-46). Hepatic macrophages (and less frequently hepatocytes) contain intralysosomal trilamellar inclusions and insoluble lipid material. The trilamellar inclusions are thought to represent unsaturated fatty acid esters and are characteristic of peroxisomal disorders. They are also seen in adrenocortical cells, brain macrophages, and other tissues (Fig. 8-47). Liver disease may be caused by toxins that accumulate because of defective peroxidation, damage by H_2O_2, and abnormal bile acid synthesis. Following Goldfischer's 1973 report,

peroxisomes were thought to be absent. Although true of the most severe cases (Fig. 8-48), in many ZS patients peroxisomes are either severely reduced or present but consist of empty vesicles without enzymes. The kidneys show cortical cysts representing cystic Bowman spaces and dilated convoluted tubules (Fig. 8-49). The adrenal cortex contains ballooned striated cells with trilamellar inclusions. The renal and adrenal abnormalities cause no clinical disease. Thirty-two percent of ZS patients have ventricular septal defects, and others have milder congenital heart abnormalities.

NEUROPATHOLOGIC CHANGES

The brain in ZS patients is frequently enlarged and shows neuronal migration abnormalities, white matter pathology, and lipid accumulation. In its full-blown state, the neuronal migration defect (NMD) is characterized by perisylvian pachygyria (Fig. 8-50) with polymicrogyria in the adjacent frontoparietal areas. The sylvian fissures are vertically oriented. The cortex in the pachygyric areas is thick (Fig. 8-51). The molecular layer is fused, thus eliminating the cerebral sulci. The superficial cortex contains large and medium-sized pyramidal cells, whereas smaller neurons that normally populate the superficial cortex are found in the deeper layers or in the subcortical white matter. The topography and cytoarchitecture of the NMD are characteristic of ZS. The cerebellum is often small in comparison to

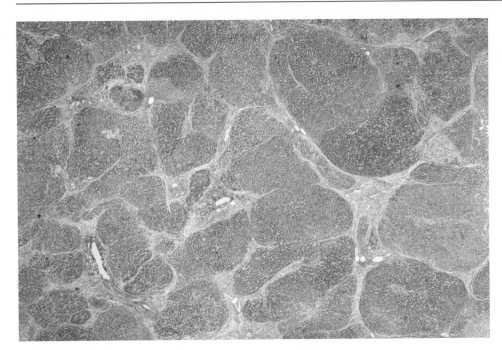

FIGURE 8-46

Hepatic fibrosis and cirrhosis in the Zellweger syndrome.

the cerebrum and shows microgyria and heterotopic islands of Purkinje and granular cells in the white matter (Fig. 8-52). The neuronal ribbons of the dentate nuclei and inferior olives lose their elaborate folding (Fig. 8-53) or are discontinuous. The main cause of the profound neurologic abnormality in ZS is the NMD. The pathogenesis of the NMD in ZS has not been explained. Alteration of neuronal membranes as a result of incorporation of abnormal fatty acids may impair the

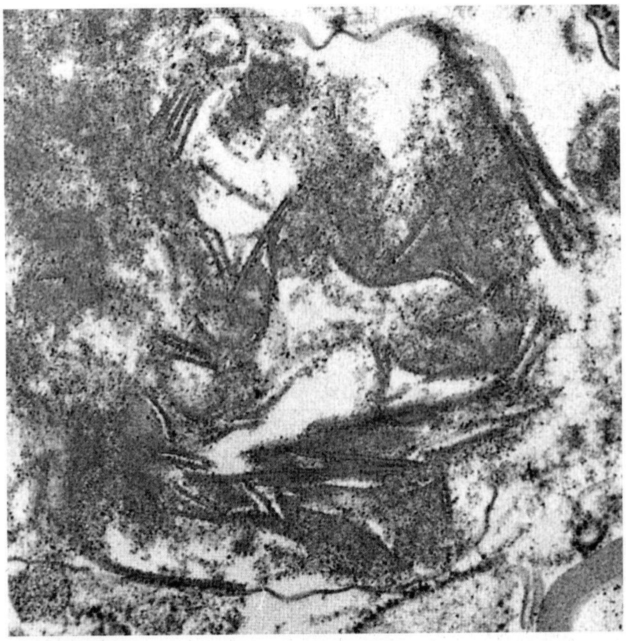

FIGURE 8-47

Trilamellar inclusions in a cerebral macrophage in the Zellweger syndrome. (Reproduced with permission of the Journal of Neuropathology and Experimental Neurology.)

cellular interactions and signaling that guide migrating neurons. Deficiencies of doublecortin and L1 CAM have also been reported.

The white matter in ZS is reduced in mass and shows deficient myelin, lipid accumulation in macrophages, and gliosis. This white matter abnormality has been loosely referred to as leukodystrophy, but it is not comparable to the classic leukodystrophies such as Krabbe's disease or metachromatic leukodystrophy. Clinical evidence of progression is lacking, perhaps because ZS patients do not live long enough for such progression to be appreciated. The decreased white matter mass is due, in part, to the cortical dysplasia. The lipid macrophages are not confined to white matter (they are more abundant in gray matter) and do not contain products of myelin degradation.

The brain in ZS is sodden with sudanophilic lipid products. These products accumulate mostly in macrophages but are also present in neurons, oligodendroglia, astrocytes, and the neuropil. Macrophages are randomly scattered in the cortex and white matter and are more abundant in the cerebral and particularly the cerebellar cortex (Fig. 8-54). They are globose and PAS positive and contain a variety of abnormal lipid products (Fig. 8-55), including cholesterol clefts, MCBs, and trilamellar inclusions. These lipid products may be gangliosides containing VLCFAs and other lipids that are present in excessive amounts and cannot be used by brain cells. Other neuropathologic findings include neuronal degeneration and loss in spinal cord nuclei and glycogen accumulation in neurons and astrocytes, findings suggestive of possible failure of cellular respiration and other metabolic pathways.

The metabolic defect in ZS begins in utero and progresses through the pregnancy. Abnormal cortical layering and lipid accumulation have been observed as early as 14 weeks of gestation.

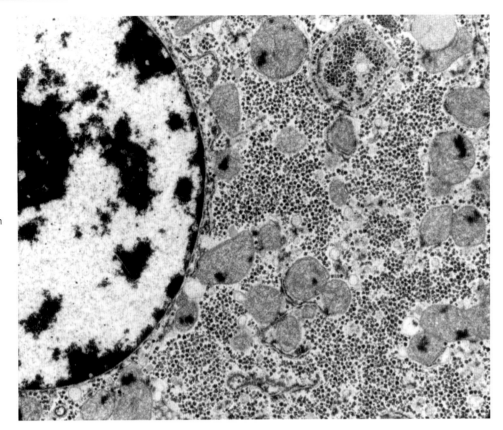

FIGURE 8-48
Hepatocyte without peroxisomes in the Zellweger syndrome.

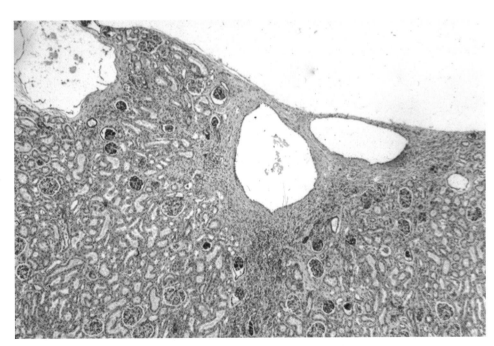

FIGURE 8-49
Cortical renal cysts in the Zellweger syndrome.

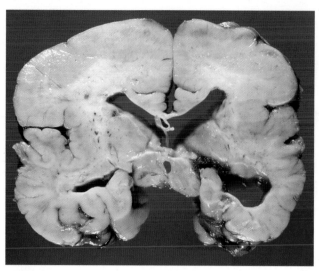

FIGURE 8-50

Pachygyria in the Zellweger syndrome. (Reproduced from *www.akron childrens.org/neuropathology* with permission of Akron Children's Hospital.)

NEONATAL ADRENOLEUKODYSTROPHY

NALD has similar, but milder, dysmorphic features and neurologic abnormalities than ZS does, and patients survive, on average, for 3 years and some of them into adolescence. Hepatic fibrosis and cirrhosis are common, and hepatocellular peroxisomes are normal or reduced. The adrenocortical atrophy with VLCFA storage in ballooned and striated adrenocortical cells is identical to that found in XALD, and macrophages with abnormal lipid contents are present in many organs. The brain shows polymicrogyria, subcortical heterotopia, and cerebellar dysplasia, but no pachygyria. Lipid-laden

CNS histiocytes and swollen neurons are less frequent than in ZS. An inflammatory demyelinative white matter disorder identical to XALD develops in NALD patients surviving longer than 3 to 5 years (Fig. 8-56).

INFANTILE REFSUM'S DISEASE (INFANTILE PHYTANIC ACID STORAGE DISEASE)

IRD is characterized by psychomotor retardation, sensorineural deafness, pigmentary degeneration of the retina, anosmia, and minor dysmorphic features. Patients survive into adolescence or adulthood. The liver is enlarged and cirrhotic, and hepatocytes contain lamellar inclusions similar to the phytol inclusions seen in chloroplasts of plant cells. This observation prompted biochemical studies that revealed elevation of phytanic acid, hence the term infantile phytanic acid storage (Refsum's) disease. Peroxisomes are absent or reduced. The adrenals are atrophic, and the adrenal cortex contains ballooned and striated cells. Magnetic resonance imaging (MRI) shows diffuse white matter atrophy. Postmortem study of a patient who died at 12 years of age revealed cerebellar atrophy and a mild diffuse decrease in axons and myelin without active demyelination.

BIOCHEMICAL ABNORMALITIES IN THE ZELLWEGER SPECTRUM

The biochemical abnormalities (Table 8-12) are the same in all ZS spectrum patients. They differ only in degree, being most severe in ZS and least severe in IRD.

The clinical and pathologic similarities of the ZS spectrum disorders are obvious. Their differences have to do, in part, with (1) the severity of the mutation and

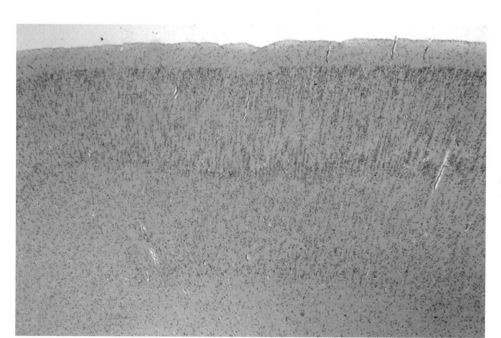

FIGURE 8-51

Thick, abnormally layered cortex in the Zellweger syndrome.

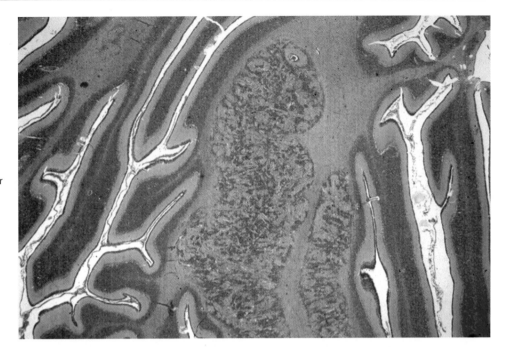

FIGURE 8-52

Heterotopic Purkinje and granular cells in the Zellweger syndrome.

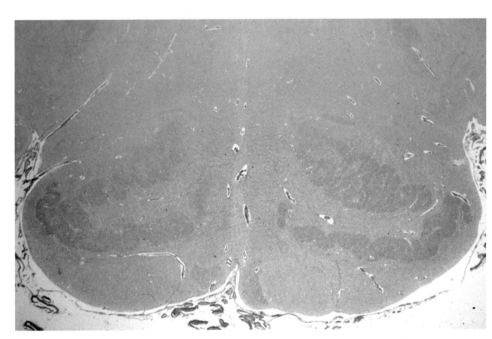

FIGURE 8-53

Inferior olive in the Zellweger syndrome: thick neuronal bands without folding.

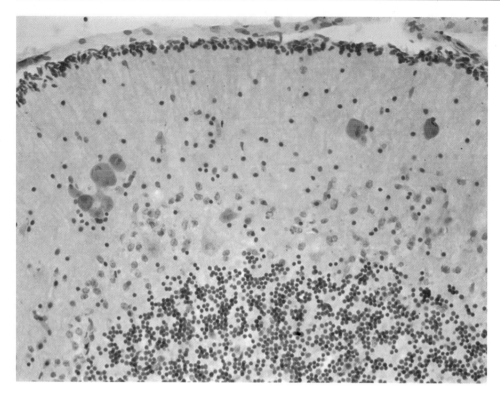

FIGURE 8-54

Lipid-filled macrophages in the cerebellum in the Zellweger syndrome (oil red O).

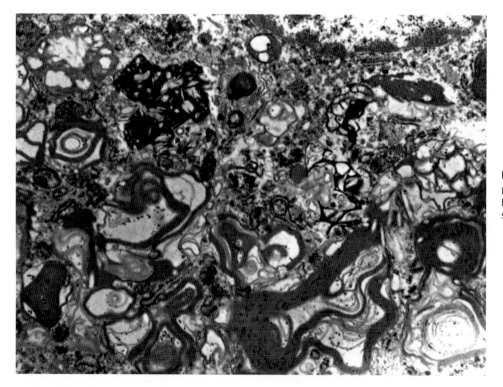

FIGURE 8-55

Diverse lipid products in a cerebral macrophage in the Zellweger syndrome.

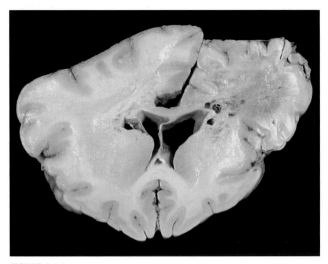

FIGURE 8-56

Extensive demyelination in a 10-year-old patient with neonatal adrenoleukodystrophy.

(2) length of survival, which is inversely related to severity. The NMD is static, and its extent depends on the severity of the mutation. Other aspects of the spectrum (cirrhosis, adrenal atrophy, white matter pathology) are progressive metabolic pathologies and are more prominent in patients with milder mutations and longer survival.

RHIZOMELIC CHONDRODYSPLASIA PUNCTATA TYPE 1

CLINICAL FINDINGS

Chondrodysplasia punctata is a genetically diverse (X-linked, autosomal recessive, and autosomal dominant) group of bone dysplasias characterized by punctate calcifications of the epiphyses and the cartilaginous skeleton (which disappear with age) and coronal clefts of the vertebrae. The only chondrodysplasia that is a peroxisomal disorder is rhizomelic chondrodysplasia punctata

TABLE 8-12

Biochemical Abnormalities in the Zellweger Spectrum

Elevated very long chain fatty acids

Elevated dihydrocholestanoic and trihydrocholestanoic acid

Elevated pristanic and phytanic acid

Elevated L-pipecolic acid

Deficient docosahexaenoic acid

Deficient plasmalogens

RHIZOMELIC CHONDRODYSPLASIA PUNCTATA TYPE 1— DISEASE FACTS AND PATHOLOGIC FEATURES

Definition

▶ A peroxisomal biogenesis disorder characterized by skeletal abnormalities, dysmorphic features, and severe psychomotor retardation

Inheritance

▶ Autosomal recessive

Gene Locus

▶ 6q22-q24

Protein Defect

▶ PEX7, the PTS2 receptor

Clinical Findings

▶ Dysmorphic features, cataracts, contractures, severe psychomotor retardation, and death by 1 year

Radiologic Features

▶ Punctate calcification of the epiphyses and cartilaginous skeleton, coronal clefts of the vertebrae

Laboratory Diagnosis

▶ Decreased plasmalogens, normal VLCFAs

Gross Findings

▶ Microcephaly, cerebellar atrophy

Microscopic Findings

▶ Cerebellar degeneration

(RCDP), which shows, in addition, severe shortening of long bones and flaring of their metaphyses. There are three types of RCDP. The most common, RCDP type 1, is autosomal recessive and is caused by mutations of *PEX7*. In addition to the skeletal abnormalities, RCDP1 patients have a dysmorphic face, cataracts, ichthyosis, joint contractures, and severe psychomotor retardation. Most cases are fatal in the first year of life. The biochemical findings in RCDP1 are decreased plasmalogens, elevated phytanic acid, and normal VLCFAs.

PATHOLOGIC CHANGES

The common denominator in the few reported autopsy cases of RCDP1 is severe microcephaly with a normal cortical cytoarchitecture and normal myelin despite the severe plasmalogen deficiency. Three chronic RCDP1 patients had severe cerebellar degeneration (Fig. 8-57). It appears that RCDP1 patients are born with microcephaly and that progressive cerebellar degeneration develops postnatally. The cause of the microcephaly is unknown. The cerebellar degeneration has been

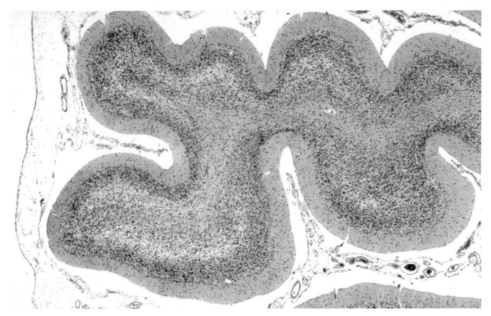

FIGURE 8-57
Cerebellar degeneration in rhizomelic chondrodysplasia punctata.

attributed to elevated phytanic acid. The severe plasmalogen deficiency does not seem to affect myelinogenesis, notwithstanding the fact that plasmalogens are the most abundant myelin lipids. However, plasmalogens are also present in all membranes, including neuronal membranes, and their deficiency may impair brain development. An analogous situation occurs in the Smith-Lemli-Opitz syndrome, in which a defect in cholesterol biosynthesis causes microcephaly and psychomotor retardation. Plasmalogen deficiency, by some unknown mechanism, probably accounts for the skeletal changes in RCDP and the ZS spectrum.

SINGLE PEROXISOMAL ENZYME DEFICIENCIES

More than 50 peroxisomal enzymes are known. Genetic deficiencies of 11 of them have been described. The two best known entities are D-bifunctional protein deficiency and adult Refsum's disease.

BIFUNCTIONAL PROTEIN DEFICIENCY

D-Bifunctional protein deficiency (DBPD), the most common among the single peroxisomal enzymopathies involving β-oxidation enzymes, phenotypically resembles the ZS spectrum. Patients have dysmorphic features similar to ZS, severe hypotonia and seizures, and no neurologic development, and most die in their first year of life. Neuropathologic studies have revealed NMDs (centrosylvian pachygyria and polymicrogyria, neuronal heterotopia); dysplasia of the cerebellar cortex, dentate nuclei, and inferior olives; and a white matter abnormality ranging from hypomyelination to inflammatory demyelinative lesions similar to NALD and XALD. The liver is enlarged and fibrotic but has normal

---

BIFUNCTIONAL PROTEIN DEFICIENCY—DISEASE FACTS AND PATHOLOGIC FEATURES

Definition
▶ An autosomal recessive deficiency of the D-bifunctional enzyme protein that resembles the Zellweger spectrum

Clinical Findings
▶ Hypotonia, seizures, psychomotor retardation

Laboratory Diagnosis
▶ Elevated VLCFAs, normal plasmalogens

Pathologic Changes
▶ Neuronal migration defects, white matter abnormalities, hepatic fibrosis

---

peroxisomes. Biochemically, DBPD patients have elevated VLCFAs and bile acid intermediates and normal plasmalogens. The pathology of DBPD reiterates the notion that the key biochemical abnormality that accounts for the NMDs and the white matter abnormality of peroxisomal disorders is probably VLCFA elevation and that plasmalogen deficiency does not cause myelin degeneration.

ADULT REFSUM'S DISEASE

Phytanic acid is derived entirely from dietary sources such as dairy products and ruminant fat. Ruminants make phytanic acid from phytol bound to chlorophyll. It can be further processed only after it is converted to pristanic acid by phytanoyl-CoA hydroxylase. Pristanic acid is then β-oxidized by other peroxisomal enzymes. Deficiency of phytanoyl-CoA hydroxylase causes an accumulation of phytanic acid and adult Refsum's disease. Phytanoyl-CoA hydroxylase is a PTS2 enzyme and is also deficient in rhizomelic chondrodysplasia punctata. Phytanic acid accumulation also occurs in the ZS spectrum of peroxisomal biogenesis disorders.

Patients with adult Refsum's disease are normal at birth. The disease is manifested by 20 years of age as symmetric sensorimotor polyneuropathy, retinitis pigmentosa, anosmia, hearing loss, ataxia, ichthyosis, skeletal abnormalities, and cardiomyopathy. Dietary restriction lowers phytanic acid and prevents or reverses the clinical manifestations.

The neuropathologic changes of untreated adult Refsum's disease are a mixed axonal and demyelinative neuropathy with hypertrophic changes (onion bulbs), lipid droplet (presumably phytanic acid) deposition in the CNS, and degeneration of white matter tracts, including the superior and middle cerebellar peduncles, corticospinal tracts, and medial lemnisci. In the retina, there is a loss of photoreceptors and decrease in neurons of the inner nuclear and ganglion cell layers. The pathogenesis of these changes is unknown but possibly has to do with cell membrane abnormalities caused by the incorporation of phytanic acid into phospholipids.

MITOCHONDRIAL DISORDERS

Mitochondria capture the energy in pyruvate and fatty acids and store it as ATP. This process, which takes place in the electron transport chain (ETC), is called oxidative phosphorylation because it combines oxidation of fuels to CO_2 and H_2O with phosphorylation of

adenosine diphosphate (ADP) to ATP. The term "mitochondrial disorders" has been applied to disorders of the respiratory chain in general or, in a narrower sense, to disorders caused by mitochondrial DNA mutations. The former definition is used for this chapter.

In addition to making ATP, mitochondria also catabolize pyruvate and perform β-oxidation of fatty acids, glycine cleavage, important steps in urea synthesis, and other functions. Genetic disorders of all these metabolic processes are, in a broader sense, mitochondrial disorders. Mitochondrial dysfunction and oxidative stress play an important role in the pathogenesis of degenerative diseases such as Alzheimer's disease, motor neuron disease, Huntington's disease, Wilson's disease, and others. Along these lines, Friedreich's ataxia and Parkinson's disease are, in essence, mitochondrial diseases.

BIOLOGY OF MITOCHONDRIA

ANATOMY

The term *mitochondrion* was used by Benda to describe the filamentous and granular morphology of these organelles. Mitochondria measure 1 to 1.5 μm, vary in shape, and are very plastic. They are located along the cytoskeleton and move about the cytoplasm and up and down axons. They can split and fuse. During cell division, mitochondria divide and are distributed in roughly equal numbers to the daughter cells. Mitochondrial division is not synchronized with the cell cycle. Mitochondria can increase in number in response to high energy demand or cell hypertrophy. In nondividing cells such as neurons and myocytes, replication replenishes damaged mitochondria.

The mitochondrion consists of a porous outer membrane, a selectively permeable, highly folded inner membrane, and two spaces, the intermembrane space and the matrix. The intermembrane space has a chemical composition similar to that of the cytosol. The matrix contains selected molecules, including enzymes that metabolize pyruvate and fatty acids to produce acetyl CoA and enzymes of the tricarboxylic acid cycle that oxidize acetyl CoA. Embedded in the inner membrane are transporter proteins and enzymes of the respiratory chain.

ENERGY PRODUCTION IN MITOCHONDRIA

Enzymes of the mitochondrial matrix convert pyruvate derived from anaerobic glycolysis and fatty acids to acetyl CoA. Acetyl CoA enters the tricarboxylic acid cycle, where it is converted to CO_2. The high-energy electrons generated in this reaction are carried by $NADH_2$ to the inner mitochondrial membrane, where they enter the ETC. The ETC consists of five complexes of transmembrane enzymes (complexes I to V). Energized by electrons passing through them, complexes I to IV pump H^+ (protons) out of the mitochondrial membrane into the intermembrane space, thereby generating a proton gradient across the inner membrane. Protons concentrated in the intermembrane space then reverse flow, return to the mitochondrial matrix, and pass through complex V (ATP synthase). Energy released during this passage is used to add one phosphate to ADP to generate ATP. This process produces 15 times as much ATP as generated from conversion of glucose to pyruvate.

MITOCHONDRIAL AND NUCLEAR DNA

Each mitochondrion contains 2 to 10 copies of the mitochondrial genome, a 16.5-kilobase double-stranded circular molecule, attached to the inner mitochondrial membrane. Most of the enzymes and other proteins in mitochondria are encoded by nuclear genes, synthesized on free ribosomes, and imported into the mitochondria by means of a specific signal sequence attached to their N-terminus. They bind to specific transporters on the outer mitochondrial membrane that recognize their signals and are translocated to the inner mitochondrial membrane or mitochondrial matrix, where they assume their folded conformation. The ETC contains 86 proteins. Seventy-three of them are made in this fashion. Thirteen proteins are encoded by mitochondrial genes and are synthesized in the mitochondria. Complex I consists of 42 subunits, 7 of which are encoded by mitochondrial DNA (mtDNA); complex II consists of 4 subunits, all of which are encoded by nuclear genes; complex III consists of 11 subunits, 1 of which is encoded by mtDNA; complex IV (cytochrome-c oxidase) consists of 13 subunits, 3 of which are encoded by mtDNA; and complex V (ATP synthase) consists of 16 subunits, 2 of which are encoded by mtDNA. In addition, mtDNA contains 2 genes coding for rRNA and 22 genes coding for tRNA. Although only about 10% of mtDNA codes for tRNA, these genes account for about 25% of mtDNA-related disease.

FREE RADICALS

Reduction of molecular oxygen to H_2O is a stepwise process in which O_2 picks up four electrons and sequentially generates superoxide, hydrogen peroxide, hydroxyl radical, and H_2O. These activated intermediate forms of O_2, which are called free radicals, are highly toxic and damage proteins, carbohydrates, lipids, and nucleic acids. A small amount of free radicals is even generated in normal cells. More free radicals are produced when the ETC malfunctions, such as occurs in mitochondrial disorders, Alzheimer's disease, Parkinson's disease, amyotrophic lateral sclerosis, and other diseases. Free radicals are produced along the inner mitochondrial membrane and damage mtDNA and matrix elements that are closest to them. This damage further impairs ETC function and causes mtDNA mutations. This vicious cycle compounds and accelerates mitochondrial and cell damage. Moreover, rupture of mitochondrial membranes and release of cytochrome-c oxidase and other inner membrane proteins activates the apoptotic cascade.

APOPTOSIS

Mitochondria play an important role in initiation of apoptosis. In damaged cells, apoptosis is initiated from within and begins with the release of cytochrome-c and other inner membrane proteins into the cytosol. Cytochrome-c activates Apaf-1, which in turn initiates the caspase apoptotic cascade. This mechanism is triggered by deficient energy production, free radical damage, or influx of calcium into the mitochondrion, which occurs in hypoxic-ischemic states.

MITOCHONDRIAL DISORDERS IN GENERAL

GENETIC ABNORMALITIES

The nuclear gene mutations that cause mitochondrial disorders affect genes that encode subunits of the ETC and non-ETC proteins involved in assembly of the ETC and maintenance of mtDNA. Most ETC subunit mutations affect complex I and cause Leigh's syndrome; a small minority affect complex II. Mutations of assembly proteins affect complexes III and IV (cytochrome-c oxidase) and cause encephalopathy, Leigh's syndrome,

MITOCHONDRIAL DISORDERS IN GENERAL— DISEASE FACTS AND PATHOLOGIC FEATURES

Nuclear and Mitochondrial DNA Mutations

▶ Nuclear and mitochondrial DNA mutations cause distinct and overlapping phenotypes

Genetics

▶ Nuclear gene mutations are transmitted along mendelian lines, and most are autosomal recessive
▶ Mitochondrial gene mutations are passed on by maternal transmission. Maternal transmission is modulated by heteroplasmy (uneven proportion of mutant and wild-type mitochondria in cells) and replicative segregation (a change in the proportion of mutant mitochondria with each cell division)

Clinical Aspects

▶ Mitochondrial disorders can affect any organ system but more severely compromise the brain and muscle, which are heavily dependent on mitochondria for energy
▶ Wide spectrum of neurologic abnormality

Pathogenesis

▶ The key factors that cause cellular injury and death are energy deficiency, free radicals, and apoptosis

Pathology

▶ The pathologic hallmark of mitochondrial disorders in muscle is the "ragged red fiber"
▶ CNS lesions include hypoxic-ischemic pathology, stroke, system degeneration, and spongy myelinopathy

Laboratory Diagnosis

▶ The key findings are elevated blood and CSF lactate levels and lactate-pyruvate ratio and ragged red fibers
▶ Biochemical analysis of the electron transport chain and DNA analysis can also be used

---

liver disease, and cardiomyopathy. Mutations of genes involved in mtDNA maintenance cause large-scale mtDNA deletions and quantitative mtDNA loss. The clinical syndromes that are most commonly associated with these findings are autosomal dominant progressive external ophthalmoplegia, mitochondrial neurogastrointestinal encephalomyopathy, and myopathy.

The mtDNA changes consist of mutations in genes encoding subunits of the ETC and mutations that affect mitochondrial protein synthesis. Mutations of individual subunits of complexes I, III, IV, and V cause deficiencies of these complexes and are associated with Leber's hereditary optic neuropathy; myopathy; mitochondrial encephalopathy, lactic acidosis, and stroke-like episodes (MELAS); neuropathy, ataxia, and retinitis pigmentosa (NARP); Leigh's syndrome; and other phenotypes. Deletions affecting one or more tRNA genes and point mutations of tRNA and rRNA genes affect protein synthesis. Such lesions have a profound effect on all ETC complexes (except II, which is encoded entirely by nuclear DNA) and cause MELAS, myoclonic

epilepsy with ragged red fibers (MERRF), chronic progressive external ophthalmoplegia, NARP, and other syndromes.

GENETIC TRANSMISSION

Nuclear gene mutations are transmitted in mendelian fashion. Most are autosomal recessive, with a few being autosomal dominant. Because the ovum has numerous mitochondria and the sperm almost none, mutations of mitochondrial genes are transmitted through the mother (maternal inheritance). Male and female offspring are equally affected, but only females transmit the disease.

The maternal transmission of mtDNA mutations is modulated by two phenomena, heteroplasmy and replicative segregation. Cells usually contain a mixture of mutant and wild-type mtDNA, a state known as heteroplasmy. During cell division, mutant and wild-type mitochondria are distributed in daughter cells in a random fashion; some cells may get many and others a few. Random distribution of mitochondria through many cycles may lead to a state in which a given cell contains mostly mutant mtDNA (replicative segregation). In heteroplasmic cells, respiratory chain function is maintained as long as there are enough wild-type mitochondria. Cellular dysfunction occurs when the proportion of mutant mtDNA exceeds a certain threshold. With some important exceptions (see "Leber's Hereditary Optic Neuropathy" later), most mtDNA mutations are heteroplasmic. Presumably, homoplasmy for mutant mtDNA would be lethal.

In nondividing cells such as myocytes and neurons, the mutation load is relatively stable. In dividing cells it may shift rapidly, depending on turnover at the stem cell level. Hematopoietic cells and cultured fibroblasts with deleterious mutations may become extinct, restoring a state of wild-type homoplasmy. This possibility should be considered when DNA testing is performed on such samples. Even in nondividing cells, mtDNA replicates and such replication may lead to a change in the level of heteroplasmy. Thus, in mtDNA mutations, the genetic defect is dynamic, and cell and tissue dysfunction is in a state of flux.

In no other group of diseases is the genotypic and phenotypic heterogeneity greater. The same phenotype may be caused by multiple nuclear DNA and mtDNA mutations involving different ETC complexes, and mutations of the same nuclear DNA or mtDNA gene can cause different phenotypes. The genetics of mitochondrial disorders is further complicated by the interaction of nuclear DNA and mtDNA. Thus, mutation of nuclear genes involved in mtDNA maintenance can cause large-scale mtDNA deletions and reduced mtDNA copy number (mtDNA depletion).

CLINICAL ASPECTS

More than 200 mitochondrial disorders are listed in the On-Line Mendelian Inheritance in Man (OMIM) database. Their combined prevalence is 11.5 per 100,000. The alphabet soup in their terminology is a small indication of their chaotic phenotypic diversity. Certain core phenotypes are well known. However, each condition has such variation in clinical expression and overlaps with others to such an extent that they appear as focal points in a widely shared phenotypic spectrum. Mitochondrial disorders can affect virtually any organ system and can cause hepatic, gastrointestinal, renal, hematopoietic, and endocrine abnormalities. However, the cells and organs that are most frequently affected are those that have the highest energy consumption, namely, the brain and skeletal and cardiac muscle (mitochondrial encephalomyopathy). Some mitochondrial disorders, such as Leber's hereditary optic neuropathy, affect a single organ. Most cause multiorgan dysfunction with prominent neurologic abnormalities and muscle disease. The neurologic abnormalities include loss of vision and hearing, headaches, seizures and myoclonus, focal neurologic deficits, encephalopathy, psychomotor retardation, ataxia, spasticity, motor neuron disease, system degeneration, and peripheral neuropathy. Almost any unexplained neurologic disorder in a child or young adult, especially if it has a component of muscle disease, could be a mitochondrial disorder.

PATHOGENESIS

Cellular dysfunction and damage in mitochondrial disorders results from (1) declining energy production, (2) chronic exposure to free radicals, and (3) apoptosis. Damage from free radicals occurs with advancing age in all cells (even in normal tissues), but it is more severe in patients with genetic mitochondrial abnormalities because they produce more free radicals. Free radicals damage mitochondrial and cell structure and introduce acquired mtDNA mutations. Acquired mtDNA muta-

tions are then propagated and amplified similar to inherited ones.

PATHOLOGIC CHANGES

The signature lesion of mitochondrial disorders is the ragged red fiber (RRF) (Fig. 8-58), a lesion that occurs in no other metabolic disease. RRFs were so named because their sarcoplasm is coarse and contains deposits that stain red with modified Gomori trichrome stain. They are usually cytochrome-c oxidase deficient and succinic dehydrogenase hyperreactive. Cytochrome-c oxidase is encoded by mtDNA, and its deficiency reflects loss of mitochondrial function. Succinic dehydrogenase is encoded by nuclear DNA, and its increase indicates proliferation of mitochondria. Cytochrome-c oxidase–positive RRFs occur in tRNA point mutations in MELAS. The red deposits are clusters of large, irregular mitochondria with unusual configurations of their cristae and other structural abnormalities (Fig. 8-59). The abnormal mitochondria often contain rectangular inclusions with a highly ordered structure, possibly crystallized mitochondrial proteins. These inclusions appear to be located in the intermembrane compartment and contain mitochondrial creatine phosphokinase. RRFs can be detected with antibodies to an inner mitochondrial membrane protein, M1168. Abnormal mitochondria occur primarily in skeletal muscle, but they have also been reported in vascular smooth muscle, choroid plexus, astrocytes, and neurons. They probably represent a reactive hyperplasia of inherently defective mitochondria. Proliferation and hypertrophy of mitochondria probably represent compensatory hypertrophy in an effort to overcome the biochemical defects of these mitochondria. RRFs occur in large deletions and point mutations of mtDNA and in mutations of nuclear genes that cause multiple mtDNA deletions or a reduction

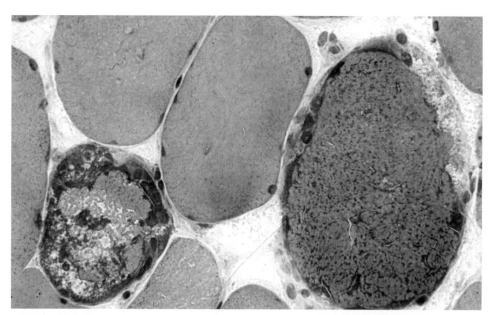

FIGURE 8-58

Ragged red fibers (Gomori trichrome stain).

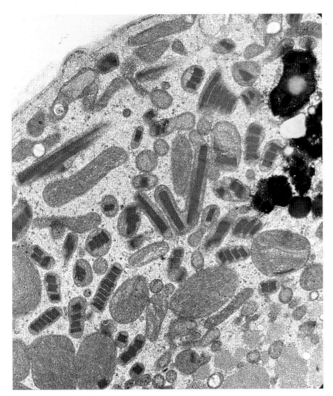

FIGURE 8-59
Abnormal mitochondria in a ragged red fiber.

in mtDNA copy number. The common denominator of these conditions is impairment of intramitochondrial protein synthesis. RRFs also arise from drug-induced mtDNA damage, such as in zidovudine treatment, and occur in inclusion body myositis and polymyalgia rheumatica, in which they are thought to be caused by mtDNA damage induced by free radicals.

Not a single characteristic CNS lesion is tied to mitochondrial disorders the way that RRFs are. Their CNS lesions (described under each entity later) affect gray and white matter. Gray matter lesions consist of hypoxic-ischemic neuronal damage affecting individual or groups of neurons (MELAS), neuronal loss (MERFF), and vacuolization and vascular proliferation of the neuropil with relative sparing of neurons (Leigh's syndrome). The white matter pathology is spongy myelinopathy, seen mainly in Kearns-Sayre syndrome.

LABORATORY DIAGNOSIS

Lactate and Pyruvate • The key laboratory test for the diagnosis of mitochondrial disorders is determination of blood and CSF lactate levels. In mitochondrial disorders, unprocessed pyruvate is converted to lactate. Both lactate and pyruvate are elevated, and the lactate-pyruvate (L/P) ratio increases. Arterial blood is preferable for lactate determination, but venous blood can be used if it is collected without stress to the patient. Elevation of blood and CSF lactate above 2.5 mM/dL and elevation of the L/P ratio above 25 occurs in all mito-

chondrial disorders except Leber's hereditary optic neuropathy.

Muscle Biopsy • Most patients with mitochondrial disorders undergo muscle biopsy. Absence of RRFs does not rule out a mitochondrial disorder. With the notable exceptions of Leigh's syndrome, Leber's hereditary optic neuropathy, and NARP, most other mitochondrial disorders have RRFs.

Enzyme Analysis of the Electron Transport Chain • One hundred to 500 mg of muscle, heart, or liver, frozen in liquid nitrogen and stored at −70° C, can be used for spectrophotometric analysis of the ETC. Polarographic analysis of ETC enzymes can also be performed on mitochondria-enriched fractions derived from fresh (not frozen) muscle tissue. For enzyme analysis of lymphocytes, 5 to 10 mL of blood should be collected and lymphocytes should be isolated within 24 hours of collection. Abnormal enzyme activity confirms an abnormality of the ETC, but normal enzyme activity does not rule it out. Normal enzyme activity may be seen in tissues that do not express the defect. Even in tissues that express the enzyme defect, activity may be normal or borderline because of heteroplasmy. The enzyme defect may be present in muscle but not in lymphocytes. Rapidly dividing hematopoietic cells may revert to normal because of replicative segregation or because leukocytes carrying the defect die. Cultured fibroblasts also tend to revert to normal enzyme activity because selection favors wild-type cells.

DNA Analysis • DNA extracted from blood (for nuclear DNA and some mtDNA gene mutations) or from muscle (for mtDNA mutations) can be used for molecular analysis. mtDNA mutations may not be detected in DNA extracted from blood.

THERAPY

The limited options for treatment of mitochondrial disorders include administration of coenzyme Q10 and other substances that have antioxidant properties and enhance mitochondrial function, such as ibotenone, menadione, riboflavin, dichloroacetate, and thiamine. Another approach for treating the myopathy is to induce myonecrosis by excessive exertion. The rationale behind this seemingly counterintuitive procedure is that regenerating muscle fibers are healthier because they are derived from satellite cells that have lower levels of the mutation.

Selected features of mitochondrial disorders are presented in Table 8-13, and the best known mitochondrial disorders are described in the following sections.

LEIGH'S SYNDROME

CLINICAL FINDINGS AND GENETICS

Leigh's syndrome, also known as subacute necrotizing encephalopathy, is one of the most frequent phenotypes

TABLE 8-13
Mitochondrial Disorders

Disorder	mtDNA/nDNA	Transmission	Mutations	RRFs
LS	nDNA, few mtDNA	Autosomal recessive	Many ETC genes and PC	No
MERRF	mtDNA	Maternal	8344, 8356 tRNA lysine	Yes
MELAS	mtDNA	Maternal	3243, 3271 tRNA leucine	Yes
KSS-PEO	mtDNA	Sporadic	mtDNA deletions and duplications	Yes
LHON	mtDNA	Maternal Male predominance	G11778A, 63460A, T14494C mutations	No

ETC, electron transport chain; KSS, Kearns-Sayre syndrome; LHON, Leber's hereditary optic neuropathy; LS, Leigh's syndrome; MELAS, mitochondrial encephalopathy with ragged-red fibers and stroke-like episodes; MERRF, myoclonic epilepsy with ragged red fibers; PC, pyruvate carboxylase; PEO, progressive external ophthalmoplegia.

of mitochondrial disorders. It becomes clinically apparent in infancy or early childhood and is characterized by hypotonia, ophthalmoplegia, nystagmus, ataxia, optic atrophy, respiratory abnormalities, failure to thrive, and developmental regression. Peripheral neuropathy is also seen. Hepatocellular dysfunction (steatosis) and hypertrophic cardiomyopathy occur in rare cases. The disease is progressive and gets worse with intercurrent infections. The mean age at death is 5 years. Funduscopic examination reveals retinitis pigmentosa. Computed tomography shows bilateral basal ganglia hypodensities. Brain MRI reveals increased T2 signal in the basal ganglia and brain stem. Blood and CSF lactate levels and the L/P ratio are elevated. Muscle biopsy shows myofiber atrophy. RRFs are usually absent.

Most cases of Leigh's syndrome are caused by nuclear DNA mutations and are autosomal recessive. A few cases are caused by mtDNA mutations, and these cases may have RRFs. All ETC complexes except complex III are affected. Leigh's syndrome is also caused by pyruvate dehydrogenase deficiency.

PATHOLOGIC CHANGES

The pathologic changes in Leigh's syndrome affect primarily the brain stem tectum and tegmentum and the basal ganglia (Fig. 8-60). Lesions are also found in the thalamus, hypothalamus, cerebellar roof nuclei, inferior olives (Fig. 8-61), and spinal cord. Affected structures show

LEIGH'S SYNDROME—DISEASE FACTS AND PATHOLOGIC FEATURES

Definition
▶ A childhood mitochondrial encephalopathy that damages primarily the brain stem and basal ganglia and causes hypotonia, ophthalmoplegia, nystagmus, and psychomotor regression

Inheritance
▶ Most cases are autosomal recessive

Molecular Defect
▶ Nuclear gene mutations affecting electron transport chain proteins and pyruvate dehydrogenase

Gross Findings
▶ Congestion, softening, and atrophy of the basal ganglia and brain stem tectum and tegmentum

Microscopic Findings
▶ Attenuation of the neuropil and vascular proliferation with relative preservation of neurons in the basal ganglia and brain stem tectum and tegmentum
▶ No ragged red fibers in most cases

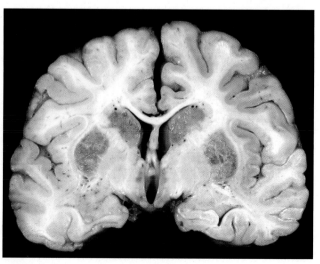

FIGURE 8-60

Necrosis of the basal ganglia and periventricular areas in Leigh's syndrome.

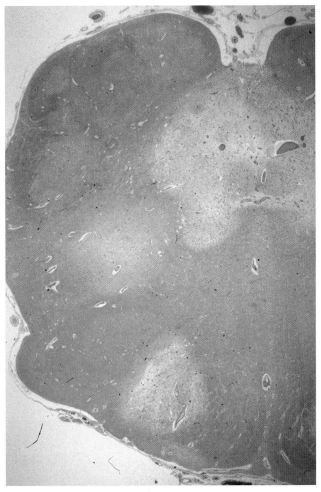

FIGURE 8-61

Hemisection of the medulla in a patient with Leigh's syndrome. The pallor of staining is due to attenuation of the neuropil. (Courtesy of Dr. Maie Herrick.)

> **MYOCLONIC EPILEPSY WITH RAGGED RED FIBERS (MERRF)—DISEASE FACTS AND PATHOLOGIC FEATURES**
>
> **Definition and Clinical Findings**
> ▶ A mitochondrial disorder characterized by myoclonus, ataxia, and dementia
>
> **Inheritance**
> ▶ Maternal
>
> **Molecular Defects**
> ▶ mtDNA mutations at positions 8344 and 8356
>
> **Pathologic Changes**
> ▶ Ragged red fibers and neuronal and tract degeneration involving multiple systems

CSF lactate levels and the L/P ratio are elevated, and muscle biopsy shows RRFs. Imaging reveals cerebral and cerebellar atrophy and bilateral hyperintense lesions of the basal ganglia and white matter. MERRF patients often have multiple lipomas in the neck, shoulders, and trunk; mild cardiomyopathy; and central hypoventilation.

MERRF is caused by mtDNA mutations and is maternally inherited. Eighty percent to 90% of cases are caused by mutations at positions 8344 and 8356 of the tRNA lysine gene, which inhibit mitochondrial protein synthesis, thus affecting multiple ETC subunits. The skeletal muscle of patients with MERRF contains 80% to 100% mutant mtDNA.

---

attenuation of the neuropil and vascular proliferation with relative preservation of neuronal perikarya (Fig. 8-62). Loosening of the neuropil and spongiosis are probably due initially to swelling and then loss of astrocytic and neuronal processes and may lead to cavitation. The histopathology and topography of the lesions, especially in the brain stem, is similar to that of Wernicke-Korsakoff syndrome, except that there is no hemorrhage and the mammillary bodies are not usually affected in Leigh's syndrome. There is also loss of Purkinje cells with torpedo-like expansions of their axons in some cases.

MYOCLONIC EPILEPSY WITH RAGGED RED FIBERS

CLINICAL FINDINGS AND GENETICS

Patients with MERRF have progressive myoclonic epilepsy, weakness, hearing loss, ataxia, and dementia beginning from late childhood to adulthood. Blood and

PATHOLOGIC CHANGES

The brain in patients with MERRF is grossly normal. Microscopic examination reveals neuronal system degeneration, most commonly involving the dentatorubral and pallidoluysian systems. There is neuronal loss in the cerebellar cortex, inferior olives, substantia nigra, and dentate nuclei. Also seen is degeneration of the superior cerebellar peduncles; the cuneate, olivocerebellar, and spinocerebellar tracts; Clarke's nuclei; and the posterior columns. These lesions resemble neurodegenerative disorders such as dentatorubral pallidoluysian atrophy and Friedreich's ataxia.

MITOCHONDRIAL ENCEPHALOPATHY WITH LACTIC ACIDOSIS AND STROKES

CLINICAL FINDINGS

Patients with MELAS are normal at birth but present in infancy, childhood, or young adulthood with unexplained strokes, migraine headaches, and seizures or with psychomotor retardation, dementia, ataxia, deaf-

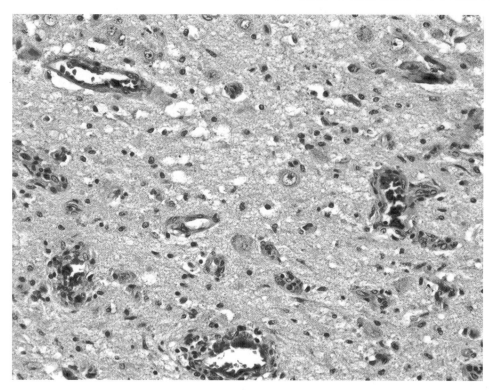

FIGURE 8-62
Spongiosis of the neuropil, vascular proliferation, and preservation of neurons in the caudate nucleus in Leigh's syndrome. (Courtesy of Dr. Maie Herrick.)

ness, and pigmentary retinopathy. Short stature is seen in some patients. Muscle pathology causes weakness, fatigability, and ophthalmoplegia. Blood and CSF lactate levels and the L/P ratio are elevated. Neuroimaging shows infarct-like lesions that more commonly involve the occipital, parietal, and posterior temporal regions. These lesions do not conform to the usual vascular patterns of thromboembolic infarcts. There is also basal ganglia mineralization. Many MELAS patients have type 2 diabetes mellitus.

MELAS is caused by mtDNA mutations and is maternally inherited. Eighty percent of cases are caused by mutations in the mitochondrial tRNA leucine gene at nucleotide positions 3243 and 3271. The muscle and brain of patients with severe manifestations contain up to 80% mutant DNA.

PATHOLOGIC CHANGES

Neuropathologic examination reveals multiple asymmetrically distributed cortical and subcortical lesions with the usual histopathologic findings and evolution of ischemic cerebral infarcts (Fig. 8-63). Pseudolaminar necrosis and basal ganglia mineralization are also seen. Mitochondrial abnormalities in vascular smooth muscle and endothelial cells have been reported in some cases, and it has been postulated that the vascular lesions, as well as ETC dysfunction, contribute to pathogenesis of the infarcts. The cerebellum shows loss of Purkinje and granular cells and cactus-like deformities of Purkinje cell dendrites similar to those seen in Menkes' kinky-hair disease.

KEARNS-SAYRE SYNDROME AND CHRONIC PROGRESSIVE EXTERNAL OPHTHALMOPLEGIA

CLINICAL FINDINGS AND GENETICS

Patients with Kearns-Sayre syndrome (KSS) often present before 20 years of age with ptosis, ophthalmoplegia, weakness, ataxia, visual and hearing loss, dementia, and seizures. CSF protein is increased above 100 mg/dL, and lactate and the L/P ratio in blood and CSF are elevated. The muscle contains RRFs. Neuroimaging

---

MITOCHONDRIAL ENCEPHALOPATHY WITH LACTIC ACIDOSIS AND STROKES (MELAS)—DISEASE FACTS AND PATHOLOGIC FEATURES

Definition and Clinical Findings
▶ A mitochondrial disorder characterized by lactic acidosis, recurrent strokes, psychomotor retardation, and other neurologic abnormalities

Inheritance
▶ Maternal

Molecular Defects
▶ mtDNA mutations at positions 3243 and 3271

Pathologic Changes
▶ Ragged red fibers and infarct-like lesions

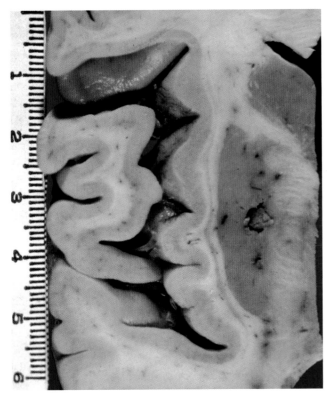

FIGURE 8-63
Small cortical infarct in MELAS.

and cerebellar white matter, as well as white matter tracts in the brain stem and spinal cord, and is similar to the myelin changes seen in amino acid disorders and organic acidemias. Additional neuropathologic changes include Purkinje cell loss with cactus-like dendritic deformities and vascular mineralization in the basal ganglia, especially the globus pallidus and thalamus.

LEBER'S HEREDITARY OPTIC NEUROPATHY

CLINICAL FINDINGS

One of the most common mitochondrial diseases, Leber's hereditary optic neuropathy (LHON) affects mostly young adult males who present with painless progressive loss of central vision. The onset may be unilateral, but the other eye is usually affected in 2 to 3 months. The visual impairment may be associated with headache, dizziness, photopsia, and eye discomfort. Visual acuity declines rapidly in the first 2 to 3 months and then remains unchanged or shows some recovery. Some LHON patients have other

shows cerebral atrophy and diffuse cerebral and cerebellar white matter hypodensity. Funduscopic examination reveals retinal degeneration and optic atrophy. The numerous non-neurologic manifestations of KSS include hypertrophic and dilated cardiomyopathy, cardiac conduction abnormalities, impaired gastrointestinal motility, diabetes mellitus and other endocrine abnormalities, short stature, and renal dysfunction. Many patients die of cardiac complications. Chronic progressive external ophthalmoplegia (CPEO) may occur as an isolated finding, usually in older patients, or in combination with other abnormalities.

Most KSS and CPEO cases are sporadic and caused by new mtDNA deletions that wipe out a large amount (up to 50%) of the mitochondrial genome, including tRNA, thus affecting mitochondrial protein synthesis. Autosomal dominant and recessive cases caused by mutations of nuclear genes involved in mtDNA maintenance have been described as well. Such mutations also result in mtDNA deletions.

PATHOLOGIC CHANGES

On external examination, the brain is usually normal. Cerebral, cerebellar, and optic nerve atrophy is rarely present. White matter shows spongy myelinopathy without gliosis or macrophage reaction. Electron microscopy reveals splitting of myelin along intraperiod lines, consistent with extracellular fluid accumulation. The spongy myelinopathy affects the diffuse cerebral

neurologic findings such as a multiple sclerosis–like picture, dystonia, pseudobulbar palsy, intellectual deterioration, and muscle weakness. Many patients have Wolff-Parkinson-White syndrome. Funduscopic examination and fluorescein angiography reveal tortuosity of the central retinal vessels and peripapillary telangiectases early on and optic atrophy in advanced disease. Visual field study shows centrocecal scotomas. Neuroimaging demonstrates white matter lesions in multiple sclerosis–like cases and bilateral striatal necrosis in cases with dystonia.

GENETICS

Most cases of LHON are caused by three homoplasmic mtDNA point mutations at nucleotide positions 11778, 3460, and 14484, which encode subunits of complex I. Only about 50% of males and 10% of females with these mutations contract the disease. LHON is maternally transmitted. Although the homoplasmic mutations are the primary genetic lesion, they are insufficient on their own to cause the disease; a modifier nuclear gene is probably involved. Male prevalence suggests that this gene may be located on chromosome X. LHON overlaps clinically with autosomal dominant optic atrophy (ADOA), which is also characterized by loss of retinal ganglion cells and optic nerve atrophy. ADOA is caused by mutations of a mitochondrial dynamin-related guanine triphosphatase that is coded by a gene on 3q28-29.

PATHOLOGIC CHANGES

Neuropathologic examination reveals loss of ganglion cells in the perifoveal region (macula densa) and degeneration of the papillomacular bundle, similar to the changes seen in tobacco-alcohol amblyopia (Fig. 8-64). There are no RRFs. Retinal ganglion cells and optic nerve axons may be damaged as a result of insufficient energy, free radical toxicity, or apoptosis. The microangiopathy suggests that vascular lesions may also play a role in its pathogenesis. Conceivably, inactivation of nitric oxide by free radicals leads to vasoconstriction and retinal ischemia.

DISORDERS OF AMINO ACID METABOLISM AND MISCELLANEOUS INHERITED METABOLIC DISORDERS

AMINO ACID DISORDERS IN GENERAL

DEFINITION, CHEMISTRY, AND GENETICS

The amino acid disorders are a group of inherited defects of the degradation of amino acids. They include

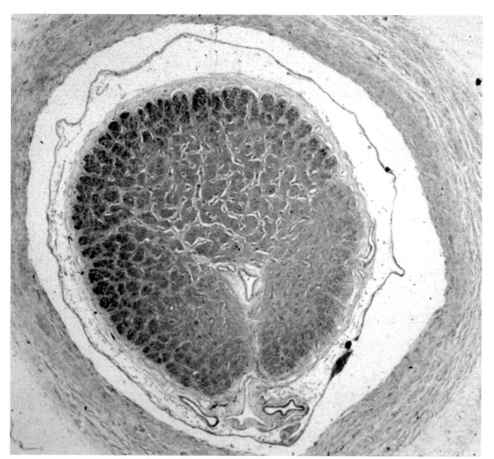

FIGURE 8-64

Myelin (and axon) loss in the optic nerve in Leber's hereditary optic neuropathy. The eccentric location of the pathology is consistent with degeneration of the papillomacular bundle.

the urea cycle disorders, in which the defect involves conversion of the amino group to urea, and many of the organic acidemias, which are caused by defects in disposal of the carbon skeletons of the branched-chain amino acids after the initial transamination step. With the exception of ornithine transcarbamylase deficiency, which is X-linked, all amino acid disorders are autosomal recessive.

CLINICAL FINDINGS

A few amino acid disorders (phenylketonuria, homocystinuria) have an insidious onset and a chronic course. Most cause a severe or fatal neonatal encephalopathy that mimics perinatal asphyxia and sepsis. Because the neonatal illness often causes respiratory depression and seizures, the primary effects of the amino acid disorders are compounded by hypoxic-ischemic encephalopathy. Survivors have psychomotor retardation and suffer from recurrent neurotoxic episodes that are triggered by hypermetabolic states such as infections. The clinical picture in older children resembles a static encephalopathy. Milder clinical phenotypes caused by less severe mutations are manifested later in life as episodes of metabolic decompensation, developmental delay, seizures, and ataxia, which are often also triggered by infections. The neurologic dysfunction is caused by the toxic effects of the accumulating amino acids and their intermediates, hyperammonemia, impairment of energy and synthetic pathways, and defective synthesis of neurotransmitters.

AMINO ACID DISORDERS IN GENERAL— DISEASE FACTS AND PATHOLOGIC FEATURES

Definition
▶ A group of inherited defects in amino acid degradation

Genetics
▶ Ornithine transcarbamylase deficiency is X-linked. All other amino acid disorders are autosomal recessive

Clinical Findings
▶ Most amino acid disorders cause severe or fatal neonatal metabolic encephalopathies and severe neurologic deficits in survivors

Pathology
▶ The key neuropathologic lesion of amino acid disorders is spongy myelinopathy

---

PATHOLOGIC CHANGES

The neuropathologic hallmark of most amino acid and organic acid disorders is a poorly understood lesion characterized by fluid-filled vacuoles in the myelin sheath. This lesion has been called spongy myelinopathy because it imparts a spongy appearance to myelinated white matter and is present mainly in the brain stem, cerebellum, and spinal cord, which are myelinated in infants (Fig. 8-65). Spongy myelinopathy involves mainly central myelin and only exceptionally has been observed in peripheral myelin. The vacuoles develop

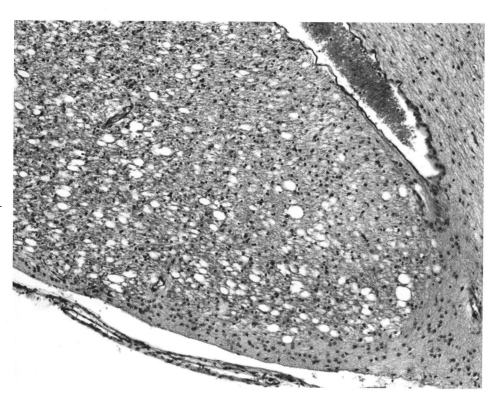

FIGURE 8-65

Spongy myelinopathy in the optic radiation in nonketotic hyperglycinemia.

by splitting of myelin lamellae along the extracellular plane (intraperiod lines). The pathogenesis of spongy myelinopathy is unknown. Impairment of synthetic pathways in amino acid disorders may conceivably disturb the lipid composition of cell membranes and result in unstable myelin. Spongy myelinopathy is not accompanied by myelin breakdown, macrophage reaction, or gliosis. It is not progressive, and it does not cause acute neonatal illness. An identical myelin lesion is seen in spongy degeneration of the nervous system (Van Bogaert-Bertrand disease), Kearns-Sayre syndrome, galactosemia, and hexachlorophene encephalopathy and in experimental triethyltin, isoniazid, and cuprizone intoxication. Some amino acid disorders show no spongy myelinopathy but have different neuropathologic lesions. Thus, Alzheimer type II astrocytes are seen in the urea cycle disorders, and vascular lesions are the key finding in homocystinuria. Agenesis of the corpus callosum occurs with high frequency in nonketotic hyperglycinemia. Hypoxic and ischemic changes (cortical and basal ganglia atrophy) are also seen in several amino acid disorders.

LABORATORY DIAGNOSIS

Newborn screening for amino acid disorders is performed on blood spots with tandem mass spectroscopy (MS/MS). A diagnosis can be made by detecting characteristic organic acid profiles in urine by gas chromatography/mass spectroscopy (GC/MS). GC/MS results may prompt additional testing such as amino acid analysis or enzyme assays in cultured fibroblasts and other cells. Prenatal diagnosis can be accomplished by detection of abnormal metabolites in amniotic fluid and by measuring enzyme activity in cultured amniocytes or CVS cells. Because multiple mutations of the affected genes occur, DNA-based diagnosis as a first step is impractical. When the actual mutation is known, DNA analysis can be used for prenatal diagnosis and carrier detection.

THERAPY

Treatment of amino acid disorders consists of dietary restriction of the offending amino acid, such as a low phenylalanine diet in phenylketonuria, a methionine-free diet with folate supplementation in homocystinuria, and restriction of branched-chain amino acids in maple syrup urine disease. Commercial dietary formulas are available for some diseases. For the urea cycle disorders, the approach is to lower ammonia in the acute phase by hemodialysis or peritoneal dialysis and treat increased intracranial pressure. Long-term management includes lowering protein intake and providing alternative pathways for disposing of ammonia. Prompt treatment of infections is important for most amino acid disorders. There is no effective therapy for nonketotic hyperglycinemia.

The genetic, clinical, and pathologic findings of the most common amino acid disorders are summarized in Table 8-14. Homocystinuria and the urea cycle disor-

TABLE 8-14

Amino Acid Disorders

Disease	Defective Enzymes	Gene Loci	Biochemical Abnormalities	Clinical Findings	Pathology
Phenylketonuria	Phenylalanine hydroxylase	12q24.1	Elevated PA	S, PMR	SM
Nonketotic hyperglycinemia	Glycine cleavage system	9p22 and other	Elevated glycine in plasma and CSF	NE, PMR	SM, ACC
Homocystinuria	CBS	21q22.3	Elevated homocysteine	Thrombosis, marfanoid habitus, dislocation of lens	Vascular abnormalities
Urea cycle disorders	5 enzymes of the urea cycle	Multiple	Hyperammonemia	NE, SX, PMR, tetraplegia	Brain swelling, Alzheimer II astrocytes
Maple syrup urine disease	Branched-chain ketoacid dehydrogenase (4 proteins)	19q13.1-q13.2 6p22-p21	Accumulation of BCAAs and their ketoacids	NE, PMR	Brain swelling, SM
Propionic and methylmalonic acidemia	Propionyl-CoA carboxylase Methylmalonyl-CoA mutase	13q, 3q21-q22 6p21	Elevated propionic and methylmalonic acid	NE, PMR	SM, basal ganglia pathology

ACC, agenesis of the corpus callosum; BCAA, branched-chain amino acid; CBS, cystathionine β-synthase; NE, neonatal encephalopathy; PA, phenylalanine; PMR, psychomotor retardation; S, spasticity; SM, spongy myelinopathy; SX, seizures.

ders, which are of special neuropathologic interest, are described in detail.

HOMOCYSTINURIA

DEFINITION AND CHEMISTRY

Homocystinuria is an inherited disorder of sulfur amino acids that is characterized by dislocation of the lens, osteoporosis, mental retardation, and thromboembolic phenomena. Homocystine is the oxidized form of homocysteine; therefore, the key abnormality is hyperhomocysteinemia. Homocysteine is a toxic amino acid that can cause DNA damage, excitotoxicity, and oxidative stress and trigger apoptosis. Most cases of homocystinuria are due to mutations of cystathionine β-synthase, which is involved in the catabolism of homocysteine to cystathionine. Homocysteine can also be converted to methionine. This reaction is catalyzed by methionine synthase and requires 5-methyltetrahydrofolic acid as a methyl donor and methylcobalamin as a cofactor. 5,10-Methylenetetrahydrofolate reductase (MTHFR) is also needed to form 5-methyltetrahydrofolic acid. Mutations of methionine synthase and MTHFR and deficiency of methylcobalamin can also cause homocystinuria.

EPIDEMIOLOGY, GENETICS, AND CLINICAL FINDINGS

The incidence of homocystinuria varies from 1 per 50,000 to 400,000 and is highest in Ireland and Italy. The gene for cystathionine β-synthase is located on 21q22.3, and more than 90 mutations have been reported. Most mutations interfere with activation of the enzyme and cause total loss of function. A few mutations affect the catalytic domain of the gene and leave some residual activity. Because methionine synthase is pyridoxine dependent, enzyme activity in partial methionine synthase deficiency can be enhanced by the administration of pyridoxine.

Patients with homocystinuria are normal at birth. Ocular, skeletal, vascular, CNS, and other abnormalities develop over a period of several years. The earliest abnormalities are upward dislocation of the lens (caused by degeneration of the zonular fibers, which are composed of the cysteine-rich protein fibrillin) and myopia. These abnormalities affect the majority of patients. Skeletal findings include a marfanoid habitus, osteoporosis, biconcave vertebrae, kyphoscoliosis, pectus excavatum or carinatum, and arachnodactyly and are probably caused by defective collagen cross-linking. Venous and arterial thrombosis, caused by endothelial damage and hypercoagulability, is frequent at all ages, including infancy. Peripheral vein thrombosis with pulmonary embolism (Fig. 8-66), ischemic stroke, and myocardial infarction are common. The risk of thromboembolic events increases with age and is higher if

other genetic and acquired risk factors are present. Premature atherosclerosis develops in heterozygotes. The neurologic abnormalities of homocystinuria include mental retardation, psychiatric disorders, seizures, and focal neurologic deficits. The focal neurologic deficits and seizures are caused by cerebral infarcts. The cause of the mental retardation and the psychiatric abnormalities is unclear.

PATHOLOGIC CHANGES

The brain in homocystinuria shows arterial and venous infarcts of varying age (Fig. 8-67). Intimal fibrosis and other vascular abnormalities, presumably secondary to endothelial injury and organized clots, have also been reported.

UREA CYCLE DISORDERS

DEFINITION AND CHEMISTRY

The urea cycle disorders are a group of inherited disorders characterized by neonatal hyperammonemia and encephalopathy. Urea synthesis occurs almost

---

HOMOCYSTINURIA—DISEASE FACTS AND PATHOLOGIC FEATURES

Definition
▶ An inherited disorder of sulfur amino acids characterized by dislocation of the lens, osteoporosis, mental retardation, and thromboembolic phenomena

Incidence
▶ 1 per 50,000 to 400,000

Genetics
▶ Autosomal recessive

Clinical Features
▶ Upward dislocation of the lens, marfanoid habitus, venous and arterial thrombosis, mental retardation, focal neurologic deficits

Radiologic Features
▶ Osteoporosis, biconcave vertebrae, kyphoscoliosis, pectus excavatum

Laboratory Diagnosis
▶ Elevated plasma methionine

Gross Findings
▶ Arterial and venous cerebral infarcts

Microscopic Findings
▶ Organizing clots, intimal fibrosis, and vascular abnormalities

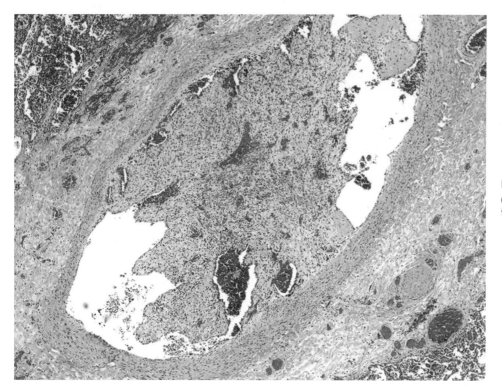

FIGURE 8-66
Organized pulmonary artery thrombus in a patient with homocystinuria.

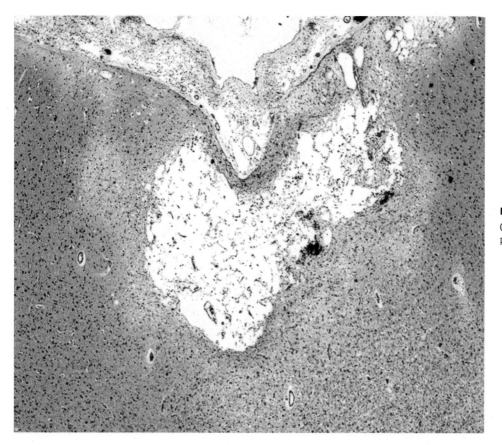

FIGURE 8-67
Old cortical infarct in a 21-year-old patient with homocystinuria.

UREA CYCLE DISORDERS—DISEASE FACTS AND PATHOLOGIC FEATURES

Definition
▶ A group of inherited disorders characterized by hyperammonemia and encephalopathy

Incidence
▶ 1 per 8200 combined, 1 per 14,000 for ornithine transcarbamylase deficiency

Genetics
▶ Ornithine transcarbamylase is X-linked. All other urea cycle disorders are autosomal recessive

Enzyme Defects
▶ Multiple (see Table 8-15)

Clinical Findings
▶ Neonatal hypotonia, irritability, seizures, coma, and high mortality
▶ Psychomotor retardation in survivors

Laboratory Diagnosis
▶ Hyperammonemia, respiratory alkalosis, decreased urea nitrogen

Gross Findings
▶ Brain swelling

Microscopic Findings
▶ Alzheimer type II astrocytes

exclusively in the liver. In addition to ridding the body of nitrogenous products, the urea cycle plays a key role in the synthesis and degradation of arginine. Consequently, in the urea cycle disorders (except arginase deficiency), arginine becomes an essential amino acid. The urea cycle enzymes and their associated disorders are presented in Table 8-15. All enzymes are expressed in the liver and kidney. Argininosuccinate synthetase

(AS), argininosuccinate lyase (AL), and arginase are also expressed in the brain.

CLINICAL FEATURES

The most common disorder in the group, ornithine transcarbamylase (OTC) deficiency, has an incidence of 1 per 14,000. The combined incidence of all urea cycle disorders has been reported to be 1 per 8200. OTC is X-linked. All other disorders are autosomal recessive. The clinical phenotype depends on the type of the mutation. Carbamoyl phosphate synthetase (CPS), OTC, AS, and AL mutations that abolish all enzyme activity cause neonatal hyperammonemia, hypotonia, irritability, poor feeding, hyperventilation, seizures, lethargy, coma, and often death. Even if promptly diagnosed and treated, survivors have psychomotor retardation. Patients with milder enzyme deficiencies are often mentally retarded but have recurrent episodes of hyperammonemia manifested as nausea, vomiting, lethargy, and seizures. These episodes resemble Reye's syndrome and are triggered by high protein intake and metabolic stress such as an infection or the postpartum state. Female OTC carriers are either asymptomatic or have an aversion to protein, cyclic vomiting, lethargy, ataxia, and seizures. The severity of these symptoms depends on the proportion of hepatocytes that carry the mutant gene on the active X chromosome. Rarely, female OTC carriers have severe disease, similar to males. Valproate may precipitate hyperammonemia in patients and previously asymptomatic carriers. Arginase deficiency has an indolent, nonspecific onset and causes progressive spastic tetraplegia beginning in the lower extremities, seizures, and psychomotor retardation.

LABORATORY DIAGNOSIS

Laboratory findings in the urea cycle disorders are marked hyperammonemia, respiratory alkalosis, ele-

---

TABLE 8-15
Urea Cycle Enzymes, Associated Disorders, and Corresponding Plasma Citrulline Levels

Enzyme and Disorder	Inheritance	Gene Locus	Enzyme Location	Plasma Citrulline
Carbamoyl phosphate synthetase (CPS) deficiency	AR	2q35	Mitochondria	Absent or trace
Ornithine transcarbamylase (OTC) deficiency	X-linked	Xp21.1	Mitochondria	Absent or trace
Argininosuccinate synthetase (AS) deficiency (citrullinemia)	AR	9q34	Cytosol	Markedly elevated
Argininosuccinate lyase (AL-argininosuccinase) deficiency (argininosuccinic aciduria)	AR	7cen-q11.2	Cytosol	Moderately elevated
Arginase deficiency (argininemia)	AR	6q23	Cytosol	Normal or reduced

vated plasma glutamine, and decreased urea nitrogen. Determination of plasma citrulline (see Table 8-15) and urinary orotic acid helps distinguish the urea cycle disorders from one another and differentiate them from other causes of hyperammonemia. Citrulline, the product of CPS and OTC, is low or undetectable in CPS and OTC deficiency and normal in the organic acidemias that can cause hyperammonemia. Urinary orotic acid is derived from diversion of excess carbamoyl phosphate to pyrimidine synthesis and is elevated in OTC deficiency but normal or low in CPS deficiency and the organic acidemias. Arginase deficiency is characterized by modest hyperammonemia (three to four times normal), marked elevation of arginine, and orotic aciduria.

PATHOLOGIC CHANGES

Patients dying in the newborn period show mainly brain swelling and Alzheimer type II astrocytes (Fig. 8-68). Additional findings such as cortical infarcts, severe cortical atrophy, neuronal loss, gliosis, calcification of the basal ganglia, spongy myelinopathy, poor myelination, ventriculomegaly, and atrophy of the cerebellar granular layer have been reported. Some of these changes are most likely the result of hypoxic and ischemic insults. Bilateral symmetric old cystic infarcts and cerebellar heterotopias have been reported in neonates with OTC deficiency, thus suggesting that the brain, in some OTC

deficiency cases, is damaged in utero. Portal fibrosis and abnormal hepatic mitochondria with swollen cristae have been reported in AL deficiency.

PATHOGENESIS

Hyperammonemia exerts its effects primarily on astrocytes. These cells express glutamine synthetase, which converts ammonia to glutamine. Osmotic attraction of water by glutamine causes astrocytic swelling and cerebral edema. The encephalopathy of the urea cycle disorders is due to increased intracranial pressure, impairment of the metabolic function of astrocytes, and probably also excitotoxicity from conversion of some ammonia to glutamate. Encephalopathy, astrocytic swelling, and cerebral edema have been reproduced in primates with experimental hyperammonemia and can be blocked by methionine sulfoximine, which prevents glutamine accumulation in astrocytes.

MENKES' DISEASE

CHEMISTRY AND GENETICS

This X-linked recessive disorder is characterized by abnormal intracellular trafficking of copper with result-

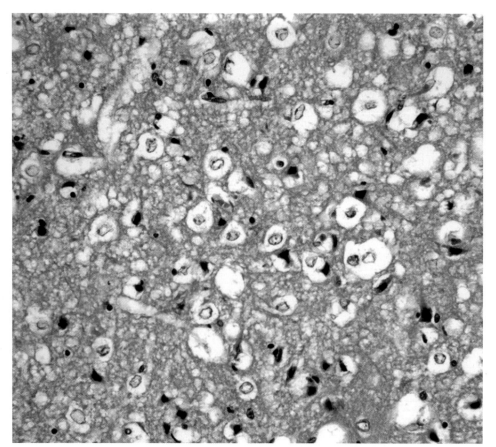

FIGURE 8-68

Alzheimer type II astrocytes in citrullinemia.

MENKES' DISEASE—DISEASE FACTS AND PATHOLOGIC FEATURES

Definition

▶ An inherited metabolic disorder of copper metabolism resulting in copper deficiency and severe neurologic manifestations

Genetics

▶ X-linked recessive

Gene Locus

▶ Xq12-q13

Enzyme Defect

▶ Copper-transporting ATPase. Failure of copper-dependent enzymes

Clinical Findings

▶ Abnormal hair, microcephaly, severe psychomotor retardation, subdural hematomas, skeletal and vascular abnormalities

Radiologic Features

▶ Wormian bones, osteoporosis, metaphyseal dysplasia, subdural hematomas, cerebral atrophy, enlarged ventricles, tortuous cerebral vessels

Laboratory Diagnosis

▶ Low serum copper and ceruloplasmin

Gross Findings

▶ Cerebral and cerebellar atrophy, subdural hematomas

Microscopic Findings

▶ Neuronal loss and gliosis in the cerebral cortex, loss of granular cerebellar neurons and Purkinje cells, and cactus-shaped Purkinje cell dendrites

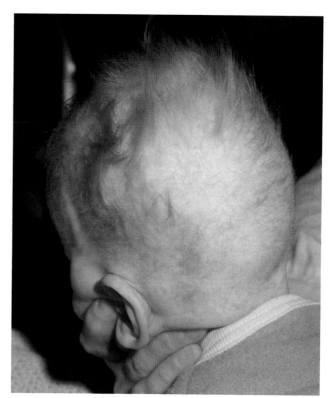

FIGURE 8-69
Abnormal hair in Menkes' disease.

ant copper deficiency in the brain and other organs. Failure of copper-dependent enzymes (which include cytochrome-*c* oxidase, superoxide dismutase-1, lysyl oxidase, tyrosinase, and dopamine hydroxylase) causes profound disruption in many metabolic pathways, including cellular respiration, antioxidant defense, collagen synthesis, neurotransmitter production, and pigment formation. The gene of Menkes' disease, *MNK* or *ATP7A* on chromosome Xq12-q13, codes for a copper-transporting ATPase. The Menkes' protein, which regulates absorption of copper in the gastrointestinal tract, delivers copper to cuproenzymes and removes excess copper from cells. A related enzyme, ATP7B, which is deficient in Wilson's disease, transports copper to ceruloplasmin and eliminates copper through bile. Menkes' disease can be regarded as copper deficiency and Wilson's disease as copper excess (and toxicosis).

CLINICAL FINDINGS

Patients with Menkes' disease are often born prematurely. The disease is manifested in the first few months of life as failure to thrive, hypothermia, hypotonia, seizures, severe psychomotor retardation, and death, usually before 2 years of age. Patients have pudgy cheeks, which imparts a characteristic "cherubic" appearance to the face, and sparse, coarse, steely, depigmented hair (Fig. 8-69) that appears twisted or broken on microscopic examination. Radiologic examination reveals wormian cranial bones, osteoporosis, and metaphyseal dysplasia. MRI shows subdural hematomas, cerebral and cerebellar atrophy, atrophy of the white matter, ventricular dilatation, and tortuous intracranial vessels. The occipital horn syndrome, a milder form of the disease previously known as X-linked cutis laxa, is characterized mainly by connective tissue abnormalities (hyperelastic skin, loose joints, skeletal abnormalities) and minor neurologic abnormalities. The phenotype of occipital horn syndrome can be explained by a deficiency of lysyl oxidase.

PATHOLOGIC CHANGES

The brain in patients with Menkes' disease shows cerebral and cerebellar atrophy (Fig. 8-70), bilateral chronic subdural hematomas (Fig. 8-71), and tortuous thin-walled arteries. The cortex shows neuronal loss, mineralized neurons, and gliosis. White matter is reduced in volume, attenuated, and gliotic. Neuronal loss and gliosis are seen in the thalamus and other subcortical nuclei. The cerebellum shows severe depletion of granular neurons and less severe loss of Purkinje cells (Fig. 8-72). The latter

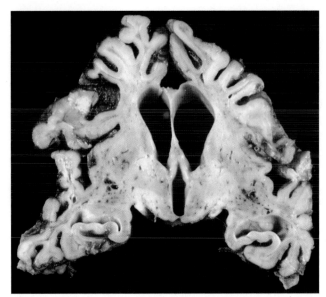

FIGURE 8-70
Cerebral atrophy in Menkes' disease. (Courtesy of Dr. Maie Herrick.)

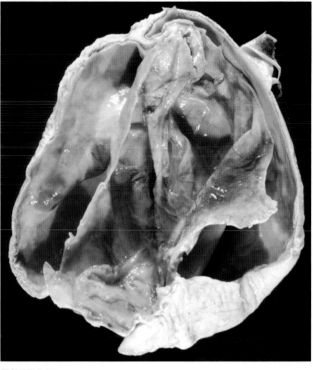

FIGURE 8-71
Bilateral old subdural hematomas in Menkes' disease. (Courtesy of Dr. Maie Herrick.)

have striking dendritic abnormalities, including star- or cactus-shaped dendrites (Fig. 8-73). Mitochondrial abnormalities in Purkinje cells have been reported. The neuronal lesions have been attributed to deficiency of cytochrome-*c* oxidase. There are frequent subdural hematomas, often bilateral, that are probably secondary to cerebral atrophy and stretching of bridging vessels.

LABORATORY DIAGNOSIS

The laboratory diagnosis of Menkes' disease is based on detection of decreased serum copper and ceruloplasmin.

However, serum copper and ceruloplasmin may be normal in the first 2 weeks of life. Plasma and CSF dihydroxyphenylalanine and dihydroxyphenylacetic acid are elevated, and norepinephrine and its derivatives are decreased. Prenatal diagnosis can be accomplished by detection of increased copper in amniocytes and CVS cells and by mutation analysis.

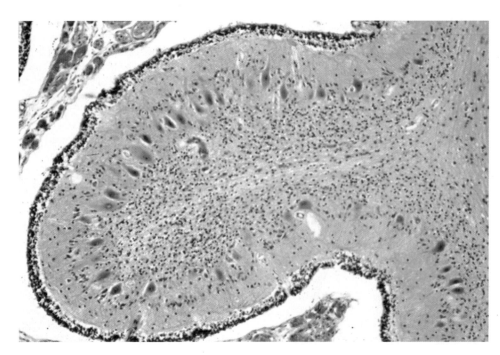

FIGURE 8-72
Cerebellar degeneration in Menkes' disease with loss of granular cells and relative preservation of Purkinje cells.

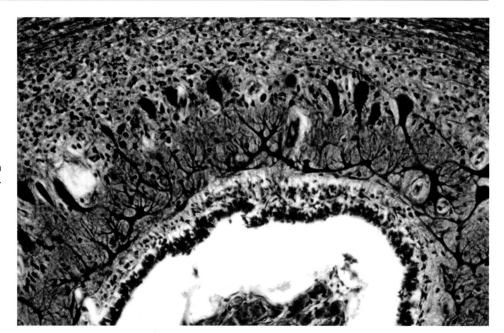

FIGURE 8-73

Abnormal Purkinje cell dendrites in Menkes' disease. (Courtesy of Dr. Richard Prayson.)

GLYCOSYLATION DISORDERS (CARBOHYDRATE-DEFICIENT GLYCOPROTEIN SYNDROMES)

CHEMISTRY AND GENETICS

The attachment of oligosaccharide chains (glycans) to glycoproteins and other glycoconjugates involves numerous enzymatic and transport steps that take place in the endoplasmic reticulum and Golgi. Impairment of glycan synthesis is the basis of a new class of inherited metabolic disorders that have begun to be reported in the 1980s. In these disorders, the oligosaccharide chains attached to glycoproteins are deficient in terminal sugars, GlcNAc, galactose, and sialic acid. Initially, these disorders were called carbohydrate-deficient glycoprotein (CDG) syndromes. They were renamed glycosylation disorders in 2000. Several entities have been described. They are multisystem diseases that severely affect the nervous system. These disorders are divided into pre-Golgi glycosylation defects (CDG type I) and Golgi glycosylation defects (CDG type II). The best known entity in the group is CDG type IA (CDG-IA), caused by deficiency of phosphomannomutase, which is encoded by a gene called *PMM2* on 16p13. CDG-IA is autosomal recessive. More than 30 mutations have been reported.

CLINICAL FINDINGS

Patients with CDG-IA have normal gestations and are normal at birth but show a succession of neurologic and physical problems that develop at different times from infancy to adolescence, after which they go into a static

---

GLYCOSYLATION DISORDERS (CARBOHYDRATE-DEFICIENT GLYCOPROTEIN SYNDROMES)—DISEASE FACTS AND PATHOLOGIC FEATURES

Definition
► Genetic disorders in which deficient glycosylation of proteins causes severe cardiac, hepatic, and neurologic disease

Genetics
► Autosomal recessive

Key Enzyme Defect
► Phosphomannomutase

Gene Locus
► 16p13

Clinical Findings
► Neonatal hypotonia, failure to thrive, hepatic failure, cardiac failure, short stature, kyphoscoliosis, ataxia, psychomotor retardation, peripheral neuropathy, stroke-like episodes

Laboratory Diagnosis
► Abnormal isoelectric focusing of serum transferrin

Gross Findings
► Cirrhosis, cerebellar atrophy

Microscopic Findings
► Hepatic steatosis, olivopontocerebellar atrophy, demyelinative neuropathy

phase. Hypotonia, weak sucking, and lethargy appear in the neonatal period. Infants fail to thrive and have delayed neurologic development. Hepatic and cardiac failure may cause death in the first few months of life but are not a problem in later stages of the disease. Non-specific dysmorphic facial features, inverted nipples, and an abnormal distribution of fat (lipodystrophy) appear by 6 months. Older children have ataxia, hypotonia, psychomotor retardation, retinal degeneration, and stroke-like episodes triggered by infections. As the disease progresses, cerebellar ataxia persists, and peripheral neuropathy, short stature, and kyphoscoliosis develop. The disease runs its course by the end of the second decade of life, and no further deterioration occurs.

PATHOLOGIC CHANGES

The neuropathologic findings consist mainly of pontocerebellar atrophy (Figs. 8-74 and 8-75). Microscopic examination reveals severe loss of Purkinje cells, subtotal loss of granular neurons, severe neuronal loss in the inferior olives, and neuronal loss in the pontine nuclei. The cerebrum is intact except in cases in which infarcts have occurred. Peripheral nerves show a demyelinative neuropathy (thin or absent myelin sheaths) with myelinoid lamellar inclusions in Schwann cells. The liver shows steatosis, fibrosis, and cirrhosis (Fig. 8-76) with lamellar lysosomal inclusions in hepatocytes. There is no specific pathology in other organs.

LABORATORY DIAGNOSIS

The diagnosis of CDG-IA and other glycosylation disorders can be made by isoelectric focusing of serum transferrin. Deficiency of terminal sialic acid causes an abnormal isoelectric focusing pattern. Other glycoproteins such as α_1-antitrypsin are affected in a similar fashion.

ACQUIRED METABOLIC DISORDERS

NEUROLOGIC COMPLICATIONS OF LIVER DISEASE

Three grades of encephalopathy resulting from liver disease are recognized: fulminant hepatic failure (FHF), hepatic encephalopathy (HE), and chronic acquired non-wilsonian hepatocerebral degeneration (CANWHCD). The most common of these disorders is HE.

FIGURE 8-74

Pontocerebellar atrophy in type I carbohydrate-deficient glycoprotein disorder. The cerebellum is atrophic with a normal cerebrum.

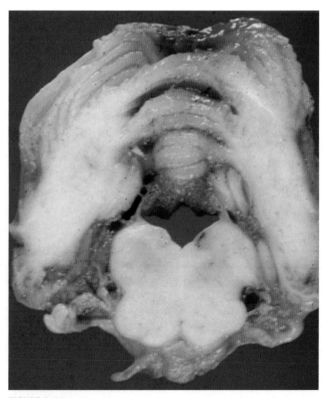

FIGURE 8-75

Cerebellar atrophy in type I carbohydrate-deficient glycoprotein disorder.

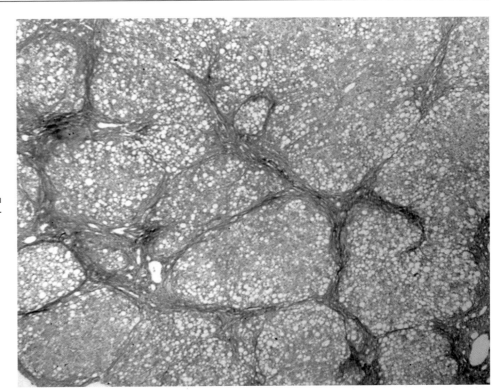

FIGURE 8-76
Hepatic steatosis and cirrhosis in type I carbohydrate-deficient glycoprotein disorder.

NEUROLOGIC COMPLICATIONS OF LIVER DISEASE— DISEASE FACTS AND PATHOLOGIC FEATURES

Definition
► A spectrum of neurologic dysfunction resulting from hepatic failure that includes three entities: fulminant hepatic failure (FHF), hepatic encephalopathy (HE) and portosystemic encephalopathy, and chronic acquired non-wilsonian hepatocerebral degeneration (CANWHCD)

Clinical Findings
► Death from increased intracranial pressure in FHF
► Reversible confusion progressing to coma in chronic HE
► Irreversible neurologic deterioration in CANWHCD

Gross Findings
► Cerebral edema and herniations in FHF
► No gross abnormalities in chronic HE

Microscopic Findings
► Alzheimer type II astrocytes in chronic HE and CANWHCD
► Pseudolaminar microcavitation and neuronal loss in the cortex and putamen in CANWHCD

Pathogenesis
► Acute increase in ammonia causes astrocytic (and cerebral) edema; a slow increase causes astrocytic dysfunction and impairs neurotransmission

---

FULMINANT HEPATIC FAILURE

FHF in acute hepatitis or failed liver transplants is characterized clinically by confusion, seizures, and coma and pathologically by cerebral edema and herniations. The edema is cytotoxic and consists of an accumulation of fluid in the astrocytic cytoplasm and foot processes. Enlargement of astrocytic nuclei (Alzheimer II astrocytes) is also seen.

HEPATIC ENCEPHALOPATHY AND PORTOSYSTEMIC ENCEPHALOPATHY

CLINICAL FINDINGS

Patients with hepatic failure have episodes of confusion, drowsiness, stupor, and coma. Asterixis (a flapping tremor that appears when the arm is extended and the hand is held in a dorsiflexed position) is seen before the patient becomes comatose. Patients may also have twitching of facial muscles, fingers, and arms; grimacing; and athetosis. MRI shows hyperintensity of the globus pallidus in some cases. The EEG is abnormal. Blood ammonia is elevated, usually above 200 μm/dL. This syndrome is precipitated by events that cause blood ammonia to rise, such as gastrointestinal hemorrhage and portosystemic shunts, including transjugular intrahepatic portosystemic shunts. The severity of symptoms correlates with the blood ammonia concentration. Untreated, HE progresses from confusion to coma within days or weeks and may be fatal. Less severe hyperammonemia causes milder clinical changes.

PATHOLOGIC CHANGES

The pathologic hallmark of HE is the Alzheimer type II astrocyte (see Fig. 8-68). Alzheimer type II astrocytes, first described in Wilson's disease, have large clear nuclei with marginated chromatin and frequent cytoplasmic invaginations that contain glycogen. The cytoplasm is not visible on hematoxylin-eosin staining. Electron microscopic studies in animals with portocaval anastomosis show cytoplasmic enlargement, increased mitochondria and other organelles, and swelling of astrocytic end-feet. No transition to gemistocytic astrocytes or fibrous gliosis occurs. There is no neuronal pathology. Groups of astrocytes are often seen and suggest astrocytic proliferation. Alzheimer type II astrocytes are found primarily in the cortex and gray matter structures, as are Bergmann astrocytes. No Alzheimer type II astrocytes are seen in patients who die even a few days after blood ammonia normalizes.

CHRONIC ACQUIRED NON-WILSONIAN HEPATOCEREBRAL DEGENERATION

Irreversible neurologic damage develops in some patients with chronic hepatic failure, sustained hyperammonemia, and repeated episodes of HE. Clinically, such patients have choreoathetosis, dysarthria, ataxia, asterixis, and dementia, which remain unchanged after lowering blood ammonia. In addition to Alzheimer II astrocytes, the brain shows pseudolaminar microcavitation in the deeper cortical layers associated with mild gliosis (Fig. 8-77). The hippocampus is spared. A similar change affects the putamen (Fig. 8-78). Identical changes are seen in Wilson's disease, thus underlining the point that the neuropathology of Wilson's disease is due to HE, not to copper accumulation.

PATHOGENESIS OF ENCEPHALOPATHIES RESULTING FROM LIVER DISEASE

Such encephalopathies are thought to be caused primarily by ammonia intoxication. Elevated manganese (which is excreted in bile) with accumulation of manganese in the brain, particularly in the globus pallidus, is also thought to contribute to the neurologic dysfunction. The manifestations of ammonia intoxication depend on the clinical setting, the ammonia concentration, and how rapidly ammonia rises. Rapid rise of ammonia causes fatal cerebral edema, a slower rise causes the reversible clinical syndrome of HE, and sustained elevation results in the permanent loss of neurologic function and irreversible structural changes that characterize CANWHCD. Ammonia is derived from the catabolism of proteins and is also produced in the colon from protein by urease-containing bacteria. In FHF, ammonia is not converted to urea. In patients with portal hypertension and portocaval shunts, ammonia bypasses the liver. Restriction of protein and suppression of bacterial activity with neomycin and kanamycin

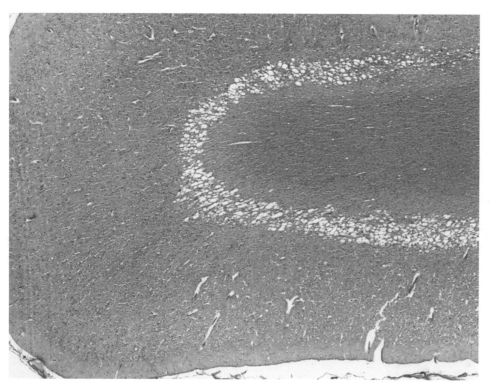

FIGURE 8-77

Pseudolaminar microcavitation of the cortex in chronic acquired non-wilsonian hepatocerebral degeneration.

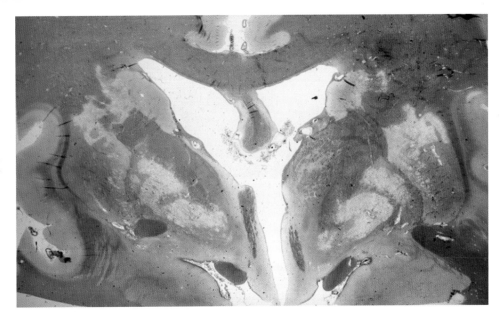

FIGURE 8-78
Chronic acquired non-wilsonian hepatocerebral degeneration: microcavitation of the basal ganglia.

or by lactulose, which acidifies the colonic contents, lowers blood ammonia and reverses the clinical findings of HE. The central role of ammonia in HE is underlined by the occurrence of coma and Alzheimer type II astrocytes in urea cycle defects in which hyperammonemia develops as a result of deficiency of hepatic enzymes that convert ammonia to urea.

Ammonia readily crosses the blood-brain barrier and is taken up by astrocytes. These cells are rich in glutamine synthetase, which converts ammonia to glutamine. The osmotic action of glutamine draws water into astrocytes and causes cytotoxic edema. Cerebral edema is present in FHF, a condition in which ammonia rises rapidly, and in some patients with urea cycle defects. In HE, hyperammonemia causes a metabolic dysfunction of astrocytes and impairs their ability to process glutamate and GABA. Buildup of glutamate and GABA and other neurotransmission aberrations explain the neurologic abnormality of chronic HE. It is not clear how Alzheimer type II astrocytes are derived or how their characteristic appearance correlates with their functional defects. No astrocytic edema is seen in patients with reversible HE. The Alzheimer type II astrocyte is thought to represent a specific reaction of astrocytes to metabolic injury. In the case of HE, this reaction is an adaptation to elevated ammonia. Alzheimer type II astrocytes are also seen in hypoxic-ischemic encephalopathy but probably arise by a different mechanism.

REYE'S SYNDROME

CLINICAL AND PATHOLOGIC FINDINGS

Reye's syndrome is a condition characterized by encephalopathy with fatty degeneration of the liver. It

is uncommon now, but in the 1970s it was a much feared, lethal, postviral encephalopathy in children. Reye's syndrome is preceded by a viral upper respiratory infection, varicella, or other infection. Five to 7 days later, vomiting (secondary to increased intracranial pressure), delirium, stupor, seizures, and coma develop. Mortality in the 1970s was 40%. Laboratory studies show a threefold elevation in serum transaminases and

---

REYE'S SYNDROME—DISEASE FACTS AND PATHOLOGIC FEATURES

Definition
▶ A postviral encephalopathy syndrome characterized by fatty degeneration of the liver. Inherited metabolic disorders can mimic Reye's syndrome

Clinical Findings
▶ Confusion and obtundation progressing to seizures, coma, and death

Gross Findings
▶ Severe cerebral edema and herniations

Microscopic Findings
▶ Microvesicular hepatocellular steatosis

Electron Microscopic Findings
▶ Swelling and dissolution of the cristae of hepatic mitochondria

Laboratory Diagnosis
▶ Threefold elevation of serum transaminases and ammonia

Pathogenesis
▶ Failure of mitochondrial function triggered by the viral illness

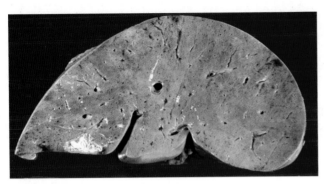

FIGURE 8-79
Fatty liver in Reye's syndrome.

ammonia, hypoprothrombinemia, and other metabolic abnormalities involving fatty acids and carnitine. The hepatic pathology consists of microvesicular hepatocellular steatosis (Figs. 8-79 and 8-80) and striking mitochondrial changes (marked distention, irregular shapes, thinning of the mitochondrial matrix, narrowing of the intercristal space, and dissolution of cristae) (Fig. 8-81). The brain is markedly swollen as a result of cytotoxic astrocytic edema and shows herniations and secondary hypoxic-ischemic encephalopathy. No Alzheimer type II astrocytes are seen.

PATHOGENESIS

Reye's syndrome is thought to be caused by a generalized impairment of mitochondrial function triggered by an unknown mechanism. There is decreased activity of all mitochondrial enzymes, including ornithine transcar-

bamylase and carbamoyl phosphate synthetase, which are responsible for the hyperammonemia. The role of aspirin in the pathogenesis of Reye's syndrome has not been clarified. The incidence of Reye's syndrome has decreased in the United States after the use of aspirin as an antipyretic for the management of febrile illness in children was discontinued, but it has also decreased in Europe, where aspirin use was never stopped.

Several inherited metabolic disorders are characterized by attacks of encephalopathy that are indistinguishable from Reye's syndrome. The most common of these disorders are the urea cycle defects, especially partial ornithine transcarbamylase deficiency, and disorders of mitochondrial fatty acid oxidation, especially medium-chain acyl-CoA dehydrogenase deficiency. Probably 50% or more of patients in whom Reye's syndrome was diagnosed in the 1960s and 1970s had inherited metabolic disorders and suffered Reye-like attacks precipitated by hypermetabolic states such as infections.

CENTRAL PONTINE MYELINOLYSIS

CLINICAL AND PATHOLOGIC FINDINGS

Central pontine myelinolysis (CPM) is symmetric demyelination of the basis pontis associated with a dysosmolar state. In the course of a severe illness treated with intravenous fluids, patients suffer flaccid quadriparesis and pseudobulbar palsy with relative preservation of sensation. They are probably conscious but in a locked-in state. Brain MRI reveals a symmetric, bat wing–shaped hypointense lesion in the basis pontis. Neuropathologic examination reveals a symmetric

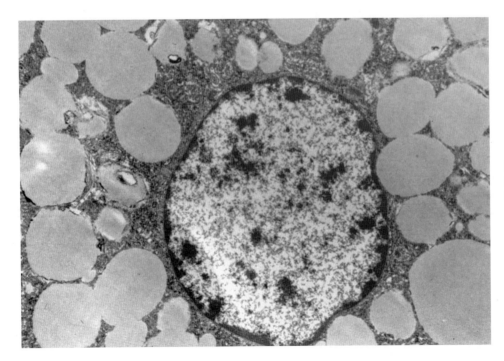

FIGURE 8-80
Microvesicular hepatocellular steatosis in Reye's syndrome.

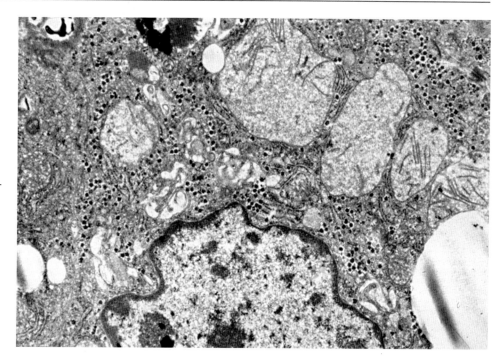

FIGURE 8-81

Distended mitochondria with dissolved cristae in Reye's syndrome.

CENTRAL PONTINE MYELINOLYSIS—DISEASE FACTS AND PATHOLOGIC FEATURES

Definition

▶ A symmetric patch of demyelination in the basis pontis seen in alcoholic and nonalcoholic patients with severe electrolyte abnormalities. Similar lesions occur in the corpus callosum and other locations

Clinical Findings

▶ Most cases are incidental autopsy findings
▶ When symptomatic, causes quadriplegia and pseudobulbar palsy

Radiologic Findings

▶ A symmetric, bat wing–shaped hypodensity in the basis pontis

Pathologic Findings

▶ Demyelination with preservation of axons and neurons in the basis pontis

Pathogenesis

▶ Caused by a disturbance in osmolality that damages oligodendroglial processes

---

swellings, and even necrosis. Lesions of some duration have macrophages, but there is no inflammation. Burned-out lesions show gliosis without macrophage activity. In rare cases, the pons is involved more extensively (Fig. 8-83), and the pathology extends beyond the pons into the midbrain, cerebellum, diencephalon, striatum, and hemispheric white matter (extrapontine myelinolysis) (Fig. 8-84). In the past, most CPM cases were diagnosed at autopsy, and many burned-out cases were found in patients without a history of a preceding illness. A parallel can be drawn between CPM and Marchiafava-Bignami disease, a rare demyelinative lesion seen in alcoholic and nonalcoholic patients that affects the corpus callosum.

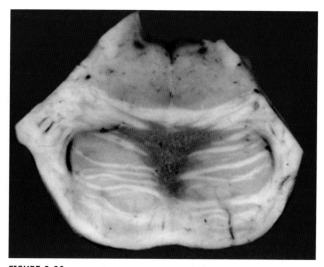

FIGURE 8-82

Old central pontine myelinosis: incidental autopsy finding.

midline patch of demyelination in the upper two thirds of the basis pontis (Fig. 8-82). The typical lesion involves the transverse fibers of the pons and corticospinal and corticobulbar tracts. It does not extend into the tegmentum or surface of the pons. Microscopic examination reveals demyelination and loss of oligodendrocytes with relative preservation of axons. Neurons of the pontine nuclei are spared. Severe cases also show axonal destruction, as evidenced by axonal

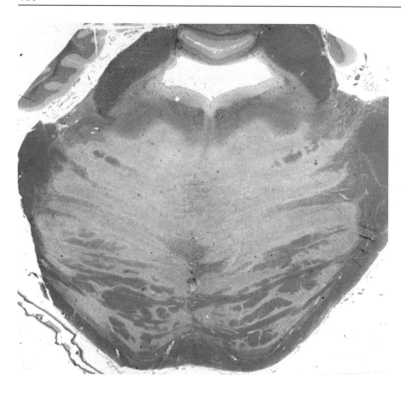

FIGURE 8-83

Severe acute central pontine myelinosis involving the basis and tegmentum. The patient was not an alcoholic.

ETIOLOGY AND PATHOGENESIS

After its original description by Adams and Victor, CPM was conceived of as a complication of alcoholism. Subsequently, it has also been reported in patients with burns, sepsis, cancer, liver disease, malnutrition, and fluid and electrolyte disorders and in other settings, including pediatric patients. CPM occurs in hyponatremic patients when hyponatremia is corrected rapidly, and it has been reproduced in dogs that were made hyponatremic and then given injections of hypertonic saline. CPM has also been reported in burned patients with severe hyperosmolality that was not preceded by

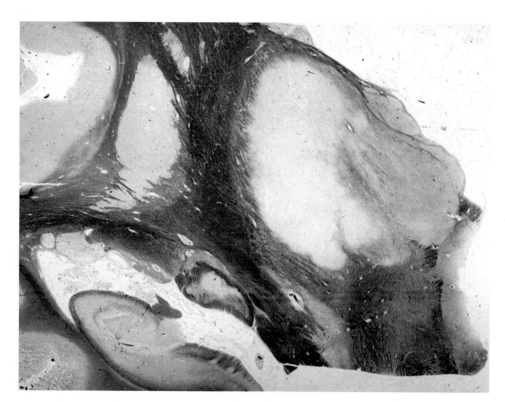

FIGURE 8-84

Extrapontine myelinosis involving the thalamus and basal ganglia.

hyponatremia. The key triggering factor is now thought to be a dysosmolar state in the course of which electrolytes and organic osmolytes move out of brain cells into the extracellular space. Any further osmotic stress at this fragile phase may cause brain shrinkage and shearing of oligodendrocyte processes, the initial stage of myelin breakdown.

NUTRITIONAL CENTRAL NERVOUS SYSTEM DISORDERS

Most nutritional CNS disorders involve vitamin deficiencies, especially vitamins of the B group, and many of them occur in the background of alcoholism. In children, protein malnutrition causes kwashiorkor (edema secondary to hypoproteinemia, ascites, hepatomegaly secondary to hepatic steatosis), and protein-calorie malnutrition causes marasmus (extreme cachexia and growth failure). Apart from apathy and lack of activity, children with these conditions have no hard neurologic findings. Animal studies and limited observations in humans show that protein-calorie malnutrition in utero and early childhood has an adverse affect on gliogenesis, synaptic branching, and myelin formation, but this effect is mild and the brains of such children show a mild reduction in weight without gross or microscopic abnormalities. Most children with protein-calorie malnutrition have normal neurologic development if proper nutrition is restored. In mature animals, calorie restriction retards the loss of cognitive and motor ability that develops with advancing age.

THIAMINE DEFICIENCY AND WERNICKE-KORSAKOFF SYNDROME

ETIOLOGY AND CLINICAL FINDINGS

The Wernicke-Korsakoff syndrome (WKS) is most common in alcoholics but is also seen in malnourished demented people, in patients with gastric cancer, in hyperemesis gravidarum, and in other malnutrition settings. The classic manifestation is a triad of eye abnormalities (nystagmus, oculomotor paralysis, paralysis of conjugate gaze), ataxia of stance and gait, and mental symptoms such as withdrawal, confusion, anterograde and retrograde amnesia, and confabulation (a tendency to fill gaps of memory with fabrications). Peripheral neuropathy (a form of beriberi disease) is seen in 80% of patients. Overt heart disease is uncommon, but subtle cardiac abnormalities (tachycardia, dyspnea, hypotension, abnormal electrocardiogram) are common. Patients may also suffer postural hypotension, syncope, and sudden death, probably as a result of autonomic involvement and pathology in brain stem cardiorespiratory centers. The syndrome may be partial, so a high index of suspicion is essential for diagnosis, especially

---

THIAMINE DEFICIENCY AND THE WERNICKE-KORSAKOFF SYNDROME—DISEASE FACTS AND PATHOLOGIC FEATURES

Definition
▶ A syndrome of oculomotor abnormalities and mental symptoms seen in malnourished alcoholic and nonalcoholic patients with thiamine deficiency

Clinical Findings
▶ Oculomotor abnormalities, mental symptoms, ataxia, and neuropathy. Some symptoms are reversed by thiamine administration

Imaging Findings
▶ Hypodense enhancing lesions in the mammillary bodies, walls of the third ventricle, periaqueductal area, and floor of the fourth ventricle

Laboratory Diagnosis
▶ Decreased blood transketolase activity

Topography and Gross Findings
▶ Mammillary bodies in the periaqueductal gray matter, floor of the fourth ventricle, and thalamus
▶ Affected areas are dusky and hemorrhagic in the acute phase
▶ Mammillary body atrophy is seen in chronic cases
▶ Midline cerebellar degeneration is seen in 30% to 50% of patients

Microscopic Findings
▶ Degeneration of the neuropil with partial preservation of neurons
▶ Pericapillary hemorrhages

Pathogenesis
▶ Thiamine is required for enzymes of glucose metabolism and energy production. Thiamine is easily depleted. Intravenous glucose administration may trigger Wernicke-Korsakoff syndrome

---

in debilitated patients with unexplained mental confusion. Administration of thiamine leads to rapid reversal of ophthalmoplegia within hours. Recovery from nystagmus and confusion is slower. Amnesia does not respond to treatment fully. The acute lesions can be detected by MRI. Reduction of blood transketolase activity (an enzyme that requires thiamine as a cofactor) is a sensitive laboratory finding in WKS.

PATHOLOGIC CHANGES AND CLINICOPATHOLOGIC CORRELATION

The histopathology and topography of the lesions of WKS are distinctive. The acute lesions consist of incomplete loss of neurons, loosening and vacuolization of the neuropil because of destruction of myelin and axons, punctate hemorrhages, vascular prominence, and endothelial proliferation. Each successive bout of WKS causes additional loss of neural tissue. In burned-out cases, the affected structures shrink and turn a brownish color because of deposition of lipofuscin and hemo-

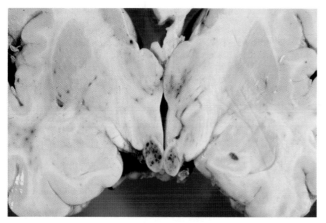

FIGURE 8-85

Acute hemorrhagic lesions of the mammillary bodies in Wernicke-Korsakoff syndrome. (Reproduced from *www.akronchildrens.org/neuropathology* with permission of Akron Children's Hospital.)

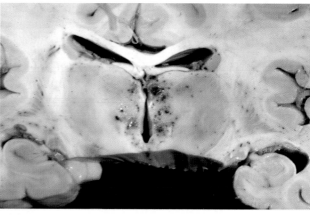

FIGURE 8-86

Hemorrhagic lesions of the walls of the third ventricle in Wernicke-Korsakoff syndrome.

siderin. The lesions affect the hypothalamus, thalamus, periaqueductal gray matter, colliculi, and floor of the fourth ventricle (Figs. 8-85 and 8-86). The mammillary bodies are involved in all cases and represent the signature pathology of WKS. Lesions of the colliculi and floor of the fourth ventricle (oculomotor nuclei, loci cerulei, dorsal motor nuclei of the vagus, vestibular nuclei) cause the oculomotor and brain stem signs. Involvement of the medial dorsal nuclei of the thalamus is responsible for the memory defect. The thalamic pathology is subtle and difficult to recognize. It is characterized by neuronal loss and gliosis without the punctate hemorrhages seen in other locations. In full-blown WKS, all these structures are involved. In less severe cases, some

may be spared. Old cases show atrophy of the mammillary bodies and dilatation of the third ventricle (Fig. 8-87). In 30% to 50% of cases the cerebellum shows degeneration of the superior vermis (see later).

PATHOGENESIS

WKS is due to thiamine deficiency. Thiamine pyrophosphate is a cofactor required for enzymes involved in glucose and amino acid metabolism and energy production. Except for involvement of the mammillary bodies, the distribution of lesions in WKS resembles Leigh's syndrome, a metabolic disorder caused by defects in the

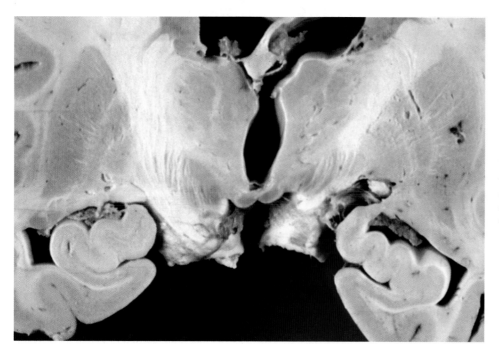

FIGURE 8-87

Shrunken mammillary bodies and dilated third ventricle in burned-out Wernicke-Korsakoff syndrome. (Reproduced from *www.akronchildrens.org/neuropathology* with permission of Akron Children's Hospital.)

pyruvate dehydrogenase complex and the respiratory chain. This suggests that damage to sensitive CNS structures in WKS is due to energy failure or lactic acidosis. Thiamine is stored in several organs (heart, kidneys, liver, brain, muscles). These stores can be depleted within a few weeks in malnourished patients. Alcohol displaces more nutritious foods from the diet, adds carbohydrates that use up thiamine, and impairs the absorption of vitamins. Intravenous glucose administration to a patient with borderline thiamine deficiency may trigger WKS. Therefore, thiamine supplementation is mandatory for patients even remotely at risk.

MIDLINE CEREBELLAR DEGENERATION

Midline cerebellar degeneration (alcoholic cerebellar degeneration) may be a component of WKS but may also occur alone. It causes postural instability, gait ataxia, and ataxia of the legs, with relative sparing of the arms. It has an insidious onset and a subacute or chronic course. There is gross atrophy of the cerebellar folia because of loss of Purkinje cells and granular neurons. In most cases the lesions are confined to the superior vermis (Fig. 8-88); in severe cases they extend symmetrically to the superior aspects of the cerebellar hemispheres. The association of midline cerebellar degeneration with WKS suggests that thiamine deficiency is an important factor in its pathogenesis.

VITAMIN B₁₂ DEFICIENCY AND SUBACUTE COMBINED DEGENERATION

ETIOLOGY

Vitamin B_{12} (cobalamin) is synthesized by microorganisms that grow in sewage, soil, and water and inhabit the intestinal lumen of animals, but not humans. Vegetables are free of vitamin B_{12} unless they are contaminated with such microorganisms. The main dietary sources of vitamin B_{12} are animal products such as meat and dairy foods. In the stomach, cobalamin is bound to intrinsic factor (a glycoprotein produced by the parietal cells of the stomach). The cobalamin–intrinsic factor complex is transported to the terminal ileum, where it binds to receptors on the brush border of enterocytes and is absorbed. Cobalamin is stored in many tissues. If cobalamin absorption ceased, body stores would probably last 3 to 4 years. The common setting of vitamin B_{12} deficiency is pernicious anemia, an autoimmune disorder caused by antibodies against gastric parietal cells and intrinsic factor. Vitamin B_{12} deficiency may also result from *Helicobacter pylori* gastritis and from surgical resection,

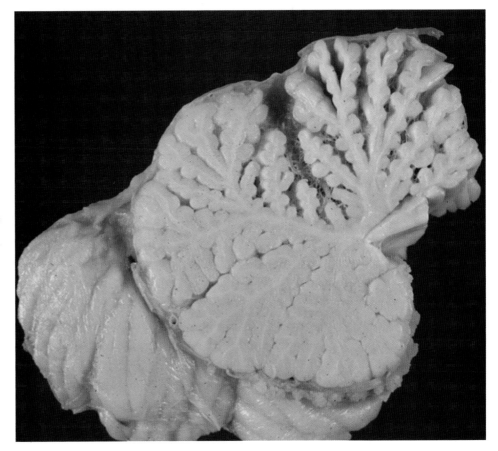

FIGURE 8-88

Degeneration of the superior vermis (midline cerebellar degeneration). The patient also had Wernicke-Korsakoff syndrome. (Reproduced from *www. akronchildrens.org/neuropathology* with permission of Akron Children's Hospital.)

tumors, and other pathology involving large parts of the stomach or lower ileum. Strict vegetarians (vegans) who omit all animal food from their diet and infants born to vegetarian mothers may also be vitamin B_{12} deficient.

CLINICAL FINDINGS

Lack of vitamin B_{12} causes hematologic abnormalities (megaloblastic anemia) and neurologic complications (subacute combined degeneration [SCD] of the spinal cord). SCD is manifested as weakness and paresthesias of the distal end of the lower extremities. As the disease progresses, weakness increases, spasticity of the lower extremities appears, and postural sensation is lost, all of which result in unsteadiness of gait. The advanced state is characterized by spastic paraplegia, contractures, ataxia, and impairment of other sensory modalities. Mental and psychiatric disturbances and visual impairment (centrocecal scotomas, optic atrophy) also occur.

PATHOLOGIC CHANGES

The earliest lesion in SCD is distention of the myelin sheaths, which imparts a spongy appearance to the affected white matter (Fig. 8-89). This change is followed by disintegration and removal of myelin by macrophages. Loss of axons and gliosis occur at a more advanced stage. The lesions initially affect the posterior and lateral (combined) columns of the upper thoracic and low cervical spinal cord. In cases with visual impairment, the optic nerves show similar changes involving the papillomacular bundle. These changes are indistinguishable from tobacco/alcohol amblyopia. Optic nerve lesions are rare in humans but are the earliest pathologic alteration seen in monkeys deprived of vitamin B_{12} (Fig. 8-90). Perivascular foci of demyelination are also seen in the central white matter. There is no conclusive evidence that pure vitamin B_{12} deficiency causes peripheral neuropathy, and no peripheral nerve pathology is seen in experimental animals with vitamin B_{12} deficiency.

PATHOGENESIS

The pathogenesis of SCD is not clear. There are two forms of cobalamin: adenosylcobalamin, a cofactor of

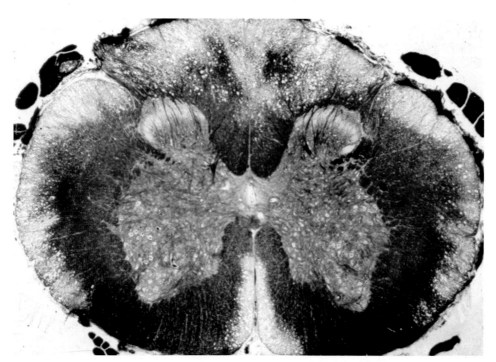

FIGURE 8-89

Extensive myelin degeneration in the spinal cord in a rhesus monkey with experimental vitamin B_{12} deficiency.

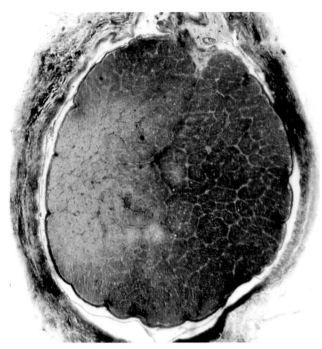

FIGURE 8-90
Optic nerve degeneration in a monkey with vitamin B$_{12}$ deficiency.

methylmalonyl-CoA mutase, and methylcobalamin, a cofactor of methionine synthase. Loss of methylmalonyl-CoA mutase activity leads to the accumulation of propionic acid, which may cause odd-chain fatty acids to be incorporated into biologic membranes and thereby result in myelin instability. Impairment of methionine synthase activity affects DNA synthesis and is the basis of the hematologic abnormalities, but it may also result in deficient methylation of myelin basic protein. Nitric oxide inactivates methionine synthase and causes megaloblastic anemia and spinal cord pathology similar to SCD. Thus, both forms of cobalamin may be potentially involved in the pathogenesis of SCD.

VITAMIN E DEFICIENCY

ETIOLOGY AND CLINICAL FINDINGS

α-Tocopherol, the active form of the lipid-soluble vitamin E, is an important antioxidant that protects cell membranes from free radical damage. Vitamin E deficiency is seen in intestinal malabsorption secondary to cystic fibrosis, celiac disease, large intestinal resections, congenital biliary atresia, and abetalipoproteinemia. A rare genetic form of isolated vitamin E deficiency is caused by mutation of a gene on 8q13 that encodes an α-tocopherol transfer protein. Vitamin E deficiency causes acanthocytosis, sensory peripheral neuropathy, ataxia, pigmentary retinopathy, myopathy, and cardiomyopathy. The full spectrum of pathology is seen in patients with abetalipoproteinemia. The clinical mani-

---

VITAMIN E DEFICIENCY—DISEASE FACTS AND PATHOLOGIC FEATURES

Etiology
▶ Lipid malabsorption

Clinical Findings
▶ Peripheral neuropathy, ataxia, pigmentary retinopathy, myopathy

Pathogenesis
▶ Loss of antioxidant activity of vitamin E

Pathologic Findings
▶ Loss of dorsal root ganglionic neurons and degeneration of their axons in the peripheral and central nervous systems

---

festations overlap with those of Friedreich's ataxia and other spinocerebellar atrophies.

PATHOLOGIC CHANGES

Vitamin E deficiency primarily affects neurons of the dorsal root ganglia and their axons in peripheral nerves and the posterior columns. Dorsal root ganglia show neuronal loss and nests of Nageotte. Peripheral nerve biopsies show loss of large myelinated axons. In the spinal cord, degeneration of the posterior columns, spinocerebellar tracts, and Clarke's nuclei occurs. Axonal spheroids are present in the gracile and cuneate nuclei. The incidental finding of spheroids in these nuclei in old people raises the issue of antioxidant deficiency. Skeletal muscle shows a vacuolar myopathy from the accumulation of lipofuscin. These changes can be reproduced in animals with experimental vitamin E deficiency.

NEUROTOXICOLOGY

- Neurotoxins are ubiquitous, and millions of people are exposed to them.
- Chronic low-grade exposure to neurotoxins has been implicated in the pathogenesis of Alzheimer's disease, Parkinson's disease, and motor neuron disease.
- Neurotoxins affect neurons, axons, myelin, and blood vessels.
- Neurotoxins cause developmental malformations.

There are probably thousands of chemicals with neurotoxic potential. They include naturally occurring substances (neurotoxins) and synthesized compounds (neurotoxicants). The generic term "neurotoxin" is used here for both. Neurotoxins are used as pesticides (fungicides, rodenticides, insecticides, herbicides), industrial solvents, therapeutic and abused drugs, food additives, and cosmetics and for other purposes. Eight hundred fifty workplace chemicals can be classified as neurotoxic. Neurotoxins have been known (and used) since ancient times. Several high-profile neurotoxicity outbreaks, including the "ginger-Jake" syndrome caused by organophosphorus compounds, the methyl mercury poisoning in Minamata Bay and Iraq, the hexachlorobenzene poisoning in Turkey, and the clioquinol neuropathy in Japan, have been well publicized. Millions of people are exposed to toxic chemicals at the workplace and at home. The risk of insidious neurologic damage from chronic low-level exposure is unknown and probably underestimated. There is mounting suspicion that neurotoxins plays a role in the pathogenesis of neurodegenerative diseases, including Alzheimer's disease, Parkinson's disease, and motor neuron disease. This suspicion has been reinforced in recent years by the story of 1-methyl-4-phenyl-1,2,3,6-tetrahydropyridine (MPTP).

Neurotoxins act on the neuronal body (neuronopathies), the axon (axonopathies), the myelin sheath (myelinopathies), and the synapses. One of the most common manifestations of neurotoxicity is peripheral neuropathy. CNS manifestations include vague neuropsychiatric complaints, ataxia, extrapyramidal syndromes, loss of vision and hearing, and spastic paralysis. Some neurotoxins cause vascular injury, cerebral edema, and acute encephalopathy. Most neurotoxins cause functional disturbances that subside if exposure is discontinued. A few cause "hard" pathologic changes that may be irreversible or fatal. Although all ages are at risk, the clinical manifestations of neurotoxicity are more evident in elderly persons, probably because of diminishing functional reserves and plasticity.

Several neurotoxins damage the developing brain and result, most commonly, in microcephaly and low IQ. In a few instances, specific pathology develops. Thus, valproate causes neural tube defects; vitamin A analogues cause microcephaly, hydrocephalus, and abnormalities in neuronal migration; warfarin causes microcephaly, the Dandy-Walker syndrome, and occipital encephalocele; and alcohol causes the fetal alcohol syndrome (see later). Experimental animals are used extensively in the investigation of neurotoxic disorders, and animal models are generally concordant with human pathology.

Detailed accounts of neurotoxins are available in the literature. Examples of neurotoxins and the type of injury that they cause are presented in Table 8-16. Two neurotoxins, lead and alcohol, are briefly described.

LEAD INTOXICATION

EXPOSURE-EPIDEMIOLOGY

Lead causes acute and chronic poisoning in children and adults and neurocognitive deficits in children with chronic exposure to low lead levels. The main source of lead in pediatric lead poisoning is leaded paint (found in houses built before the 1960s) ingested by children with pica. Children absorb lead through the gastrointestinal tract more readily than adults do. Adults are exposed to lead-containing fumes from burning or smelting of lead (painting, pottery glazing, battery burning, auto repair, welding), ingest lead contained in illicit liquor, or inhale lead by sniffing gasoline.

TABLE 8-16

Neurotoxic Disorders

Neuronopathy	Axonopathy and Peripheral Neuropathy	Myelinopathy	Impaired Neurotransmission	Vascular Injury	Developmental Neurotoxicity
Aluminum	Acrylamide	Amiodarone	Domoic acid	Lead	Alcohol
Bismuth	Arsenic	Hexachlorophene	Kainate	Cadmium	Lead
Lead	Carbon disulfide	Perhexiline	Organophosphates	Thallium	Mercury
Manganese	Chlordecone (Kepone)	Trimethyltin	and carbonates	Trimethyltin	Retinoids
Mercury (inorganic and methyl mercury)	Clioquinol	Toluene			Valproate
	Colchicine				Warfarin
	Dimethylaminoproprionitrile				
	Doxorubicin				
Methanol	Hexane				
MPTP	Methyl-*n*-butyl ketone				
Trimethyltin	Organophosphates				
	Vincristine				

MPTP, 1-methyl-4-phenyl-1,2,3,6-tetrahydropyridine.

LEAD INTOXICATION—DISEASE FACTS AND PATHOLOGIC FEATURES

Exposure

▶ Children get acute lead poisoning by eating paint chips from old houses. Adults are exposed to different sources of lead

Clinical Findings

▶ Hematologic abnormalities
▶ Increased intracranial pressure in acute lead poisoning in children
▶ Motor neuropathy in chronic lead poisoning in adults
▶ Low IQ and neurobehavioral abnormalities with chronic low-level exposure in children

Pathologic Changes

▶ Cerebral edema in acute lead poisoning
▶ Axonal neuropathy in adults with chronic lead poisoning

Laboratory Diagnosis

▶ Basophilic stippling of red blood cells, elevated δ-aminolevulinic acid and coproporphyrin, elevated lead levels in blood

Absorbed lead is tightly bound to bone but loosely bound to RBCs, soft tissues, and liver. Lead interferes with the action of enzymes containing sulfhydryl groups and impairs heme biosynthesis by preventing the conversion of δ-aminolevulinic acid to porphobilinogen. It binds with calmodulin and interferes with the action of calcium as a second messenger. This action impairs neurotransmission.

CLINICAL AND PATHOLOGIC FINDINGS

The early manifestations of acute lead poisoning in children are irritability, listlessness, vomiting, and abdominal pain, which develop insidiously over a period of several weeks. If lead poisoning is not recognized, intracranial pressure rises. Seizures, papilledema, and drowsiness appear within days and progress to coma and death. Changes in homeostasis occurring during acute illness in infants and children may trigger lead encephalopathy by mobilizing loosely bound lead into the blood. The manifestations of lead encephalopathy may be mistaken as symptoms of the underlying illness. Laboratory studies show basophilic stippling of RBCs and bone marrow normoblasts, increased urinary δ-aminolevulinic acid and coproporphyrin, and lead lines in the metaphyses of long bones. Immediate chelation is recommended if the blood lead concentration exceeds 70 μm/dL, but acute lead encephalopathy may develop with much lower levels. The basis of acute lead poisoning in children is vascular injury and increased vascular permeability. The brain is massively swollen (Fig. 8-91) and shows pools of perivascular proteinaceous material (Fig. 8-92) and few perivascular mononuclear cells.

Acute lead poisoning is rare in adults. The main symptoms of lead poisoning in adults are colic, anemia, and a predominantly motor polyneuropathy that characteristically involves the radial nerve and causes bilateral wristdrop. Lower extremity involvement with footdrop and other peripheral nerve involvement may also occur. Segmental demyelination has been empha-

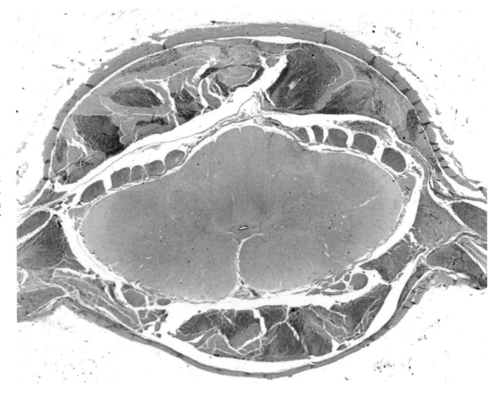

FIGURE 8-91

Acute lead poisoning. Massive cerebral edema caused cerebellar tonsillar herniation with fragmentation and displacement of the cerebellar tonsils around the spinal cord.

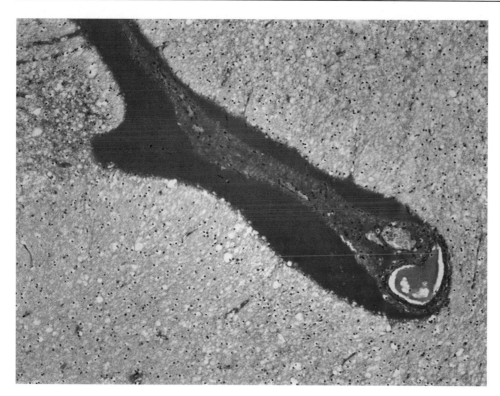

FIGURE 8-92
Perivascular proteinaceous material in acute lead poisoning.

sized in experimental lead poisoning, but human lead neuropathy is primarily axonal.

LOW-LEVEL EXPOSURE IN CHILDREN

The most pervasive form of lead poisoning in recent years is that resulting from chronic low-level exposure in children. Numerous studies show that these children have low IQ, attention deficits, increased aggression, and antisocial behavior. On the basis of this evidence, the Agency for Toxic Substances and Disease Registry recommended that the lead threshold for neurobehavioral toxicity be lowered to 10 to 15 µg/dL. No pathologic changes have been detected in children with low lead exposure, but interference with neurotransmission is a probable mechanism.

TOXIC EFFECTS OF ALCOHOL ON THE NERVOUS SYSTEM

- Alcohol damages the nervous system indirectly. Direct damage has been postulated on clinical and imaging grounds but is not supported by pathology.
- Alcohol damages the developing brain by causing the fetal alcohol syndrome.
- The fetal alcohol syndrome is characterized by intrauterine growth retardation, dysmorphic facial features, and low IQ. Varied and nonspecific neuropathologic changes have been reported.

"ALCOHOLIC DEMENTIA"

The clinical effects of alcohol intoxication and alcohol withdrawal are explained by the pharmacology and physiology of alcohol and are reversible. The metabolic and nutritional complications of alcoholism (hepatic encephalopathy, Wernicke-Korsakoff syndrome, etc.) are indirect. It has been proposed that alcohol also damages the CNS directly by causing "alcoholic dementia" and "alcoholic cerebral atrophy." The terms "alcoholic deteriorated state," "chronic alcoholic psychosis," and "organic brain syndrome due to alcohol" have been used in the psychiatric literature to designate this syndrome. The clinical profile of this syndrome is nonspecific and encompasses physical, personality, and psychosocial deterioration associated with alcoholism. There are no "hard" neurologic findings that could not be attributed to Korsakoff's psychosis or some other medical complication. The pathologic changes are also nonspecific and include decreased brain weight, frontal atrophy, dilatation of the lateral ventricles, leptomeningeal thickening, increased lipofuscin, neuronal loss, and other findings. The cortical atrophy detected by imaging is probably age related, and dilatation of the lateral ventricles is reversible on cessation of drinking.

FETAL ALCOHOL SYNDROME

Although direct structural damage to the CNS by alcohol is questionable, there is no question that alcohol injures the developing brain by causing fetal alcohol syndrome (FAS). Alcohol readily crosses the placenta and exerts its embryotoxic and teratogenic effects either directly or through its metabolite acetaldehyde. At an incidence of 1.9 per 1000 live births, FAS is thought to be the leading cause of mental retardation in the United States and Europe.

Infants with the FAS have intrauterine growth retardation and characteristic craniofacial dysmorphic features (short palpebral fissures, epicanthal folds, low nasal bridge, short nose, flat face, indistinct philtrum, and thin upper lip). Neonatal mortality is high. Children with FAS have psychomotor retardation and behavioral abnormalities that are often diagnosed as attention-deficit/hyperactivity disorder.

No single malformation or characteristic malformation complex has been described in the few cases of FAS in which neuropathology has been reported. The neuropathologic changes are varied and nonspecific and include microcephaly; hydrocephalus; leptomeningeal, white matter, and periventricular neuroglial heterotopia; agenesis of the corpus callosum and the cerebellar vermis; incomplete holoprosencephaly; and neural tube defects. The majority of patients have no gross abnormalities.

The brain abnormalities seen in FAS probably arise in the first trimester, but the mechanism of action of alcohol and the amount of alcohol needed to produce these lesions are unclear. Poor neurologic functioning, microcephaly, and midfacial abnormalities have been reported in animal models of FAS.

ACKNOWLEDGMENTS

I thank Helen Snow for typing the manuscript, Theresa Moles and Sara Dowey for scanning the illustrations, and Drs. Irwin Jacobs, Robert Eiben, Robert Novak, Haynes Robinson, and Roger Lebo for reviewing the manuscript. Figures 8-61, 8-62, 8-70, and 80-71 were provided by Dr. Maie Herrick and Figure 8-73 by Dr. Richard Prayson.

SUGGESTED READINGS

Lysosomal Storage Disorders

Colodny EH: Niemann-Pick disease. Curr Opin Hematol 2000;7:48-52.

Cooper JD: Progress towards understanding the neurobiology of Batten disease or neuronal ceroid lipofuscinosis. Curr Opin Neurol 2003;16:121-128.

Feldt-Rasmussen U, Rasmussen AK, Mersebach H, et al: Fabry disease. A metabolic disorder with a challenge for endocrinologists? Horm Res 2002;58:259-265.

Folkerth RD, Alroy J, Bhan I, et al: Infantile G(M1) gangliosidosis: Complete morphology and histochemistry of two autopsy cases, with particular reference to delayed central nervous system myelination. Pediatr Dev Pathol 2000;3:73-86.

Garver WS, Heidenreich RA: The Niemann-Pick C proteins and trafficking of cholesterol through the last endosomal/lysosomal system. Curr Mol Med 2002;2:485-505.

Haltia M: The neuronal ceroid-lipofuscinoses. J Neuropathol Exp Neurol 2003;62:1-13.

Hesselink R, Wagenmakers A, Drost M, et al: Lysosomal dysfunction in muscle with special reference to glycogen storage disease type II. Biochim Biophys Acta 2003;1637:164-170.

Jolly RD, Walkley SN: Lysosomal storage diseases of animals: An essay in comparative pathology. Vet Pathol 1997;34:527-548.

Meikle PJ, Hopwood JJ, Clagne AE, et al: Prevalence of lysosomal storage diseases. JAMA 1999;281:249-254.

Raben N, Plotz P, Byrne B: Acid alpha-glucosidase deficiency (glycogenosis type II, Pompe disease). Curr Mol Med 2002;2:145-166.

Suzuki K, Suzuki K: Lysosomal diseases. In Graham DI, Lantos PI (eds): Greenfield's Neuropathology, 7th ed. London, Arnold, 2002, pp 653-735.

Walkley SN: Cellular pathology of lysosomal storage disorders. Brain Pathol 1998;8:175-193.

Walkley S: Neurobiology and cellular pathogenesis of glycolipid storage diseases. Philos Trans R Soc Lond B Biol Sci 2003;358:893-904.

Zhao H, Grabowski GA: Human genome diseases: Review. Gaucher disease: Perspectives on a prototype lysosomal disease. Cell Mol Life Sci 2002;59:694-707.

Peroxisomal Disorders

Agamanolis DP, Novak RW: Rhizomelic chondrodysplasia punctata: Report of a case with review of the literature and correlation with other peroxisomal disorders. Pediatr Pathol Lab Med 1995;15:503-513.

Baumgartner MR, Saudubray JM: Peroxisomal disorders. Semin Neonat 2002;7:85-94.

Brosius U, Gartner J: Cellular and molecular aspects of Zellweger syndrome and other peroxisome biogenesis disorders. Cell Mol Life Sci 2002;59:1058-1069.

Depreter M, Espeel M, Roels F: Human peroxisomal disorders. Microsc Res Tech 2003;61:203-223.

Goldfischer S, Moore CL, Johnson AB: Peroxisomal and mitochondrial defects in the cerebro-hepato-renal syndrome. Science 1973;182:62-64.

Gould SJ, Raymond GV, Valle D: The peroxisome biogenesis disorders. In Scriver C, Beaudet A, Sly W, Valle D (eds): The Metabolic and Molecular Bases of Inherited Disease. New York, McGraw-Hill, 2001, pp 3181-3217.

Gould SJ, Valle D: Peroxisome biogenesis disorders: Genetics and cell biology. Trends Genet 2000;16:340-345.

Jansen GA, Wanders RJA, Watkins PA, et al: Phytanoyl-coenzyme A hydroxylase deficiency: The enzyme defect in Refsum's disease. N Engl J Med 1997;337:133-134.

Moser HW: Peroxisomal disorders. Semin Pediatr Neurol 1996;3:298-304.

Powers J, DeVivo DC: Peroxisomal and mitochondrial disorders. In Graham DI, Lantos PL (eds): Greenfield's Neuropathology, 7th ed. London, Arnold, 2002, pp 738-797.

Powers JM, Moser HW: Peroxisomal disorders: Genotype, phenotype, major neuropathologic lesions, and pathogenesis. Brain Pathol 1998;8:101-120.

Wanders RJA, Barth PG, Heymans HSA: Peroxisomal disorders. In Rimoin DL, Connor JM, Pyeritz RE, Corf BR (eds): Emery and Rimoin's Principles and Practice of Medical Genetics. London, Churchill Livingstone, 2002, pp 2753-2787.

Watkins PA, Chen WW, Harris CJ, et al: Peroxisomal bifunctional enzyme deficiency. J Clin Invest 1989;83:771-777.

Mitochondrial Disorders

Bernier FP, Boneh A, Dennett X, et al: Diagnostic criteria for respiratory chain disorders in adults and children. Neurology 2002;59:1406-1411.

Bindoff L: Mitochondria and the heart. Eur Heart J 2003;24:221-224.

Biousse V, Newman NJ: Neuro-ophthalmology of mitochondrial disorders. Semin Neurol 2001;21:275-291.

Bouillot S, Martin-Negrier ML, Vital A, et al: Peripheral neuropathy associated with mitochondrial disorders: 8 cases and review of the literature. J Peripher Nerv Syst 2002;7:213-220.

Chinnery PF: Mitochondrial disorders overview. http://www.genclinics.org, 2002.

DiMauro S: Lessons from mitochondrial DNA mutations. Semin Cell Dev Biol 2001;12:397-405.

Man PYW, Turnbull DM, Chinnery PF: Leber hereditary optic neuropathy. J Med Genet 2002;39:162-169.

Oldfors A, Tulinius M: Mitochondrial encephalomyopathies. J Neuropathol Exp Neurol 2003;62:217-227.

Schapira AHV, DiMauro S: Mitochondrial disorders. In Neurology 2. Boston, Butterworth-Heinemann, 2002.

Smeitink J, van der Heuvel L, DiMauro S: The genetics and pathology of oxidative phosphorylation. Nat Rev 2001;2:342-352.

Tanji K, Kuninutsu T, Vu TH, et al: Neuropathological features of mitochondrial disorders. Semin Cell Dev Biol 2001;12:429-439.

Wallace DC: Mitochondrial diseases in man and mouse. Science 1999;283:1482-1488.

Amino Acid and Miscellaneous Inherited Metabolic Disorders

Agamanolis DP: Disorders of amino acid metabolism. In Golden JA, Harding B (eds): Pathology and Genetics. Developmental Neuropathology. Basel, ISN Neuropath Press, 2004, pp 303-310.

Agamanolis DP, Potter JL, Lundgren DW: Neonatal glycine encephalopathy: Biochemical and neuropathologic findings. Pediatr Neurol 1993;9:140-143.

Agamanolis DP, Potter JL, Naito HK, et al: Lipoprotein disorder, cirrhosis, and olivopontocerebellar degeneration in two siblings. Neurology 1986;36:674-681.

Dobyns WB: Agenesis of the corpus callosum and gyral malformations are frequent manifestations of nonketotic hyperglycemia. Neurology1989;39:817-820.

Filloux F, Townsend JJ, Leonard C: Ornithine transcarbamylase deficiency: Neuropathologic changes acquired in utero. J Pediatr 1986;108:942-945.

Friede RL: Developmental Neuropathology, 2nd ed. New York, Springer-Verlag, 1989, pp 524-533.

Hagberg BA, Blennow G, Kristiansson B, et al: Carbohydrate-deficient glycoprotein syndromes: Peculiar group of new disorders. Pediatr Neurol 1993;9:255-262.

Harding BN, Dunger DB, Grant DB, et al: Familial olivopontocerebellar atrophy with neonatal onset: A recessively inherited syndrome with systemic and biochemical abnormalities. J Neurol Neurosurg Psychiatry 1988;51:385-390.

Harding BN, Surtees R: Metabolic and neurodegenerative diseases of childhood. In Graham DI, Lantos PI (eds): Greenfield's Neuropathology, 7th ed. London, Arnold, 2002, pp 485-517.

Hawkins RA, Jessy J: Hyperammonaemia does not impair brain function in the absence of net glutamine synthesis. Biochem J 1991;277:697-703.

Horn N, Tonnesen T, Tumer Z: Menkes disease: An X-linked neurological disorder of the copper metabolism. Brain Pathol 1992;2:351-362.

Marquardt T, Denecke J: Congenital disorders of glycosylation: Review of their molecular bases, clinical presentations and specific therapies. Eur J Pediatr 2003;162:359-379.

Menkes JH: Menkes disease and Wilson disease: Two sides of the same copper coin. Part I: Menkes disease. Eur J Paediatr Neurol 1999;3:147-158.

Mudd SH, Levy HL, Kraus JP: Disorders of transsulfuration. In Scriver C, Beaudet A, Sly W, Valle D (eds): The Metabolic and Molecular Bases of Inherited Disease. New York, McGraw-Hill, 2001, pp 2007-2056.

Shuman RM, Leech RW, Scott CR: The neuropathology of the nonketotic and ketotic hyperglycinemias: Three cases. Neurology 1978;28:139-146.

Volpe JJ: Neurology of the Newborn, 4th ed. Philadelphia, WB Saunders, 2001, pp 547-595.

Welch GN, Loscalzo J: Homocysteine and atherothrombosis. N Engl J Med 1998;338:1042-1050.

Wilcox SI, Sederbaum SD: Amino acid metabolism. In Rimoin DL, Connor JM, Pyeritz RE, Corf BR (eds): Emery and Rimoin's Principles and Practice of Medical Genetics. London, Churchill Livingstone, 2002, pp 2405-2440.

Nutritional, Acquired Metabolic, and Toxic Disorders

Agamanolis DP, Chester EM, Victor M, et al: Neuropathology of experimental vitamin B_{12} deficiency in monkeys. Neurology 1976;26:905-914.

Blair PG, Harris JB (eds): Medical Neurotoxicology. London, Arnold, 1999.

Brown D: Osmotic demyelination disorders: Central pontine and extrapontine myelinolysis. Curr Opin Neurol 2000;13:691-697.

Butterworth RF: Pathophysiology of hepatic encephalopathy: A new look at ammonia. Metab Brain Dis 2000;217:221-227.

Filley CM, Halliday W, Kleinschmidt-DeMasters BK: The effects of toluene on the nervous system. J Neuropathol Exp Neurol 2004;63:1-12.

Jalan R, Shawcross D, Davies N: The molecular pathogenesis of hepatic encephalopathy. Int J Biochem Cell Biol 2003;35:1175-1181.

Jones EA: Ammonia, the GABA neurotransmitter system, and hepatic encephalopathy. Metab Brain Dis 2002;17:275-281.

Harper C: The neuropathology of alcohol-specific brain damage, or does alcohol damage the brain? J Neuropathol Exp Neurol 1998;57:101-110.

Hazell AS, Butterworth RFB: Hepatic encephalopathy: An update of pathophysiologic mechanisms. Proc Soc Exp Biol Med 1999;222:99-112.

Lampl C, Yazdi K: Central pontine myelinolysis. Eur Neurol 2002;47:3-10.

Laureno R: Central pontine myelinolysis following rapid correction of hyponatremia. Ann Neurol 1983;13:232.

Layrargues GP, Rose C, Spahr L, et al: Role of manganese in the pathogenesis of portal-systemic encephalopathy. Metab Brain Dis 1998;13:311-317.

Mendola P, Selevan SG, Gutter S, et al: Environmental factors associated with a spectrum of neurodevelopmental deficits. Ment Retard Dev Disabil Res Rev 2002;8:188-197.

Norenberg MD: Astroglial dysfunction in hepatic encephalopathy. Metab Brain Dis 1998;13:319-335.

Rama RKV, Jayakumar AR, Norenberg DM: Ammonia neurotoxicity: Role of the mitochondrial permeability transition. Metab Brain Dis 2003;18:113-127.

Scalabrino G: Subacute combined degeneration one century later. The neurotrophic action of cobalamin (vitamin B_{12}) revisited. J Neuropathol Exp Neurol 2001;60:109-120.

Surtees R: Biochemical pathogenesis of subacute combined degeneration of the spinal cord and brain. J Inherit Metab Dis 1993;16:762-770.

Tanyel MC, Mancano LD: Neurologic findings in vitamin E deficiency. Am Fam Physician 1997;55:197-201.

Thomson AD: Mechanisms of vitamin deficiency in chronic alcohol misusers and the development of the Wernicke-Korsakoff syndrome. Alcohol Alcohol Suppl 2000;35(Suppl 1):2-7.

Victor M, Adams RD, Collins G: The Wernicke-Korsakoff Syndrome. Philadelphia, FA Davis, 1971.

9 Glial and Glioneuronal Tumors

Arie Perry

Gliomas and glioneuronal tumors constitute the largest and most heterogeneous group of primary central nervous system (CNS) tumors. Normal glia includes astrocytes, oligodendrocytes, and ependyma; gliomas are analogously designated as astrocytomas, oligodendrogliomas, and ependymomas to reflect the non-neoplastic cell types that they most closely resemble. The actual histogenesis is mostly speculated rather than proven. The term "astrocytoma" has been applied broadly, but the four most common types include diffuse astrocytoma, pilocytic astrocytoma, pleomorphic xanthoastrocytoma, and subependymal giant cell astrocytoma. Each has a distinct localization, histology, and natural history, with the first representing an infiltrative form and the latter three representing more circumscribed and prognostically favorable tumors. Diffuse astrocytoma (grade II), anaplastic astrocytoma (grade III), and glioblastoma (grade IV) form a malignancy continuum for the diffusely infiltrating astrocytomas. The term "diffuse glioma" is also commonly used to encompass astrocytomas, oligodendrogliomas, and mixed oligoastrocytomas (grades II to IV), all infiltrative and malignant gliomas with overlapping clinical, radiographic, and histologic features. Glioneuronal tumors also contain neuronal elements, and a growing list of rare entities are being recognized. In this chapter, the two most common forms are discussed: ganglioglioma/ganglion cell tumor and dysembryoplastic neuroepithelial tumor.

DIFFUSE (FIBRILLARY) ASTROCYTOMAS

CLINICAL FEATURES

Diffuse astrocytomas (grades II to IV) account for roughly 40% of primary intracranial tumors, with an

▶ Most arise in the cerebral hemispheres with a subcortical epicenter, but they may be seen anywhere along the neural axis, including the brain stem, cerebellum, and spinal cord

Gender and Age Distribution

▶ Slight male preponderance (M/F ratio of 3:2)
▶ Can occur at any age, although the incidence increases with advancing age
▶ Older patients are more likely to have higher-grade gliomas, especially glioblastoma

Clinical Features

▶ Manifestations dependent on location of tumor
▶ Focal neural deficits (e.g., motor, cranial nerve, sensory, visual), increased intracranial pressure, and seizures are most common
▶ Generalized neurologic signs and symptoms of increased intracranial pressure include headaches, nausea/vomiting, and papilledema
▶ Rapid onset and progression suggest high grade (III or IV), whereas a protracted history is more consistent with low grade (II)

Radiologic Features

▶ Astrocytomas (WHO grade II) are typically nonenhancing masses with increased signal on T2-weighted (see Fig. 9-1A) and FLAIR MRI sequences
▶ Anaplastic astrocytomas (WHO grade III) are typically nonenhancing or focally enhancing
▶ Glioblastomas (a.k.a. glioblastoma multiforme or GBM; WHO grade IV) are usually ring enhancing and may be a "butterfly lesion" crossing the corpus callosum (see Fig. 9-1B)
▶ "Multifocal gliomas" usually show separate foci of enhancement, with or without discernible nonenhancing signal abnormalities in between
▶ In treated gliomas, foci of radiation necrosis may appear virtually identical to that of tumor recurrence or progression (or both) (see Fig. 9-1C)

Prognosis and Treatment

▶ Patient age: powerful predictor, with survival inversely proportional to patient age
▶ Histologic grade: survival averages 5 to 10 years for grade II, 2 to 3 years for grade III, and 1 year for grade IV
▶ Histologic cell type: Pure astrocytomas have a worse prognosis than mixed oligoastrocytomas and oligodendrogliomas do
▶ Preoperative performance status: measure of neurologic function, with greater impairment associated with a poorer prognosis
▶ Extent of resection: gross total resection/debulking may be beneficial
▶ Radiotherapy often used to treat subtotally resected and higher-grade gliomas
▶ Chemotherapy often used in high-grade (III or IV) or oligodendroglial tumors, the latter being more chemosensitive than their astrocytic counterparts

annual incidence of 4 per 100,000 person-years. They occur at all ages, although the median age is 30 to 40 for astrocytoma (grade II), 40 to 50 for anaplastic astrocytoma (grade III), and 50 to 60 years for glioblastoma multiforme (grade IV). Glioblastomas are the most frequent, with low-grade examples being comparatively uncommon, particularly in the elderly. The clinical manifestations vary according to the site of involvement, but most common are new-onset seizures, motor deficits, and signs/symptoms of increased intracranial pressure (e.g., headaches, nausea/vomiting, papilledema). High-grade (III and IV) astrocytomas tend to have short histories with rapid progression, whereas low-grade (II) examples are more indolent, often with an insidious onset and a long, protracted clinical course. Radiographically, grade II astrocytomas are most commonly nonenhancing, ill-defined deep-seated or predominantly subcortical cerebral hemispheric masses, best appreciated on T2-weighted or fluid-attenuated inversion recovery (FLAIR) magnetic resonance imaging (MRI) sequences (Fig. 9-1A). Because of their infiltrative nature, there are often foci of microscopic disease beyond the suspected "tumor margins." Secondary signs of mass effect include midline shift, ventricular compression, and sulcal effacement. Anaplastic astrocytomas may be radiographically identical or may show faint punctate or irregular foci of contrast enhancement. Glioblastomas are typically ring enhancing with central low-density regions of necrosis surrounded by an irregular, variable-thickness rim of contrast enhancement (see Fig. 9-1B). Those that cross the corpus callosum are often referred to as "butterfly lesions" because of involvement of the white matter in the centrum semiovale bilaterally. Other diagnostic considerations include CNS lymphoma and multiple sclerosis. In treated gliomas, foci of radiation necrosis are radiographically and grossly very similar to glioblastoma and may produce considerable neurologic worsening as a result of a mass effect (see Figs. 9-1C and 9-2B). Therefore, the differential diagnosis of tumor recurrence/progression versus radiation necrosis is a common problem. Special techniques such as positron emission tomography and single-photon emission computed tomography may be useful for further distinguishing these two diagnostic considerations, although they are both imperfect and biopsy is sometimes necessary.

PATHOLOGIC FEATURES

Grossly, low-grade and anaplastic tumors are ill defined and subtly discolored with secondary mass effects

---

DIFFUSE (FIBRILLARY) ASTROCYTOMAS—PATHOLOGIC FEATURES

Gross Findings

▶ Borders are ill defined, and there are often foci of tumor involvement that are grossly invisible, particularly in gliomatosis cerebri (see the subsequent section)

▶ Tumor epicenter most common in white matter or deep gray matter (e.g., thalamus or basal ganglia) (see Fig. 9-2A)
▶ Blurring of corticomedullary and other gray-white junctions
▶ Mass effect with a midline shift, blunting of sulci, compression of ventricles, or any combination of these effects
▶ A variegated appearance with foci of necrosis and hemorrhage suggests glioblastoma (see Fig. 9-2A)
▶ Foci of radiation necrosis may appear grossly similar to glioblastoma multiforme (Fig. 9-2B)

Microscopic Features

▶ Hypercellularity with intermingling of neoplastic and non-neoplastic elements (i.e., infiltrative)
▶ Hyperchromatic oval to spindled nuclei with irregular contours (see Fig. 9-3A)
▶ Mild to moderate nuclear atypia
▶ Either no discernible cytoplasm ("naked nuclei") or eosinophilic cytoplasmic processes
▶ Secondary structures of Scherer (e.g., subpial condensation, perineuronal satellitosis, perivascular aggregation) are less common than in oligodendrogliomas, but occasionally prominent (see Fig. 9-3B)
▶ See Table 9-1 for histologic variants of diffuse astrocytoma (see Figs. 9-3C and 9-5)
▶ Mitotic figures/increased proliferation present in grades III and IV (see Fig. 9-3D)
▶ Endothelial hyperplasia or necrosis (or both) present in glioblastoma (grade IV) (see Fig. 9-3E and F)

Ultrastructural Features

▶ Electron-dense cells with prominent cytoplasmic intermediate filaments corresponding to GFAP

Immunohistochemical Features

▶ GFAP—usually positive, but sometimes difficult to distinguish brain from tumor immunoreactivity
▶ S-100 protein—positive; less specific, but more sensitive than GFAP for glial lineage
▶ Cytokeratins—negative, but may get false-positive result with AE1/AE3 cocktail
▶ Epithelial membrane antigen (EMA)—negative
▶ HMB-45, melan A, leukocyte common antigen (LCA)—negative
▶ Neurofilament highlights entrapped axons, consistent with an infiltrative growth pattern
▶ p53 protein positive in more than half
▶ MIB-1 (Ki-67) labeling index roughly proportional to grade (see Fig. 9-3D)

Genetics

▶ Mutations of *p53* gene in 40% to 50% of astrocytomas, anaplastic astrocytomas, and secondary glioblastomas (i.e., those arising from a lower-grade precursor)
▶ Amplification of epidermal growth factor receptor (*EGFR*) gene in 30% to 40% of primary (i.e., de novo) glioblastomas and in 70% to 80% of the small cell variant of glioblastomas
▶ Monosomy 10 or 10q deletions/loss of heterozygosity in the majority of glioblastomas
▶ Loss of p16 gene or other members of the retinoblastoma regulatory pathway in most anaplastic astrocytomas and glioblastomas

Differential Diagnosis

▶ Oligodendroglioma/mixed oligoastrocytoma (see Figs. 9-5F, 9-17, and 9-18)
▶ Metastatic carcinoma or melanoma
▶ CNS lymphoma
▶ Radiation necrosis (see Fig. 9-4)
▶ Reactive gliosis

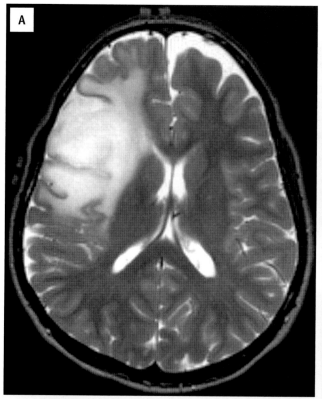

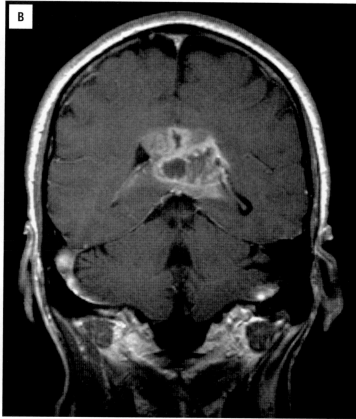

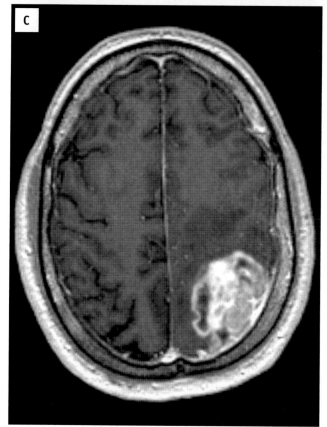

FIGURE 9-1

Representative MRI from patients with diffuse astrocytoma, glioblastoma, and radiation necrosis. **A**, Diffuse astrocytoma, grade II. A T2-weighted image shows ill-defined margins and increased signal in the white matter and cortex. **B**, Glioblastoma. A T1-weighted image with gadolinium contrast shows a deep-seated, ring-enhancing mass that crossed the corpus callosum. **C**, Radiation necrosis in a treated glioblastoma patient (difficult to distinguish from tumor recurrence). A T1-weighted image with gadolinium contrast shows a heterogeneously enhancing mass.

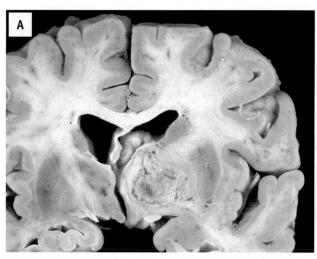
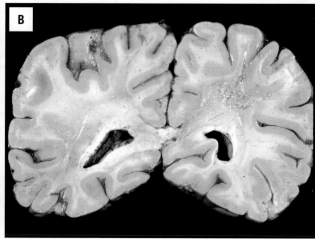

FIGURE 9-2

Similar gross appearance of glioblastoma (**A**) and radiation necrosis (**B**) with variegated necrotic masses.

identical to those seen radiographically. As described earlier, there are typically foci of microscopic disease beyond the grossly suspected borders that are invisible to the naked eye. Glioblastomas are classically variegated with foci of necrosis and hemorrhage (Fig. 9-2A).

Diffuse astrocytomas may have a wide spectrum of cell types in pure or mixed form (see Table 9-1), although the fibrillary variant is the prototype; this variant is composed of elongated, irregular hyperchromatic nuclei, often with no discernible cytoplasm ("naked nuclei"), but embedded in a dense fibrillary matrix (Fig. 9-3). Alternatively, these cells may have visible eosinophilic cytoplasmic processes. Other cellular variants include gemistocytic (eccentric bellies of cytoplasm) (see Fig. 9-3C), protoplasmic (wispy cobweb-like processes), giant cell (large mononucleated and multinucleated cells with abundant cytoplasm) (see Fig. 9-5A), and small cell (monomorphic oval nuclei with minimal cytoplasm) (see Fig. 9-5E). Diffuse astrocytomas are characterized by invasive growth such that non-neoplastic cells are often intermixed and may even predominate in some areas. The secondary structures of Scherer are less commonly encountered than they are in oligodendrogliomas but include subpial condensation, perineuronal satellitosis, and perivascular aggregation (see Fig. 9-3B). The extreme end of the infiltrative spectrum is known as gliomatosis cerebri; it involves multiple lobes of the brain, often bilaterally and frequently extending into the brain stem, cerebellum, and even the spinal cord. A number of grading schemes have been applied, although most pathologists today use the World Health Organization (WHO) scheme. Adopted from a simple St. Anne–Mayo approach, four criteria are used, the "AMEN criteria" of atypia, mitoses, endothelial hyperplasia, and necrosis. Grade II astrocytomas have atypia only. Anaplastic astrocytomas (grade III) additionally have mitotic activity, and glioblastomas (grade IV) have endothelial hyperplasia or necrosis, usually both. The number of mitoses necessary for anaplasia has been debated, but probably one is enough

in a small biopsy (e.g., stereotactic needle) specimen, whereas more are needed in resection specimens. Vascular proliferation often includes glomeruloid vessels (i.e., multiple lumina), although endothelial hyperplasia is probably best defined by multilayering (see Fig. 9-3E). The necrosis may be bland and infarct-like, but it is most commonly geographic or serpentine with associated nuclear pseudopalisading (i.e., tumor hypercellularity at the edge of the necrosis) (see Fig. 9-3F).

By immunohistochemistry, most astrocytomas are positive for glial fibrillary acidic protein (GFAP), although the degree of cytoplasmic positivity is highly variable and some astrocytomas have minimal discernible cytoplasm. In addition, it may be difficult to distinguish positivity in native non-neoplastic tissue or reactive astrocytes from that belonging to the tumor. S-100 protein is a less specific glial marker but is positive in most gliomas, particularly those in which GFAP is negative or equivocal. Neurofilament is also useful because it highlights entrapped axons, thus calling attention to the infiltrative growth pattern. Many diffuse astrocytomas are strongly p53 positive. Although not lineage specific, this characteristic is occasionally useful for supporting a neoplastic designation in the differential diagnosis of grade II astrocytoma versus a reactive process. Finally, MIB-1 (Ki-67) is useful for estimating the proliferative index, which is roughly proportional to the histologic grade (see Fig. 9-3D).

DIFFERENTIAL DIAGNOSIS

The most common and difficult diagnostic considerations in diffuse astrocytomas are other diffuse gliomas, including oligodendrogliomas and mixed oligoastrocytomas. The primary distinction for oligodendroglial differentiation is cytologic, including rounded regular nuclei, bland chromatin, small nucleoli, and clear perinuclear haloes. In poorly differentiated cases, metasta-

---

TABLE 9-1
Diffuse Astrocytomas—Variants

Fibrillary Astrocytoma (see Fig. 9-3)

Prototype of diffuse astrocytomas

Cells with inconspicuous cytoplasm embedded in a densely fibrillary matrix ("naked nuclei") or with thin GFAP-positive cytoplasmic processes

Enlarged elongated hyperchromatic nuclei with irregular nuclear contours

Hypocellular examples may be difficult to distinguish from reactive gliosis

Gemistocytic Astrocytoma (see Fig. 9-3C)

Eccentrically placed eosinophilic, GFAP-positive cytoplasm with short, polar cytoplasmic processes, round, variably hyperchromatic nuclei, and asymmetric distribution of tumor cells (unlike reactive gemistocytes)

Associated perivascular inflammation

Rare mitoses, but high-grade examples frequently associated with proliferating small cell astrocytes

High rate of malignant progression to glioblastomas

Protoplasmic Astrocytoma

Thin, wispy processes creating a cobweb-like growth pattern

Oval, mildly hyperchromatic nuclei

Less widely infiltrative than other variants

Usually low-grade (WHO grade II)

Not accepted as a distinct variant by all pathologists because of some overlapping features with oligodendrogliomas and pilocytic astrocytomas

Giant Cell Astrocytoma/GBM (see Fig. 9-5A-C)

Mononucleate and multinucleate giant cells with abundant cytoplasm and bizarre nuclei

Often deceptively circumscribed grossly

Usually grade IV

Previously known as "monstrocellular glioblastomas"

Gliosarcoma (Feigin's tumor) (see Fig. 9-5D)

Grade IV tumor with both astrocytic and sarcomatous components

Thought to represent a form of mesenchymal metaplasia in a gliomas, analogous to carcinosarcoma arising in epithelial sites

The sarcomatous element is usually fibrosarcoma or malignant fibrous histiocytoma, but may show bone, cartilage, or muscle differentiation

Often superficial and deceptively circumscribed

Prognosis and response to therapy do not differ significantly from conventional glioblastoma

Small Cell Astrocytoma/GBM (see Fig. 9-5E)

Small cells with minimal cytoplasm and oval, mildly hyperchromatic nuclei

Deceptively bland chromatin and perinuclear haloes mimics oligodendroglioma

Brisk mitotic/proliferative indices

Usually grade IV

Gliomatosis Cerebri

Clinicopathologic diagnosis requiring extensive involvement of multiple lobes or brain compartments (sometimes the whole neuraxis)

Usually resembles fibrillary astrocytoma, grade II or III, but rare cases show oligodendroglial features

Long, thin, mildly hyperchromatic "microglia-like" astrocytoma nuclei are typical

Secondary structures (subpial or subependymal condensation, perivascular aggregates, perineuronal satellitosis) are common

Brain stem involvement common

May be associated with multiple foci of dedifferentiation to GBM

GBM, glioblastoma multiforme; GFAP, glial fibrillary acidic protein; WHO, World Health Organization.

---

tic carcinoma and melanoma enter the differential diagnosis. The latter tumors are GFAP negative, being highlighted instead by cytokeratin and melanocytic markers (HMB-45, melan A), respectively. One caveat to keep in mind is that keratin cocktails, such as AE1/AE3, often cross-react with GFAP and may lead to false-positive results with astrocytomas. Generally, low-molecular-weight keratins such as CAM 5.2 do not suffer this problem and are thus preferable in this differential. As stated earlier, neurofilament is also helpful for highlighting the infiltrative nature of astrocytomas as opposed to metastases, which tend to push axon-rich parenchyma to the side rather than infiltrate. CNS lymphomas are similarly infiltrative, but are characterized by angiocentricity and immunoreactivity for lym-phocytic (CD45) and B-cell (CD20) markers. In post-treated astrocytomas, a common differential diagnosis is that of tumor recurrence/progression versus radiation necrosis. Histologically, there is often a combination of each with some suggestion that the prognosis is improved when radiation necrosis predominates. Although it is not always possible to distinguish radiation necrosis from tumor necrosis, the former is typified by large geographic zones of infarct-like necrosis unassociated with nuclear pseudopalisading, with or without dystrophic calcification. Other radiation effects consist of parenchymal rarefaction and vascular changes, including telangiectasia, hyalinization, and fibrinoid necrosis of vessel walls (Fig. 9-4). In patients with

Text continued on p. 433

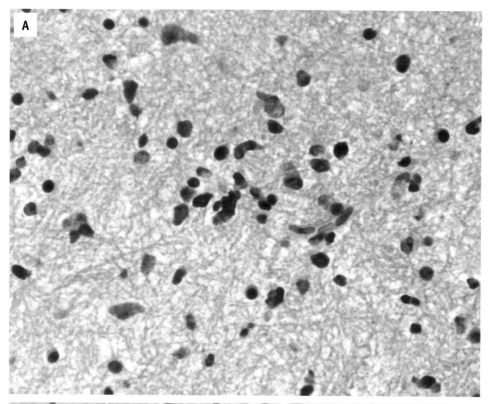

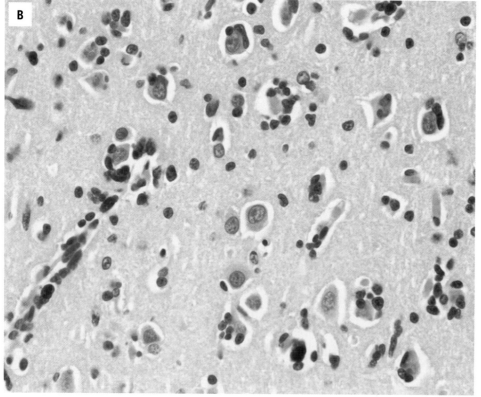

FIGURE 9-3

Diffuse astrocytomas. **A**, Cluster of mildly enlarged, elongated or irregular, hyperchromatic "naked nuclei" intermingled with native nonneoplastic cells in a grade II astrocytoma. **B**, Secondary structures of Scherer with perineuronal satellitosis and perivascular aggregation of tumor cells.

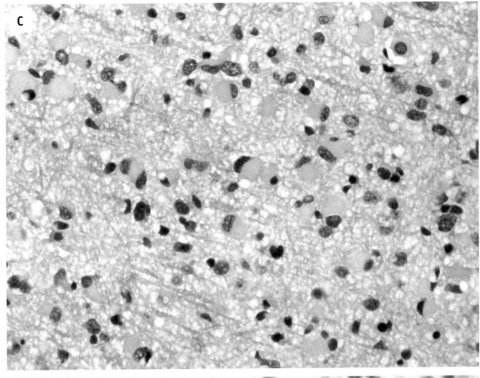

FIGURE 9-3, cont'd
C, Gemistocytic component in a grade II astrocytoma. **D**, MIB-1 (Ki-67) immunostain showing increased labeling index in an anaplastic astrocytoma, WHO grade III.

Continued

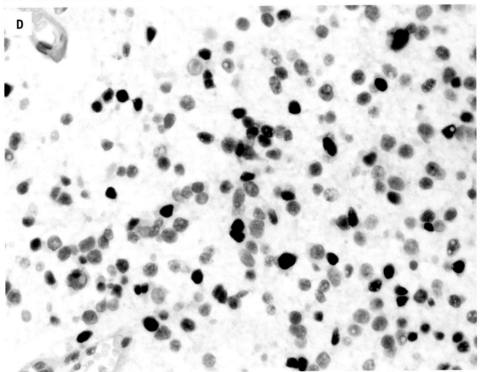

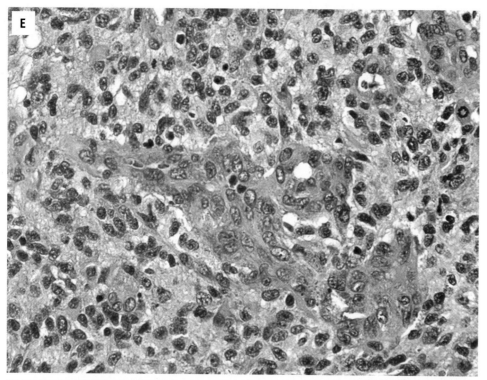

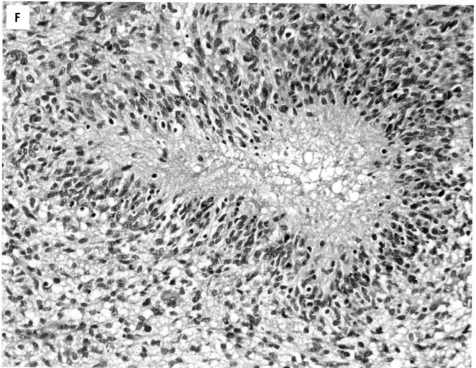

FIGURE 9-3, cont'd
E, Endothelial hyperplasia in a glioblastoma. **F**, Pseudopalisading necrosis in a glioblastoma.

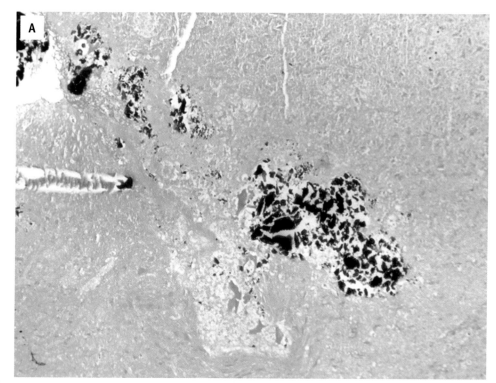

FIGURE 9-4

Radiation necrosis and radiation changes. **A**, Large zones of coagulative necrosis with dystrophic calcification and no adjacent tumor hypercellularity or pseudopalisading. **B-D**, Vascular changes such as fibrinoid necrosis (**B**),

Continued

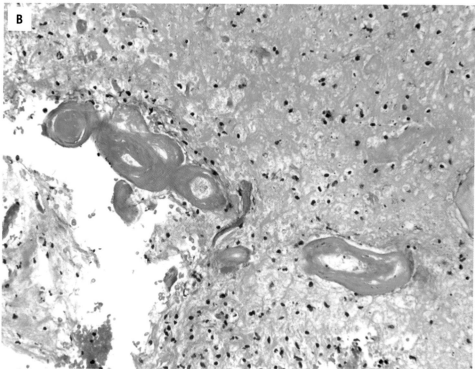

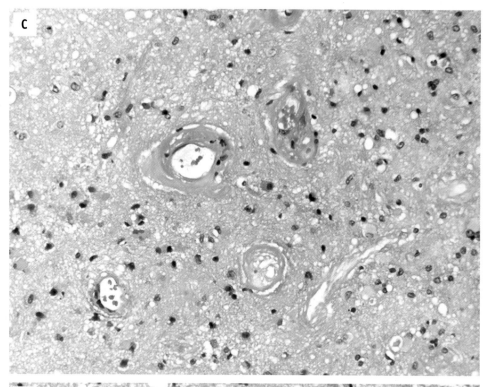

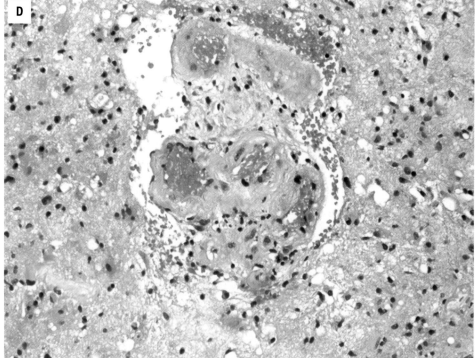

FIGURE 9-4, cont'd
hyalinization (**C**), and telangiectasia (**D**).

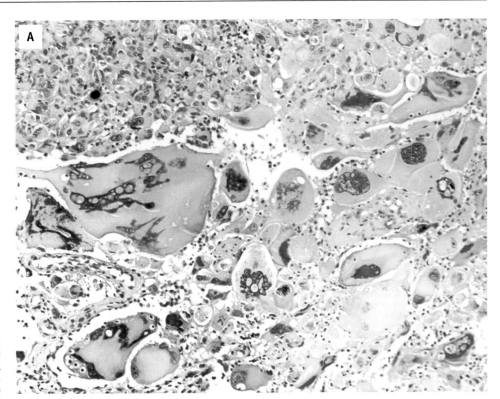

FIGURE 9-5

Glioblastoma variants, including giant cell glioblastoma multiforme (GBM) (**A-C**), gliosarcoma (**D**), small cell GBM (**E**), and GBM with oligodendroglial features (**F**). **A**, Huge mononucleated and multinucleated giant tumor cells. **B**, Most of the proliferative activity is in the intervening small tumor cells, but some of the giant cell nuclei are also stained with MIB-1.   *Continued*

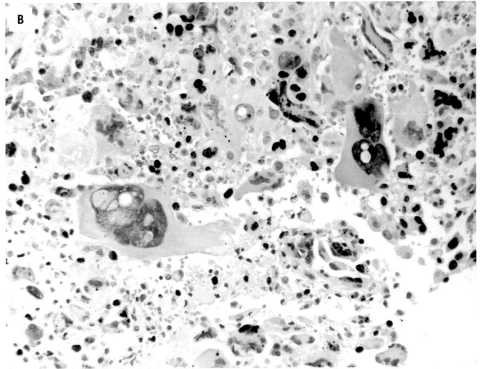

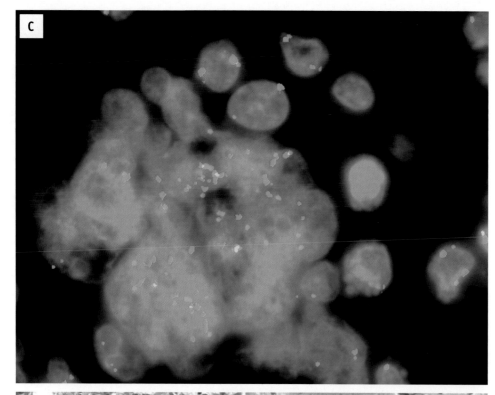

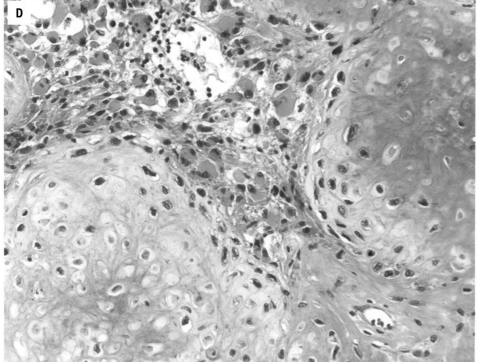

FIGURE 9-5, cont'd

C, Marked polysomy 9 (i.e., chromosomal gains) in a multinucleated giant cell determined with FISH markers (centromere 9 in green and the p16 gene in red). Note that the intervening small cells have the normal two copies (*right*). **D**, Gliosarcoma with extensive cartilaginous differentiation in the sarcomatous element. The glial component is predominantly gemistocytic in this example.

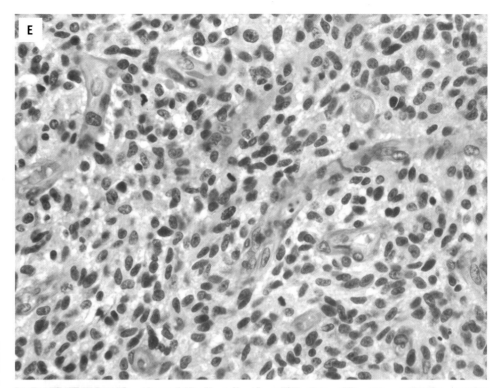

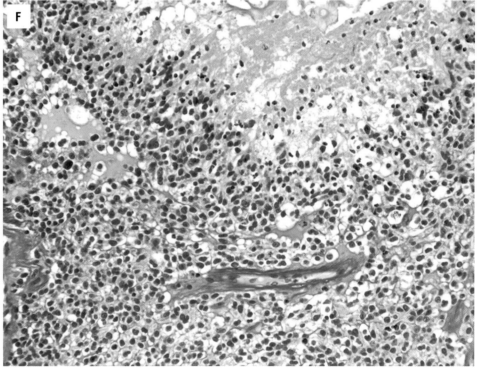

FIGURE 9-5, cont'd

E, Small cell glioblastoma with monomorphous, deceptively bland oval nuclei, chicken wire–like vessels, and a high mitotic index. This is often mistaken for an oligodendroglial component (**F**), although the latter tends to have rounder nuclei and mucin-filled microcystic spaces.

low-grade (WHO grade II) astrocytomas with low cellularity and minimal atypia, distinction from reactive gliosis may be difficult. Findings supportive of neoplasia include radiographic features of diffuse glioma, nuclear enlargement/hyperchromasia, nuclear clustering, increased MIB-1 proliferative index, and p53 immunoreactivity.

PROGNOSIS AND THERAPY

The biologic behavior of diffuse astrocytic neoplasms is highly variable, although all are considered malignant. The two most powerful prognostic variables are patient age and histologic grade. Age is inversely proportional to survival time such that younger patients live significantly longer than elderly patients with the same diagnosis. Average survival times by grade are 5 to 10 years, 2 to 3 years, and 1 year for grades II, III, and IV, respectively. Less powerful prognostic variables include Karnofsky performance status (degree of neurologic impairment) and extent of surgical resection.

PILOCYTIC ASTROCYTOMA

CLINICAL FEATURES

Overall, pilocytic astrocytomas account for only about 2% of primary CNS tumors, but in children they represent the most common glioma. They account for roughly 10% of cerebral and 85% of cerebellar astrocytomas

overall. Besides the cerebellum, they are particularly common in the optic nerves/chiasm, hypothalamus, dorsal aspect of the brain stem, and spinal cord. Vague clinical terms such as cerebellar astrocytoma, optic pathway glioma, tectal glioma, and dorsal exophytic brain stem or medullary glioma generally refer to pilocytic astrocytomas, although they should be clarified whenever possible because diffuse astrocytomas may also involve these sites, albeit considerably less often. Although generally considered a pediatric tumor, they may also be seen in adults of virtually any age. Some of these tumors have probably been present in the patient in an asymptomatic form for years to decades. Most pilocytic astrocytomas are sporadic, but patients with neurofibromatosis type 1 (NF1) are known to be predisposed to this tumor type, particularly in the optic pathway and to a lesser extent the brain stem and other sites. On neuroimaging studies, the majority of these tumors appear well circumscribed, and they may be cystic with an enhancing mural nodule (Fig. 9-6). In the optic pathway, they usually appear solid and expand the optic nerves, the chiasm, or both.

PATHOLOGIC FEATURES

Pilocytic astrocytomas typically appear well demarcated grossly, although there is nearly always some microscopic evidence of infiltration, usually at the edges. Cystic degeneration is common.

Microscopically, the classic pilocytic astrocytoma has a biphasic appearance with alternating dense and

---

PILOCYTIC ASTROCYTOMA—FACT SHEET

Definition
► Benign astrocytic neoplasm with piloid (hair-like) processes and a relatively circumscribed growth pattern

Incidence and Location
► Accounts for approximately 2% of primary intracranial neoplasms
► Annual incidence rate of roughly 0.3 per 100,000 person-years
► Most arise in the cerebellum, optic pathway ("optic gliomas"), hypothalamus/third ventricle, dorsal brain stem ("tectal glioma," "dorsal medullary glioma"), and spinal cord, but may be seen in the cerebral hemisphere as well

Gender and Age Distribution
► No major association with gender
► Can occur at any age, although encountered predominantly in children
► Median age of 13 years at diagnosis

Clinical Features
► Manifestations dependent on location of tumor
► Typically slow or insidious onset of symptoms
► Increased incidence in NF1 patients with neurofibromatosis type 1 (NF1), particularly in the optic pathway and brain stem

Radiologic Features (see Fig. 9-6)
► Cyst with an enhancing mural nodule is most common
► Well-demarcated (i.e., noninfiltrative) appearance
► Diffuse or fusiform enlargement of the optic nerve(s), optic chiasm, or both in the "optic gliomas"

Prognosis and Treatment
► Excellent prognosis, with a roughly 80% 20-year survival rate
► Most are surgically curable
► Radiation therapy may be used for subtotally resected or recurrent cases
► No consistently efficacious chemotherapy at this time

PILOCYTIC ASTROCYTOMA—PATHOLOGIC FEATURES

Gross Findings
► Cystic and well demarcated
► May appear spongy because of microcysts or hypervascularity (or both)

Microscopic Features (see Fig. 9-7)
► Biphasic dense and loose appearance, although only one component may be present in some
► Relatively sharply circumscribed, although some degree of infiltration nearly always seen microscopically
► Piloid astrocytic cells with long thin hair-like processes
► Round to oval nuclei with bland chromatin
► Oligodendroglioma-like cells may be seen or even predominate in rare cases
► Rosenthal fibers and PAS-positive eosinophilic granular bodies are characteristic
► Glomeruloid and hyalinized vessels common
► Mitotic figures uncommon
► Infarct-like necrosis seen in 5% to 10% of cases

Ultrastructural Features
► Electron-dense cells with prominent cytoplasmic intermediate filaments corresponding to GFAP

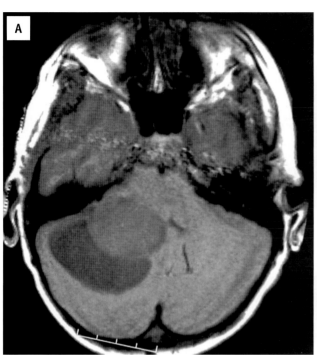

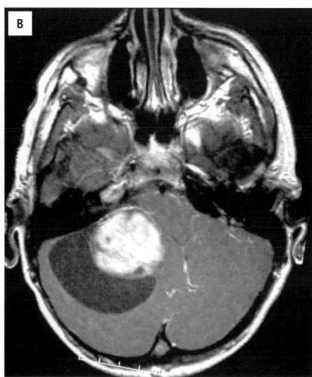

FIGURE 9-6
Pilocytic astrocytoma of the cerebellum. T1-weighted MRI without (**A**) and with (**B**) contrast shows a cyst with an enhancing mural nodule.

Immunohistochemical Features

▶ GFAP—usually strongly and nearly diffusely positive

▶ S-100 protein—positive

▶ Neurofilament-positive axons may be seen at the periphery, but solid axon-lacking components are also present

Genetics

▶ Reduced expression of neurofibromin (protein product of the *NF1* gene) is seen in NF1-associated but not sporadic pilocytic astrocytomas

▶ Gain of chromosomes 6 to 10 is common, but otherwise there are no signature alterations

Differential Diagnosis

▶ Diffuse astrocytoma (see Fig. 9-3)

▶ Oligodendroglioma/mixed oligoastrocytoma (see Figs. 9-17 to 9-20)

▶ Pleomorphic xanthoastrocytoma (see Fig. 9-11)

▶ Ganglioglioma (see Fig. 9-26)

▶ Monomorphous pilomyxoid astrocytoma

▶ Dysembryoplastic neuroepithelial tumor (see Fig. 9-27)

▶ Reactive pilocytic gliosis

loose/microcystic components (Fig. 9-7). In some cases, only one of the two patterns is encountered. The dense regions often resemble fibrillary astrocytoma, except that the cytoplasmic processes are particularly long and hair-like (i.e., "piloid" as indicated by the tumor's name). The latter is best appreciated on cytologic specimens such as

intraoperative smears. They also differ from fibrillary astrocytoma by a typically more solid growth pattern (e.g., lack of neurofilament-positive entrapped axons) and, in most cases, the presence of corkscrew-shaped brightly eosinophilic Rosenthal fibers (see Fig. 9-7B and C). The loose component sometimes looks remarkably similar to oligodendroglioma, although the long thin cellular processes are often highlighted with a GFAP immunostain. Additionally, this component frequently harbors mulberry-shaped eosinophilic granular bodies (EGBs), which may be numerous or rare (see Fig. 9-7D). In the latter scenario, staining with periodic acid–Schiff (PAS) and diastase may help draw attention to these structures. The nuclei of pilocytic astrocytomas are typically oval with bland chromatin, but significant atypia (perhaps degenerative in nature) may occasionally be seen and is generally unassociated with increased mitotic/proliferative activity. Multinucleated forms may also be visualized. Glomeruloid vessels with multiple lumina are also typical and should not be mistaken for the multilayered endothelial hyperplasia of diffuse gliomas. Nevertheless, the latter may be encountered in pilocytic astrocytomas as well and does not have the ominous significance that it does in diffuse gliomas. Bland infarct-like necrosis is encountered in roughly 5% of pilocytic astrocytomas and, similarly, has no clinical significance. Likewise, extension into the subarachnoid space is quite common and does not alter the prognosis. In contrast, pseudopalisading necrosis and foci of hyper-cellularity with increased proliferative activity should prompt consideration of an alternative diagnosis or

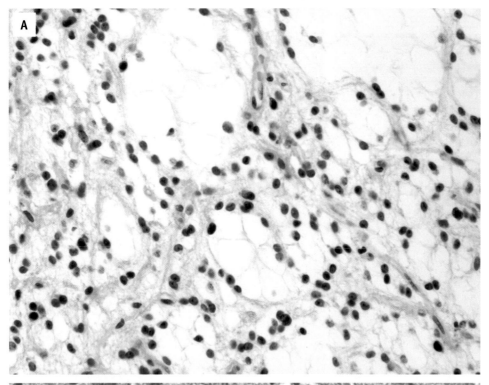

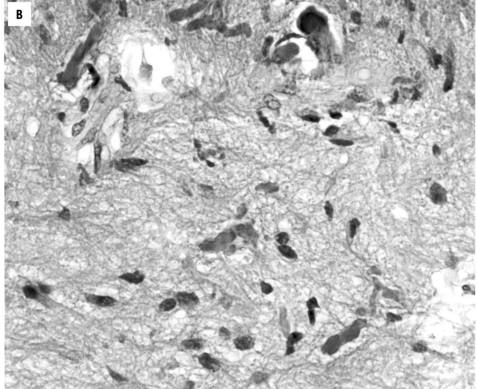

FIGURE 9-7

Pilocytic astrocytomas with spindled astrocytes containing long thin processes, loose microcystic foci (**A**), dense foci with Rosenthal fibers (**B** and **C**),

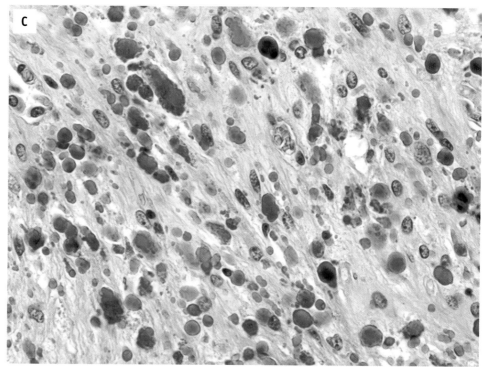

FIGURE 9-7, cont'd
and abundant eosinophilic granular bodies (**D**).

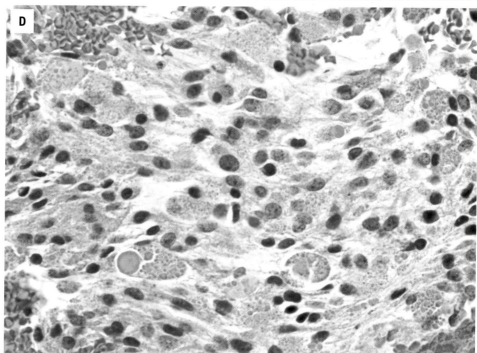

malignant transformation, an exceptionally rare complication in pilocytic astrocytomas with most examples being encountered after radiation therapy.

DIFFERENTIAL DIAGNOSIS

The most common differential diagnosis is that of a diffuse astrocytoma or oligodendroglioma. However, the unique clinical, radiographic, and microscopic features help distinguish these tumor types. Given the rare finding of endothelial hyperplasia and necrosis, one may even find oneself in the unsettling differential diagnosis of glioblastoma multiforme. A predominantly solid growth pattern with a neurofilament stain, low MIB-1 labeling index, and lack of p53 protein positivity help rule out this possibility. Although neither Rosenthal fibers nor EGBs are entirely specific for pilocytic astrocytoma, they generally suggest a benign or slowly evolving process such as pilocytic astrocytoma, pleomorphic xanthoastrocytoma, and ganglioglioma, all representing more favorable tumor types, often with similar radiographic features. However, pleomorphic xanthoastrocytoma has greater pleomorphism, mesenchymal-like spindled elements, vacuolated cells, and reticulin-rich foci not seen in pilocytic astrocytomas, whereas gangliogliomas have a neuronal component characterized by dysmorphic ganglion cells. A rare entity known as monomorphous pilomyxoid astrocytoma was recently described and has many overlapping features. However, this tumor is typically found in the hypothalamic/third ventricular region of infants, produces abundant mucin/myxoid stroma, and generally lacks Rosenthal fibers and EGBs. Dysembryoplastic neuroepithelial tumors most often resemble oligodendrogliomas, but they may have areas resembling pilocytic astrocytoma as well. A temporal lobe predilection, patterned mucinous nodules, and floating neurons serve to distinguish this entity. Finally, Rosenthal fibers are also often encountered in a piloid form of reactive gliosis, most often next to craniopharyngiomas, ependymomas, hemangioblastomas, developmental cysts, and syringomyelia. Pilocytic gliosis is typically less cellular and does not have a microcystic component. Additional sampling and attention to the clinical/radiographic features generally allows one to avoid this pitfall.

PROGNOSIS AND THERAPY

Pilocytic astrocytomas are benign (WHO grade I) neoplasms treated primarily with surgery. However, they occasionally produce significant morbidity and mortality, depending on the tumor's location. Therefore, subtotally resected cases may undergo radiotherapy for enhanced local control. Rare examples, particularly those arising from the hypothalamic region, may disseminate through the cerebrospinal fluid (CSF). Some of these patients may have stable or slowly progressive disease despite metastatic meningeal deposits, presumably because of their slow growth.

SUBEPENDYMAL GIANT CELL ASTROCYTOMA

CLINICAL FEATURES

Subependymal giant cell astrocytoma (SEGA) is a benign intraventricular tumor encountered nearly exclusively in the setting of tuberous sclerosis. It is typically located in the lateral or third ventricle (or both ventricles) near the foramen of Monro and comes to clinical attention because of obstructive hydrocephalus. Radiographically, it appears solid, enhancing, well demarcated, and often calcified (Fig. 9-8). Since it may be the first detected manifestation of this familial

---

SUBEPENDYMAL GIANT CELL ASTROCYTOMA—FACT SHEET

Definition

▶ Benign or hamartomatous astrocytic and partially neuronal intraventricular tumor

Incidence and Location

▶ Accounts for <1% of primary intracranial neoplasms
▶ Involves the lateral or third ventricle (or both ventricles) near the region of the foramen of Monro

Gender and Age Distribution

▶ No major association with gender
▶ Mostly children and young adults

Clinical Features

▶ Signs and symptoms of obstructive hydrocephalus with increased intracranial pressure
▶ Almost exclusively seen in the setting of tuberous sclerosis, although this may be the initial manifestation
▶ Some believe that "sporadic" cases represent a forme fruste of tuberous sclerosis

Radiologic Features (see Fig. 9-8)

▶ Enhancing intraventricular mass
▶ Well demarcated (i.e., noninfiltrative)
▶ Often calcified
▶ Other features of tuberous sclerosis may be present (e.g., tubers, candle gutterings, gray matter heterotopia)

Prognosis and Treatment

▶ Excellent prognosis
▶ Most are surgically curable

---

disorder, other characteristic features should be sought, including cortical tubers, candle gutterings (smaller masses along the ventricular lining resembling wax drippings), and gray matter heterotopia. Extracranial manifestations include facial cutaneous angiofibromas, renal angiomyolipoma, pulmonary lymphangioleiomyomatosis, subungual fibroma, cardiac rhabdomyoma, intestinal polyps, and visceral cysts. Many believe that cases of SEGA without these other manifestations represent a forme fruste of tuberous sclerosis.

PATHOLOGIC AND GROSS FINDINGS

Grossly, SEGA is a solid, well-demarcated mass, often with zones of dense calcification. Candle gutterings are smaller versions that are more widely distributed along the ventricular surface. They are otherwise identical microscopically.

Histologically, SEGA is a noninfiltrative mass composed of spindled and epithelioid cells arranged in sweeping fascicles or even perivascular pseudorosettes, such as those encountered in ependymomas (Fig. 9-9A).

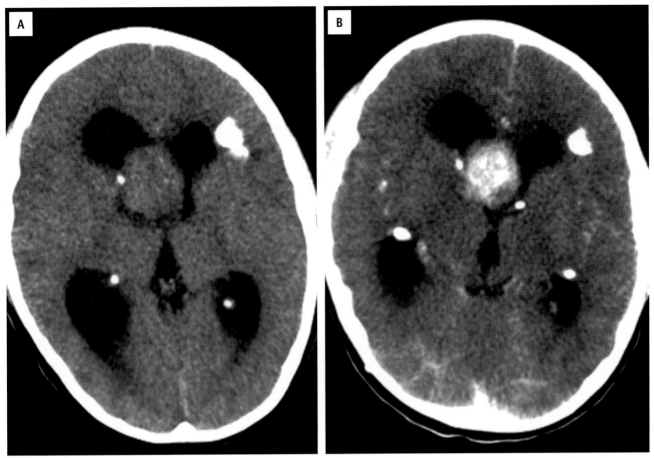

FIGURE 9-8

Computed tomography scans without (**A**) and with (**B**) contrast from a patient with a subependymal giant cell astrocytoma showing an enhancing intraventricular mass near the foramen of Monro with obstructive hydrocephalus. Also note the calcified tuber in the left frontal lobe of this patient with tuberous sclerosis. (Courtesy of Dr. Robert McKinstry, Washington University, St. Louis.)

SUBEPENDYMAL GIANT CELL ASTROCYTOMA— PATHOLOGIC FEATURES

Gross Findings

- ▶ Solid and well demarcated
- ▶ Often calcified
- ▶ Candle gutterings represent smaller, histologically similar lesions that grossly resemble wax drippings throughout the ventricular surface

Microscopic Features (see Fig. 9-9)

- ▶ Epithelioid, gemistocyte-like, or spindled cells (or all three) arranged in sweeping fascicles
- ▶ Dysmorphic cells with neuron-like nuclei (i.e., vesicular chromatin, prominent nucleoli) and astrocyte-like cytoplasm (i.e., eccentrically placed and eosinophilic)
- ▶ Overlying ependymal cells sometimes evident
- ▶ Perivascular pseudorosettes common
- ▶ Mitotic figures and necrosis uncommon

Ultrastructural Features

- ▶ Electron-dense cells with prominent cytoplasmic intermediate filaments corresponding to GFAP

- ▶ Rare neuronal features such as dense core granules

Immunohistochemical Features

- ▶ GFAP—usually positive in a subset of cells, but may be surprisingly weak
- ▶ S-100 protein—positive
- ▶ Neuronal markers may be positive in a subset of cells (e.g., synaptophysin, neurofilament, NeuN, chromogranin)

Genetics

- ▶ No consistent alterations known

Differential Diagnosis

- ▶ Gemistocytic astrocytoma (see Fig. 9-3C)
- ▶ Ependymoma (see Fig. 9-21)
- ▶ Intraventricular meningioma (clinically)
- ▶ Central neurocytoma (clinically)
- ▶ Subependymoma (clinically)

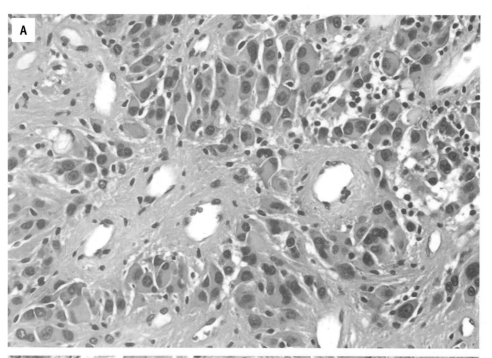

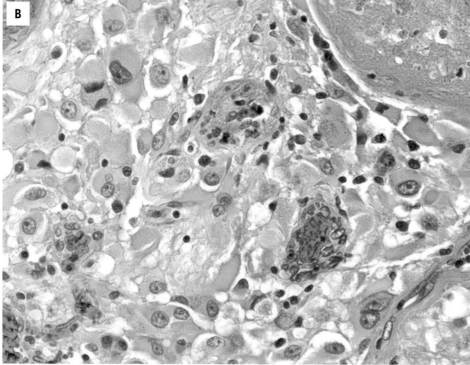

FIGURE 9-9

Examples of subependymal giant cell astrocytoma highlighting perivascular pseudorosettes (**A**) and typical cytologic features (**B**), including neuronal-like nuclei and astrocyte-like cytoplasm.

The cells often have a mixed glioneuronal appearance with brightly eosinophilic cytoplasm resembling that of astrocytes and large vesicular nuclei and prominent nucleoli similar to those of ganglion cells (see Fig. 9-9B). Mitoses and necrosis are uncommon and do not have a negative impact on prognosis. Immunostains reveal GFAP positivity in a subset of tumor cells. Neuronal marker immunoreactivity may also be seen in some cells, sometimes in the same cells that are GFAP positive. Other cells are negative for both. Because of the mixed glioneuronal features, some prefer the term "subependymal giant cell tumor" rather than SEGA.

DIFFERENTIAL DIAGNOSIS

SEGA resembles gemistocytic astrocytoma, but it does not grow in an infiltrative pattern, it expresses GFAP less intensely, and it is found within the ventricle rather than the parenchyma. The perivascular pseudorosettes raise the possibility of ependymoma, although in ependymoma they are typically intraparenchymal rather than intraventricular when they are supratentorial. Furthermore, the ganglion-like and gemistocyte-like cytology is not typical of ependymoma. Clinically, other intraventricular tumors in the differential diagnosis include intraventricular meningioma, central neurocytoma, and subependymoma, although these tumors' histologic characteristics are quite different.

PROGNOSIS AND THERAPY

SEGAs are benign tumors (WHO grade I) and probably represent hamartomatous rather than neoplastic proliferations. Rare examples recur but do not undergo malignant progression. Despite its benign nature, SEGA has significant prognostic implications for patients and their families because of this tumor's nearly universal association with tuberous sclerosis.

PLEOMORPHIC XANTHOASTROCYTOMA

CLINICAL FEATURES

Pleomorphic xanthoastrocytoma (PXA) is a specialized variant of astrocytoma with a predilection for the superficial cortex, particularly in the temporal lobe. Patients are typically young and often have a chronic seizure disorder. Radiographically, some appear as cysts with an enhancing mural nodule (Fig. 9-10), but they may also be solid or attached to the dura and mimic a meningioma.

PATHOLOGIC FEATURES

Grossly, PXAs appear well demarcated and firm. Cystic components and calcifications are seen in some.

Histologically, they are characterized by foci of pleomorphic astrocytes and spindled mesenchymal-like cells arranged in fascicles or a storiform pattern (Fig. 9-11). Multinucleated cells are common. Lipidized astrocytes ("xanthoastrocytes") are seen in roughly a fourth of cases (see Fig. 9-11A). Despite the pleomorphism, the mitotic/proliferative index is low in most cases (see Fig. 9-11B). EGBs are typical (see Fig. 9-11C), and Rosenthal fibers may also be seen, particularly at the edges of the tumor. Unlike diffuse astrocytomas, there is increased intercellular reticulin deposition, either diffusely or in a patchy fashion (see Fig. 9-11D). The latter corresponds to basal lamina ultrastructurally, which is why PXA has been speculated to arise from a specialized subpial astrocyte with basal lamina production. Occasional cases are mixed with classic ganglioglioma, intratumoral ganglion

cells, or lesser forms of neuronal differentiation such as synaptophysin or neurofilament positivity in otherwise astrocytic-looking cells. Subsets of tumor cells are GFAP positive, but the fraction is highly variable. The definition of anaplasia is controversial, although ironically, there is less pleomorphism with an overall resemblance to high-grade diffuse astrocytomas, including frequent mitoses, endothelial hyperplasia, pseudopalisading necrosis, or any combination of these findings.

DIFFERENTIAL DIAGNOSIS

Because of the prominent nuclear pleomorphism and mesenchymal-like foci, the most common differential diagnoses are glioblastoma multiforme, gliosarcoma, and pleomorphic sarcoma. However, EGBs are not found in any of these entities, and foci of reticulin deposition help exclude glioblastoma. PXA has significant overlap with ganglioglioma, and both entities may combine to form a composite neoplasm. In general, however, ganglioglioma has less pleomorphism, a more obvious neuronal component, and no lipidized astrocytes. Similarly, pilocytic astrocytomas may have bizarre, atypical/pleomorphic nuclei, but intercellular deposition of reticulin does not occur.

PLEOMORPHIC XANTHOASTROCYTOMA—PATHOLOGIC FEATURES

Gross Findings

▶ Solid and rubbery; may have a cystic component
▶ Seemingly demarcated
▶ Often calcified

Microscopic Features (see Fig. 9-11)

▶ Pleomorphic with mixed glial and mesenchymal-like features
▶ Spindled and atypical gemistocyte-like or epithelioid cells
▶ PAS-positive eosinophilic granular bodies in the vast majority
▶ Increased intercellular reticulin deposition, either focally or diffusely
▶ Rosenthal fibers may be seen, particularly at the periphery of the tumor
▶ Xanthomatous (clear and foamy) astrocytes in roughly a fourth of cases
▶ Mitotic figures and necrosis are uncommon, except in cases with malignant progression (grade III)
▶ Foci of anaplastic (grade III) PXA show less pleomorphism and resemble anaplastic fibrillary astrocytoma or glioblastoma
▶ PXA may be mixed with ganglioglioma in rare cases

Ultrastructural Features

▶ Electron-dense cells with prominent cytoplasmic intermediate filaments corresponding to GFAP

▶ Pericellular basal lamina
▶ Rare neuronal features such as dense core granules

Immunohistochemical Features

▶ GFAP—usually positive in a subset of cells
▶ S-100 protein—positive
▶ Neuronal markers may be positive in a subset of cells, sometimes despite a lack of neuron-like morphology (e.g., synaptophysin, neurofilament, NeuN, chromogranin)
▶ The MIB-1 (Ki-67) labeling index is typically low, except in anaplastic examples

Genetics

▶ No consistent alterations known, although alterations in fibrillary astrocytoma are uncommon in PXA

Differential Diagnosis

▶ Glioblastoma/gliosarcoma (see Figs. 9-3E and F and 9-5D)
▶ Malignant fibrous histiocytoma/pleomorphic sarcoma
▶ Ganglioglioma (see Fig. 9-26)
▶ Pilocytic astrocytoma with increased atypia (see Fig. 9-7)
▶ Meningioma (clinically)

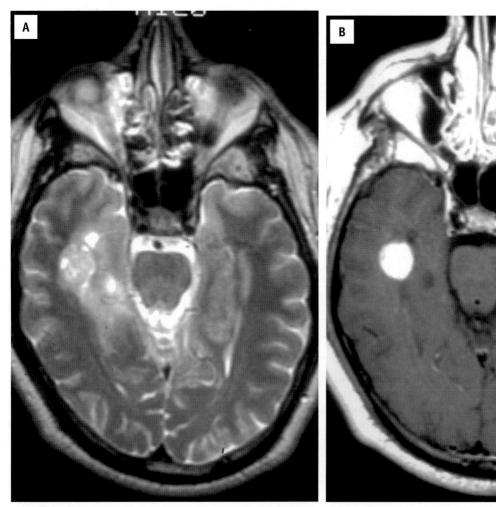

FIGURE 9-10

MRI in a patient with pleomorphic xanthoastrocytoma. T2-weighted (**A**) and T1-weighted images with contrast (**B**) show a well-demarcated, partially cystic, enhancing right temporal lobe mass.

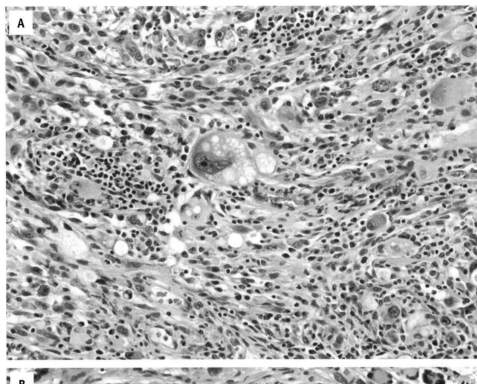

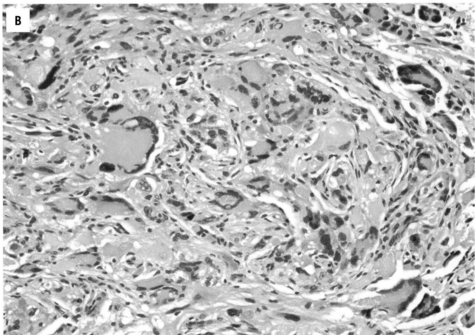

FIGURE 9-11

Examples of pleomorphic xanthoastrocytoma with spindled cells and lipidized astrocytes (**A**), pleomorphism with multinucleated giant cells (**B**),   *Continued*

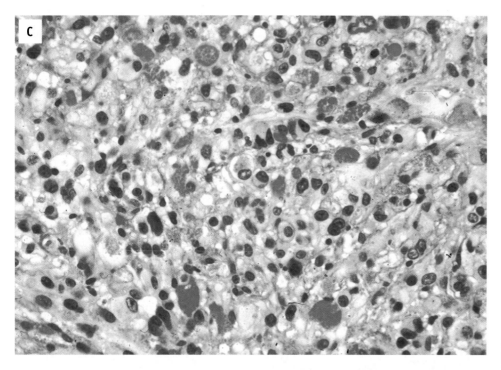

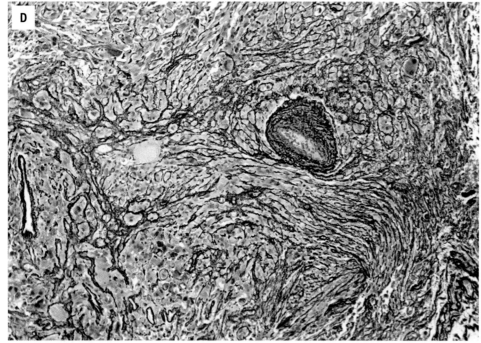

FIGURE 9-11, cont'd

PAS-positive eosinophilic granular bodies (**C**), and a dense intercellular reticulin network (**D**).

PROGNOSIS AND THERAPY

PXA generally has a favorable prognosis, with many cases curable by surgery alone. Nevertheless, it is recognized that 15% to 20% undergo malignant progression, which along with a somewhat less predictable behavior than that of pilocytic astrocytoma and ganglioglioma, accounts for the WHO grade II designation assigned to these tumors. Those with histologic foci of anaplasia are considered grade III. Some of these tumors are associated with aggressive behavior and shortened survival, although others still do better than diffuse astrocytomas of similar grade.

ASTROBLASTOMA

CLINICAL FEATURES

Astroblastoma is a rare, usually cerebral glioma of unknown histogenesis. Most occur in children and young adults. Radiologically, they are well-demarcated, enhancing masses that may be cystic or necrotic.

PATHOLOGIC FEATURES

Grossly, astroblastomas appear well demarcated and may be cystic.

Histologically, they have mixed astrocytoma-like and ependymoma-like features (Fig. 9-12). Like ependymomas, they grow in a relatively circumscribed fashion and have perivascular pseudorosettes. However, the cells are more epithelioid or cuboidal with broader perivascular processes (see Fig. 9-12B-D). Characteristically, abundant vascular hyalinization is evident (see Fig. 9-12A). Papillary foci are common, and the tumor cells are usually strongly GFAP positive (see Fig. 9-12C and D).

DIFFERENTIAL DIAGNOSIS

The main differential diagnosis is ependymoma, and distinction between the two is made primarily by the presence of broader processes associated with the perivascular pseudorosettes. Diffuse astrocytomas may also look similar, but they are more infiltrative. Those with a prominent papillary growth pattern may resemble another rare entity known as papillary glioneuronal tumor, but the latter has a discernible neuronal element. Because of the sharp circumscription, metastatic disease may also be considered, but metastases are not GFAP positive.

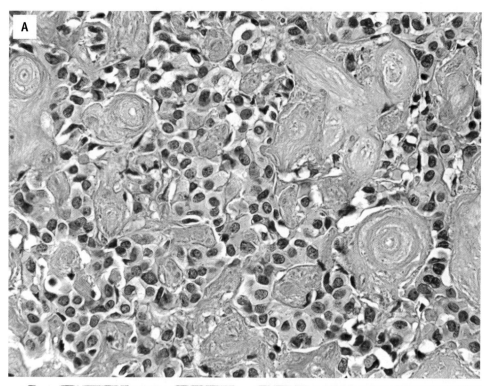

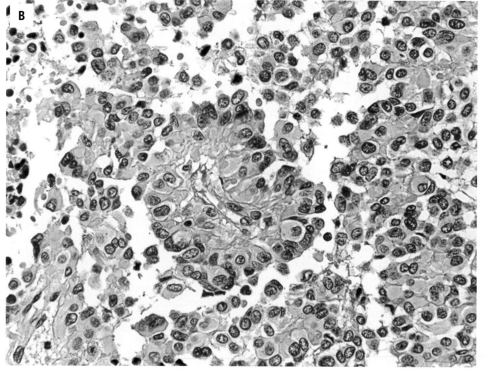

FIGURE 9-12

Astroblastoma. **A**, Epithelioid cytology and extensive perivascular and stromal hyalinization. **B**, Perivascular pseudorosette with broad tumoral cell processes.

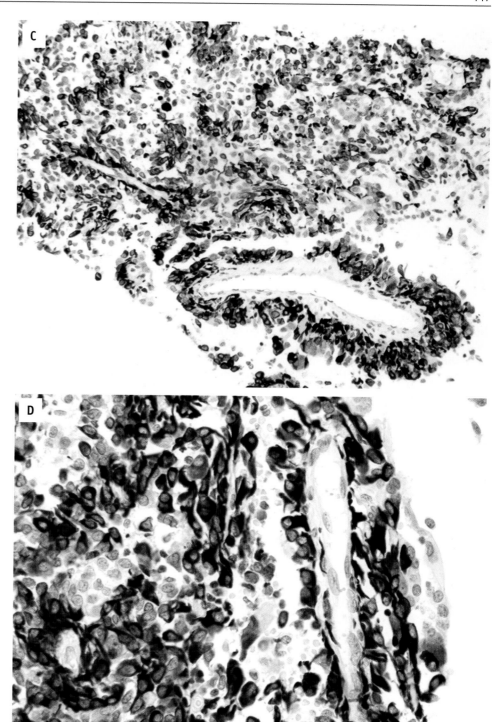

FIGURE 9-12, cont'd
C and **D**, Strong GFAP expression with broad tumoral processes surrounding vessels.

PROGNOSIS AND THERAPY

Because of the rarity of this tumor type, little clinical experience has accrued. Currently, they are divided into low-grade and anaplastic types, the latter more likely to recur or lead to patient death.

DESMOPLASTIC INFANTILE ASTROCYTOMA/GANGLIOGLIOMA

CLINICAL FEATURES

Desmoplastic infantile ganglioglioma (DIG) and its related ganglion cell–deficient entity desmoplastic infantile astrocytoma (DIA) are benign CNS tumors that develop virtually exclusively in infants younger than 2 years, often as a remarkably large solid and cystic hemispheric mass that may replace much of the brain on one side (Fig. 9-13). Increased head circumference

and bulging fontanelles are the most common initial clinical signs, although seizures, hyperreflexia, and cranial nerve palsies may also be encountered. Because of this dramatic manifestation, a malignancy is often expected.

PATHOLOGIC FEATURES

Grossly, both DIG and DIA appear largely cystic, with a firm to rubbery superficial cortical/meningeal solid component. The latter may also be attached to the dura.

Histologically, the first impression is often that of a mesenchymal neoplasm such as a fibroma or malignant fibrous histiocytoma because of the dense collagen deposition and prominent spindled elements arranged

---

DESMOPLASTIC INFANTILE ASTROCYTOMA/ GANGLIOGLIOMA—FACT SHEET

Definition
▶ Rare form of glial (DIA) or glioneuronal (DIG) neoplasm of infancy with prominent desmoplasia, a large cystic component, and a favorable prognosis despite often alarming clinical and pathologic features

Incidence and Location
▶ Account for <1% of primary intracranial neoplasms
▶ Most involve the superficial cerebral hemispheres, meninges, and dura

Gender and Age Distribution
▶ M/F ratio of 1.7:1
▶ Infants younger than 2 years

Clinical Features
▶ Increased head circumference with bulging fontanelles
▶ Seizures, hyperreflexia, or cranial nerve palsies in some (or any combination of these features)

Radiologic Features (see Fig. 9-13)
▶ Large to massive cystic hemispheric mass
▶ Enhancing solid component, superficial and often attached to the dura

Prognosis and Treatment
▶ Excellent prognosis in most cases
▶ WHO grade I
▶ Gross total resection associated with long-term survival

DESMOPLASTIC INFANTILE ASTROCYTOMA/GANGLIOGLIOMA— PATHOLOGIC FEATURES

Gross Findings
▶ Large cystic component
▶ The superficial solid component is firm to rubbery, tan-white, often attached to the dura, and may merge imperceptibly with adjacent cortex

Microscopic Features (see Fig. 9-14)
▶ Spindled cells arranged in a storiform or fascicular architecture
▶ Small inconspicuous gemistocyte-like cells
▶ Small to large neuronal cells in DIG, often a minor subset
▶ Desmoplastic stroma highlighted with reticulin and trichrome stains
▶ PNET-like foci common, but do not alter the grade or prognosis

Ultrastructural Features
▶ Electron-dense astrocytic cells with surrounding basal lamina
▶ Fibroblasts with abundant rough endoplasmic reticulum and well-developed Golgi bodies
▶ Neuronal cells with dense core granules in DIG

Immunohistochemical Features
▶ GFAP-positive astrocytes
▶ Neuronal markers (e.g., synaptophysin, neurofilament, NeuN, chromogranin) positive in DIG
▶ MIB-1 (Ki-67) may be high in PNET-like foci

Genetics
▶ No consistent alterations known

Differential Diagnosis
▶ Fibrous histiocytoma
▶ Fibrosarcoma/malignant fibrous histiocytoma
▶ Fibrous meningioma
▶ Supratentorial PNET
▶ Malignant glioma

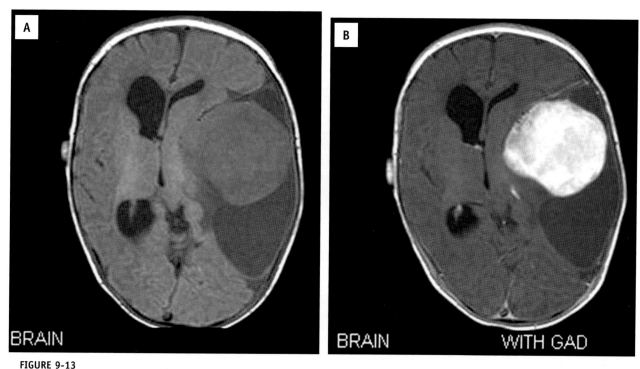

FIGURE 9-13

T1-weighted MRI without (**A**) and with (**B**) contrast in a patient with desmoplastic infantile ganglioglioma. A massive, superficial cystic mass with an enhancing nodule is apparent. (Courtesy of Dr. Beth Levy, St. Louis University.)

in fascicular and storiform patterns (Fig. 9-14A). Meningeal and dural involvement is also common, thus further contributing to the perception of a mesenchymal derivation. The glial elements are often inconspicuous and range from small gemistocyte-like to spindled cells (see Fig. 9-14B). Neuronal components are also present in DIG and typically take the form of small ganglion-like cells. These cells are similarly enmeshed in a spindled, reticulin-rich desmoplastic background (see Fig. 9-14C) and are subtle on hematoxylin-eosin stain. Primitive neuroectodermal tumor (PNET)-like foci are common and consist of hypercellular foci with small round cells, increased mitotic activity, or necrosis (or any combination of these characteristics). Occasionally, foci of conventional-appearing ganglioglioma may also be seen, particularly at the edge of the tumor. Immunostains are useful for highlighting both GFAP-positive astrocytes (see Fig. 9-14D) and synaptophysin-positive neurons (see Fig. 9-14E). The MIB-1 labeling index is typically low, except in PNET-like foci, where it may be markedly elevated.

DIFFERENTIAL DIAGNOSIS

Because of the desmoplasia, spindled morphology, and frequent dural attachment, the differential diagnosis includes benign and malignant mesenchymal tumors, as well as fibrous meningioma. Careful inspection and immunohistochemistry reveal the glial and, in the case of DIG, the neuronal elements. The presence of small

blue cells with increased proliferative activity raises the differential diagnosis of PNET, although the more differentiated histologic elements and characteristic desmoplasia are also present. Malignant gliomas similarly lack this desmoplasia, a neuronal component, and the characteristic clinicoradiologic features.

PROGNOSIS AND THERAPY

DIG and DIA are considered benign (WHO grade I) neoplasms, and the majority of patients enjoy an excellent prognosis despite the alarming clinical features, large tumor size, and PNET-like foci. In cases in which gross total resection is possible, the risk of recurrence is substantially reduced.

CHORDOID GLIOMA

CLINICAL FEATURES

Chordoid glioma is a rare, low-grade intraventricular glioma that typically involves the anterior portion of the third ventricle. Patients are usually adults, with women outnumbering men three to one. Because of their location, the initial signs and symptoms are most often those

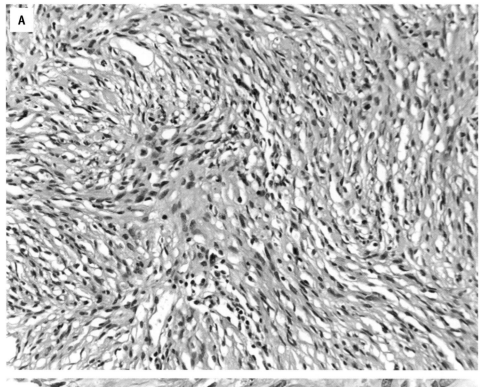

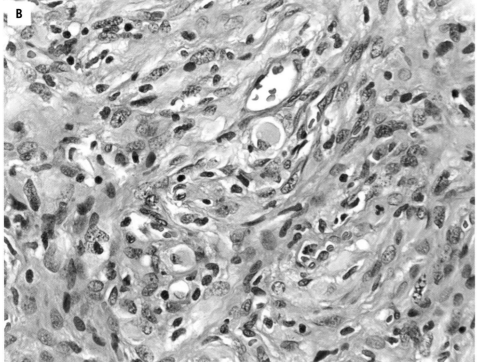

FIGURE 9-14

Desmoplastic infantile ganglioglioma with spindled cells arranged in a storiform pattern (**A**), small gemistocyte-like cells (**B**),

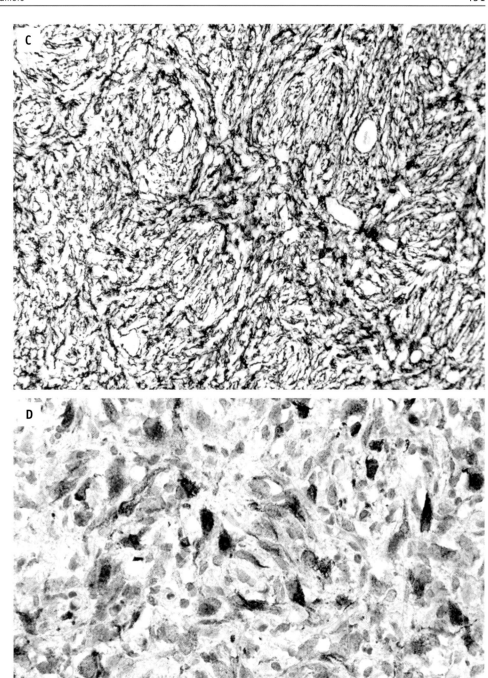

FIGURE 9-14, cont'd
a dense reticulin network (**C**), patchy
GFAP immunoreactivity (**D**),
Continued

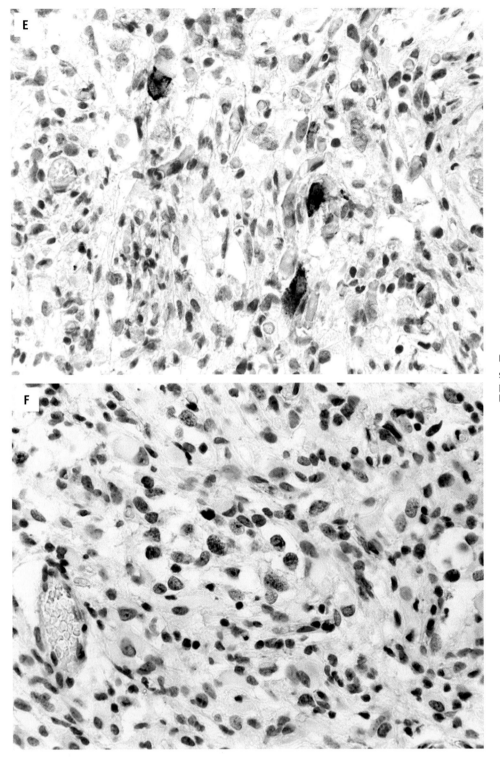

FIGURE 9-14, cont'd
scattered small synaptophysin-positive ganglion cells (**E**), and rare NeuN-positive cells (**F**).

of obstructive hydrocephalus. However, hypothyroidism and visual field losses have also been described and are presumably caused by compression of the hypothalamus and optic chiasm, respectively. Some have also suffered psychiatric symptoms, possibly from compression of medial temporal lobe structures. Radiographically, they appear as solid, well-demarcated masses of the third ventricular region.

PATHOLOGIC FEATURES

Grossly, chordoid gliomas are soft and mucoid.

Histologically, they resemble chordoma of the bone, with epithelioid cells arranged in ribbons/trabeculae and a mucin-rich stroma (Fig. 9-15). Stromal vacuolation further masquerades as physaliferous cells. A

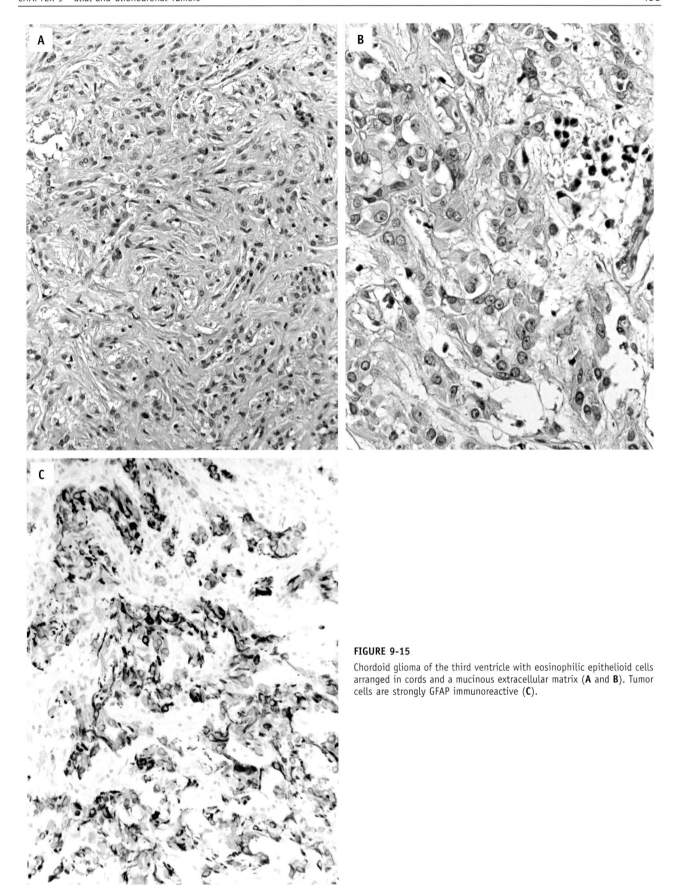

FIGURE 9-15

Chordoid glioma of the third ventricle with eosinophilic epithelioid cells arranged in cords and a mucinous extracellular matrix (**A** and **B**). Tumor cells are strongly GFAP immunoreactive (**C**).

CHORDOID GLIOMA—FACT SHEET

Definition
▶ Rare glioma of the third ventricle with chordoma-like histology

Incidence and Location
▶ Accounts for <1% of primary intracranial neoplasms
▶ Exclusively found in the anterior portion of the third ventricle

Gender and Age Distribution
▶ Female preponderance; F/M ratio of 3:1
▶ Adult patients, typically older than 30 years
▶ Mean age of 46 years at diagnosis

Clinical Features
▶ Most have signs and symptoms of obstructive hydrocephalus (e.g., headache, ataxia, nausea/vomiting, papilledema)
▶ Hypothyroidism and visual field losses from compression of the hypothalamus and optic chiasm
▶ Psychiatric disturbances in some, presumably from compression of the temporal lobes

Radiologic Features
▶ Enhancing, usually solid-appearing mass in the anterior portion of the third ventricle
▶ Attachment to the hypothalamus/suprasellar structures in some

Prognosis and Treatment
▶ Slow growth, but complete resection often precluded by location
▶ WHO grade II
▶ Role of adjuvant therapy unclear because of insufficient experience

---

CHORDOID GLIOMA—PATHOLOGIC FEATURES

Gross Findings
▶ Solid, mucin-rich mass

Microscopic Features (see Fig. 9-15)
▶ Clusters and cords of epithelioid cells embedded in a mucin-rich stroma
▶ Vacuolation in stroma imparts a resemblance to physaliferous cells
▶ Lymphoplasmacytic infiltrate with Russell bodies
▶ Occasional cells with overt glial features, including fibrillary processes
▶ Mitoses, endothelial hyperplasia, and necrosis are rare

Ultrastructural Features
▶ Electron-dense glial cells with abundant intermediate filaments
▶ Focal basal lamina formation
▶ Microvilli may be present, but more definitive ependymal features such as desmosomes and cilia are lacking

Immunohistochemical Features
▶ GFAP—positive
▶ S-100 protein—variably positive
▶ Neuronal markers negative
▶ Focal EMA positivity in some
▶ Cytokeratin negative
▶ MIB-1 (Ki-67) labeling index typically very low

Genetics
▶ No consistent alterations known

Differential Diagnosis
▶ Chordoid meningioma
▶ Pituitary adenoma
▶ Craniopharyngioma
▶ Pilocytic astrocytoma (see Fig. 9-7)
▶ Ependymoma (see Fig. 9-21)
▶ Chordoma (but excluded by location)

---

lymphoplasmacytic infiltrate with Russell bodies is also common. More typical glial-appearing cells are occasionally found, but are not prominent. Mitoses, endothelial hyperplasia, and necrosis are rare. Immunohistochemically, tumor cells are strongly GFAP positive (see Fig. 9-15C) and show a low MIB-1 labeling index. Focal EMA reactivity has been described in a few.

DIFFERENTIAL DIAGNOSIS

The resemblance to chordoma is often striking and accounts for the naming of this tumor. However, these tumors do not involve bone, and the glial rather than notochordal epithelial derivation is highlighted by GFAP. Nevertheless, the histogenesis of this recently described entity has been controversial. Its intraventricular location and the ultrastructural finding of microvilli have suggested the possibility of ependymal rather than astrocytic histogenesis. However, more compelling ependymal features are not usually found ultrastructurally. Similarly, chordoid meningioma has overlapping features and may be intraventricular, although the lack of desmosomes and extensive GFAP immunoreactivity exclude this possibility. Papillary craniopharyngioma and pituitary adenoma may occur in the same location, but they do not have the mucinous background and GFAP immunoreactivity. Recent studies have suggested potential origins from either tanycytes or secretory ependymal cells of the subcommissural organ of the anterior aspect of the third ventricle.

PROGNOSIS AND THERAPY

Chordoid gliomas are generally slow-growing, low-grade gliomas; nevertheless, a WHO grade of II has been assigned on the basis of documented recurrences, considerable morbidity, and death in some patients.

Therapy is primarily surgical, although there has been insufficient experience to date to make recommendations regarding ancillary therapy in subtotally resected cases.

"NASAL GLIOMA"

CLINICAL FEATURES

The term "nasal glioma" is a confusing misnomer because these lesions are not gliomas, but rather heterotopic glial or glioneuronal tissue encountered in the nasal region. As such, they are probably congenital or developmental abnormalities rather than true neoplasms. They typically develop in infants or young children with nasal obstruction or deformity. The most important radiologic task is to rule out a small connection with the intracranial contents such that a CSF leak is not created during surgical removal of the glioma. If a connection is found, it represents a form of frontal encephalocele rather than heterotopia. Nasal gliomas are rare and generally sporadic and not associated with other malformations or familial syndromes.

PATHOLOGIC FEATURES

These lesions are grossly solid or polypoid masses that are nonpulsatile endoscopically. They have a tan-gray appearance similar to that of normal brain.

Histologically, they are composed of mature glial or glioneuronal tissue, which may appear disorganized and intermixed with fibrovascular stroma (Fig. 9-16). Overlying respiratory mucosa is often evident. The CNS nature of this tissue may be highlighted with GFAP immunostain. There is minimal proliferation as evidenced by MIB-1 immunostain.

DIFFERENTIAL DIAGNOSIS

The primary differential diagnostic consideration is that of a frontal encephalocele. Since this entity is histologically identical, it is primarily the radiologist's job to make this distinction.

PROGNOSIS AND TREATMENT

"Nasal gliomas" are benign and generally surgically curable. Rare recurrences have been described in incompletely resected examples.

"NASAL GLIOMA"—FACT SHEET

Definition
- ► Congenital/developmental abnormality with glial or glioneuronal heterotopia in the nasal region. Given a lack of neoplastic potential, the term "glioma" is a misnomer

Incidence and Location
- ► Rare and unassociated with other anomalies or familial syndromes
- ► Intranasal, without a demonstrable connection to the intracranial cavity

Gender and Age Distribution
- ► No major sex predilection
- ► Infants or young children

Clinical Features
- ► The initial clinical manifestation is nasal obstruction or deformity

Radiologic Features
- ► Intranasal or perinasal mass
- ► Unlike a frontal encephalocele, there is no demonstrable connection to intracranial structures

Prognosis and Treatment
- ► Benign and surgically curable
- ► May rarely recur if incompletely resected

"NASAL GLIOMA"—PATHOLOGIC FEATURES

Gross Findings
- ► Firm, nonpulsatile (in vivo) polypoid mass
- ► Tan-gray mass resembling brain tissue

Microscopic Features (see Fig. 9-16)
- ► Nests of mature glial or glioneuronal tissue intermixed with fibrovascular stroma
- ► Overlying respiratory epithelium

Ultrastructural Features
- ► Mature neuroglial elements

Immunohistochemical Features
- ► GFAP—positive
- ► MIB-1 (Ki-67) labeling index very low

Genetics
- ► No alterations known

Differential Diagnosis
- ► Frontal encephalocele

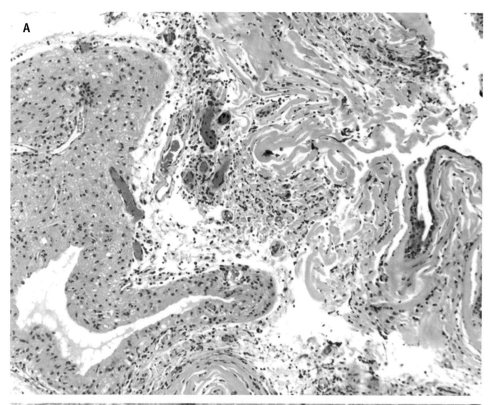

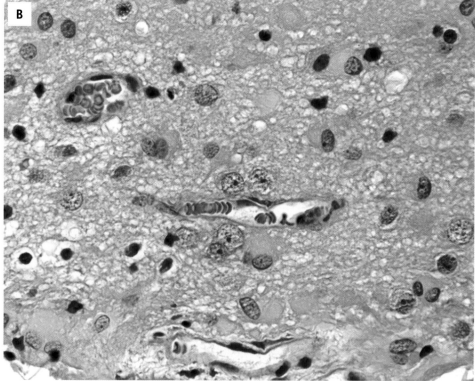

FIGURE 9-16

"Nasal glioma" showing nests of mature CNS tissue (*left* side of **A**) adjacent to respiratory mucosa (*right* side of **A**). At higher magnification, astrocytes and clusters of ganglion cells are evident (**B**).

OLIGODENDROGLIOMA

CLINICAL FEATURES

Oligodendroglioma represents the second major category of diffuse glioma. In contrast to astrocytomas, most of which are high grade at the time of diagnosis, more than half of oligodendrogliomas become clinically apparent at the grade II stage and typically affect young to middle-aged adults. They are distinctly uncommon in children. Most are hemispheric masses, mainly in the frontal lobe, followed in frequency by the parietal and temporal lobes. Brain stem, cerebellum, and spinal cord examples are distinctly unusual. Because of a notable corticotropism, seizure disorder is a particularly common manifestation. Radiologically, the low-grade (WHO II) cases are typically nonenhancing intra-axial masses, often with foci of calcification best appreciated on computed tomography (CT). Anaplastic (WHO grade III) oligodendrogliomas are nearly always enhancing, most commonly in either an irregular or diffuse fashion.

OLIGODENDROGLIOMA—FACT SHEET

Definition

▶ Diffusely infiltrative glioma displaying predominantly oligodendroglial features

Incidence and Location

▶ Accounts for 10% to 25% of diffuse gliomas
▶ Annual incidence rate of roughly 0.6 per 100,000 person-years
▶ Most arise in the cerebral hemispheres with prominent corticotropism
▶ More than half occur in the frontal lobes
▶ Extremely rare in the brain stem, cerebellum, and spinal cord

Gender and Age Distribution

▶ Slight male preponderance (M/F ratio of 3:2)
▶ Can occur at any age, although peak at 40 to 45 years
▶ Rare in children

Clinical Features

▶ Manifestations dependent on location of tumor
▶ Focal neural deficits, increased intracranial pressure, and seizures are the most common symptoms
▶ Generalized neurologic signs and symptoms of increased intracranial pressure include headaches, nausea/vomiting, and papilledema
▶ Rapid onset and progression suggest anaplastic (III), whereas a protracted history (e.g., chronic seizure disorder) is more consistent with low-grade (II) tumor

Radiologic Features

▶ Oligodendrogliomas (WHO grade II) are typically nonenhancing masses with increased signal on T2-weighted and FLAIR MRI sequences
▶ Anaplastic oligodendrogliomas (WHO grade III) are typically enhancing
▶ Intratumoral calcifications are common

Prognosis and Treatment

▶ Patient age: powerful predictor, with survival inversely proportional to patient age
▶ Grade: survival averages 10 to 15 years for grade II and 3 to 5 years for grade III
▶ Histologic cell type: oligodendrogliomas have a better prognosis than astrocytomas do
▶ Preoperative performance status: measure of neurologic function, with greater impairment associated with a poorer prognosis
▶ Extent of resection: gross total resection/debulking may be beneficial
▶ Radiotherapy often used to treat patients with subtotal resection, anaplasia, or older age (e.g., >40 years)
▶ Chemotherapy often used in oligodendroglial tumors, particularly those with chromosome 1p and 19q deletions

---

PATHOLOGIC FEATURES

Oligodendrogliomas are often superficial with extensive cortical involvement. Like other diffuse gliomas, they have ill-defined tumor borders with blurring of gray-white junctions, although some appear deceptively circumscribed grossly. There may also be zones of microscopic disease that are only notable grossly because of secondary mass effects such as ventricular compression, midline shift, and sulcal effacement. Calcifications are grossly evident in some.

The most classic histologic features include uniformly round nuclei, bland chromatin with sharply defined nuclear membranes, clear perinuclear haloes imparting a "fried-egg" appearance, and a rich branching capillary network reminiscent of "chicken wire" (Fig. 9-17A and B). Less specific findings include cortical involvement, microcalcifications, mucin-rich microcystic spaces, and secondary structures such as perineuronal satellitosis (see Fig. 9-17B), perivascular aggregation, and subpial condensation. Although helpful in diagnosis, the "fried-egg" appearance is a formalin fixation artifact that is neither necessary for diagnosis nor encountered in frozen sections or rapidly fixed specimens. The morphologic spectrum includes two strongly GFAP-positive cells: minigemistocytes or microgemistocytes and gliofibrillary oligodendrocytes. The former are gemistocyte-like cells with small bellies of eosinophilic cytoplasm, round nuclei resembling those of classic oligodendroglioma, and no cytoplasmic processes (see Fig. 9-17C). Gliofibrillary oligodendrocytes are histologically identical to classic oligodendroglioma cells on hematoxylin-eosin stain, but they have a thin perinuclear rim of strong GFAP immunoreactivity (see Fig. 9-17D).

Anaplastic oligodendroglioma (grade III) is defined by hypercellularity, numerous mitoses (Fig. 9-18A) (e.g., ≥6/10 high-power fields in a recent study), and/or microvascular proliferation (see Fig. 9-18B). These tumors also commonly have a more epithelioid cytology with increased cytoplasm, sharper cytoplasmic borders, and prominent nucleoli (see Fig. 9-18C). Occasional cases display distinct nodules of anaplasia in otherwise

Text continued on p. 462

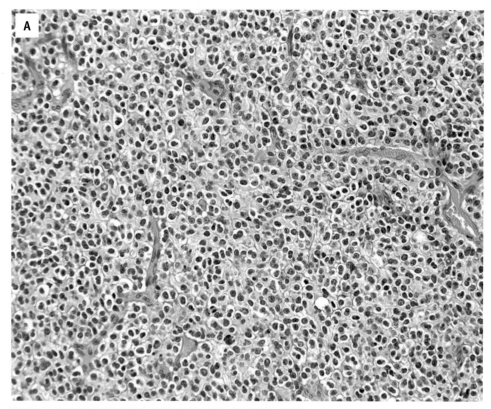

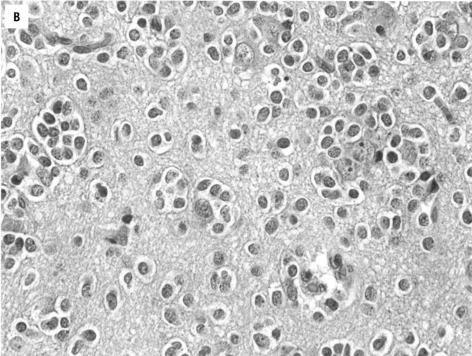

FIGURE 9-17

Oligodendroglioma with a chicken wire–like branching capillary network, uniformly rounded nuclei, and clear perinuclear haloes imparting a "fried-egg" or honeycomb-like pattern (**A**). Perineuronal satellitosis is evident in regions of cortical infiltration (**B**).

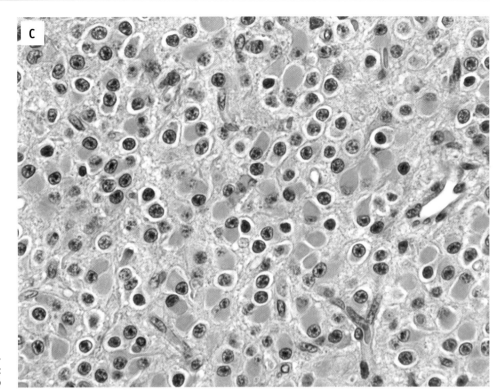

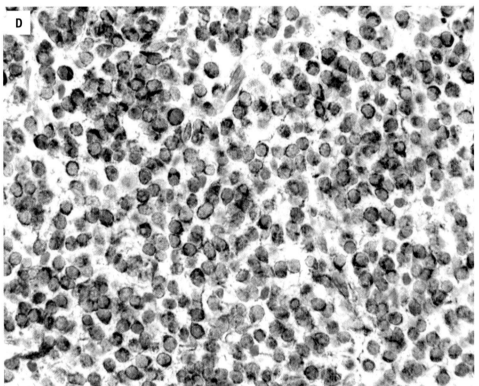

FIGURE 9-17, cont'd

Minigemistocytes have small rounded eccentric bellies of eosinophilic cytoplasm with nuclei identical to those of adjacent classic oligodendroglial cells (**C**). Gliofibrillary oligodendrocytes are characterized by thin perinuclear rims of GFAP positivity, sometimes with a short tadpole-like cytoplasmic tail (**D**).

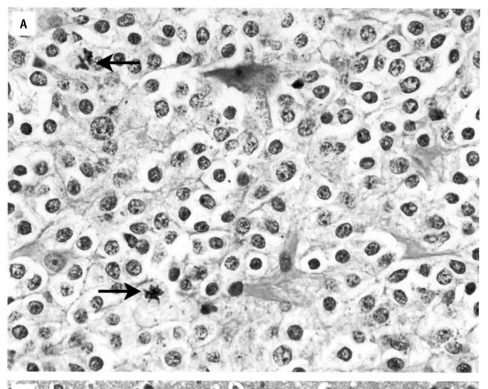

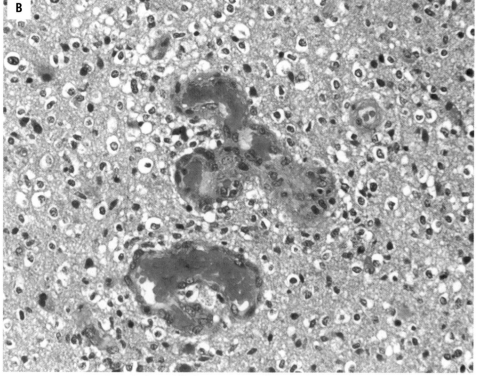

FIGURE 9-18

Anaplastic oligodendrogliomas (WHO grade III) are characterized by increased mitotic activity (**A**, *arrows*), endothelial hyperplasia (**B**), and

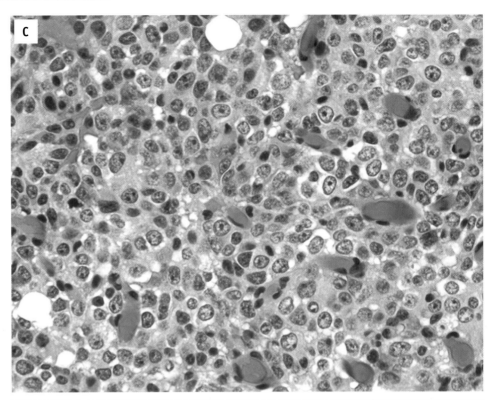

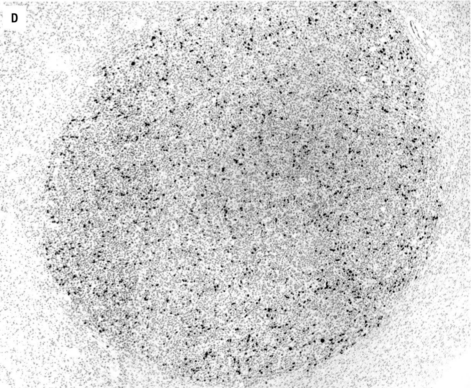

FIGURE 9-18, cont'd

increased pleomorphism with epithelioid cytology and prominent nucleoli (**C**). Some otherwise low-grade examples are characterized by focal nodules of anaplastic transformation, including increased MIB-1 proliferative activity (**D**).

OLIGODENDROGLIOMA—PATHOLOGIC FEATURES

Gross Findings

- ▶ Borders are ill defined and there are often foci of tumor involvement that are grossly invisible
- ▶ Rare cases of gliomatosis cerebri are histologically oligodendroglial
- ▶ Tumor epicenter most commonly in the cortex or corticomedullary junction
- ▶ Blurring of corticomedullary and other gray-white junctions
- ▶ Mass effect with a midline shift, blunting of sulci, compression of ventricles, or any combination of these findings
- ▶ A variegated appearance with foci of necrosis and hemorrhage suggests anaplasia

Microscopic Features (see Figs. 9-17 and 9-18)

- ▶ Hypercellularity with intermingling of neoplastic and non-neoplastic elements (i.e., infiltrative), but may have solid-appearing foci as well
- ▶ Uniformly round to oval nuclei with bland chromatin and, often, small nucleoli
- ▶ Clear perinuclear haloes impart a "fried-egg" appearance (formalin fixation artifact)
- ▶ Minigemistocytes maintain the nuclear features, but contain small rounded bellies of eosinophilic cytoplasm
- ▶ Mucin-rich microcystic spaces common
- ▶ Microcalcifications common and may be extensive in some
- ▶ Rich branching capillary network resembling "chicken wire"
- ▶ Secondary structures (e.g., subpial condensation, perineuronal satellitosis, perivascular aggregation) and tumor clusters or hypercellular nodules common
- ▶ Anaplastic (grade III) examples have frequent mitoses, endothelial hyperplasia, or both, often with increased pleomorphism and epithelioid cytology
- ▶ Existence of a grade IV oligodendroglioma is debated, but typically has all the features of glioblastoma multiforme, including pseudopalisading necrosis, yet maintains oligodendroglial cytology; often referred to as "glioblastoma with oligodendroglial features"

Ultrastructural Features

- ▶ Electron-lucent organelle-poor cells with minimal accumulations of intermediate filaments, except in minigemistocytes and gliofibrillary oligodendrocytes

Immunohistochemical Features

- ▶ GFAP—usually negative in classic cells, but strongly positive in two cell types: minigemistocytes (rounded eccentric cytoplasmic belly) and gliofibrillary oligodendrocytes (thin rim of perinuclear staining, with or without a thin cytoplasmic tail)
- ▶ S-100 protein—positive
- ▶ Cytokeratins—negative, but may get false-positive result with an AE1/AE3 cocktail
- ▶ EMA—negative
- ▶ HMB-45, melan A, LCA—negative
- ▶ Neurofilament highlights entrapped axons, consistent with an infiltrative growth pattern
- ▶ p53 protein usually negative
- ▶ MIB-1 labeling index typically elevated in anaplastic examples

Genetics (see Fig. 9-19A and B)

- ▶ Codeletion of one 1p and one 19q arm in 50% to 80% of cases and associated with enhanced survival and therapeutic responsiveness
- ▶ Mutations of p53 gene uncommon in oligodendrogliomas
- ▶ Losses of p16 gene or other members of the retinoblastoma regulatory pathway primarily seen in anaplastic or recurrent oligodendrogliomas (or in both types)
- ▶ EGFR amplifications and 10q deletions are rare even in anaplastic cases

Differential Diagnosis

- ▶ Astrocytoma/mixed oligoastrocytoma (see Figs. 9-3 and 9-20)
- ▶ Small cell glioblastoma (see Figs. 9-5E and 9-19C and D)
- ▶ Dysembryoplastic neuroepithelial tumor (see Fig. 9-27)
- ▶ Pilocytic astrocytoma (see Fig. 9-7)
- ▶ Clear cell ependymoma (see Fig. 9-23B)
- ▶ Central neurocytoma
- ▶ Extraventricular neurocytoma
- ▶ Metastatic clear cell carcinoma
- ▶ CNS lymphoma
- ▶ Clear cell meningioma

low-grade oligodendrogliomas (see Fig. 9-18D). The significance of focal versus diffuse anaplasia has yet to be elucidated. Similarly, the existence of a "grade IV" oligodendroglioma is controversial, although some cases of classic textbook oligodendroglioma clearly progress to a tumor containing all the features of glioblastoma multiforme, including pseudopalisading necrosis, and many use the term "glioblastoma with oligodendroglial features" for such cases (see Fig. 9-5F). The differential diagnosis in these cases often includes the small cell variant of glioblastoma (see Fig. 9-5E). Furthermore, some oligodendrogliomas have regions that overlap significantly with diffuse astrocytoma, particularly in previously frozen, cauterized, or poorly preserved regions (best to avoid such regions). Unfortunately, no specific oligodendroglioma markers are currently available.

Genetic characterization of oligodendrogliomas has provided important clues in the diagnosis and treatment of diffuse gliomas. A characteristic codeletion of chromosomal arms 1p and 19q is found in 50% to 80% of cases, particularly those with the most classic histology (Fig. 9-19A and B). Furthermore, this genetic signature is associated with both prolonged survival and a favorable response to PCV (procarbazine, CCNU, vincristine) chemotherapy or radiation therapy (or both therapies). Based on these findings, ancillary testing for 1p and 19q status has become routine in some medical centers. The most commonly used techniques include fluorescence in situ hybridization (FISH) and loss of heterozygosity (LOH), each with advantages and disadvantages. Similar to their astrocytic counterparts, p16 deletions are common progression-associated alterations. However, p53 mutation, EGFR gene amplification, and chromosome 10 losses are uncommon and suggest the possibility of an astrocytic rather than an oligodendroglial neoplasm.

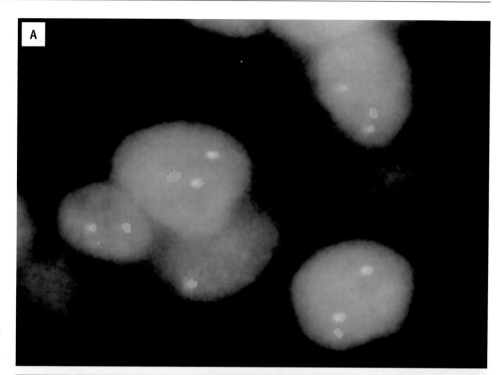

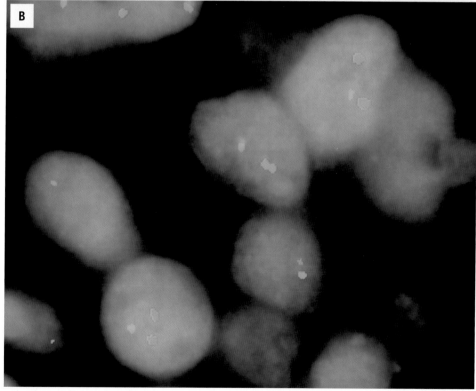

FIGURE 9-19

Dual-color fluorescence in situ hybridization (FISH) with DAPI nuclear counterstain (blue) in an oligodendroglioma with chromosome 1p (**A**) and 19q (**B**) deletions and a morphologically similar small cell glioblastoma with EGFR amplification (**C**) and chromosome 10q deletion (**D**). **A**, 1p32 probe = green (mostly one signal per tumor nucleus), 1q42 = red (mostly two signals). **B**, 19p13 = green (mostly two signals), 19q13 = red (mostly one signal).

Continued

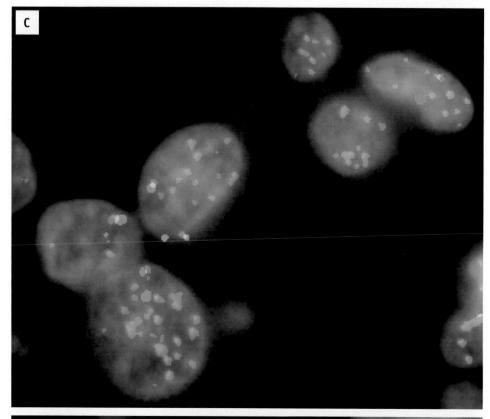

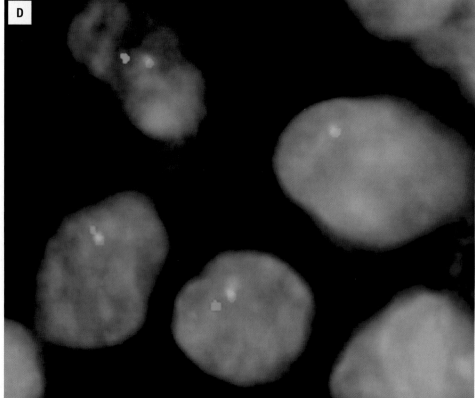

FIGURE 9-19, cont'd

C, Chromosome 7 centromere = green (mostly two or three signals), *EGFR* gene = red (many signals). **D**, *PTEN* gene (10q23) = green (mostly one signal), *DMBT1* gene (10q25-q26) = red (mostly one signal).

DIFFERENTIAL DIAGNOSIS

Since rounded nuclei and clear haloes may be seen in many entities, the differential diagnosis for oligodendroglioma is long. The overlap with astrocytoma has already been discussed and is a common problem. In fact, the small cell variant of glioblastoma in particular may have many overlapping features, including monomorphic deceptively bland nuclei, clear haloes, a "chicken wire" capillary network, and microcalcifications. However, the nuclei tend to be oval or elongated rather than round, there is a surprisingly brisk proliferative index given the bland chromatin, mucin-filled microcystic spaces are generally absent, and GFAP immunostain often reveals long cytoplasmic processes in tumor cells. Additionally, there may be more conventional fibrillary or gemistocytic astrocytic elements elsewhere in the tumor, and neuroimaging often reveals a ring-enhancing mass. Finally, these tumors are genetically characterized by *EGFR* gene amplification ($\approx$70%) and chromosome 10 loss (>90%) rather than 1p and 19q codeletions (see Fig. 9-19C and D).

On a small biopsy sample, dysembryoplastic neuroepithelial tumor may be totally indistinguishable from oligodendroglioma but shows the typical mucin-rich patterned intracortical nodules and floating neurons in larger biopsy and resection specimens. Similarly, the loose component of pilocytic astrocytoma may look remarkably similar to oligodendroglioma but usually has EGBs, Rosenthal fibers, a less infiltrative growth pattern, GFAP-positive processes, and a completely different clinical manifestation, including sites of predilection, radiologic appearance, and age at onset. Given that dysembryoplastic neuroepithelial tumor and pilocytic astrocytoma are benign, it is particularly important prognostically and therapeutically to accurately distinguish these entities from oligodendroglioma.

The clear cell variant of ependymoma shares the haloes and rounded nuclei but has the sharp interface with adjacent parenchyma typical of ependymoma in general. Perivascular pseudorosettes may be less conspicuous than in other variants, but they are usually present. Central neurocytoma is distinguished by its intraventricular location, neurocytic rosettes, and diffuse synaptophysin immunoreactivity. Extraventricular neurocytomas are considerably rarer but are also diffusely synaptophysin immunoreactive and display rosettes or neuropil-rich islands. Rare cases of oligodendroglioma with neurocytic differentiation and 1p/19q codeletions in both components have been reported recently, thus suggesting that there may be greater overlap between these two entities than previously suspected. Metastatic clear cell carcinomas such as renal cell carcinoma are discrete or noninfiltrative tumors and are positive for epithelial rather than glial markers. CNS lymphoma may show haloes but is associated with greater nuclear irregularities than oligodendroglioma is and is positive for lymphoid and B-cell markers. Clear cell meningioma is distinguished by both location and histology. It is an extra-axial rather than parenchymal tumor with a predilection for the spinal cord and posterior fossa. As opposed to oligodendroglioma, there is pronounced vascular and interstitial collagenization, PAS-positive glycogen-rich cytoplasm, and EMA immunoreactivity.

PROGNOSIS AND THERAPY

The prognosis for grade II oligodendrogliomas is significantly better than that for grade II astrocytomas, with average survival times of 10 to 15 years. Patients with the genetically favorable (1p/19q deleted) variant may survive even longer. As with astrocytomas, however, there is considerable individual variability in time to progression and overall survival. The average survival for anaplastic (grade III) oligodendrogliomas is 3 to 5 years, although similarly, some patients with the genetically favorable subset may survive 10 years or longer despite the high-grade histology. Genetically favorable oligodendrogliomas have been shown to be more likely to respond to chemotherapy, including the PCV regimen and, more recently, temozolomide. They are similarly more responsive to radiation therapy. Patients are often stratified into therapeutic groups according to age, extent of resection, tumor grade, and 1p/19q status. Therefore, genetic parameters are often used both for prognosis and for guiding patient management, although there is still much debate over the optimal therapeutic approaches and timing of various therapeutic modalities.

MIXED OLIGOASTROCYTOMA

CLINICAL FEATURES

The clinical features of mixed oligoastrocytoma (MOA) are essentially identical to those of pure astrocytomas and pure oligodendrogliomas of similar grade (see the fact sheet and previous descriptions).

PATHOLOGIC FEATURES

The WHO recognizes two types of MOA, a biphasic (compact) variant with anatomically separate areas resembling oligodendroglioma and astrocytoma and an intermixed (diffuse) variant in which the two elements are intermingled. The intermixed form is the more common and diagnostically challenging type and often displays nuclei with intermediate or ambiguous features, as well as the more classic forms (Fig. 9-20). Therefore, it is not surprising that MOAs are associated with the least diagnostic concordance and reproducibility of all gliomas. Genetically, most have astrocytoma-like or oligodendroglioma-like alterations, but not both.

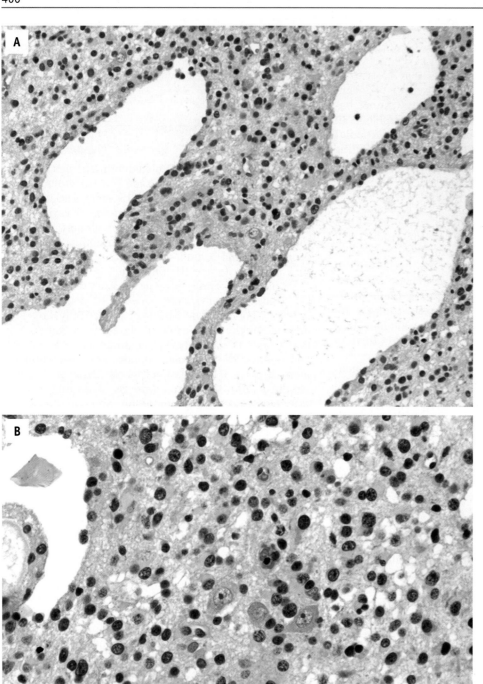

FIGURE 9-20

Mixed oligoastrocytoma with micro-cystic spaces (**A**), mild to moderate nuclear pleomorphism, and inter-mixed oligodendroglioma-like cells, including minigemistocytes and astrocytoma-like cells with irregular hyperchromatic nuclei (**B**).

MIXED OLIGOASTROCYTOMA—FACT SHEET

Definition

► Diffusely infiltrative glioma displaying both oligodendroglial and astrocytic features, either in geographically distinct zones (biphasic or compact variant) or intermixed (intermingled or diffuse variant)

Incidence and Location

► Accounts for 5% to 15% of diffuse gliomas
► Annual incidence rate of roughly 0.4 per 100,000 person-years
► Most arise in the cerebral hemispheres
► Extremely rare in the brain stem, cerebellum, and spinal cord

Gender and Age Distribution

► Slight male preponderance (M/F ratio of 3:2)
► Can occur at any age, although peak at 40 to 45 years
► Rare in children

Clinical Features

► Manifestations dependent on location of tumor
► Focal neural deficits, increased intracranial pressure, and seizures are the most common symptoms
► Generalized neurologic signs and symptoms of increased intracranial pressure include headaches, nausea/vomiting, and papilledema
► Rapid onset and progression suggest anaplastic (III), whereas a protracted history (e.g., chronic seizure disorder) is more consistent with low-grade (II) tumor

Radiologic Features

► Oligoastrocytomas (WHO grade II) are typically nonenhancing masses with increased signal on T2-weighted and FLAIR MRI sequences
► Anaplastic oligoastrocytomas (WHO grade III) are typically enhancing
► Intratumoral calcifications are common

Prognosis and Treatment

► Patient age: powerful predictor, with survival inversely proportional to patient age
► Grade: survival averages 5 to 10 years for grade II and 2 to 4 years for grade III
► Histologic cell type: mixed oligoastrocytomas have a prognosis intermediate between that of pure oligodendrogliomas and astrocytomas
► Preoperative performance status: measure of neurologic function, with greater impairment associated with a poorer prognosis
► Extent of resection: gross total resection/debulking may be beneficial
► Radiotherapy often used to treat patients with subtotal resection, anaplasia, or older age (e.g., >40 years)
► Chemotherapy often used as in pure oligodendrogliomas, particularly those with chromosome 1p and 19q deletions

MIXED OLIGOASTROCYTOMA—PATHOLOGIC FEATURES

Gross Findings

► Borders are ill defined, and there are often foci of tumor involvement that are grossly invisible
► Generally indistinguishable from other forms of diffuse glioma
► Blurring of corticomedullary and other gray-white junctions
► Mass effect with a midline shift, blunting of sulci, compression of ventricles, or any combination of these findings
► A variegated appearance with foci of necrosis and hemorrhage suggests anaplasia

Microscopic Features (see Fig. 9-20)

► Hypercellularity with intermingling of neoplastic and non-neoplastic elements (i.e., infiltrative), but may have solid-appearing foci as well
► Same features as pure astrocytomas and oligodendrogliomas, but both present
► Intermixed variant more common than the biphasic variant, and some nuclei may have features intermediate between those of astrocytoma and oligodendroglioma
► Anaplastic (grade III) examples have frequent mitoses or endothelial hyperplasia, or both, often with increased pleomorphism
► Existence of a grade IV oligoastrocytoma is debated, but it typically has all the features of glioblastoma multiforme, including pseudopalisading necrosis, yet maintains at least some foci with oligodendroglial cytology; often referred to as "glioblastoma with oligodendroglial features"

Ultrastructural Features

► Same as those for pure astrocytomas and oligodendrogliomas, but both present

Immunohistochemical Features

► Same as those for pure astrocytomas and oligodendrogliomas, but both present

Genetics

► Most cases are either genetically similar to pure astrocytomas (e.g., p53 mutations, monosomy 10, EGFR gene amplification) or pure oligodendrogliomas (1p/19q deletions) throughout the tumor regardless of regional differences in histology (i.e., monoclonal); some cases have none of these alterations
► Codeletion of one 1p and one 19q arm in roughly 20% of intermixed and 50% of biphasic examples; yet to be determined whether the same prognostic implications apply as they do with pure oligodendrogliomas

Differential Diagnosis

► Diffuse astrocytoma (see Fig. 9-3)
► Oligodendroglioma (see Fig. 9-17)
► Dysembryoplastic neuroepithelial tumor (see Fig. 9-27)

The same clonal aberrations are found throughout the entire tumor, regardless of the morphologic component being examined. For this reason, some believe that MOA is a wastebasket diagnosis and that only the pure gliomas exist. Nonetheless, it remains a viable category based on pathologic features and has an intermediate prognosis between that encountered in the two pure gliomas. Grading of MOAs is identical to that used for oligodendrogliomas, with the two major categories being low grade (WHO II) and anaplastic (WHO III). As with pure oligodendrogliomas, the existence of a "grade IV" variant is controversial, with many still using the term "glioblastoma with oligodendroglial features" for such cases. Studies suggest that 25% to 50% of biphasic MOAs have the 1p/19q codeletion whereas the intermixed variant shows this pattern much less frequently ($\approx$10%).

DIFFERENTIAL DIAGNOSIS

As discussed earlier, the diagnoses to exclude include pure astrocytoma, pure oligodendroglioma, and all the other differential considerations associated with these two entities.

PROGNOSIS AND THERAPY

The prognosis for MOAs is generally intermediate between that of pure astrocytoma and oligodendroglioma of similar grade, although there is great individual variability. Average survival is 5 to 10 years and 2 to 4 years for grades II and III, respectively. Treatment recommendations are usually identical to those given to patients with pure oligodendroglioma of similar grade. A recent FISH study showed that MOAs with genetic alterations typically associated with astrocytoma progression (e.g., 10q deletion, *EGFR* amplification, 9p or p16 deletion) had poor survival (average of 16 months) whereas those with 1p/19q codeletion, solitary 19q deletion, or none of the listed alterations had favorable survival times (average of 7 to 8 years). Nevertheless, patient age and histologic grade remained the two most powerful predictors of outcome in this cohort.

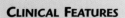

EPENDYMOMA

CLINICAL FEATURES

Ependymomas account for 3% to 9% of all brain tumors and are the third most common CNS tumors in children. They may occur at any age, but in children, the peak incidence is in the first decade. Ninety percent of tumors are in the brain, with an infratentorial site twice as common as a supratentorial site. Roughly 10% are in the spinal cord, most often in adults. In the spinal cord, ependymoma is the most common glioma subtype (accounting for 50% to 60%). The typical infratentorial ependymoma fills the fourth ventricle, and obstructive hydrocephalus is a common complication. Some are periventricular or may not have any obvious association with native ependyma (e.g., spinal cord or cerebral hemispheres). Supratentorial cases are more often cystic and anaplastic. Otherwise, neuroimaging typically shows a solid, well-demarcated enhancing mass. A

sausage-shaped mass is typical of spinal examples, often with an associated syrinx.

PATHOLOGIC FEATURES

Grossly, ependymomas are usually solid, well-demarcated, soft tan-red masses. In the posterior fossa, they are often intraventricular (fourth ventricle), whereas spinal tumors are intraparenchymal. Supratentorial cases are usually periventricular or superficial and

EPENDYMOMA—PATHOLOGIC FEATURES

Gross Findings

▶ Well-circumscribed, soft tan-red mass
▶ Hemorrhage and necrosis may be present
▶ Associated syrinx in some spinal examples

Microscopic Features (see Fig. 9-21)

▶ Sharp demarcation from adjacent CNS parenchyma
▶ Most characteristic feature is perivascular pseudorosette
▶ True ependymal rosettes and canals seen in 5% to 10%
▶ Cytology ranges from astrocyte-like to epithelioid
▶ Nuclei typically round to oval with small nucleoli
▶ Clear vacuoles in signet ring cells represent enlarged intracellular lumina
▶ Hypercellularity, frequent mitoses, and endothelial hyperplasia in anaplastic (WHO grade III) ependymomas
▶ See Table 9-2 for histologic variants

Ultrastructural Features (see Fig. 9-22D)

▶ One of the few remaining tumors in which electron microscopy remains a diagnostic gold standard
▶ Long, zipper-like desmosomes/intercellular junctions
▶ Intracytoplasmic lumina
▶ Intraluminal or surface cilia and microvilli
▶ Intracytoplasmic intermediate filaments (GFAP)

Immunohistochemical Features (see Fig. 9-22A-C)

▶ GFAP—usually positive and highlights the tapering process in perivascular pseudorosettes
▶ S-100 protein—usually positive
▶ Cytokeratins—usually negative, but focal positivity in rare cases
▶ EMA—highlights intracytoplasmic lumina in a minority of cases
▶ CD99—highlights surface membranes and intracytoplasmic lumina in most
▶ Neurofilament highlights axons pushed to the periphery, consistent with a noninfiltrative growth pattern
▶ MIB-1 labeling index typically elevated in anaplastic examples

Genetics

▶ Limited data available
▶ Greater degrees of aneuploidy in lower grades (I and II)
▶ Increased susceptibility for spinal ependymomas in NF2 patients
▶ NF2 gene mutations common in spinal but not intracranial ependymomas
▶ 22q losses and 1q gains are common
▶ Usually lack the alterations typically found in astrocytomas and oligodendrogliomas

Differential Diagnosis

▶ Diffuse astrocytoma (see Fig. 9-3)
▶ Astroblastoma (see Fig. 9-12)
▶ Oligodendroglioma (versus clear cell ependymoma) (see Fig. 9-17)
▶ Medulloblastoma/PNET (versus cellular ependymoma)
▶ Choroid plexus papilloma (versus papillary ependymoma)
▶ Pilocytic astrocytoma (versus tanycytic ependymoma) (see Fig. 9-7)
▶ Schwannoma (versus tanycytic ependymoma)
▶ Paraganglioma (versus myxopapillary ependymoma)
▶ Adenocarcinoma (versus myxopapillary ependymoma)
▶ Chordoma (versus myxopapillary ependymoma)

are frequently cystic. Secondary hemorrhage, necrosis, or calcifications may be seen in some cases, and an associated syrinx is common in spinal examples.

Microscopically, ependymomas are also remarkably well circumscribed and tend to compress rather than infiltrate the adjacent parenchyma (Fig. 9-21A). The latter may be highlighted with neurofilament immunostains, which show axons displaced to the periphery rather than entrapped within the tumor. Cerebral examples are often cystic. Ependymomas are usually arranged in sheets of spindled, astrocyte-like, epithelioid, and signet ring–shaped (containing large intracytoplasmic lumina appearing as clear vacuoles) cells with round to oval nuclei containing small nucleoli. The architecture is interrupted by perivascular rosettes (i.e., nuclear free zones around central blood vessels) (see Fig. 9-21B-D). True ependymal rosettes (i.e., containing a central lumen) and canals (i.e., slit-like structures resembling small ventricles) are more specific, but encountered in only about 10% of cases (see Fig. 9-21C). Most ependymomas are considered WHO grade II, although the myxopapillary ependymoma variant is grade I by definition. Anaplastic ependymoma (grade III) is diagnosed by the presence of hypercellularity, increased mitotic activity, and microvascular proliferation (see Fig. 9-21D). Regions of infarct-like necrosis are fairly common in otherwise low-grade–appearing tumors and are thus not a reliable grading criterion. In fact, the predictive value of histologic grading of ependymomas is questionable because its prognostic significance has not been consistent in reported series. Unfortunately, there are no specific immunohistochemical markers for ependymal differentiation. GFAP may be particularly helpful in highlighting the thin cytoplasmic processes radiating toward the vessels in these pseudorosettes (Fig. 9-22A). A small subset displays membrane-pattern EMA positivity, including positivity within small intracytoplasmic lumina, which yields a characteristic dot-like pattern (see Fig. 9-22B). Recently, CD99 has been reported to show a similar staining pattern with higher sensitivity (see Fig. 9-22C). A number of histologic variants exist and are described in Table 9-2.

Given the limitations of immunohistochemistry, ependymoma is one of the few remaining tumors for which ultrastructural examination is the diagnostic gold standard in atypical or challenging cases. Electron microscopy shows a combined glial and epithelial-like appearance, including abundant intermediate filaments (GFAP), microvilli, zipper-like intercellular junctions, intracellular lumina, and cilia and their basal attachments, known as basal bodies or blepharoplasts (see Fig. 9-22D).

Ependymomas are often aneuploid with complex, albeit nonspecific alterations. Chromosome 22q deletions are among the most common, with associated *NF2* mutations primarily restricted to spinal examples, a fact that fits with the spinal localization of most ependymomas in NF2 patients. Additional tumor suppressors are also suspected on 22q and other chromosomal sites, and there is some evidence that other protein 4.1 family members may also be involved.

Text continued on p. 474

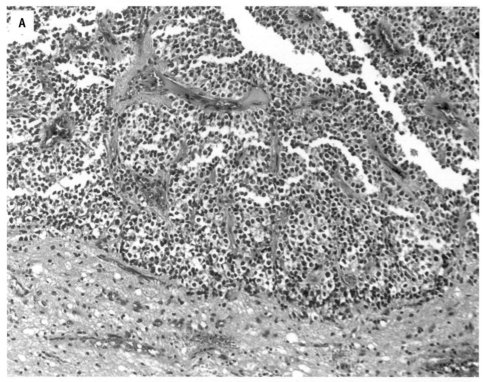

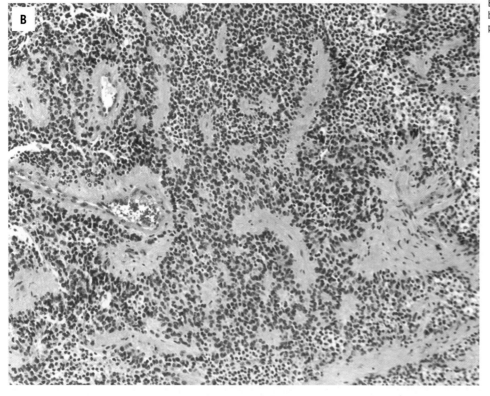

FIGURE 9-21

Ependymomas with a sharp tumor-to-brain interface (**A**), perivascular pseudorosettes (**B-D**), and

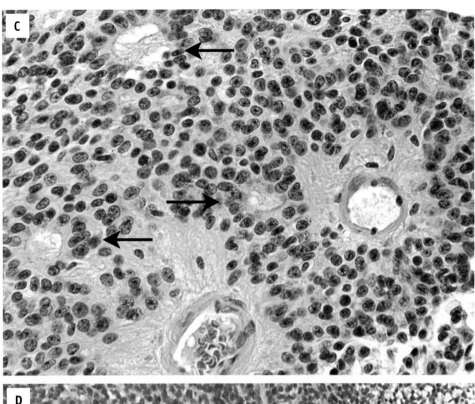

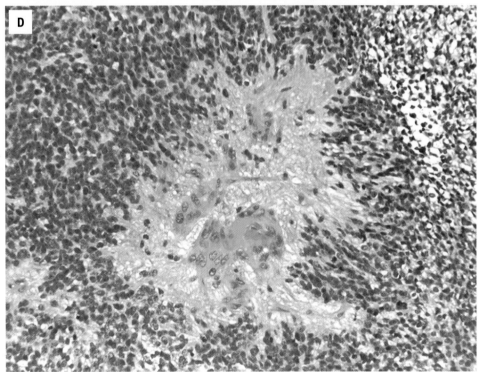

FIGURE 9-21, cont'd

true ependymal rosettes (**C**, *arrows*). **D**, Anaplastic ependymoma with hypercellularity, a high mitotic index, and endothelial hyperplasia.

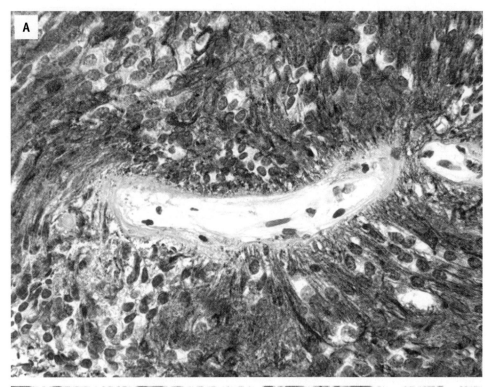

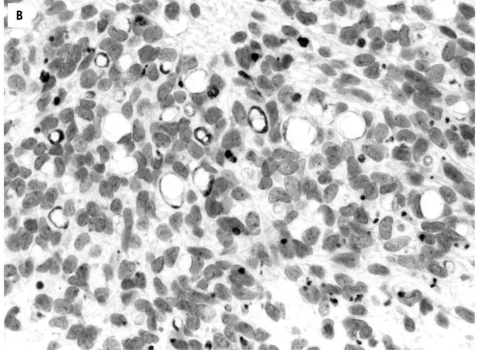

FIGURE 9-22

Immunohistochemistry and electron microscopy in ependymomas. **A**, GFAP stain highlighting thin tumoral processes radiating toward a central vessel. **B**, Epithelial membrane antigen showing membrane staining of signet ring–like cells and smaller intracellular lumina yielding a dot-like pattern.

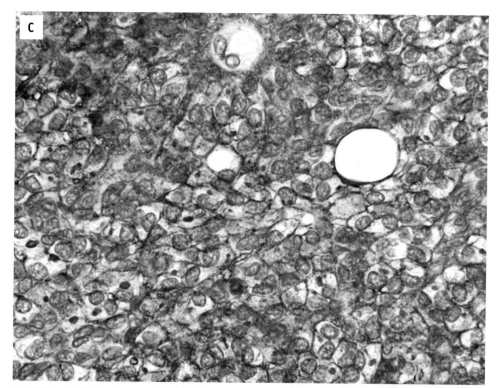

FIGURE 9-22, cont'd

C, CD99 shows a similar pattern of staining, but stronger and more diffuse. **D**, Electron micrograph showing a long, zipper-like intercellular junction (*right central*) and a collection of microvilli and cilia (*left central*).

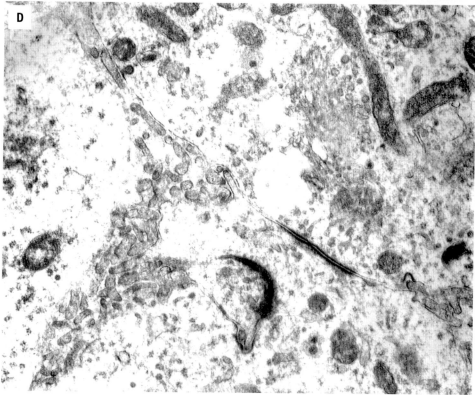

TABLE 9-2

Ependymoma—Variants

Conventional Ependymoma (see Fig. 9-21)	Often supratentorial, cystic, and in a child
Described in text	Can be grade II, but most fulfill criteria for anaplasia (grade III)
Cellular Ependymoma	**Tanycytic Ependymoma** (see Fig. 9-23C)
Same as above, but arranged predominantly in hypercellular sheets	Associated with long thin processes, similar to pilocytic astrocytoma or schwannoma
Presence of perivascular pseudorosettes distinguishes it from medulloblastoma and PNET	Most are located in the spinal cord
Most are WHO grade II and lack associated endothelial hyperplasia and high mitotic/proliferative indices	Perivascular pseudorosettes present, but often more subtle than other variants
Papillary Ependymoma (see Fig. 9-23A)	Most are WHO grade II
Discohesive growth pattern with pseudopapillae	**Myxopapillary Ependymoma** (see Fig. 9-23D-F)
Gliovascular rather than the fibrovascular cores seen in choroid plexus tumors	Prominent vascular hyalinization with perivascular mucoid degeneration
Typically multilayered papillae, as opposed to the single layer of choroid plexus papilloma	Nearly exclusively found in the region of the filum terminale
WHO grade II, unless anaplastic (grade III) criteria fulfilled	Rare cases encountered intracranially or in soft tissue of the sacral region
Clear Cell Ependymoma (see Fig. 9-23B)	WHO grade I tumor with an excellent prognosis, particularly if resected intact
Mimics oligodendroglioma because of prominent perinuclear haloes	If the capsule is breached and mucoid material spilled intraoperatively, the risk or recurrence increases
Sharply demarcated, unlike oligodendrogliomas	A subset of the soft tissue examples metastasize to lung or other organs
Perivascular pseudorosettes present, but often more subtle than other variants	

PNET, primitive neuroectodermal tumor; WHO, World Health Organization.

DIFFERENTIAL DIAGNOSIS

The potential differential diagnosis for ependymoma is extensive, although most cases are quite classic by histology alone. Most of the diagnostic difficulties result from specific variants that mimic other tumor types (see Table 9-2). Cellular ependymoma may mimic medulloblastoma or PNET, although pseudorosettes are often well developed and no neuronal features are detected by histology, immunohistochemistry, or electron microscopy. Papillary ependymomas superficially resemble choroid plexus papillomas, but they contain gliovascular rather than fibrovascular cores, they are multilayered, and the papillary architecture results more from discohesiveness than from true papillary growth (Fig. 9-23A). Clear cell ependymoma is characterized by rounded cells with clear cytoplasm mimicking oligodendroglioma (see Fig. 9-23B). The perivascular pseudorosettes are sometimes subtle, but nearly always present, and the typical childhood onset and noninfiltrative growth pattern are important clues. Tanycytic ependymoma is a rare variant encountered predominantly in the spinal cord. It is often misdiagnosed as either pilocytic astrocytoma or schwannoma because of

its spindled morphology with long thin processes (see Fig. 9-23C). Unlike the former, Rosenthal fibers and EGBs are absent within the tumor, whereas schwannomas are distinguished by their diffuse pericellular basement membrane pattern (reticulin or collagen IV stains) and absent to minimal GFAP immunoreactivity. Myxopapillary ependymomas are nearly always located in the filum terminale and have a distinctive perivascular mucinous/myxoid degeneration that separates them from paraganglioma, adenocarcinoma, and chordoma (see Fig. 9-23D-F).

PROGNOSIS AND THERAPY

Most ependymomas behave as low-grade malignancies (WHO grade II). Because of their circumscribed growth pattern, some tumors may be surgically curable, and the extent of resection constitutes a much more important prognostic variable in ependymomas than in diffuse gliomas. Age and location are also important, such that children younger than 3 years have a worse prognosis and those with spinal ependymomas do considerably better. In contrast, histologic grading is a much less

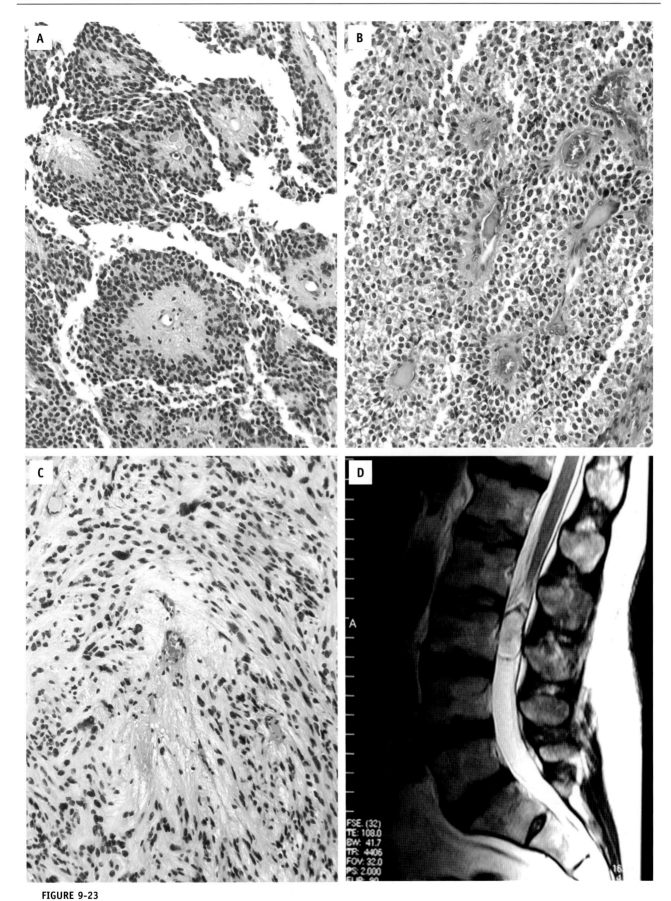

FIGURE 9-23

Ependymoma variants, including papillary (**A**), clear cell (**B**), tanycytic (**C**), and myxopapillary (**D-F**) subtypes. Myxopapillary ependymoma (WHO grade I) involves the filum terminale (**D-F**).   *Continued*

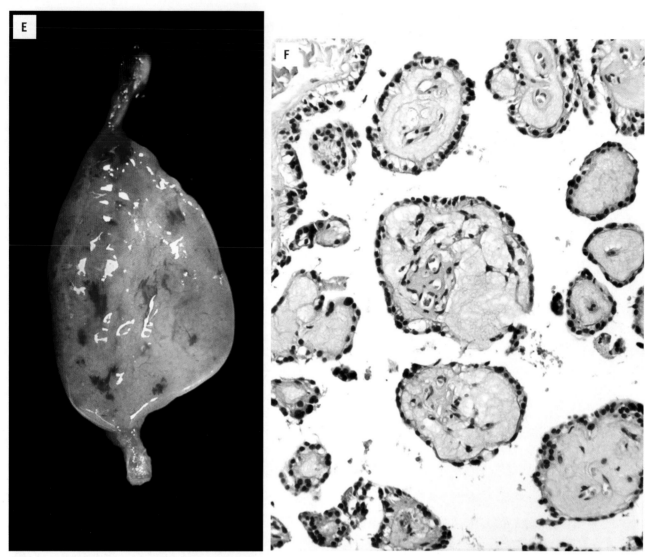

FIGURE 9-23, cont'd

reliable prognostic variable in ependymomas than in the other gliomas. The main clinical problem is that of local failure/recurrence rather than dissemination. Therefore, localized irradiation is a common form of adjuvant therapy. Nonetheless, ependymomas in contact with CSF pathways may seed the subarachnoid spaces and generate drop metastases in approximately 5% of cases. This finding is associated with a poor prognosis.

SUBEPENDYMOMA

CLINICAL FEATURES

Subependymomas are slow-growing, benign intraventricular tumors that are being detected with increasing

frequency by MRI in the absence of clinical manifestations. Ninety percent of subependymomas occur in adults, in whom they are small and incidental. In children, subependymomas are more likely to be large and symptomatic. They are most common in the lateral ventricles (50% to 60%), with the fourth ventricle being the second most common (30% to 40%). Rare cases involve the spinal cord. Radiologically, they are nonenhancing, nodular, often calcified masses.

PATHOLOGIC FEATURES

Subependymomas appear as glistening, pearly white, lobulated, intraventricular protuberances. Large tumors may obstruct the ventricle and cause hydrocephalus.

Microscopically, they are characterized by clusters of bland, rounded nuclei embedded in a fibrillary matrix

SUBEPENDYMOMA—FACT SHEET

Definition

▶ Benign (WHO grade I) intraventricular/subependymal glioma with clusters of ependymal-like nuclei embedded in a dense fibrillary matrix. Suggested cells of origin include ependymal cells and subependymal glia or astrocytes

Incidence and Location

▶ Accounts for <1% of primary brain tumors
▶ Most common in the fourth ventricle (50% to 60%)
▶ Also common in the lateral ventricles (30% to 40%)
▶ Rare examples in the spinal cord

Gender and Age Distribution

▶ Slight male predilection
▶ Occur at any age, but encountered most often in middle-aged to elderly

Clinical Features

▶ Most often asymptomatic and detected incidentally
▶ May be manifested as obstructive hydrocephalus and signs and symptoms of increased intracranial pressure, including headaches and nausea/vomiting
▶ Spinal tumors: motor and sensory deficits

Radiologic Features

▶ Usually nonenhancing nodular intraventricular mass
▶ Foci of calcification, hemorrhage, or both common
▶ Spinal tumors are intra-axial sausage-shaped expansions of cord, sometimes associated with adjacent syrinx

Prognosis and Treatment

▶ Benign tumor with an excellent prognosis
▶ Mixed ependymoma-subependymomas have malignant potential and should be graded and treated as pure ependymomas

SUBEPENDYMOMA—PATHOLOGIC FEATURES

Gross Findings

▶ Firm, well-circumscribed, nodular or lobulated tan-red mass
▶ Hemorrhage and calcifications may be evident
▶ Associated syrinx in some spinal examples

Microscopic Features (see Fig. 9-24)

▶ Sharp demarcation from adjacent CNS parenchyma
▶ Microcystic spaces and hyalinized vessels common
▶ Round to oval ependymal-like nuclei arranged in cellular clusters
▶ Dense fibrillary matrix
▶ Normal ependymal lining often seen overlying the tumor
▶ Mitoses and necrosis uncommon, but may have endothelial proliferation
▶ Foci of classic ependymoma in mixed ependymoma-subependymoma
▶ Rare cases have been reported with malignant components, including rhabdomyosarcoma

Ultrastructural Features

▶ Combined ependymal and astrocytic features, including cilia, microvilli, and accumulations of intermediate filaments

Immunohistochemical Features

▶ GFAP—usually positive
▶ S-100 protein—usually positive
▶ MIB-1 labeling index typically very low

Genetics

▶ No consistent alterations reported

Differential Diagnosis

▶ Ependymoma
▶ Diffuse astrocytoma

with microcysts and foci of calcification (Fig. 9-24). The proliferative index is typically low. Rare cases contain foci of classic ependymoma and are referred to as mixed ependymoma/subependymoma. These cases are graded and treated according to the potentially more aggressive ependymoma component. The histogenesis of subependymomas is still a matter of debate, with candidates including subependymal glia, astrocytes, ependymal cells, or some mixture of these cells.

DIFFERENTIAL DIAGNOSIS

The main differential considerations include ependymoma and astrocytoma. Subependymoma is more demarcated than the latter and differs from the former by forming nuclear clusters rather than perivascular pseudorosettes.

PROGNOSIS AND TREATMENT

Subependymomas are benign (WHO grade I) tumors with an excellent prognosis.

GANGLIOGLIOMA/GANGLION CELL TUMORS

CLINICAL FEATURES

Ganglioglioma (with a glial element) and gangliocytoma (without a glial element) represent the prototype of mature neuronal tumors of the CNS. Such a distinction is artificial and probably does not have any clinical significance. Therefore, they are frequently lumped together under the inclusive designation "ganglion cell tumor." In this text, they are used interchangeably as

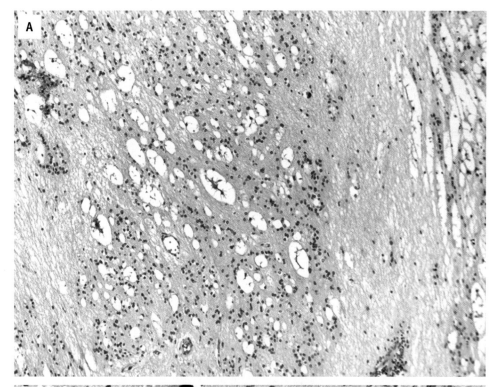

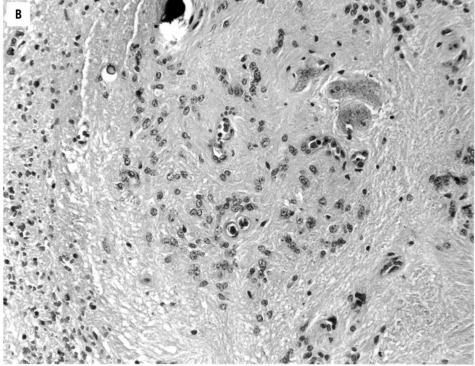

FIGURE 9-24

Subependymoma with nodularity, microcystic spaces (**A**), and clusters of ependymoma-like nuclei embedded in a dense fibrillary matrix (**B**).

GANGLIOGLIOMA/GANGLION CELL TUMOR—FACT SHEET

Definition

▶ Mature glioneuronal neoplasm with dysmorphic ganglion cells either alone (gangliocytoma) or in combination with a glial element resembling either pilocytic or fibrillary astrocytoma (ganglioglioma)

Incidence and Location

▶ Account for <2% of primary brain tumors
▶ Annual incidence rate of roughly 0.2 per 100,000 person-years
▶ May occur anywhere, but most common in the superficial temporal lobe
▶ Dysplastic cerebellar gangliocytoma (Lhermitte-Duclos disease)—associated with Cowden's syndrome

Gender and Age Distribution

▶ No major sex predilection
▶ Can occur at any age, although most develop in children and young adults

Clinical Features

▶ Manifestations dependent on location of tumor
▶ Chronic seizure disorder particularly common

Radiologic Features (see Fig. 9-25)

▶ Highly variable, but cystic mass with enhancing mural nodule common
▶ Calcifications are frequent
▶ Minimal mass effect and surrounding edema in most

Prognosis and Treatment

▶ Vast majority are benign (WHO grade I)
▶ Anaplasia (grade III) is rare and not always predictive of aggressive clinical behavior
▶ Therapy is primarily surgical, but may include radiation in subtotal or anaplastic cases

GANGLIOGLIOMA/GANGLION CELL TUMOR—PATHOLOGIC FEATURES

Gross Findings

▶ Well-circumscribed, firm intracortical mass
▶ Cystic component common
▶ Heavy calcification in some

Microscopic Features (see Fig. 9-26)

▶ Dysmorphic, haphazardly arranged ganglion cells
▶ Binucleate neurons in some cases
▶ Eosinophilic granular bodies
▶ Rosenthal fibers in some
▶ Perivascular lymphocytic infiltrates
▶ Increased interstitial reticulin and collagen
▶ Intermixed glioma in ganglioglioma; most often resembles pilocytic or fibrillary astrocytoma
▶ Foci of cortical dysplasia may be seen at the edges
▶ Mitoses, endothelial hyperplasia, and necrosis rare, except in foci of anaplasia

Ultrastructural Features

▶ Well-developed neuronal features, including dense core granules, synaptic vesicles, processes with microtubules, neurofilaments, etc.
▶ Subset of cells with astrocytic features in ganglioglioma

Immunohistochemical Features

▶ Neuronal markers—positive in the ganglion cell component, including synaptophysin, chromogranin, and neurofilament
▶ NeuN is usually negative in the neoplastic neurons but positive in adjacent or entrapped non-neoplastic cortical neurons
▶ GFAP—positive in the astrocytic elements of ganglioglioma
▶ S-100 protein—positive
▶ MIB-1 labeling index typically very low, but elevated in anaplastic examples

Genetics

▶ No consistent alterations reported

Differential Diagnosis

▶ Pilocytic astrocytoma (see Fig. 9-7)
▶ Pleomorphic xanthoastrocytoma (see Fig. 9-11)
▶ Diffuse astrocytoma with entrapped cortical neurons (see Fig. 9-3B)
▶ Dysembryoplastic neuroepithelial tumor (see Fig. 9-27)
▶ Cortical dysplasia

synonymous terms. Most gangliogliomas occur before the age of 21 and account for 4% to 8% of pediatric brain tumors. They grow slowly, most commonly in the temporal lobe, and seizures are a typical initial finding. In fact, ganglioglioma is one of the most common tumors encountered in surgical specimens obtained for epilepsy. Other lobes of the cerebral hemispheres, cerebellum, and spinal cord are less often affected. Radiographically, they are often cystic with an enhancing mural nodule, but more solid forms may also be encountered (Fig. 9-25). They frequently extend to the surface of the brain or may even attach to the dura and mimic a meningioma clinically.

PATHOLOGIC FEATURES

Grossly, they are often partially cystic, and the solid portions are firm, gray, and gritty as a result of calcific deposits.

Microscopically, portions of the tumor may resemble a low-grade astrocytoma, either pilocytic or fibrillary in nature. However, unlike native entrapped neurons within an infiltrative glioma, some of the tumor ganglion cells have a dysmorphic appearance, as evidenced by their lack of polarity and by their clustering, cytoplasmic vacuolation, increased nuclear pleomorphism, or multinucleation (Fig. 9-26A and B). Binucleate or multinucleate neurons are particularly helpful, when present. Otherwise, the most useful features in the distinction from diffuse gliomas include relative circumscription and EGBs. Perivascular lymphocytic cuffing, microcystic spaces, and fibrosis with collagen deposition

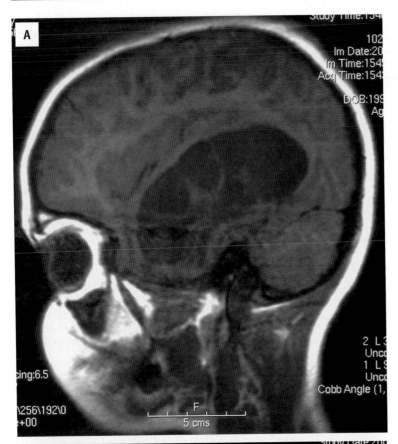

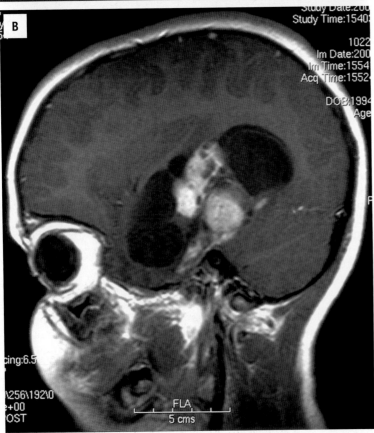

FIGURE 9-25

T1-weighted MRI without (**A**) and with (**B**) contrast in a patient with ganglioglioma. A well-demarcated, cystic, enhancing temporal lobe mass is apparent.

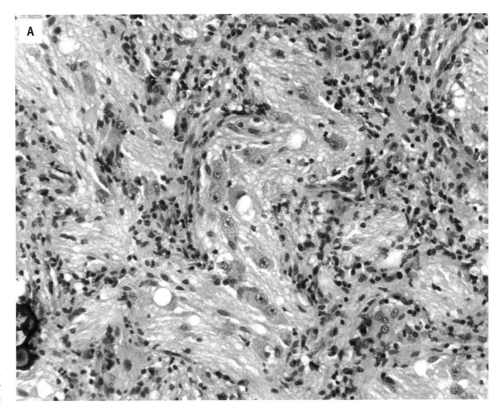

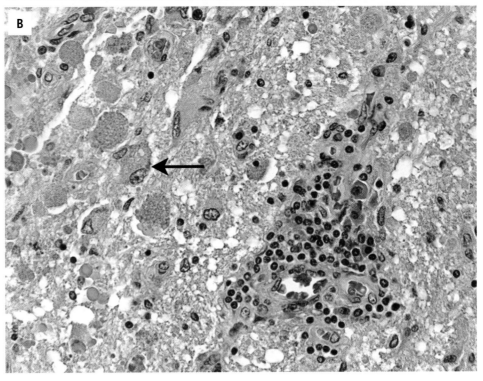

FIGURE 9-26

Ganglioglioma with abnormally clustered ganglion cells (**A**), perivascular lymphocytic cuffing, eosinophilic granular bodies, and dysmorphic neurons, including binucleate forms (**B**, *arrow*). *Continued*

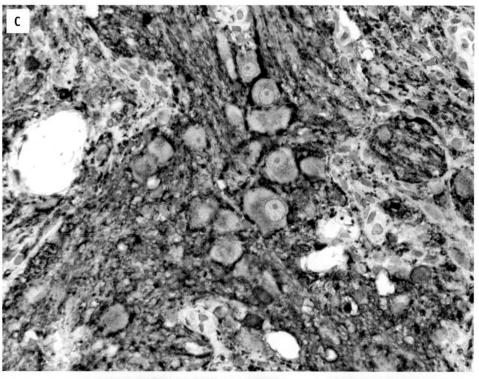

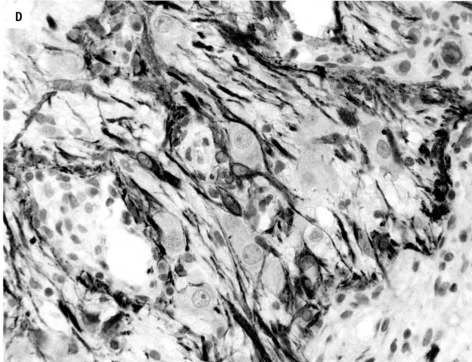

FIGURE 9-26, cont'd
The neuronal and glial components
are highlighted with immunostains
for synaptophysin (**C**) and GFAP (**D**),
respectively.

are other common findings. Rosenthal fibers are also
found in many cases, particularly at the edges of the
lesion. Cortical dysplasia has likewise been described
adjacent to ganglioglioma, although it is sometimes difficult to distinguish this dysplasia from foci of tumor
infiltration with certainty. Rare cases demonstrate signs
of anaplasia (grade II or III), most often in the glial component, but the grading criteria and their predictive

value have yet to be firmly established. GFAP activity is
abundant in the astrocytic component, whereas the ganglion cell component expresses most markers of mature
neurons, such as synaptophysin, chromogranin, and
neurofilament (see Fig. 9-26C and D). In most cases,
NeuN is negative in the neoplastic ganglion cells, but
positive in the adjacent native cortical neurons. Ultrastructural evidence of neuronal differentiation includes

dense core granules, synaptic vesicles, cell processes rich in microtubules, and intermediate filaments corresponding to neurofilament.

DIFFERENTIAL DIAGNOSIS

The clinical, radiologic, and pathologic features of ganglioglioma overlap significantly with both pilocytic astrocytoma and pleomorphic xanthoastrocytoma. However, only ganglioglioma has a well-developed neuronal component that is evident on routine hematoxylin-eosin staining. Another common and more critical differential is that of a diffusely infiltrating glioma with entrapped native neurons. Unlike ganglioglioma, these neurons are cytologically normal and architecturally well organized. Neoplastic ganglion cells tend to have greater degrees of cell body or membrane immunoreactivity (or both) for synaptophysin, chromogranin, and neurofilament, although these markers are not 100% reliable. The native cortical architecture is often highlighted at low magnification by an immunostain for NeuN, whereas neoplastic ganglion cells are often negative by comparison. Dysembryoplastic neuroepithelial tumor may also enter the differential diagnosis clinically and pathologically, although the neurons in this entity appear cytologically normal and are frequently embedded or appear to be floating in a mucin-rich stroma. In addition, the glial element of dysembryoplastic neuroepithelial tumor usually resembles oligodendroglioma rather than astrocytoma. Finally, there is often a great deal of overlap with cortical dysplasia, although ganglioglioma is distinguished by the formation of a mass lesion rather than the simple presence of dysmorphic ganglion cells in the cortex and white matter. The presence of cystic spaces, perivascular inflammation, and EGBs also favors ganglioglioma over cortical dysplasia.

PROGNOSIS AND THERAPY

The vast majority of gangliogliomas behave in a benign fashion (WHO grade I), although rare cases of malignant progression have been reported. In most cases therapy is limited to surgery, and control of seizures often improves after resection.

DYSEMBROPLASTIC NEUROEPITHELIAL TUMOR

CLINICAL FEATURES

Dysembryoplastic neuroepithelial tumor (DNT) is a benign, quasi-hamartomatous glial or glioneuronal tumor. DNTs occur throughout childhood and early

---

DYSEMBRYOPLASTIC NEUROEPITHELIAL TUMOR—FACT SHEET

Definition
▶ Quasi-hamartomatous intracortical glioneuronal tumor with mucin-rich nodules, floating neurons, oligodendroglia-like cells, and a temporal lobe predilection

Incidence and Location
▶ Accounts for <1% of primary brain tumors, but relatively common tumor type reported in epilepsy surgical series
▶ May occur anywhere, but most common in the mesial temporal lobe
▶ Rare cases reported in the caudate nuclei, third ventricular region, cerebellum, and brain stem

Gender and Age Distribution
▶ Slight male predilection
▶ Can occur at any age, although most develop in children and young adults

Clinical Features
▶ Manifestations dependent on location of tumor
▶ Chronic seizure disorder particularly common

Radiologic Features
▶ Intracortical low-density lesion, sometimes with appreciable nodularity
▶ Most are nonenhancing, but some enhancement seen in roughly a third
▶ Molding of the overlying calvaria common
▶ Minimal mass effect and surrounding edema

Prognosis and Treatment
▶ Benign (WHO grade I) tumor with an excellent prognosis
▶ Therapy is primarily surgical for diagnosis and control of seizures
▶ Recurrences rare, even in subtotally resected cases

---

adulthood, with the mean age at onset being 9 years. They are usually supratentorial and intracortical in location and are often associated with a long history of intractable seizures. The temporal lobe is the most common location for DNTs, although histologically similar tumors have been described in rarer sites such as the basal ganglia, thalamus, lateral ventricle, septum pellucidum, and brain stem. Radiographically, they are well-demarcated, usually nonenhancing, multinodular low-density intracortical lesions. Molding of the overlying calvaria is common, and there is typically minimal mass effect and surrounding edema. Like ganglioglioma, it is one of the most commonly encountered tumors in surgical series for chronic seizure disorder.

PATHOLOGIC FEATURES

Grossly, DNTs are mucin-rich intracortical expansions, sometimes with a discernibly nodular growth pattern (Fig. 9-27A).

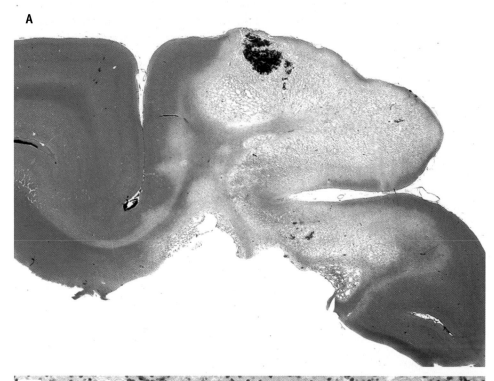

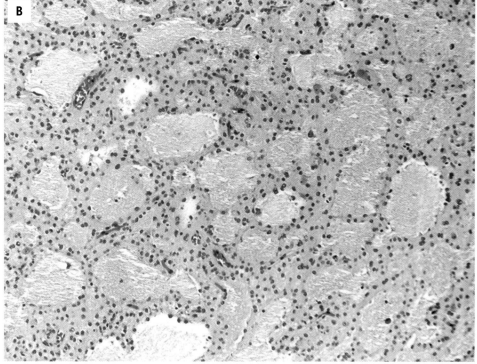

FIGURE 9-27

Dysembryoplastic neuroepithelial tumor with predominantly cortical localization (**A**), patterned mucin-rich cortical nodules (**A-C**),

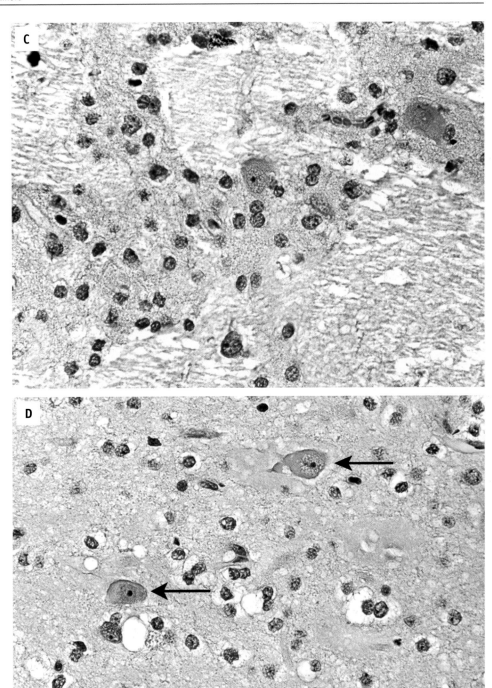

FIGURE 9-27, cont'd
and an intervening diffuse glioma-like "specific glioneuronal component" with oligodendroglioma-like cells and floating neurons (**D**, *arrows*).

DYSEMBRYOPLASTIC NEUROEPITHELIAL TUMOR—PATHOLOGIC FEATURES

Gross Findings

▶ Soft mucoid intracortical mass
▶ Nodularity evident in some

Microscopic Features (see Fig. 9-27)

▶ Patterned, intracortical mucin-rich nodules
▶ Internodular "specific glioneuronal component" with floating mature-appearing neurons and columns of oligodendroglia-like cells
▶ Oligodendroglioma-like cells with perinuclear haloes, but lack of prominent secondary structures such as perineuronal satellitosis
▶ Adjacent cortical dysplasia in some
▶ Foci resembling pilocytic astrocytoma or ganglioglioma seen in rare cases
▶ Mitoses, endothelial hyperplasia, and necrosis are rare

Ultrastructural Features

▶ Most oligodendroglial-like cells resemble those encountered in oligodendrogliomas
▶ Well-developed neuronal features only rarely encountered in the oligodendroglial-like cells, but present in the ganglion cells

Immunohistochemical Features

▶ Neuronal markers—positive in the ganglion cell component, including synaptophysin, chromogranin, and neurofilament
▶ GFAP—usually negative
▶ S-100 protein—positive in oligodendroglial-like cells
▶ MIB-1 labeling index typically very low

Genetics

▶ No consistent alterations reported

Differential Diagnosis

▷ Oligodendroglioma (see Fig. 9-17)
▷ Ganglioglioma (see Fig. 9-26)
▷ Pilocytic astrocytoma (see Fig. 9-7)

Histologically, there is a wide range of appearances, although the most characteristic features include patterned (i.e., with ribbons or arcades) mucin-rich cortical nodules (see Fig. 9-27B and C) and "floating neurons," the latter consisting of ganglion cells that appear to float within a lacune-like mucin-filled space (see Fig. 9-27D). In between the patterned nodules is the "specific glioneuronal component" that often resembles a diffuse glioma, particularly oligodendroglioma. Foci resembling pilocytic astrocytoma or ganglioglioma may also be encountered in rare examples. Cortical dysplasia may be seen at the edges of the tumor. Little is known regarding the genetic basis of this tumor, although recent studies suggest that they do not carry the 1p and 19q deletions typical of oligodendrogliomas.

DIFFERENTIAL DIAGNOSIS

On a small biopsy sample it may be virtually impossible to distinguish DNT from oligodendroglioma, but the presence of diffuse cortical invasion, clear white matter involvement, and prominent perineuronal satellitosis on larger samples argues against a diagnosis of DNT. Ganglioglioma and pilocytic astrocytoma typically appear as more sharply demarcated masses with prominent EGBs, Rosenthal fibers, dysmorphic ganglion cells, or any combination of these constituents.

PROGNOSIS AND THERAPY

DNT is a benign (WHO grade I) tumor with an excellent prognosis. In most cases, therapy is limited to surgery, and control of seizures often improves after resection.

SUGGESTED READINGS

General

CBTRUS: Statistical report: Primary brain tumors in the United States, 1995-1999. Central Brain Tumor Registry of the United States. 2002.
Kleihues P, Cavenee WK (eds): World Health Organization Classification of Tumours. Pathology and Genetics of Tumours of the Nervous System. Lyon, France, IARC Press, 2000.

Diffuse (Fibrillary) Astrocytomas

Burger PC, Pearl DK, Aldape K, et al: Small cell architecture—a histological equivalent of EGFR amplification in glioblastoma multiforme? J Neuropathol Exp Neurol 2001;60:1099-1104.
Giannini C, Scheithauer BW, Burger PC, et al: Cellular proliferation in pilocytic and diffuse astrocytomas. J Neuropathol Exp Neurol 1999;58:46-53.
Kitange GJ, Templeton KL, Jenkins RB: Recent advances in the molecular genetics of primary gliomas. Curr Opin Oncol 2003;15:197-203.
Maher EA, Furnari FB, Bachoo RM, et al: Malignant glioma: Genetics and biology of a grave matter. Genes Dev 2001;15:1311-1333.
Perry A: Pathology of low-grade gliomas. An update of emerging concepts. Neuro-Oncology 2003;5:168-178.
Pignatti F, van den Bent M, Curran D, et al: Prognostic factors for survival in adult patients with cerebral low-grade glioma. J Clin Oncol 2002;20:2076-2084.
Scott JN, Rewcastle NB, Brasher PMA, et al: Which glioblastoma multiforme patient will become a long-term survivor? A population-based study. Ann Neurol 1999;46:183-188.
Shafqat S, Hedley-Whyte ET, Henson JW: Age-dependent rate of anaplastic transformation in low-grade astrocytoma. Neurology 1999;52:867-869.

Pilocytic Astrocytoma

Chan M-Y, Foong AP, Heisey DM, et al: Potential prognostic factors of relapse-free survival in childhood optic pathway glioma: A multivariate analysis. Pediatr Neurosurg 1998;29:23-28.
Cummings TJ, Provenzale JM, Hunter SB, et al: Gliomas of the optic nerve: Histological, immunohistochemical (MIB-1 and p53), and MRI analysis. Acta Neuropathol 2000;99:563-570.

Fernandez C, Figarella-Branger D, Girard N, et al: Pilocytic astrocytoma in children: Prognostic factors. A retrospective study of 80 cases. Neurosurgery 2003;53:544-555.

Forsyth PA, Shaw E, Scheithauer BW, et al: Supratentorial pilocytic astrocytomas. Cancer 1993;72:1335-1342.

Giannini C, Scheithauer BW: Classification and grading of low-grade astrocytic tumors in children. Brain Pathol 1997;7:785-798.

Komotar RJ, Burger PC, Carson BS, et al: Pilocytic and pilomyxoid hypothalamic/chiasmatic astrocytomas. Neurosurgery 2004;54:72-80.

Subependymal Giant Cell Astrocytoma

Cuccia V, Zuccaro G, Sosa F, et al: Subependymal giant cell astrocytoma in children with tuberous sclerosis. Childs Nerv Syst 2003;19:232-243.

Hirose T, Scheithauer BW, Lopes MBS, et al: Tuber and subependymal giant cell astrocytoma associated with tuberous sclerosis: An immunohistochemical, ultrastructural, and immunoelectron microscopic study. Acta Neuropathol 1995;90:387-399.

Lopes MBS, Altermatt HJ, Scheithauer BW, et al: Immunohistochemical characterization of subependymal giant cell astrocytomas. Acta Neuropathol 1996;91:368-375.

Pleomorphic Xanthoastrocytoma

Giannini C, Scheithauer BW, Burger PC, et al: Pleomorphic xanthoastrocytoma. What do we really know about it? Cancer 1999;85:2033-2045.

Giannini C, Scheithauer BW, Lopes MBS, et al: Immunophenotype of pleomorphic xanthoastrocytoma. Am J Surg Pathol 2002;26:479-485.

Kaulich K, Blaschke B, Numann A, et al: Genetic alterations commonly found in diffusely infiltrating cerebral gliomas are rare or absent in pleomorphic xanthoastrocytomas. J Neuropathol Exp Neurol 2002;61:1092-1099.

Kepes JJ: Pleomorphic xanthoastrocytoma: The birth of a diagnosis and a concept. Brain Pathol 1993;3:269-274.

Korshunov A, Golanov A: Pleomorphic xanthoastrocytomas: Immunohistochemistry, grading and clinico-pathologic correlations. An analysis of 34 cases from a single institute. J Neurooncol 2001;52:63-72.

Perry A, Giannini C, Scheithauer BW, et al: Composite pleomorphic xanthoastrocytoma and ganglioglioma: Report of four cases and review of the literature. Am J Surg Pathol 1997;21:763-771.

Astroblastoma

Bonnin JM, Rubinstein LJ: Astroblastomas: A pathological study of 23 tumors, with a postoperative follow-up in 13 patients. Neurosurgery 1989;25:6-13.

Brat DJ, Hirose Y, Cohen KJ, et al: Astroblastoma: Clinicopathologic features and chromosomal abnormalities defined by comparative genomic hybridization. Brain Pathol 2000;10:342-352.

Mierau GW, Tyson RW, McGavran L, et al: Astroblastoma: Ultrastructural observations on a case of high-grade type. Ultrastruct Pathol 1999;23:325-332.

Thiessen B, Finlay J, Kulkarni R, Rosenblum MK: Astroblastoma: Does histology predict biologic behavior? J Neurooncol 1998;40:59-65.

Desmoplastic Infantile Astrocytoma/Ganglioglioma

Kros JM, Delwel EJ, Rob de Jong TH, et al: Desmoplastic infantile astrocytoma and ganglioglioma: A search for genomic characteristics. Acta Neuropathol 2002;104:144-148.

Tamburrini G, Colosimo C, Giangaspero F, et al: Desmoplastic infantile ganglioglioma. Childs Nerv Syst 2003;19:292-297.

VandenBerg SR: Desmoplastic infantile ganglioglioma and desmoplastic cerebral astrocytoma of infancy. Brain Pathol 1993;3:275-281.

Chordoid Glioma

Brat DJ, Scheithauer BW, Staugaitis SM, et al: Third ventricular chordoid glioma: A distinct clinicopathologic entity. J Neuropathol Exp Neurol 1998;57:283-290.

Cenacchi G, Roncaroli F, Cerasoli S, et al: Chordoid glioma of the third ventricle. An ultrastructural study of three cases with a histogenetic hypothesis. Am J Surg Pathol 2001;25:401-405.

Pasquier B, Peoc'h M, Morrison AL, et al: Chordoid glioma of the third ventricle. A report of two new cases, with further evidence supporting an ependymal differentiation, and review of the literature. Am J Surg Pathol 2002;26:1330-1342.

Reifenberger G, Weber T, Weber RG, et al: Chordoid glioma of the third ventricle: Immunohistochemical and molecular genetic characterization of a novel tumor entity. Brain Pathol 1999;9:617-626.

Sato K, Kubota T, Ishida M, et al: Immunohistochemical and ultrastructural study of chordoid glioma of the third ventricle: Its tanycytic differentiation. Acta Neuropathol 2003;106:176-180.

"Nasal Glioma"

Rahbar R, Resto VA, Robson CD, et al: Nasal glioma and encephalocele: Diagnosis and management. Laryngoscope 2003;113:2069-2077.

Roy S, Gungor A: Pathology quiz case. Heterotopic neuroglial tissue (nasal glioma). Arch Otolaryngol Head Neck Surg 2002;128:721-722.

Oligodendroglioma

Bauman GS, Ino Y, Ueki K, et al: Allelic loss of chromosome 1p and radiotherapy plus chemotherapy in patients with oligodendrogliomas. Int J Radiat Oncol Biol Phys 2000;48:825-830.

Burger PC: Controversies in neuropathology: What is an oligodendroglioma? Brain Pathol 2002;12:257-259.

Cairncross JG, Ueki K, Zlatescu MC, et al: Specific genetic predictors of chemotherapeutic response and survival in patients with anaplastic oligodendroglioma J Natl Cancer Inst 1998;90:1473-1479.

Giannini C, Scheithauer BW, Weaver AL, et al: Oligodendrogliomas: Reproducibility and prognostic value of histologic diagnosis and grading. J Neuropathol Exp Neurol 2001;60:248-262.

Perry A: Oligodendroglial neoplasms: Current concepts, misconceptions, and folklore. Adv Anat Pathol 2001;8:183-199.

Perry A, Fuller CE, Banerjee R, et al: Ancillary FISH analysis for 1p and 19q status: Preliminary observations in 287 gliomas and oligodendroglioma mimics. Front Biosci 2003;8:a1-a9.

Raghavan R, Balani J, Perry A, et al: Pediatric oligodendrogliomas: A study of molecular alterations on 1p and 19q using fluorescence in-situ hybridization. J Neuropathol Exp Neurol 2003;62:530-537.

Shaw EG, Scheithauer BW, O'Fallon JR, et al: Oligodendrogliomas: The Mayo experience. J Neurosurg 1992;76:428-434.

Smith JS, Perry A, Borell TJ, et al: Alterations of chromosome arms 1p and 19q as predictors of survival in oligodendrogliomas, astrocytomas, and mixed oligoastrocytomas. J Clin Oncol 2000;18:636-645.

Mixed Oligoastrocytoma

Fuller CE, Schmidt RE, Roth KA, et al: Clinical utility of fluorescence in situ hybridization (FISH) in morphologically ambiguous gliomas with hybrid oligodendroglial/astrocytic features. J Neuropathol Exp Neurol 2003;62:1118-1128.

Jeuken JWM, Sprenger SHE, Boerman RH, et al: Subtyping of oligo-astrocytic tumours by comparative genomic hybridization. J Pathol 2001;194:81-87.

Maintz D, Fiedler K, Koopmann J, et al: Molecular genetic evidence for subtypes of oligoastrocytomas. J Neuropathol Exp Neurol 1997;56:1098-1104.

Mueller W, Hartmann C, Hoffmann A, et al: Genetic signature of oligoastrocytomas correlates with tumor location and denotes distinct molecular subsets. Am J Pathol 2002;161:313-319.

Shaw EG, Scheithauer BW, O'Fallon JR, Davis DH: Mixed oligoastrocytomas: A survival and prognostic factor analysis. Neurosurgery 1994;34:577-582.

Ependymoma

Choi Y-L, Chi JG, Suh Y-L: CD99 immunoreactivity in ependymoma. Appl Immunohistochem Mol Morphol 2001;9:125-129.

Ebert C, von Haken M, Meyer-Puttlitz B, et al: Molecular genetic analysis of ependymal tumors. NF2 mutations and chromosome 22q loss occur preferentially in intramedullary spinal ependymomas. Am J Pathol 1999;155:627-632.

Fouladi M, Helton K, Dalton J, et al: Clear cell ependymoma: A clinicopathologic and radiographic analysis of 10 patients. Cancer 2003;98:2232-2244.

Kawano N, Yagishita S, Oka H, et al: Spinal tanycytic ependymomas. Acta Neuropathol 2001;101:43-48.

Min K-W, Scheithauer BW: Clear cell ependymoma: A mimic of oligodendroglioma: Clinicopathologic and ultrastructural considerations. Am J Surg Pathol 1997;21:820-826.

Rosenblum MK: Ependymal tumors: A review of their diagnostic surgical pathology. Pediatr Neurosurg 1998;28:160-165.

Singh PK, Gutmann DH, Fuller CE, et al: Differential involvement of protein 4.1 family members, DAL-1 and NF2 in intracranial and intraspinal ependymomas. Mod Pathol 2002;15:526-531.

Sonneland PRL, Scheithauer BW, Onofrio BM: Myxopapillary ependymoma. A clinicopathologic and immunocytochemical study of 77 cases. Cancer 1985;56:883-893.

van Veelen-Vincent MLC, Pierre-Kahn A, Kalifa C, et al: Ependymoma in childhood: Prognostic factors, extent of surgery, and adjuvant therapy. J Neurosurg 2002;97:827-835.

Vege KDS, Giannini C, Scheithauer BW: The immunophenotype of ependymomas. Appl Immunohistochem Mol Morphol 2000;8:25-31.

Subependymoma

Lombardi D, Scheithauer BW, Meyer FB, et al: Symptomatic subependymoma: A clinicopathological and flow cytometric study. J Neurosurg 1991;75:583-588.

Shimada S, Ishizawa K, Horiguchi H, et al: Subependymoma of the spinal cord and review of the literature. Pathol Int 2003;53:169-173.

Ganglioglioma/Ganglion Cell Tumor

Blumcke I, Wiestler OD: Gangliogliomas: An intriguing tumor entity associated with focal epilepsies. J Neuropathol Exp Neurol 2002;61:575-584.

Prayson RA, Khajavi K, Comair YG: Cortical architectural abnormalities and MIB1 immunoreactivity in gangliogliomas: A study of 60 patients with intracranial tumors. J Neuropathol Exp Neurol 1995;54:513-520.

Wolf HK, Muller MB, Spanle M, et al: Ganglioglioma: A detailed histopathological and immunohistochemical analysis of 61 cases. Acta Neuropathol 1994;88:166-173.

Dysembryoplastic Neuroepithelial Tumor

Daumas-Duport C: Dysembryoplastic neuroepithelial tumours. Brain Pathol 1993;3:283-295.

Honavar M, Janota I, Polkey CE: Histological heterogeneity of dysembryoplastic neuroepithelial tumour: Identification and differential diagnosis in a series of 74 cases. Histopathology 1999;34:342-356.

Prayson RA, Castilla EA, Hartke M, et al: Chromosome 1p allelic loss by fluorescence in situ hybridization is not observed in dysembryoplastic neuroepithelial tumors. Am J Clin Pathol 2002;118:512-517.

10 Non-Glial Tumors

Richard A. Prayson

Non-glial tumors constitute the bulk of neoplasms encountered in the central nervous system (CNS). They include a wide variety of tumor types and a spectrum of behavior ranging from benign to highly malignant. This chapter discusses some of the more commonly encountered non-glial tumors of the CNS.

MENINGIOMAS

CLINICAL FEATURES

Meningiomas account for approximately 13% to 26% of primary intracranial tumors. Lesions arise from arachnoidal cap cells, which are generally situated proximal to the meninges and dura. Occasionally, arachnoidal cap cell nests may be found in unusual locations, thus accounting for some of the more unusual sites of origin for these tumors (intraventricular region, head, and neck). The lesion has a clear female preponderance, although high-grade meningiomas are more commonly encountered in males. Meningiomas may arise at any age, but the peak incidence is in elderly adults. There is a known association of meningiomas with neurofibromatosis type 2, previous radiation therapy, and certain gynecologic malignancies such as breast carcinoma. Radiographically, tumors are circumscribed, generally dural-based lesions that may have a wedge-shaped extension of tumor at the edge, referred to as the dural tail. The radiographic appearance may be altered by calcification, bone and cartilage formation, and hypervascularity.

PATHOLOGIC FEATURES

Grossly, tumors are well demarcated and generally compress the adjacent parenchyma (Fig. 10-1A). Occasional tumors grow in a flat, en plaque pattern. A subset of atypical and malignant meningiomas may invade neural parenchyma. Hyperostosis of the overlying skull may be encountered.

The majority of meningiomas are of the syncytial, fibrous, or transitional types and are World Health

---

MENINGIOMAS—FACT SHEET

Definition

▶ Generally slow-growing, dural-based tumors derived from meningothelial (arachnoid cap) cells

Incidence and Location

▶ Account for about 13% to 26% of primary intracranial neoplasms
▶ Annual incidence rate of approximately 6 per 100,000 persons
▶ Most arise proximal to the dura within the intracranial, orbital, and intravertebral cavities
▶ Most common sites of origin—parasagittal region, cavernous sinus, tuberculum sellae, lamina cribrosa, foramen magnum, torcular zone

Gender and Age Distribution

▶ Female preponderance (F/M ratio of 3:2)
▶ Can occur at any age
▶ Most common in middle-aged and elderly patients, peak during the sixth and seventh decades
▶ Atypical and malignant meningiomas more common in males

Clinical Features

▶ Manifestations dependent on location of tumor
▶ Focal neural deficits, increased intracranial pressure, and seizures are the most common symptoms
▶ May cause hyperostosis of the overlying skull

Radiologic Features

▶ Circumscribed isodense dural masses that enhance with contrast
▶ May show evidence of calcification, bone or cartilage
▶ Dural tail—wedge-shaped extension of tumor at the edge, contrast enhancing
▶ Malignant and brain invasive tumors associated with cerebral edema

Prognosis and Treatment

▶ Most variants have an excellent prognosis and are curable by gross total resection
▶ Major predictor of recurrence is the extent of surgical resection
▶ Rare, more aggressive variants (papillary, chordoid, rhabdoid, clear cell, atypical, and anaplastic tumors) are more likely to recur and in some cases metastasize
▶ Recurrence rates: WHO grade I, 7% to 20%; WHO grade II, 29% to 40%; WHO grade III, 50% to 78%
▶ Higher cell proliferative labeling indices correlate with increased risk of recurrence
▶ Radiotherapy used to treat higher-grade and aggressive tumors

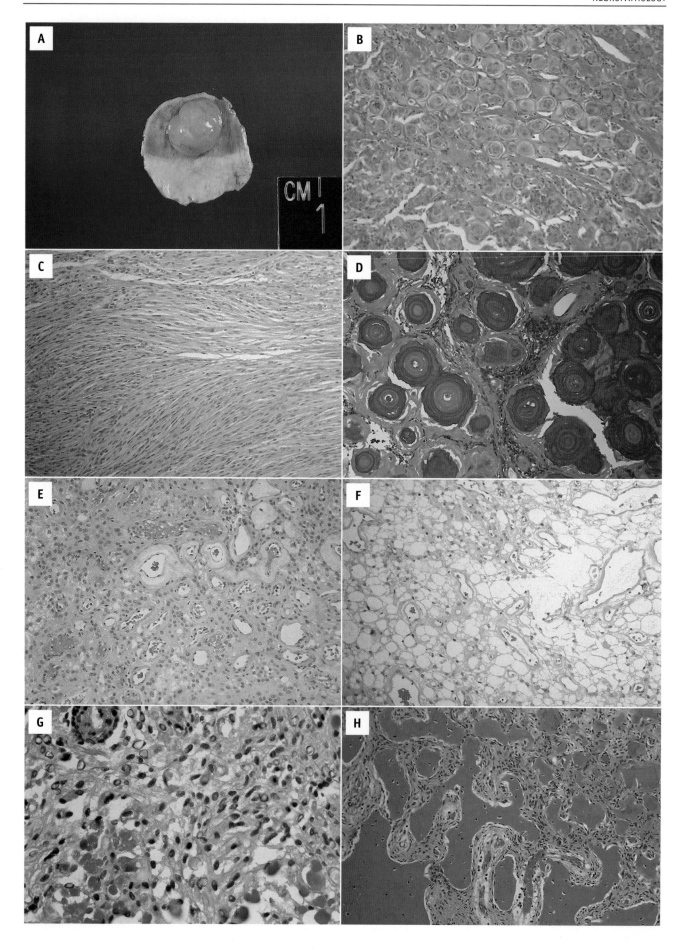

FIGURE 10-1

A, Gross appearance of a typical meningioma showing a well-circumscribed, tan-yellow mass attached to the dura. **B,** Syncytial meningioma (WHO grade I) marked by lobules of cells separated by fibrovascular septa. Whorling of cells in the lobules is common. **C,** Fibrous meningioma (WHO grade I) characterized by a proliferation of monomorphic spindled cells. **D,** Numerous laminated calcified structures mark a psammomatous meningioma (WHO grade I). **E,** Angiomatous meningioma (WHO grade I) showing prominent numbers of blood vessels. **F,** Microcystic meningioma characterized by a loose cystic background (WHO grade I). **G,** Secretory meningioma (WHO grade I) characterized by the presence of intracellular eosinophilic lumina (so-called pseudopsammoma bodies). **H,** Metaplastic meningioma (WHO grade I) marked by the presence of bone formation—osseous differentiation.

Organization (WHO) grade I tumors (Table 10-1). Specific histologic subtypes that have been associated with more aggressive behavior include chordoid and clear cell tumors (WHO grade II) (Fig. 10-2A and B) and papillary and rhabdoid tumors (WHO grade III) (Fig. 10-3A and B). Histologic grading of tumors into atypical (WHO grade II) and anaplastic (malignant) (WHO grade III) categories is based on mitotic activity, degree of cellularity, small cell change, prominent nucleolation, sheet-like growth pattern, necrosis, brain invasion, and lack of differentiation.

By immunohistochemistry, approximately 80% of meningiomas stain with epithelial membrane antigen (EMA). Approximately 20% to 40% of tumors are

---

TABLE 10-1

Meningiomas—Histologic Variants

Syncytial (Meningotheliomatous) (see Fig. 10-1B)

WHO grade I

Cells arranged in lobules separated by collagenous septa

Fibrous (Fibroblastic) (see Fig. 10-1C)

WHO grade I

Cells spindled and arranged in interlacing bundles

Psammoma bodies and whorling of cells around vessels common

Transitional (Mixed)

WHO grade I

Demonstrates features of both syncytial and fibrous types

Psammomatous (see Fig. 10-1D)

WHO grade I

Abundant psammoma bodies

Particularly common in the spinal cord

Angiomatous (see Fig. 10-1E)

WHO grade I

Numerous blood vessels in the background of an ordinary meningioma

Microcystic (see Fig. 10-1F)

WHO grade I

Cells with elongated processes arranged against a loose, mucoid background

Secretory (see Fig. 10-1G)

WHO grade I

Intracellular lumina with eosinophilic, PAS-positive material (pseudopsammoma bodies)

Lymphoplasmocyte-Rich

WHO grade I

Extensive chronic inflammatory infiltrates

Metaplastic (see Fig. 10-1H)

WHO grade I

Focal mesenchymal differentiation (bone, cartilage, adipose, xanthomatous)

Chordoid (see Fig. 10-2A)

WHO grade II

Areas resembling chordoma with trabeculae of eosinophilic and vacuolated cells arranged against a myxoid background

Clear Cell (see Fig. 10-2B)

WHO grade II

Polygonal cells with glycogen-rich, clear cytoplasm

Atypical (see Fig. 10-2C-E)

WHO grade II

Tumor marked by either increased mitotic activity (4 or more mitotic figures per 10 high-power fields—0.16 mm^2) or 3 or more of the following: increased cellularity, small cell change, prominent nucleoli, sheet-like growth pattern, necrosis, brain invasion

Papillary (see Fig. 10-3A)

WHO grade III

Perivascular pseudopapillary pattern

Rhabdoid (see Fig. 10-3B)

WHO grade III

Presence of "rhabdoid cells" with eccentric nuclei and prominent eosinophilic cytoplasmic inclusions of intermediate filaments

Anaplastic (malignant) (see Fig. 10-3C)

WHO grade III

Tumor marked by either 20 or more mitotic figures per 10 high-power fields (0.16 mm^2) or excessive malignant cytology with an appearance similar to sarcoma, carcinoma, or melanoma

---

PAS, periodic acid–Schiff; WHO, World Health Organization.

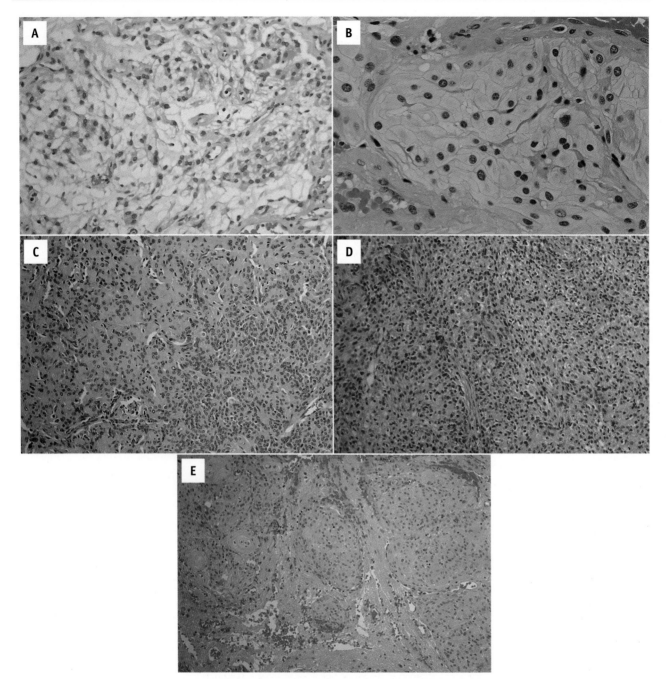

FIGURE 10-2

A, Chordoid meningioma (WHO grade II) marked by the arrangement of meningothelial cells in the cords and trabeculae against a chondromyxoid background, reminiscent of a chordoma. **B**, Clear cell meningioma (WHO grade II) composed of polygonal cells with abundant clear, glycogen-rich cytoplasm. **C**, Atypical meningioma (WHO grade II) demonstrating small cell change with a disorderly architectural pattern. **D**, Atypical meningioma marked by a disorderly architectural pattern associated with increased mitotic activity, increased cellularity, and prominent nucleoli. **E**, Atypical meningioma (WHO grade II) demonstrating parenchymal infiltration by tumor. Historically, many of these tumors were previously categorized as anaplastic or malignant meningiomas.

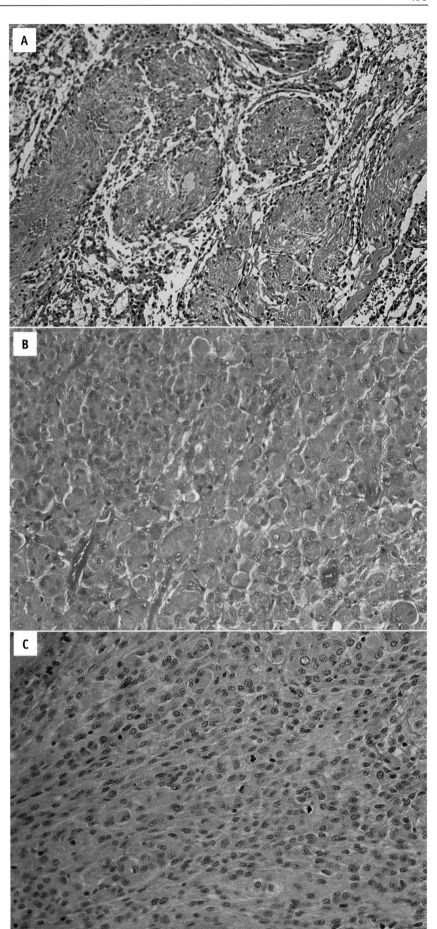

FIGURE 10-3

A, Papillary meningioma (WHO grade III) marked by a pseudopapillary architectural pattern with meningothelial cells arranged around vascular or fibrovascular cores. **B**, Rhabdoid meningioma (WHO grade III) characterized by the presence of large cells with eccentric nuclei and prominent eosinophilic cytoplasmic inclusions resembling cells seen in rhabdoid tumors. **C**, Anaplastic malignant meningioma (WHO grade III) characterized by extremely high mitotic activity and malignant cytology.

MENINGIOMAS—PATHOLOGIC FEATURES

Gross Findings

▶ Dural-based, sharply demarcated, rubbery or firm mass that compresses adjacent brain parenchyma
▶ Appearance may be altered by lipid content, cystic change, metaplastic components, vascularity, and calcification
▶ Meningioma en plaque—flat growth pattern, most common along the sphenoid wing

Microscopic Features

▶ Monomorphic cells arranged in a syncytium
▶ Nuclei oval to round with inconspicuous nucleoli
▶ Intranuclear pseudoinclusions (cytoplasmic invaginations)
▶ Psammoma bodies common
▶ See Table 10-1 for histologic variants

Ultrastructural Features

▶ Prominent intermediate filaments, interdigitating cell processes, and desmosomal intercellular functions

Immunohistochemical Features

▶ Vimentin—almost all are positive
▶ EMA—about 80% focally positive
▶ CEA, cytokeratins—focally positive in a minority of tumors; S-100 protein—20% to 40% focal positivity
▶ GFAP—negative

Genetics

▶ Most common abnormality—deletion on chromosome 22q
▶ Mutations in the neurofibromatosis 2 gene in 60% of sporadic tumors

Differential Diagnosis

▶ Schwannoma
▶ Metastatic carcinoma
▶ Astrocytoma
▶ Sarcoma
▶ Solitary fibrous tumor

immunoreactive to S-100 protein. Focal positivity with antibodies to carcinoembryonic antigen (CEA) and cytokeratins may be observed. Structural examination of the tumor is marked by the presence of prominent numbers of intermediate filaments, interdigitating cell processes, and desmosomal intercellular junctions.

DIFFERENTIAL DIAGNOSIS

Differential diagnostic considerations are numerous, given the phenotypic variability of these tumors. The fibrous variant of meningioma can be particularly problematic because of its bland spindled cell composition. Distinction of this lesion from schwannoma, especially in the cerebellopontine angle region, may be difficult. Schwannomas demonstrate diffuse S-100 protein immunoreactivity, Verocay body formation, biphasic Antoni A and Antoni B patterns, and a lack of psammoma

body formation. Solitary fibrous tumors are generally CD34 positive and marked by collagen material deposited between individual cells (Fig. 10-4). Meningioangiomatosis is a rare lesion characterized by perivascular collars of meningothelial cells extending into the parenchyma (Fig. 10-5), but it lacks the other worrisome histologic features that mark most brain invasive meningiomas. The other group of meningiomas that tend to be problematic with regard to the differential diagnosis includes the anaplastic tumors. According to WHO criteria, these tumors have areas that resemble carcinoma, melanoma, or sarcoma. Distinction of high-grade meningiomas from these various lesions may be challenging. In general, carcinomas demonstrate more widespread cytokeratin immunoreactivity. Melanomas are S-100, HMB-45, and melan A positive. Differentiation of nondescript high-grade sarcomas from spindled, high-grade meningiomas may be difficult and requires ultrastructural evaluation in certain cases. Occasionally, high-grade astrocytomas may also have a spindled cell or sarcomatous appearance (gliosarcomas). Most gliomas demonstrate some degree of glial fibrillary acidic protein (GFAP) immunoreactivity.

PROGNOSIS AND THERAPY

Overall, the majority of meningiomas behave in a benign clinical fashion and are amenable to surgical resection. Grade II tumors are more likely to recur in a shorter interval after subtotal resection, whereas malignant or anaplastic tumors are more likely to recur as well as metastasize. Radiotherapy may be used in managing the high-grade tumors and lesions that are particularly aggressive and associated with multiple recurrences.

MESENCHYMAL TUMORS

CLINICAL FEATURES

Mesenchymal tumors may arise at any age and generally show no gender predilection. They run the gamut from benign lesions such as lipoma to malignant tumors such as sarcomas. Manifestations are primarily dependent on location and may include focal neural deficits, symptoms related to increased intracranial pressure, and seizures. Imaging studies tend to be nonspecific and are dependent on the tissue types present. Sarcomas tend to be locally infiltrative and destructive lesions. There is an association of previous irradiation and the development of sarcoma.

PATHOLOGIC FEATURES

Benign lesions tend to be well circumscribed, in contrast to sarcomas, which are often infiltrative. Sarcomas may

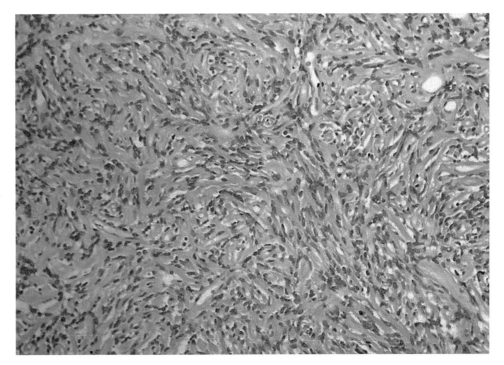

FIGURE 10-4

Solitary fibrous tumors may resemble a fibrous meningioma. In contrast to fibrous meningioma, solitary fibrous tumors are marked by abundant collagen material deposited between individual cells and CD34 immunoreactivity.

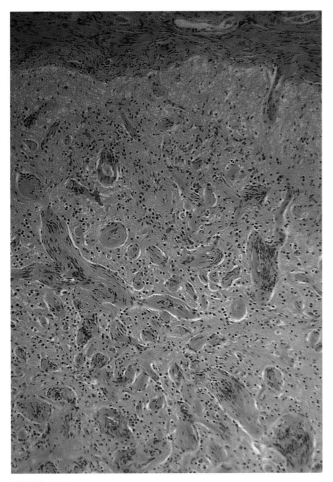

FIGURE 10-5

Meningioangiomatosis is characterized by a proliferation of meningothelial cells and vessels. Collars of meningothelial cells surround parenchymal vessels.

MESENCHYMAL TUMORS—FACT SHEET

Definition

▶ Tumors of mesenchymal origin that arise in the CNS or dura, including benign (leiomyoma, lipoma) and malignant (sarcomas, including hemangiopericytoma) neoplasms

Incidence and Location

▶ Lipoma is the most common of benign tumors—0.4% of intracranial tumors; sarcomas represent 2.5% of intracranial tumors, with hemangiopericytoma being the most common type
▶ More commonly dural than parenchymal based
▶ Most supratentorial
▶ Lipomas usually midline, rhabdomyosarcomas more often infratentorial, chondrosarcomas skull based

Gender and Age Distribution

▶ Occur at any age; rhabdomyosarcoma more common in children, hemangiopericytoma more common in adults
▶ Generally no gender predilection; hemangiopericytomas show a slight male preponderance (M/F ratio of 1.4:1)

Clinical Features

▶ Manifestations dependent on location and most commonly include focal neural deficits, increased intracranial pressure, and seizures

Radiologic Features

▶ Imaging appearances generally nonspecific
▶ Lipomas with high-signal intensity on T1-weighted magnetic resonance imaging (MRI)
▶ Sarcomas may be associated with lytic destruction of adjacent bone

Prognosis and Treatment

▶ Benign tumors can be completely resected with a favorable prognosis
▶ Sarcomas have a high incidence of recurrence and metastasis with a poor outcome despite aggressive irradiation and chemotherapy

---

MESENCHYMAL TUMORS—PATHOLOGIC FEATURES

Gross Findings

▶ Depend on tumor type
▶ Benign lesions tend to be circumscribed
▶ Sarcomas may be grossly well delineated with a firm and fleshy cut surface; necrosis and hemorrhage are common

---

Microscopic Features

▶ Benign lesions resemble normal tissue types
▶ Sarcomas demonstrate features by light microscopy, immunohistochemistry, or ultrastructural examination that indicate their lineage
▶ Sarcomas are marked by increased cellularity, nuclear atypia, mitotic activity, and necrosis
▶ Hemangiopericytomas are composed of randomly oriented plump cells with scant cytoplasm and a prominent "staghorn" vascular pattern

---

Ultrastructural Features

▶ Depend on tumor type
▶ Hemangiopericytoma cells contain small bundles of intermediate filaments and lack desmosomes or gap junctions

---

Immunohistochemical Features

▶ Depend on tumor type
▶ Hemangiopericytoma—vimentin, factor XIIIa, Leu-7, and CD34 positive; EMA and S-100 protein negative

---

Genetics

▶ Hemangiopericytomas are genetically distinct from meningiomas

---

Differential Diagnosis

▶ Gliomas with mesenchymal differentiation, including gliosarcoma
▶ Meningioma
▶ Metastatic carcinoma and melanoma

---

have a fleshy appearance on sectioning and are frequently marked by areas of necrosis and hemorrhage.

Microscopically, a myriad of tumor types fall into this general category. The most commonly encountered sarcoma type in childhood is rhabdomyosarcoma. In adults, hemangiopericytomas are the most frequently encountered sarcoma type (Fig. 10-6A and B). These latter tumors are marked by randomly oriented cells with scant cytoplasm and a prominent staghorn vascular pattern. By immunohistochemistry, hemangiopericytomas are generally CD34 positive and negative for EMA and S-100 protein. Criteria for subtyping sarcoma in the CNS should follow the rules for subtyping sarcoma elsewhere in the body (Fig. 10-7A and B). Many of these tumors represent metastasis from extra-CNS sites.

DIFFERENTIAL DIAGNOSIS

Differential diagnostic considerations include metastatic spindled carcinomas or melanomas, anaplastic meningiomas, and gliosarcoma. In contrast to the

majority of sarcomas, metastatic carcinomas demonstrate some degree of cytokeratin immunoreactivity, whereas melanomas demonstrate S-100, melan A, and HMB-45 immunoreactivity. Nondescript high-grade sarcomas may be difficult to distinguish from meningiomas if no differentiating features are evident; ultrastructural evaluation to look for characteristic features of meningioma may be required to delineate these entities. Gliosarcomas contain a glioblastomatous component that is GFAP immunoreactive.

PROGNOSIS AND THERAPY

Benign tumors may be completely resected with a favorable prognosis. Sarcomas have a high risk of recurrence and metastasis despite extensive surgical debulking and the use of adjuvant radiation therapy, chemotherapy, or both.

HEMANGIOBLASTOMA

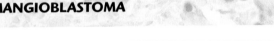

CLINICAL FEATURES

Historically, hemangioblastoma used to be considered a subtype of meningioma. In more recent years, it has been

---

HEMANGIOBLASTOMA—FACT SHEET

Definition

▶ Tumor of uncertain histogenesis composed of stromal cells and abundant capillaries

---

Incidence and Location

▶ Relatively uncommon tumor, 1% to 3% of intracranial tumors
▶ Most commonly arise in the cerebellum; rarely arise in the brain stem, spinal cord, and supratentorium

---

Gender and Age Distribution

▶ Slight male preponderance
▶ Peak incidence at 25 to 40 years of age
▶ von Hippel–Lindau tumors typically develop at a younger age

---

Clinical Features

▶ Symptoms related to CSF obstruction—increased intracranial pressure
▶ 10% with secondary polycythemia

Radiologic Features

▶ Contrast-enhancing nodule associated with a cyst or syrinx

Prognosis and Treatment

▶ WHO grade I tumor
▶ Good prognosis, curable with gross total resection
▶ Radiotherapy may be of limited use in recurrent or nonresectable tumors
▶ Increased risk of multiple/multifocal tumors in von Hippel–Lindau disease

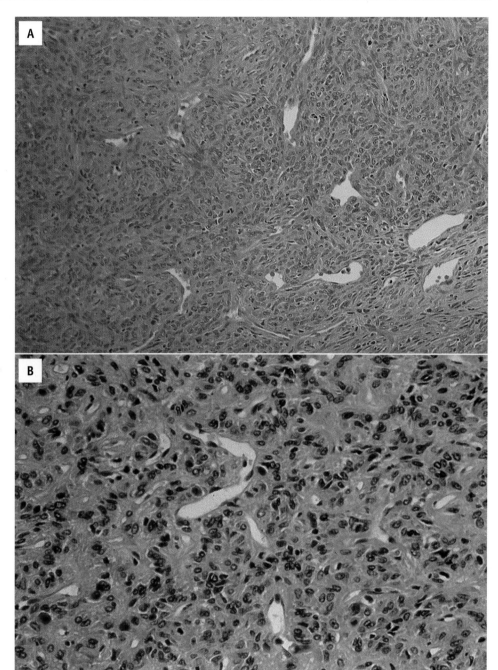

FIGURE 10-6

A, Hemangiopericytoma with marked hypercellularity and a staghorn vascular pattern. **B**, Nuclear atypia and a vascular pattern typical of hemangiopericytoma.

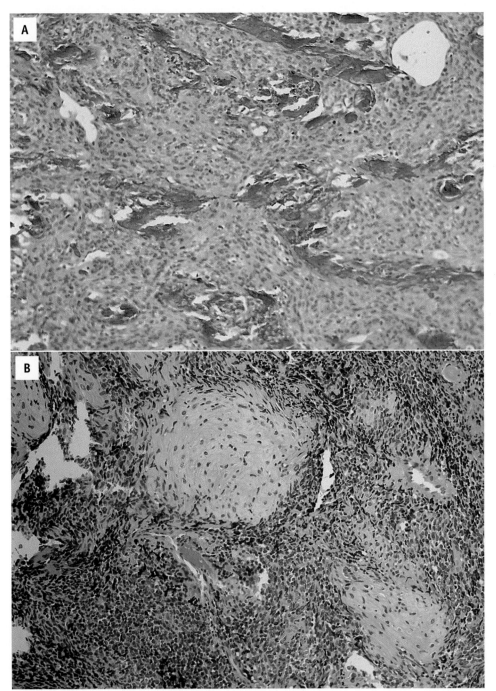

FIGURE 10-7

A, Abundant bone formation for the diagnosis of osteosarcoma. **B**, Focal chondroid differentiation in the background of otherwise undifferentiated tumor characterizes mesenchymal chondrosarcoma.

classified as a distinct tumor. The lesion may arise at any age, although it has a peak incidence during the third and fourth decades. There is a slight male preponderance and well-known association with von Hippel–Lindau disease (about a quarter of patients). Most tumors arise in the cerebellar region and commonly cause symptoms related to obstruction of cerebrospinal fluid (CSF). Approximately 10% of tumors produce an erythropoietin-like protein that results in secondary polycythemia vera. Radiographically, tumors demonstrate a cyst with an enhancing mural nodule configuration.

PATHOLOGIC AND GROSS FINDINGS

Tumors are often generally cystic with a mural nodule or nodules. Lesions are generally well circumscribed but not encapsulated.

Histologically, tumors consist of a prominent capillary vasculature with intermingled stromal cells (Fig. 10-8A and B). The stromal cells generally have a vacuolated or slightly eosinophilic cytoplasm. Nuclear pleomorphism is often focally prominent but is of no prognostic significance. Prominent mitotic activity and necrosis are not generally seen. It is not unusual to find a considerable number of Rosenthal fibers at the periphery of the tumor. The derivation of the stromal cells is not known.

DIFFERENTIAL DIAGNOSIS

From a clinical and radiographic standpoint, pilocytic astrocytomas can resemble hemangioblastomas; however, the tumors look very different histologically. Occasionally, a biopsy sample taken at the edge of a hemangioblastoma with numerous Rosenthal fibers and piloid gliosis may be confused with pilocytic astrocytoma. Metastatic clear cell carcinoma of renal origin can also resemble hemangioblastoma. This resemblance is particularly problematic in the setting of von Hippel–Lindau syndrome, where both lesions are more likely to appear. In general, renal cell carcinomas are EMA positive and may demonstrate areas of necrosis and mitotic activity.

PROGNOSIS AND THERAPY

Hemangioblastomas are considered benign lesions (WHO grade I) and are amenable to gross total resection. Patients with von Hippel–Lindau disease have a propensity for the development of multiple tumors.

MELANOCYTIC LESIONS

CLINICAL FEATURES

Melanocytic lesions may be found at any age, with melanocytosis being most common during childhood, melanocytoma peaking during the fifth decade, and melanoma primarily present in adults. As primary conditions in the CNS, these lesions are relatively uncommon. Melanocytosis might be manifested as seizures, psychiatric problems, and symptoms related to increased intracranial pressure. Melanocytomas and primary malignant melanomas are characterized by increased intracranial pressure and focal neural deficits. Radiographically, melanocytosis may be marked by diffuse thickening and enhancement of the leptomeninges. Melanocytomas and melanomas may have variable findings radiographically, depending on the amount of hemorrhage and melanin contained within the tumor.

HEMANGIOBLASTOMA—PATHOLOGIC FEATURES

Gross Findings
- ▶ Well-circumscribed tumor with a cystic component and red (vascular) nodule(s)
- ▶ May be yellow if lipid-rich

Microscopic Features
- ▶ Two components: prominent capillary vasculature and stromal cells with vacuolated or lightly eosinophilic cytoplasm
- ▶ Stromal cells may demonstrate focal nuclear pleomorphism
- ▶ Mitoses and necrosis unusual
- ▶ Adjacent parenchyma gliotic with Rosenthal fibers

Ultrastructural Features
- ▶ Abundant cytoplasmic lipid droplets in stromal cells
- ▶ Stromal cell histogenesis not known

Immunohistochemical Features
- ▶ Focal vimentin positive; weak GFAP positivity of uncertain significance may be present
- ▶ Stromal cells generally negative with factor VIII–related antigen, EMA, neurofilament, and keratin antibodies

Genetics
- ▶ von Hippel–Lindau cases (about 25% of tumors) associated with tumor suppressor gene on chromosome 3p25-26

Differential Diagnosis
- ▶ Metastatic clear cell carcinoma (especially renal cell carcinoma in the setting of von Hippel–Lindau disease)
- ▶ Pilocytic astrocytoma

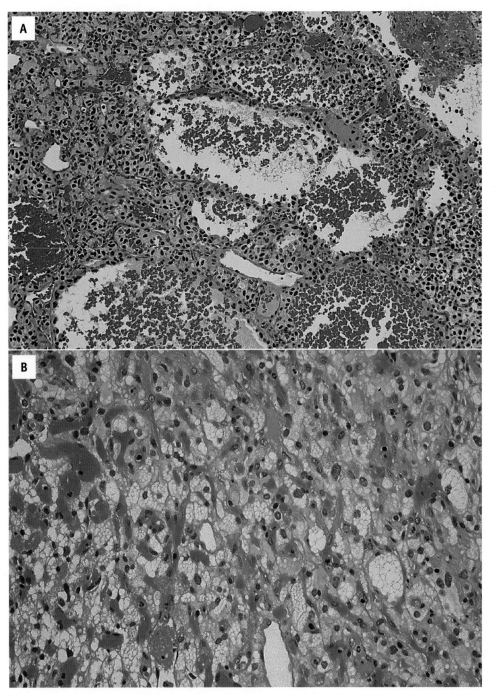

FIGURE 10-8

A, Large cystic pools with abundant vessels mark this hemangioblastoma. **B**, Hemangioblastoma characterized by the presence of abundant small vessels and stromal cells with clear, vacuolated cytoplasm.

MELANOCYTIC LESIONS—FACT SHEET

Definition

▶ Diffuse or localized, benign or malignant tumors arising from leptomeningeal melanocytes. Includes three main entities: diffuse melanocytosis, melanocytoma, and melanoma

Incidence and Location

▶ Melanocytosis and primary melanoma are very rare entities
▶ Melanocytoma—0.06% to 0.1% of brain tumors; annual incidence, 1 per 10 million population
▶ Melanocytosis is a leptomeningeal-associated process
▶ Melanocytoma most common in the posterior fossa and thoracic spinal cord

Gender and Age Distribution

▶ Melanocytosis most common in childhood
▶ Melanocytoma develops at any age, with a peak in the fifth decade and a M/F ratio of 2:1
▶ Primary melanoma occurs mostly in adults

Clinical Features

▶ Melanocytosis is manifested as seizures, psychiatric problems, and increased intracranial pressure
▶ Melanocytomas and melanomas are characterized by increased intracranial pressure and focal neural deficits

Radiologic Features

▶ Melanocytosis—diffuse thickening and enhancement of the leptomeninges
▶ Melanocytoma—isodense with gray matter, hyperintense on T1-weighted MRI, hypointense on T2-weighted MRI
▶ Melanoma—variable depending on the amount of hemorrhage
▶ Melanin deposits—highlighted by hyperintensity on short–repetition time/short–echo time MRI

Prognosis and Treatment

▶ Melanocytosis (despite its histologic appearance) and melanoma have a poor outcome
▶ Melanoma is radioresistant and readily metastasizes
▶ Melanocytoma—variable survival, prone to recur locally and invade local structures

---

MELANOCYTIC LESIONS—PATHOLOGIC FEATURES

Gross Findings

▶ Melanocytosis—black-pigmented meninges
▶ Melanocytoma and melanoma—single circumscribed lesions with variable pigmentation

Microscopic Features

▶ Melanocytosis—diffuse or multifocal proliferation of uniform, polygonal nevoid cells in the leptomeninges, may focally extend into Virchow-Robin spaces
▶ Melanocytoma—monomorphic cells (spindle to polygonal) with round vesicular nuclei, prominent nucleoli, and cytoplasmic melanin
▶ Melanoma—more pleomorphism, mitotic activity, necrosis, and parenchymal infiltration than occurs with melanocytoma

Ultrastructural Features

▶ Melanosomes in cytoplasm, no junctions, no interdigitating cytoplasmic processes

Immunohistochemical Features

▶ Positive for S-100 protein, melan A, HMB-45, vimentin
▶ Negative for GFAP, EMA, cytokeratins, and neurofilament protein

Genetics

▶ Neurocutaneous melanosis (combination of midline cutaneous nevi and melanocytosis) suggests a genetic basis for a subset of melanocytosis cases

Differential Diagnosis

▶ Metastatic melanoma
▶ Meningioma
▶ Melanocytic differentiation in other primary CNS neoplasms (gliomas, medulloblastoma, schwannoma)

PATHOLOGIC FEATURES

Grossly, melanocytosis is characterized by black pigmentation of the leptomeninges. Melanocytomas and melanomas are relatively circumscribed lesions with variable degrees of pigmentation. Melanoma may also be marked by variable amounts of hemorrhage and necrosis.

Histologically, melanocytosis is characterized by a diffuse proliferation of nevoid cells in the leptomeninges (Fig. 10-9A). Focally, extension into the Virchow-Robin spaces may be present. Melanocytomas are marked by a proliferation of monomorphic-appearing cells that may be polygonal or spindled in configuration with round vesicular nuclei, prominent nucleoli, and a variable degree of cytoplasmic melanin (see Fig. 10-9B). Melanomas, in contrast to melanocytomas, are generally more pleomorphic, have increased mitotic activity and an infiltrative growth pattern, and more frequently demonstrate evidence of necrosis (see Fig. 10-9C). Ultrastructurally, all lesions are marked by the presence of melanosomes and a lack of junctions. By immunohistochemistry, all lesions are positive for S-100 protein, melan A, and HMB-45.

DIFFERENTIAL DIAGNOSIS

Differentiating melanin-poor melanocytomas and melanomas from other tumors may at times be difficult. The immunohistochemical profile is somewhat distinctive and can be helpful in excluding most other tumor types. A variety of other primary CNS neoplasms, including gliomas, medulloblastomas, and schwannomas, may focally contain melanin pigmentation.

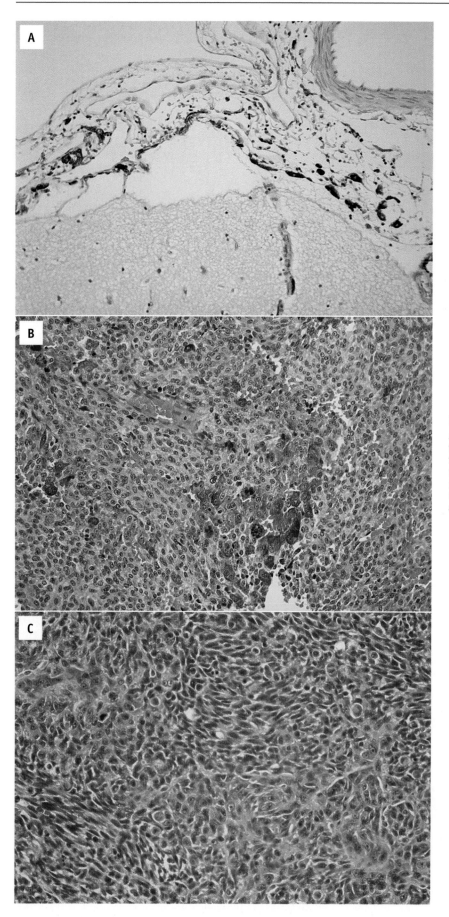

FIGURE 10-9

A, Proliferation of nevoid cells in the leptomeninges marks melanocytosis. **B**, Melanocytoma characterized by a proliferation of monomorphic-appearing cells and abundant melanin deposition. **C**, Markedly hypercellular malignant melanoma with prominent nuclear atypia and mitotic figures.

PROGNOSIS AND THERAPY

Despite its rather bland histologic appearance, melanocytosis is often associated with a poor prognosis. Melanomas have a poor outcome, are generally refractory to radiotherapy, and have a propensity to readily metastasize. The prognosis of melanocytomas is somewhat more variable; a subset of these tumors recur locally.

CHORDOMA

CLINICAL FEATURES

Chordomas are relatively uncommon tumors that may arise at any age but are most commonly encountered in adults. The majority of tumors are located in either the sacrococcygeal or the clivus/spheno-occipital region. Sacral tumors are marked by signs and symptoms related to sphincter disturbance, neurologic deficits secondary to involvement of nerve roots, or pain. Tumors arising at the base of the skull are associated with headaches, diplopia, and cranial nerve palsies. Radiographically, tumors are generally osseodestructive and infiltrate adjacent tissues.

PATHOLOGIC FEATURES

Grossly, chordomas are infiltrative, lobulated masses with a mucoid appearance on sectioning. Focal areas of cartilaginous differentiation (chondroid chordoma) may be observed (Fig. 10-10A).

Histologically, tumors are marked by a lobulated architectural pattern with fibrovascular septa. Epithelioid cells are arranged in cords or rows (see Fig. 10-10B). Many of the cells may have a prominently vacuolated cytoplasm (physaliphorous cells) (see Fig. 10-10C), and occasional mitotic figures and mild nuclear pleomorphism may be present. Ultrastructurally, the tumors are characterized by abundant cytoplasmic mucus vacuoles and desmosomal junctions. Tumors stain positively with antibodies to vimentin, cytokeratin, EMA, and S-100 protein.

CHORDOMA—FACT SHEET

Definition
▶ Tumor derived from notochord remnants

Incidence and Location
▶ Relatively uncommon tumor
▶ Most common sites: sacrococcygeal region (about half), clivus or spheno-occipital region (a third), and associated with articulating vertebrae

Gender and Age Distribution
▶ Any age, more common in adults

Clinical Features
▶ Sacral tumors are marked by pain, sphincter disturbance, and neural deficits secondary to involvement of nerve roots
▶ Base of skull tumors are characterized by headaches, diplopia, and cranial nerve palsies

Radiologic Features
▶ Osseodestructive mass with infiltration into adjacent soft tissue

Prognosis and Treatment
▶ Wide surgical resection recommended; local recurrence with subtotal resection
▶ Radiotherapy for subtotally resected tumors
▶ Minority of tumors metastasize to the lung, nodes, and skin
▶ Minority of tumors degenerate or dedifferentiate into sarcoma
▶ Younger patients have a better prognosis

CHORDOMA—PATHOLOGIC FEATURES

Gross Findings
▶ Infiltrative, bone-based, lobulated mass
▶ Mucoid appearance
▶ Cartilaginous tissue in the chondroid variant

Microscopic Findings
▶ Lobulated architecture with fibrovascular septa
▶ Epithelioid cells arranged in cords or rows against mucoid stroma
▶ Physaliphorous cells with "bubble-like" vacuolated cytoplasm
▶ Occasional mitotic figures and mild nuclear pleomorphism
▶ Focal cartilaginous differentiation (chordoid chordoma)

Ultrastructural Features
▶ Abundant cytoplasmic mucus vacuoles and desmosomal junctions

Immunohistochemical Features
▶ Positive with antibodies to vimentin, cytokeratins, EMA, and S-100 protein

Genetics
▶ No salient genetic alterations

Differential Diagnosis
▶ Chondrosarcoma
▶ Chordoid meningioma
▶ Metastatic mucinous adenocarcinoma

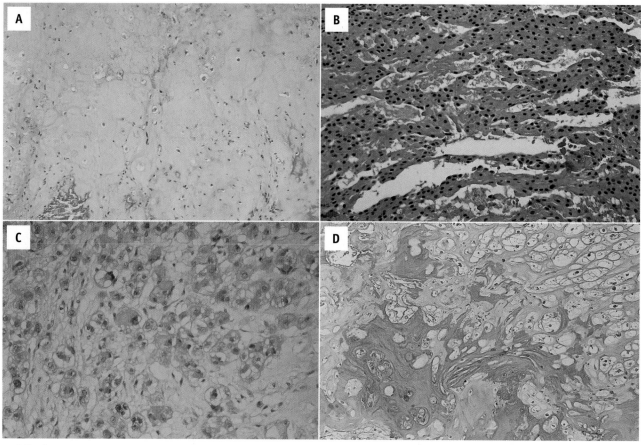

FIGURE 10-10

A, An area of chondroid differentiation in a chondroid chordoma. **B**, Cords and nests of epithelioid cells in a chordoma. **C**, Epithelioid cells with markedly vacuolated cytoplasm, so-called physaliphorous cells. **D**, Chondrosarcoma marked by atypical nuclei, in contrast to the bland nuclei of chondroid chordoma.

DIFFERENTIAL DIAGNOSIS

Metastatic mucinous adenocarcinoma may resemble chordoma but generally does not stain with S-100 protein. Chordoid meningiomas may superficially resemble chordoma, although they typically arise in other locations and do not usually demonstrate prominent cytokeratin positivity. In tumors with a chondroid component, differentiation from chondrosarcoma may be an issue. In general, the cartilaginous component in chondrosarcoma appears malignant with large pleomorphic nuclei (see Fig. 10-10D). Chondrosarcomas are cytokeratin negative.

PROGNOSIS AND THERAPY

Treatment of chordomas is wide excision because subtotally resected tumors tend to recur locally. A minority of tumors metastasize to distant sites, including the lung, lymph nodes, and skin. Radiotherapy is often used in the management of subtotally resected, recurrent tumors. Rare tumors dedifferentiate into high-grade sarcomas and have a particularly poor prognosis.

CHOROID PLEXUS TUMORS

CLINICAL FEATURES

Choroid plexus tumors account for less than 1% of all brain tumors and approximately 2% to 4% of brain tumors in children. Approximately 80% of choroid plexus tumors arise in children, with the majority being situated in the lateral ventricles. There is no definite gender predilection for choroid plexus neoplasms. Because of their intraventricular location, they are most commonly associated with signs and symptoms related to hydrocephalus and increased intracranial pressure. Radiographically, they are hyperintense, contrast-enhancing lesions.

CHOROID PLEXUS TUMORS—FACT SHEET

Definition

▶ Papillary, intraventricular neoplasm derived from choroid plexus epithelium

Incidence and Location

▶ 0.4% to 0.6% of all brain tumors
▶ 2% to 4% of all brain tumors in children
▶ Average annual incidence of 0.3 per 1,000,000
▶ Choroid plexus papilloma-to-carcinoma ratio of 5:1
▶ Intraventricular location: 50% lateral ventricle, 5% third ventricle, and 40% fourth ventricle

Gender and Age Distribution

▶ 80% of choroid plexus tumors arise in children
▶ 80% of lateral ventricle tumors develop in the first 2 decades; fourth ventricle tumors seen in all age groups
▶ M/F ratio for lateral ventricle tumors, 1:1; for fourth ventricle tumors, 3:2

Clinical Features

▶ Signs and symptoms related to hydrocephalus and increased intracranial pressure

Radiologic Features

▶ Hyperdense, contrast-enhancing tumor with hydrocephalus

Prognosis and Treatment

▶ Papillomas are low grade (WHO grade I) and curable by surgery
▶ Carcinoma (WHO grade III) has a poor outcome with a 40% survival rate at 5 years
▶ Gross total resection is the treatment of choice for carcinoma
▶ Poor prognosis associated with mitosis, necrosis, brain invasion, and absent/decreased transthyretin and S-100 immunostaining

CHOROID PLEXUS TUMORS—PATHOLOGIC FEATURES

Gross Findings

▶ Papillomas—intraventricular, circumscribed papillary masses
▶ Carcinomas—infiltrative solid mass with necrosis

Microscopic Findings

▶ Papillomas marked by fibrovascular papillary cores lined by stratified epithelial cells
▶ Minimal cytologic atypia and mitotic activity in papillomas
▶ Rare papillomas may demonstrate oncocytic and mucinous change, melanin, tubular architecture, and metaplastic cartilage or bone
▶ Carcinomas marked by nuclear pleomorphism, increased mitotic activity, increased cellularity, necrosis, and brain invasion

Ultrastructural Features

▶ Interdigitating membranes, microvilli, tight junctions, and some cells with cilia

Immunohistochemical Features

▶ Positive for vimentin, keratin, and S-100 protein; subset focally positive for GFAP and transthyretin

Genetics

▶ SV40 DNA sequences in about 50% of tumors
▶ Hyperdiploidy with genes on chromosomes 7, 9, 12, 15, 17, and 18

Differential Diagnosis

▶ Metastatic carcinoma
▶ Ependymoma

PATHOLOGIC FEATURES

Grossly, papillomas are somewhat circumscribed papillary masses. In contrast, choroid plexus carcinomas are solid masses frequently punctuated with necrosis and an infiltrative margin.

Histologically, choroid plexus papillomas are characterized by a proliferation of bland choroid plexus epithelial cells lining fibrovascular cores (Fig. 10-11A). Minimal mitotic activity and cytologic atypia are present. In contrast, carcinomas are marked by nuclear atypia, increased mitotic activity, increased cellularity, necrosis, and brain invasion (see Fig. 10-11B). Ultrastructurally, choroid plexus tumor cells are characterized by microvilli, tight junctions, and interdigitating membranes. By immunohistochemistry, tumors generally stain with antibodies to keratin and S-100 protein. Focal GFAP immunoreactivity and immunostaining with transthyretin may also be observed.

DIFFERENTIAL DIAGNOSIS

Particularly in children, differentiation of papillary ependymoma from choroid plexus papilloma may at times be problematic. In general, papillary ependymomas have a gliovascular core, demonstrate more widespread GFAP immunoreactivity, and are marked by the formation of perivascular pseudorosettes and true ependymal rosettes. Metastatic papillary carcinomas are in the differential diagnosis of choroid plexus carcinomas. Distinction of these two tumor types may be quite difficult on occasion. Most metastatic carcinomas occur in older aged patients.

PROGNOSIS AND THERAPY

Choroid plexus papillomas are low-grade lesions (WHO grade I) that are potentially curable by surgical excision. Choroid plexus carcinomas are higher-grade lesions (WHO grade III) with a poor outcome and a 40% 5-year survival rate. Gross total resection is the therapeutic modality of choice for carcinomas and may be followed by radiation therapy, chemotherapy, or both.

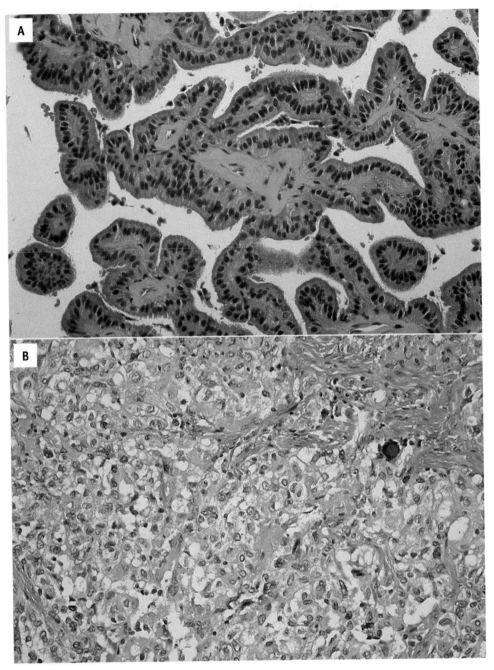

FIGURE 10-11

A, Choroid plexus papilloma marked by hyperplasia of bland choroid plexus epithelial cells on fibrovascular stalks. **B**, Choroid plexus carcinoma characterized by a sheet-like proliferation of atypical cells resembling carcinoma.

NEUROCYTOMA

CLINICAL FEATURES

Neurocytomas can arise at any age but have a peak incidence between the third and fifth decades. Classically, these tumors are located in the lateral ventricles near the foramen of Monro and show no obvious gender predilection. Symptoms are usually related to increased intracranial pressure. Radiographically, these tumors appear as contrast-enhancing or isointense lesions on computed tomography (CT) and may be calcified or focally cystic.

PATHOLOGIC FEATURES

Grossly, these intraventricular tumors are somewhat circumscribed, soft, and friable with variable amounts of calcification, hemorrhage, and cystic change (Fig. 10-12A).

Histologically, the neoplasm is marked by a proliferation of rounded cells with scant cytoplasm; the cells are

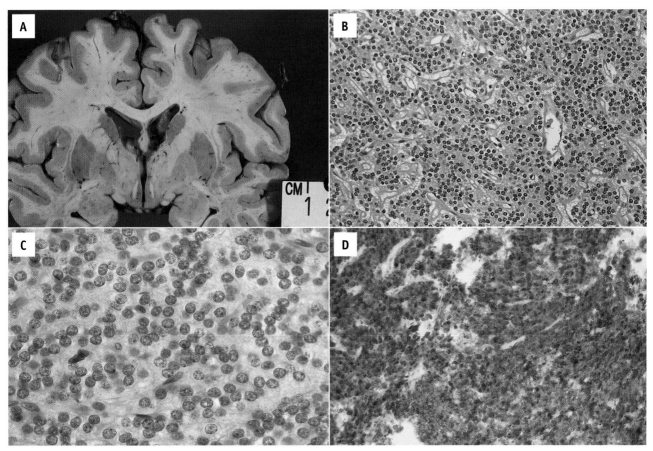

FIGURE 10-12

A, Coronal section showing a lateral ventricular mass typical of a central neurocytoma. **B**, Central neurocytoma characterized by a proliferation of rounded cells with a prominent vasculature somewhat reminiscent of oligodendroglioma. **C**, Higher-magnification appearance of cells in neurocytoma showing a finely speckled chromatin pattern. **D**, Diffuse synaptophysin immunoreactivity in a central neurocytoma.

NEUROCYTOMA—FACT SHEET

Definition

▶ Low-grade, neuronally differentiated neoplasm, typically in an intraventricular location

Incidence and Location

▶ 0.25% to 0.5% of intracranial tumors
▶ Most located in the lateral ventricles near the foramen of Monro; rare cases are extraventricular

Gender and Age Distribution

▶ Equal gender distribution
▶ Age range: infancy to seventh decade, peak incidence between 20 and 40 years of age

Clinical Features

▶ Symptoms related to increased intracranial pressure
▶ Short duration of symptoms before diagnosis

Radiologic Features

▶ On CT—isodense, contrast enhancing, may be calcified or cystic
▶ On MRI—normal to high signal intensity, enhances with gadolinium

Prognosis and Treatment

▶ Typically benign clinical course
▶ May recur locally with incomplete excision
▶ Cerebrospinal dissemination unusual
▶ Treatment of choice—surgical excision; possible role for radiotherapy in recurrent, subtotally excised tumors

---

arranged against a fibrillary background (see Fig. 10-12B). Nuclei have a finely speckled chromatin pattern (see Fig. 10-12C). The tumor is often accompanied by an arcuate capillary vascular pattern and may be calcified. By ultrastructural examination and immunohistochemistry, these neoplasms are marked by evidence of neural differentiation in the form of immunoreactivity to antibodies such as synaptophysin (see Fig. 10-12D), neuron-specific enolase, and class III β-tubulin. Ultrastructurally, these tumors demonstrate neurofilaments, neurotubule formation, and neurosecretory granules. Immunoreactivity to GFAP is unusual.

NEUROCYTOMA—PATHOLOGIC FEATURES

Gross Findings

▶ Intraventricular, gray friable tumors with variable calcification, cystic change, and hemorrhage

Microscopic Findings

▶ Sheets of uniform-appearing round cells with a fibrillary background
▶ Nuclei with a finely speckled chromatin pattern
▶ Arborizing capillary vascular pattern with calcification in about half the tumors
▶ Rare Homer Wright rosettes or ganglion cells
▶ Rare tumors with anaplastic features (increased mitoses, vascular proliferation, necrosis)—potentially more aggressive behavior

Ultrastructural Features

▶ Evidence of neural differentiation (neurotubules and neurofilaments, neurosecretory granules)

Immunohistochemical Features

▶ Positive for synaptophysin, neuron-specific enolase, class III β-tubulin, tau protein, MAP2
▶ Generally negative (or rare positivity) for GFAP and chromogranin antibody

Genetics

▶ No genetic alteration consistently recognized

Differential Diagnosis

▶ Oligodendroglioma
▶ Clear cell ependymoma
▶ Dysembryoplastic neuroepithelial tumor

DIFFERENTIAL DIAGNOSIS

Morphologically, these tumors resemble intraventricular oligodendrogliomas. Except for minor differences in the nuclear chromatin pattern, the two may be indistinguishable by casual light microscopic evaluation. Whenever a diagnosis of intraventricular oligodendroglioma is being considered, immunostaining with neural antibodies is warranted to exclude neurocytoma. Rare examples of clear cell ependymoma have also been described. These tumors generally have other areas with a more typical ependymoma appearance consisting of rosettes and perivascular pseudorosettes. Ependymomas do not stain with markers of neural differentiation and are ultrastructurally characterized by microvilli, cilia, and cell junctions. Dysembryoplastic neuroepithelial tumors are parenchymal-based lesions that are typically multinodular and cortical based and frequently arise in children in the setting of chronic epilepsy.

PROGNOSIS AND THERAPY

Central neurocytomas are regarded as low-grade lesions (WHO grade II) with an excellent prognosis. Surgical resection is curative. Rare cases of subtotally resected tumors recur locally. Radiation therapy is reserved for tumors that are problematic in terms of multiple recurrences.

EMBRYONAL TUMORS

CLINICAL FEATURES

Embryonal tumors include a constellation of neoplasms that most commonly arise during childhood. The prototypical tumor is medulloblastoma. The nomenclature is, in part, dependent on the location of the lesion. Cerebellar tumors, which are most commonly manifested as truncal ataxia and gait disturbances and with symptoms related to increased intracranial pressure, are generally medulloblastomas. Cerebral lesions resembling medulloblastoma are referred to as neuroblastomas; they are mostly commonly associated with symptoms related to focal cranial nerve deficits, headaches, and seizures. There is a slight male preponderance for medulloblastomas and atypical teratoid/rhabdoid tumors. On MRI, most tumors show decreased intensity on T1-weighted images and decreased density or isodensity on T2-weighted images with gadolinium enhancement. The most common genetic defect observed in medulloblastoma involves chromosome 17. A particularly distinctive feature of atypical teratoid/rhabdoid tumors is a deletion on chromosome 22.

PATHOLOGIC FEATURES

Most of these tumors, because of their marked cellularity, are soft, fleshy masses that appear somewhat circumscribed, although microscopically they are found to be infiltrative. Necrosis and hemorrhage are fairly common gross findings.

Histologically, medulloblastomas and neuroblastomas have similar histology and are marked by a proliferation of small cells with a high nuclear-to-cytoplasmic ratio (Fig. 10-13A). The tumors are associated with prominent mitotic activity and apoptosis. Some tumors contain large or even multinucleated cells (see Fig. 10-13B). Homer Wright pseudorosettes are evident in about a third of medulloblastomas. Some tumors may demonstrate evidence of ganglionic or glial cell differentiation, and rare examples of the tumors with muscle differentiation or melanin pigmentation

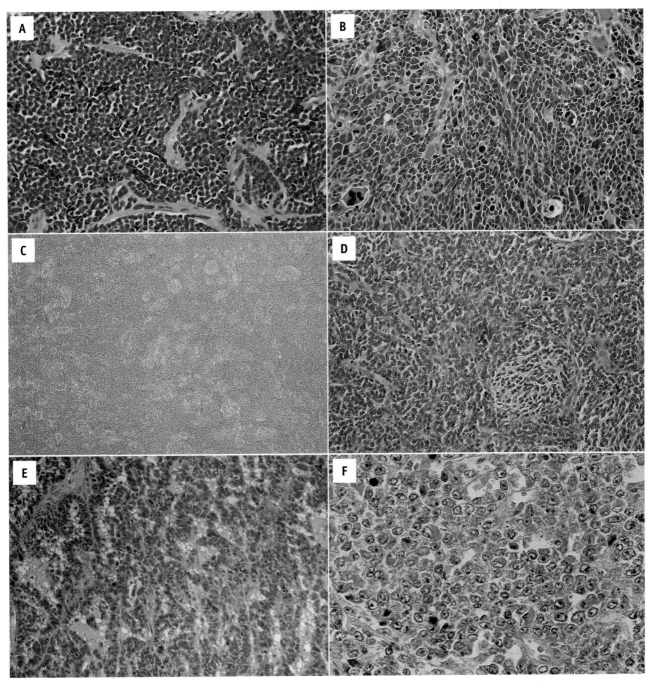

FIGURE 10-13

A, Medulloblastoma marked by a sheet-like proliferation of small blue cells. **B**, Large cell variant of medulloblastoma characterized by a sub-population of cells with increased size and occasional multinucleation. **C**, Low-magnification appearance of a desmoplastic medulloblastoma punctuated by scattered pale-staining islands. **D**, Higher-magnification appearance of a desmoplastic medulloblastoma marked by islands of loosely arranged cells arranged against a typical medulloblastoma background. **E**, Cords and trabeculae of epithelial cells in a medulloepithelioma. **F**, Atypical teratoid/rhabdoid tumor characterized by cells with eosinophilic cytoplasmic inclusions.

Continued

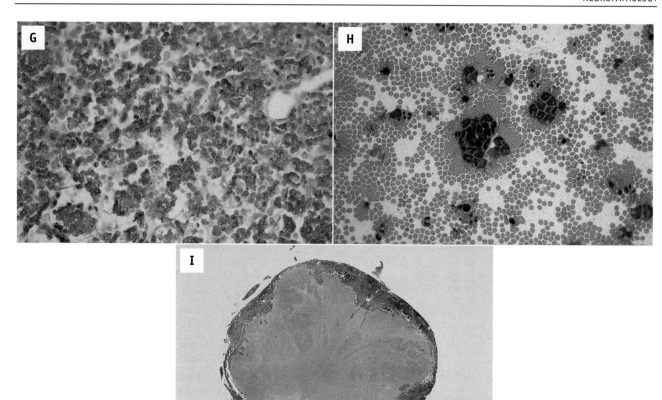

FIGURE 10-13, cont'd

G, Diffuse synaptophysin immunoreactivity in a medulloblastoma. **H**, Wright-stained cerebrospinal fluid cytology showing several exfoliated cells from a medulloblastoma, which has a predilection for seeding cerebrospinal fluid. **I**, Medulla encased by leptomeningeal, metastatic medulloblastoma.

EMBRYONAL TUMORS—FACT SHEET

Definition

▶ Group of round cell tumors capable of demonstrating divergent patterns of differentiation. Includes entities such as myoepithelioma, medulloblastoma, neuroblastoma, ependymoblastoma, pineoblastoma, and atypical teratoid/rhabdoid tumor

Incidence and Location

▶ Medulloblastomas have an incidence of 0.5 per 100,000 children
▶ Other types are less common
▶ Locations are somewhat type dependent: medulloblastoma—cerebellum; atypical teratoid/rhabdoid tumor—posterior fossa > supratentorial; neuroblastoma—supratentorial; pineoblastoma—pineal gland; ependymoblastoma—supratentorial; medulloepithelioma—supratentorial > infratentorial

Gender and Age Distribution

▶ Vast majority arise in pediatric patients, with a peak in the first decade
▶ Medulloblastoma and atypical teratoid/rhabdoid tumor have a slight male preponderance

Clinical Features

▶ Depends on location

▶ Cerebellar tumors, medulloblastoma—truncal ataxia, gait disturbances, increased intracranial pressure
▶ Noncerebellar tumors—head tilt, cranial nerve palsies, headaches, focal neural deficits, seizures
▶ High-grade tumors with a propensity to disseminate throughout the CNS axis

Radiologic Features

▶ On CT, typically solid, homogeneously contrast-enhancing masses; may have cystic or necrotic foci
▶ On MRI, decreased density on T1-weighted images and decreased density or isodensity on T2-weighted images, enhancement with gadolinium

Prognosis and Treatment

▶ Prognosis somewhat dependent on tumor type
▶ Medulloblastomas have a 50% to 85% 5-year survival rate; neuroblastomas, 30% 5-year survival rate
▶ Poor prognostic features for medulloblastoma: age younger than 3 years, metastases at initial evaluation, subtotal surgical resection, large cell variant, GFAP expression (glial differentiation), *myc* gene amplification
▶ Favorable prognostic features for medulloblastoma: desmoplastic variant (?), TrkC receptor expression
▶ Atypical teratoid/rhabdoid tumor with a very poor prognosis; most die within 1 year of diagnosis

EMBRYONAL TUMORS—PATHOLOGIC FEATURES

Gross Findings

▶ Variably soft and circumscribed, necrosis common, hemorrhage may occur

Microscopic Findings

▶ Medulloblastomas and neuroblastoma have similar histology—small blue cell neoplasms with a high nuclear-to-cytoplasmic ratio, prominent mitotic activity, and apoptosis (necrosis)
▶ Homer Wright rosettes in about a third of cases
▶ May demonstrate ganglionic cell or glial differentiation
▶ Rare tumors with muscle differentiation (medullomyoblastoma) or melanin pigment (melanotic medulloblastoma)
▶ The desmoplastic medulloblastoma variant has nodular, reticulin-free zones
▶ The large cell medulloblastoma variant has large pleomorphic nuclei with prominent nucleoli and more abundant cytoplasm
▶ Ependymoblastoma is marked by multilayered rosettes
▶ Medulloepitheliomas are characterized by a papillary, tubular, or trabecular arrangement of neuroepithelium
▶ Atypical teratoid/rhabdoid tumor has rhabdoid cells with eccentric nuclei, prominent nucleoli, and cytoplasmic pink body inclusion

Ultrastructural Features

▶ Neurally differentiated cells with neurite cytoplasmic processes, microtubules, synapses, and dense-core vesicles
▶ Glial differentiation marked by intermediate cytoplasmic filaments
▶ The cytoplasmic pink body inclusion of atypical teratoid/rhabdoid tumor consists of a whorled collection of intermediate filaments

Immunohistochemical Features

▶ Medulloblastoma positive for synaptophysin; variably positive for nestin, neuron-specific enolase, GFAP, vimentin, and S-100 protein; positive for Trk and nerve growth factor
▶ Muscle markers (myoglobin, desmin) positive in medullomyoblastoma
▶ Atypical teratoid/rhabdoid tumors are EMA and vimentin positive; variably positive for smooth muscle actin, GFAP, and keratin

Genetics

▶ Medulloblastoma—most common defects involve chromosome 17; less commonly, chromosome 1, 7, 10, and 11 abnormalities
▶ Atypical teratoid/rhabdoid tumors—90% with deletion on chromosome 22 (hSNF5/INI1 genes)

Differential Diagnosis

▶ Small cell carcinoma
▶ High-grade gliomas
▶ Sarcoma

have been described. The desmoplastic variant of medulloblastoma is marked by nodular areas of reticulin-free zones (see Fig. 10-13C and D). This subtype tends to be located in the more lateral aspects of the cerebellum and has been reported by some to have a better prognosis.

Medulloepitheliomas have a papillary, tubular, or trabecular arrangement of neuroepithelial cells, often intermixed with areas that look more like conventional medulloblastoma (see Fig. 10-13E). Pineoblastomas have histologic features similar to those of medulloblastoma but arise in the pineal gland. Ependymoblastoma resembles medulloblastoma but is accompanied by somewhat distinctive multilayered rosettes. Atypical teratoid/rhabdoid tumors are characterized by the presence of rhabdoid-type cells with eccentric nuclei, prominent nucleoli, and cytoplasmic eosinophilic body inclusions (see Fig. 10-13F).

By immunohistochemistry, most embryonal tumors demonstrate evidence of neural differentiation (see Fig. 10-13G). Atypical teratoid/rhabdoid tumors are characteristically positive for a variety of markers, including EMA, smooth muscle actin, cytokeratin, and GFAP.

Ultrastructurally, the tumors of this group demonstrate evidence of neural differentiation in the form of synaptic-type structures, dense secretory granules, and neural tubules. Atypical teratoid/rhabdoid tumors consist of cytoplasmic collections of intermediate-molecular-weight filaments.

DIFFERENTIAL DIAGNOSIS

The most common differential diagnostic consideration is high-grade gliomas (astrocytomas and ependymomas). Most high-grade gliomas show some evidence of GFAP immunoreactivity and generally do not stain with neural markers. Rare cases of metastatic small cell carcinoma may be confused with embryonal tumors. Most small cell carcinomas arise in adults, and their immunohistochemical profiles may overlap. Evidence of Homer Wright rosettes or glial differentiation supports a diagnosis of CNS embryonal tumor. Rare examples of small cell sarcoma have also been described; these tumors do not demonstrate evidence of neural differentiation by immunohistochemistry.

PROGNOSIS AND TREATMENT

The prognosis is somewhat dependent on tumor type. Medulloblastomas are associated with much better survival now than they historically used to be. In contrast, neuroblastomas still do fairly poorly, with a 30% 5-year survival rate. Of particular note is that atypical teratoid/rhabdoid tumors have a very poor prognosis, with most patients succumbing to their tumor within 1 year of diagnosis. Poor prognostic features in medulloblastoma include young age at diagnosis (<3 years), metastasis at initial evaluation, subtotal surgical resection (see Fig. 10-13H and I), large cell variants, glial differentiation by immunohistochemical evaluation, and myc gene amplification.

SCHWANNOMAS

CLINICAL FEATURES

Schwannomas may arise at any age, but most occur in adults; there is a known association with neurofibromatosis type 2. Most tumors are manifested as a symptomatic mass. Occasionally, patients have evidence of pain, cord compression, or cranial nerve deficits. Cranial nerve VIII (acoustic neuroma) is the most common cranial nerve involved by schwannoma. Radiographically, tumors are heterogeneously enhancing, well circumscribed, and sometimes cystic.

PATHOLOGIC FEATURES

Grossly, schwannomas are circumscribed, frequently encapsulated masses that are generally light tan (Fig. 10-14A). Histologically, they are biphasic lesions consisting of Antoni A areas of compactly arranged cells and

---

SCHWANNOMA—FACT SHEET

Definition

▶ Benign tumor derived from Schwann cells; also known as neurilemoma, acoustic neuroma

Incidence and Location

▶ Most frequently arise in association with peripheral nerves, most commonly in the head and neck region and on the extremities
▶ 8% of intracranial and 29% of spinal tumors (extramedullary)
▶ Association with neurofibromatosis type 2

Gender and Age Distribution

▶ No gender predilection except for intracranial tumors (F/M ratio of 2:1)
▶ Any age, peak between the fourth and sixth decades

Clinical Features

▶ Most commonly occur as asymptomatic masses
▶ Occasionally with pain, cord compression
▶ Cranial nerve VIII tumors—hearing loss, facial paresthesias, tinnitus

Radiologic Features

▶ Well-circumscribed, heterogeneously enhancing, sometimes cystic mass

Prognosis and Treatment

▶ Excellent prognosis (WHO grade I), only rarely undergoes malignant degeneration
▶ Curable with surgical resection

SCHWANNOMA—PATHOLOGIC FINDINGS

Gross Findings

▶ Circumscribed masses, frequently encapsulated, sometimes cystic
▶ Light tan color; may be yellow (macrophages) or red (hemorrhagic)

Microscopic Findings

▶ Cells with spindled nuclei, tapered ends
▶ Biphasic cellularity: compact cellular Antoni A pattern and loose microcystic Antoni B pattern
▶ Nuclear palisading—Verocay bodies
▶ Occasional mitotic figures and nuclear pleomorphism acceptable
▶ Cellular variant—hypercellular, predominantly Antoni A pattern
▶ Melanotic schwannoma—may have psammoma bodies (associated with Carney's complex)
▶ Plexiform variant—multinodular associated with neurofibromatosis type 2

Ultrastructural Features

▶ Cells with convoluted cytoplasmic processes lined by continuous basal lamina

Immunohistochemical Features

▶ S-100 positive, can be focally GFAP positive

Genetics

▶ NF2 gene (merlin protein) associated with sporadic schwannomas (60%)
▶ Subset with chromosome 22q losses

Differential Diagnosis

▶ Fibrous meningioma
▶ Neurofibroma
▶ Sarcoma (especially malignant peripheral nerve sheath tumor)
▶ Glioma

Antoni B areas with a looser, more microcystic appearance (see Fig. 10-14B). Cells generally have elongated nuclei with tapered, pointed ends. The arrangement of cells in a palisade, referred to as a Verocay body, is a common finding (see Fig. 10-14C). Occasional tumors demonstrate nuclear pleomorphism (so-called ancient change) that is of no clinical significance (see Fig. 10-14D). The cellular variant of schwannoma is marked by a predominantly hypercellular Antoni A pattern (see Fig. 10-14E). Melanotic schwannomas frequently have melanin pigment and psammoma bodies and are associated with the Carney complex (see Fig. 10-14F). Rare plexiform schwannomas have been described in association with neurofibromatosis type 2.

By immunohistochemistry, all schwannomas demonstrate diffuse strong positivity with antibody to S-100 protein. Ultrastructurally, cells are marked by convoluted cytoplasmic processes and have a continuous basal lamina.

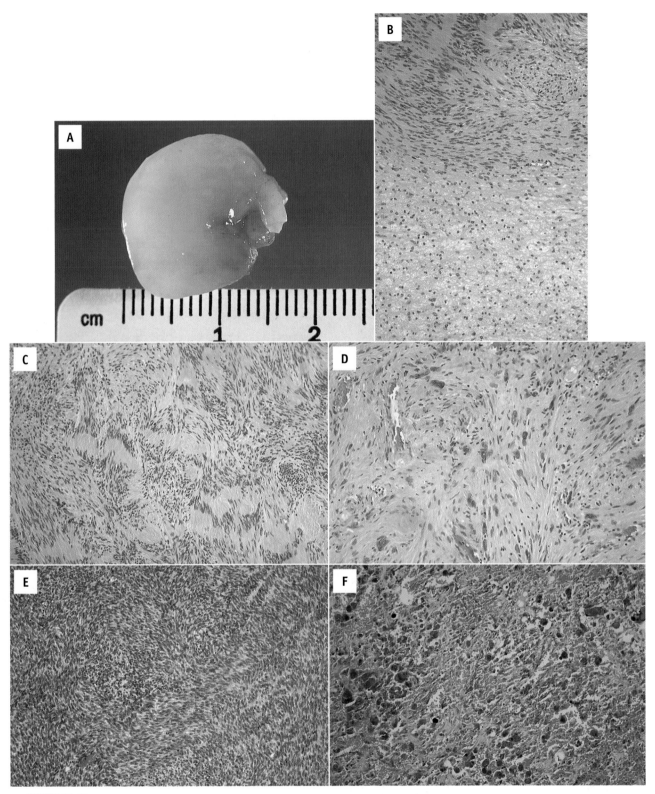

FIGURE 10-14

A, Well-circumscribed, yellow-tan schwannoma. **B**, Juxtaposition of the compact Antoni A pattern and the looser Antoni B pattern in a schwannoma. **C**, Verocay body formation in a schwannoma. **D**, Prominent nuclear pleomorphism in a schwannoma. Ancient change does not affect the prognosis. **E**, Marked hypercellularity in a cellular schwannoma. **F**, Prominent melanin pigment in a melanotic schwannoma associated with the Carney complex.

DIFFERENTIAL DIAGNOSIS

As previously mentioned, differentiation of schwannoma from fibrous meningioma may be easily accomplished with immunohistochemistry. Neurofibromas at times resemble the Antoni A pattern of a schwannoma. Sarcomas, particularly malignant peripheral nerve sheath tumors, are often more cellular than the usual schwannoma and are characterized by prominent mitotic activity. Rare spindled gliomas may also superficially resemble schwannomas, but they usually demonstrate GFAP immunoreactivity.

PROGNOSIS AND THERAPY

Schwannomas have a good prognosis (WHO grade I neoplasm) and are curable with surgical resection. Only rare cases of malignant degeneration have been documented.

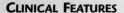

LYMPHOMA

CLINICAL FEATURES

Primary CNS lymphoma is one tumor that appears to be increasing in incidence worldwide. There is a well-known association of CNS lymphoma with immunocompromised states, particularly infection with human immunodeficiency virus (HIV). Many of these tumors have Epstein-Barr virus (EBV) as an underlying cause. In tumors arising outside the setting of an immunocompromised state, the peak incidence is in the sixth and seventh decades with a slight male preponderance. Patients typically have focal neural deficits related to the lesion. A significant subset of patients may also initially have ophthalmologic-related symptoms. Radiographically, tumors are hyperintense or isodense with variable degrees of enhancement. Periventricular extension of tumor is a common finding.

PATHOLOGIC FEATURES

Tumors may be either single or multiple. Primary CNS lymphomas tend to be parenchymal based, in contrast to secondary involvement of the brain by extra-CNS disease, which is more commonly leptomeningeal based (Fig. 10-15A). Tumors may be firm and are frequently friable, focally necrotic, and hemorrhagic.

Histologically, primary CNS lymphoma is marked by a perivascular proliferation of atypical lymphoid cells (see Fig. 10-15B). The angiocentric distribution of cells

LYMPHOMA—FACT SHEET

Definition
▶ Primary CNS lymphomas represent extranodal malignant lymphomas presumably arising in the CNS without obvious evidence of tumor outside the CNS at the time of diagnosis

Incidence and Location
▶ Incidence appears to be increasing worldwide
▶ Incidence rates of between 0.8% and 6.6% of primary intracranial neoplasms
▶ Associated with acquired immunodeficiency syndrome (AIDS) (EBV-related tumors); primary CNS lymphoma develops in 2% to 12% of AIDS patients
▶ Approximately 10% to 12% of post-transplant lymphoproliferative disorders are confined to the CNS
▶ About 60% of primary CNS lymphomas involve the supratentorial space; the frontal lobe is the most common single location
▶ About 25% to 50% of tumors are multifocal, with more than 50% occurring in AIDS and post-transplant patients
▶ 30% to 40% of primary CNS lymphomas spread to the leptomeninges

Gender and Age Distribution
▶ All ages affected, with a peak incidence during the sixth and seventh decades
▶ M/F ratio of 3:2

Clinical Features
▶ Majority of patients initially have focal neurologic deficits; minority of patients have neuropsychiatric symptoms, symptoms related to intracranial pressure, and seizures
▶ Approximately 5% to 20% of patients initially have evidence of eye involvement

Radiologic Features
▶ Solid or multiple hyperdense or isodense lesions with variable amounts of enhancement

Prognosis and Treatment
▶ Better prognostic factors include a single lesion, absence of meningeal or periventricular tumor, immunocompetent individual, age younger than 60 years, and preoperative Karnofsky score greater than 70
▶ Current therapy involves radiation and chemotherapy. Two-year survival rate of 40% to 70% and 5-year survival rate of 25% to 45%
▶ Tumors are often initially steroid responsive, which may make a diagnosis on biopsy samples difficult after initiation of steroids
▶ Tumors arising in immunocompromised individuals have a worse prognosis, with median survival of less than 1 year

is often associated with concentric perivascular reticulin deposits. With time, tumors can become confluent, marked by sheets of atypical lymphoid cells. Histologically and by immunohistochemistry, the vast majority of primary CNS lymphomas are diffuse large B-cell tumors (see Fig. 10-15C). A small percentage of T-cell lymphomas have been described. In the setting of organ

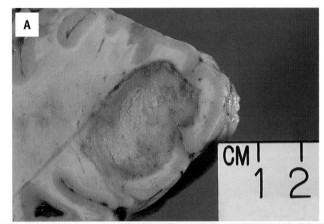

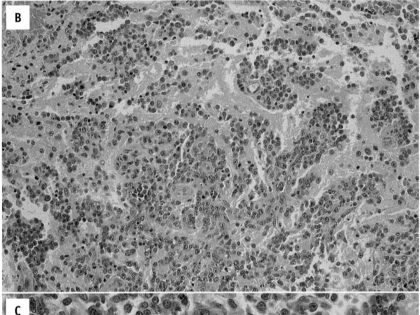

FIGURE 10-15

A, Grossly circumscribed, partially necrotic, parenchymal-based primary CNS lymphoma. **B**, Angiocentric arrangement of tumor cells in primary CNS lymphoma. **C**, Most primary CNS lymphomas are morphologically diffuse large cell lymphomas with a B-cell immunophenotype.

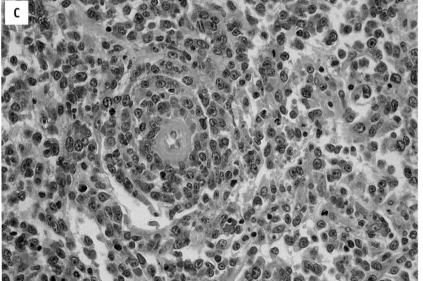

LYMPHOMAS—PATHOLOGIC FEATURES

Gross Findings

▶ Single or multiple masses in the cerebral hemispheres
▶ Tumors may be firm, friable, focally necrotic, and hemorrhagic
▶ Meningeal involvement may not be apparent grossly

Microscopic Features

▶ Proliferation of discohesive, diffusely infiltrating atypical lymphoid cells
▶ Cells often arranged in an angiocentric pattern with concentric perivascular reticulin deposits
▶ Vast majority of tumors are diffuse large B-cell lymphomas (CD20⁺ and CD79a⁺) with a variable number of associated small benign tumor-infiltrating T lymphocytes
▶ Approximately 2% of CNS lymphomas are of the T-cell type
▶ Angiotrophic large cell lymphomas or intravascular lymphomas are marked by tumor cells confined to the vascular spaces, frequently associated with infarcts related to vascular occlusion
▶ Hodgkin's disease rare in the CNS, morphologically resembles extra-CNS disease with CD30⁺ Reed-Sternberg cells
▶ Rare examples of low-grade B-cell MALT lymphomas of the dura, usually associated with a follicular growth pattern and germinal center formation

Ultrastructural Features

▶ Cells marked by a lack of specific ultrastructural features, i.e., lack of intermediate filaments, specific organelles, and intercellular junctions

Immunohistochemical Features

▶ Tumors generally stain with leukocyte common antigen (LCA) (CD45RB). Evaluation of tumor with B-cell lymphoid markers (such as CD20 and CD79a) and T-cell marker (CD3) is useful

Genetics

▶ No genetic predisposition to primary CNS lymphoma is recognized
▶ A significant subset of tumors in immunocompromised individuals have an associated EBV genome present in the tumor cells
▶ Gene rearrangement studies may be useful in confirming the diagnosis of lymphoma

Differential Diagnosis

▶ Secondary involvement of the CNS by lymphoma (more commonly leptomeningeal and dural based)
▶ Metastatic carcinoma
▶ Small cell glioblastoma multiforme
▶ Non-neoplastic inflammatory lesions, including infection, vasculitis, and demyelinating disorders

transplantation, the development of a lymphomatous-type process prompts use of the terminology post-transplant lymphoproliferative disorder, since only a subset of these tumors represent true lymphomas. Rarely, other types of lymphoma have been reported to involve the CNS, including angiotrophic large cell lymphomas (intravascular lymphoma), Hodgkin's disease, and MALT (mucosal-associated lymphoid tissue) lymphoma of the dura.

DIFFERENTIAL DIAGNOSIS

Distinction of primary CNS lymphoma from secondary spread of extra-CNS lymphoma generally requires correlation with the clinical history and demonstration of lymphoma elsewhere in the body. Distinction of lymphoma from non-neoplastic inflammatory conditions, particularly infection, vasculitis, and demyelinating disease, can be problematic. Non-neoplastic lesions generally lack the prerequisite cytologic atypia that marks lymphoma. Immunohistochemical staining with lymphoid markers such as CD20 or CD45RB is helpful in distinguishing lymphoma from other small cell malignant neoplasms, particularly metastatic small cell carcinoma and the small cell variant of glioblastoma multiforme.

PROGNOSIS AND THERAPY

Primary CNS lymphomas have a poor prognosis with 5-year survival rates of 25% to 45%. In immunocompromised patients, survival rates are much worse. These tumors are often initially quite steroid responsive, and it is generally recommended that the lesion undergo biopsy before the commencement of steroid therapy. Periventricular or leptomeningeal spread is also associated with a poor prognosis.

HISTIOCYTIC TUMORS

CLINICAL FEATURES

A wide spectrum of histiocytic lesions can be manifested as tumoral masses. As a group, these lesions are relatively uncommon. Langerhans cell histiocytosis generally occurs in the pediatric population and may be associated with signs related to hypothalamic dysfunction, increased intracranial pressure, cranial nerve symptoms, and seizures. Bone-based osteolytic lesions are not uncommon. Non–Langerhans cell histiocytosis is more common intracranially, may be dural based, and is frequently multifocal.

PATHOLOGIC FEATURES

Langerhans cell histiocytosis is marked by a mixed inflammatory cell infiltrate (Fig. 10-16A) and a proliferation of Langerhans-type histiocytes with eccentric, convoluted nuclei, conspicuous nucleoli, and abundant pale to lightly eosinophilic cytoplasm (see Fig. 10-16B). These cells stain with antibodies to S-100 protein and CD1a and are ultrastructurally characterized by

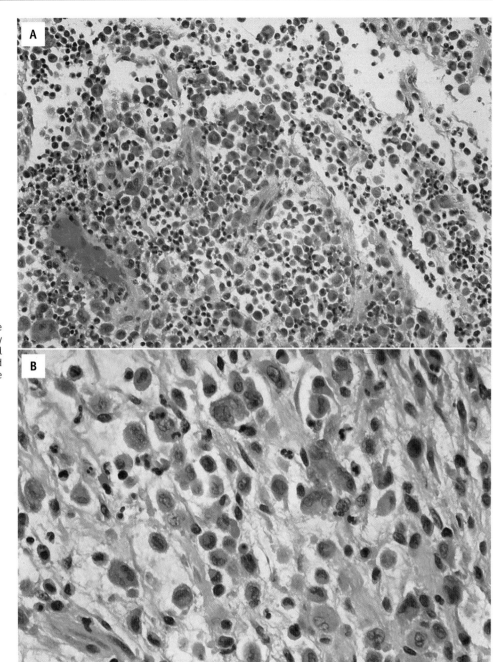

FIGURE 10-16

A, Typical heterogeneous mixture of acute and chronic inflammatory cells in histiocytosis X. **B**, Atypical histiocytic cells with convoluted nuclei typical of Langerhans-type histiocytes in histiocytosis X.

HISTIOCYTIC TUMORS—FACT SHEET

Definition

▶ Histiocytic tumors represent a heterogeneous group of tumor-like lesions composed primarily of histiocytes—either macrophage type or dendritic Langerhans cell type

Incidence and Location

▶ Incidence of Langerhans cell histiocytosis of approximately 0.2 to 0.5 per 100,000 population in children younger than 15 years
▶ Non–Langerhans cell histiocytosis less common; Langerhans cell histiocytosis frequently associated with bone lesions involving the skull or spine with occasional involvement of the CNS by direct extension
▶ Non–Langerhans cell histiocytosis more commonly intracranially or dural based, frequently multifocal lesions

Gender and Age Distribution

▶ Most Langerhans cell histiocytosis occurs in children, with no gender predilection
▶ Non–Langerhans cell histiocytosis may arise at any age, depending on type

Clinical Features

▶ Langerhans cell histiocytosis most commonly associated with diabetes insipidus, evidence of hypothalamic dysfunction, increased intracranial pressure, cranial nerve palsies, seizures, and visual disturbances
▶ Similar manifestations may be observed with non–Langerhans cell histiocytosis

Radiologic Features

▶ Osteolytic changes in bone
▶ Non–Langerhans cell lesions may show variable enhancement and may be manifested as dural-based masses (Rosai-Dorfman disease)

Prognosis and Treatment

▶ Survival rate for unifocal Langerhans cell histiocytosis at 5 years is 88% with minimal treatment (surgical resection)
▶ Multifocal or systemic disease has higher mortality rates and may be resistant to systemic therapy

---

HISTIOCYTIC TUMORS—PATHOLOGIC FEATURES

Gross Findings

▶ Langerhans cell histiocytosis and some non–Langerhans cell histiocytosis may be manifested as discrete dural-based masses marked by variable degrees of infiltration

Microscopic Features

▶ Langerhans cell histiocytosis marked by a proliferation of Langerhans-type histiocytes and a mixed inflammatory response consisting of macrophages, lymphocytes, plasma cells, eosinophils, and granulomas
▶ Langerhans cells associated with eccentric, convoluted nuclei with inconspicuous nucleoli and abundant pale to eosinophilic cytoplasm
▶ Rosai-Dorfman disease characterized by nodules of histiocytic cells with vacuolated, eosinophilic cytoplasm; frequently associated with emperipoiesis (lymphocytes and plasma cells within the cytoplasm of histiocytes)
▶ Erdheim-Chester disease marked by lipid-laden histiocytes with small nuclei, Touton giant cells, and scant numbers of lymphocytes and eosinophils
▶ Hemophagocytic lymphohistiocytosis marked by lymphocytes and macrophages and hemophagocytosis

Ultrastructural Features

▶ Langerhans cell histiocytes are characterized by Birbeck granules (34-nm-wide wedge-shaped or tennis racquet–shaped, intracytoplasmic pentilaminar structures)

Immunohistochemical Features

▶ Langerhans cell histiocytes are S-100 protein positive, vimentin positive, and characteristically CD1a positive
▶ Histiocytes of Rosai-Dorfman disease are CD1a negative, CD11c positive, CD68 positive, and S-100 protein positive
▶ The histiocytic cells of Erdheim-Chester disease are CD1a negative, CD68 positive, and S-100 protein negative
▶ The histiocytic cells of hemophagocytic lymphocytosis are variably CD1a and S-100 protein positive, CD11c positive, and CD68 positive

Genetics

▶ Most of these disorders do not have a known genetic abnormality associated with them. Genes responsible for hemophagocytic lymphohistiocytosis may be located on chromosomes 19q and 10q

Differential Diagnosis

▶ Lymphoma
▶ Non-neoplastic reactive inflammatory lesions, including infection and demyelinating disorders

---

the presence of Birbeck granules. Many of the non-Langerhans histiocytoses are marked by a proliferation of more conventional-appearing histiocytic cells, generally do not stain with CD1a antibody, and frequently demonstrate CD68 immunoreactivity.

DIFFERENTIAL DIAGNOSIS

Distinction of these lesions from non-neoplastic reactive or inflammatory conditions associated with increased numbers of macrophages, such as infection or demyelinating disorders, is the main challenge. In most cases, the clinical history is helpful, and in the case of Langerhans cell histiocytosis, immunohistochemical staining with CD1a antibody can be particularly useful. Rarely, immunohistochemistry may be required to differentiate these lesions from a lymphomatous process.

PROGNOSIS AND THERAPY

Survival rates for Langerhans cell histiocytosis are generally good, with 5-year rates of approximately 88%

in patients with unifocal disease. Those with more widespread systemic disease or multifocal disease tend to have higher mortality rates.

CYSTS

CLINICAL FEATURES

A variety of cysts can arise throughout the neuraxis, the clinical manifestations of which are somewhat depend-

ent on the location of the cyst. The details regarding specific cyst types are outlined on the fact sheet.

PATHOLOGIC FEATURES

Gross and histologic appearances are dependent on the type of cyst (Fig. 10-17). These details are presented in the box describing the pathologic features of cysts.

CYSTS—FACT SHEET

Definition
- ▶ Benign cystic lesions lined by epithelial or neuroglial tissue

Incidence and Location
- ▶ Colloid cyst near the foramen of Monro
- ▶ Rathke's cleft cyst situated at the interface between the anterior and posterior lobes of the pituitary gland
- ▶ Endodermal cyst—intracranial and intraspinal locations
- ▶ Ependymal cyst—proximal to the ventricular system and central canal
- ▶ Choroid plexus cyst—associated with choroid plexus epithelium
- ▶ Epidermoid and dermoid cysts—most epidermoid cysts are intracranial and arise in the cerebellopontine angle region; dermoid cysts are midline masses
- ▶ Arachnoid cyst associated with the meninges, the temporal lobe region being the favored site

Gender and Age Distribution
- ▶ Most cysts have no gender predilection
- ▶ Cyst types may arise at any age

Clinical Features
- ▶ Colloid cysts classically produce symptoms, including headache, sudden paralysis of the lower extremities, incontinence, personality changes, dementia, and rarely, sudden death
- ▶ Rathke's cleft cysts are frequently asymptomatic; if large enough they may become symptomatic and produce visual symptoms or abnormalities in pituitary function
- ▶ Many endodermal cysts, ependymal cysts, and choroid plexus cysts are asymptomatic
- ▶ Symptoms associated with epidermoid cysts, dermoid cysts, and arachnoid cysts are related to location and size of the lesions

Radiologic Features
- ▶ Colloid and Rathke's cleft cysts marked by increased signal on unenhanced T1-weighted MRI because of a high protein content of these cysts
- ▶ Epidermoid and dermoid cysts with variable radiointensity related to the lipid and hair content of the cyst

Prognosis and Treatment
- ▶ All cysts are benign lesions that can be managed by surgical resection if symptomatic

---

CYSTS—PATHOLOGIC FEATURES

Gross Findings
- ▶ Colloid and Rathke's cleft cysts have a thin-walled lining with cloudy, thick fluid
- ▶ Endodermal cysts are thin walled with mucoid material
- ▶ Epidermoid and dermoid cysts are marked by keratinaceous debris and hair (dermoid cysts)
- ▶ Arachnoid cysts are thin walled with clear or slightly discolored fluid

Microscopic Features
- ▶ Colloid cysts are lined by a single layer of columnar ciliated or goblet cells and filled with brightly eosinophilic, colloid-like fluid (Fig. 10-17A).
- ▶ Rathke's cleft cysts are lined by columnar epithelial cells with ciliated and goblet cells (see Fig. 10-17B)
- ▶ Endodermal cysts are lined by columnar cells with variable ciliation and mucus-filled cells; squamous cell metaplasia may be present. Some lesions have respiratory- or gastrointestinal-type lining (see Fig. 10-17C).
- ▶ Ependymal cysts are lined by ciliated epithelial lining similar to ependymal cells
- ▶ Choroid plexus cysts are lined by choroid plexus–type epithelium
- ▶ Epidermoid cysts are lined by squamous-type epithelium filled with keratinaceous material (see Fig. 10-17D)
- ▶ Dermoid cysts are lined by squamous epithelium and associated adnexal structures (see Fig. 10-17E)
- ▶ Arachnoid cysts are lined by arachnoid cap cells (see Fig. 10-17F)

Ultrastructural Features
- ▶ Ultrastructural features not routinely used in classifying these lesions; many of the epithelial-lined cysts show features of epithelial cells
- ▶ Some cyst types such as colloid cysts consist of six different epithelial cell types

Immunohistochemical Features
- ▶ Many of the epithelial-lined cysts are positive for cytokeratins or EMA
- ▶ Focal immunoreactivity of colloid cysts with CEA and S-100 protein
- ▶ Occasional endocrine cells that may stain with pituitary hormones are associated with the lining of Rathke's cleft cyst
- ▶ Choroid plexus cyst associated with transthyretin positivity
- ▶ Arachnoid cyst typically EMA positive and negative for CEA and GFAP

Genetics
- ▶ No known genetic abnormality associated with the development of cysts
- ▶ Rare form of choroid plexus cyst may be associated with trisomy 18

Differential Diagnosis
- ▶ Typically involves distinguishing one cyst from another
- ▶ Distinction of epidermoid and dermoid cysts from cystic craniopharyngioma

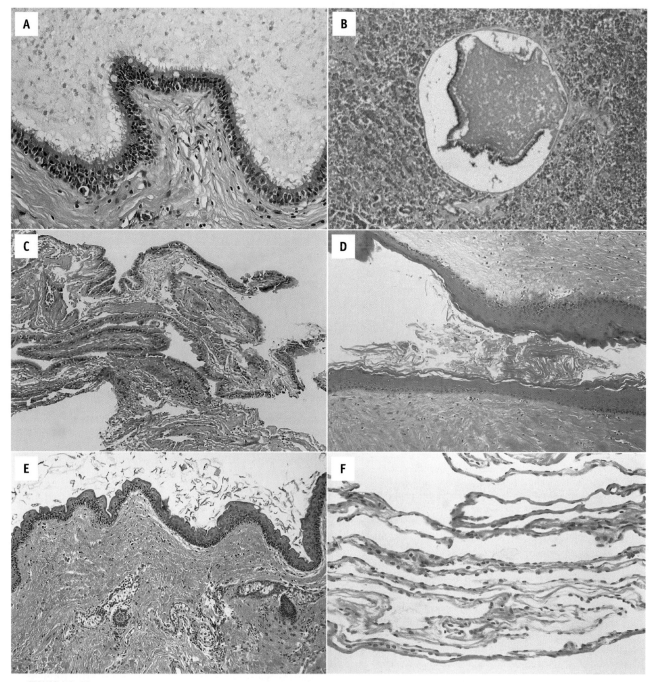

FIGURE 10-17

A, Colloid cyst marked by columnar ciliated epithelium. **B**, Columnar epithelial-lined Rathke's cleft cyst arising in the pituitary gland. **C**, Endodermal cyst lined by cuboidal to columnar epithelium. **D**, Epidermoid cyst lined by benign-appearing squamous epithelium and filled with keratinous material. **E**, Squamous epithelial–lined dermoid cyst with adnexal structures in the cyst wall. **F**, Thin-walled arachnoid cyst lined by arachnoid cap (meningothelial) cells.

DIFFERENTIAL DIAGNOSIS

The differential diagnosis usually focuses on distinguishing one cyst from another. Occasionally, distinction of epidermoid cysts from cystic craniopharyngioma may be an issue. Keratohyaline granules are not a feature of craniopharyngiomas. In addition, prominent inflammatory reactions with cholesterol cleft formation, microcalcifications, and "machine oil–like" fluid in the cyst are not characteristic of epidermoid cysts.

PROGNOSIS AND TREATMENT

All these cysts are benign lesions that can be managed surgically if symptomatic and are not generally prone to malignant degeneration.

GERM CELL TUMORS

CLINICAL FEATURES

The vast majority of germ cell neoplasms arising in the CNS are midline lesions in pediatric-aged patients. There appears to be a male preponderance in the cases that have been reported. The region around the third ventricle and the pineal gland area are often the sites of origin for these neoplasms, with the most common clinical manifestations including signs and symptoms related to CSF obstruction and intracranial hypertension. Many of these tumors secrete proteins that can be assayed in CSF. Radiographically, most of the tumors appear to be isodense or hyperdense solid neoplasms.

PATHOLOGIC FEATURES

Germ cell tumors are generally solid and may have a cystic component. Necrosis or hemorrhage is more commonly associated with higher-grade patterns of germ cell tumor, most notably in embryonal carcinoma, yolk sac tumor, and choriocarcinoma. Microscopically, these tumors resemble their counterparts in the ovary and testis. Occasionally, with a small biopsy specimen of a pineal gland mass, one might observe only granulomas, a finding highly suspicious for germinoma. At times, immunohistochemistry may be helpful in sorting out the germ cell tumor types that may be present. Germinomas may demonstrate placental alkaline phosphatase immunoreactivity. Yolk sac tumors commonly stain positively with antibody to α-fetoprotein. Embryonal carcinomas classically show immunoreactivity to CD30.

GERM CELL TUMORS—FACT SHEET

Definition
▶ Neoplasms that morphologically resemble germ cell lesions arising in the ovary or testis, including germinoma, teratoma, yolk sac tumor, embryonal carcinoma, and choriocarcinoma

Incidence and Location
▶ Account for approximately 0.3% to 0.5% of primary intracranial neoplasms in adults and 3% of intracranial tumors in children
▶ Most are midline lesions, with 80% or more arising in or around the third ventricle region and pineal gland

Gender and Age Distribution
▶ Approximately 90% of tumors arise in patients younger than 20 years
▶ M/F ratio of 2:1 to 2.5:1

Clinical Features
▶ Pineal-based tumors often associated with CSF obstruction and intracranial hypertension; less common manifestations include paralysis of upward gaze and convergence (Parinaud's syndrome), visual field defects, disruption of the hypothalamic/pituitary axis, and precocious puberty
▶ Serum and CSF assay for certain proteins generated by tumors (α-fetoprotein, β-HCG, placental alkaline phosphatase) may be helpful in preoperative diagnosis and postoperative monitoring

Radiologic Features
▶ Most lesions appear solid (except teratomas), either isodense or hyperdense relative to adjacent gray matter
▶ Most lesions show some degree of contrast enhancement

Prognosis and Treatment
▶ The histologic subtype is most important for prognosis
▶ Pure germinomas have an excellent prognosis and are radiosensitive with a 5-year survival rate ranging from 65% to 95%
▶ Gross total resection of noninvasive teratomas usually results in a good outcome
▶ Most tumors of the mixed germ cell type have a poor outcome

---

Choriocarcinomas demonstrate immunoreactivity to human chorionic gonadotropin (HCG).

DIFFERENTIAL DIAGNOSIS

In most cases, the differential diagnosis involves distinguishing one germ cell type from another. Mixed germ cell tumors, similar to those in the testis and ovary, are well recognized. Occasionally, distinguishing embryonal carcinoma or yolk sac tumors from metastatic carcinoma or high-grade glioma may be a consideration. Many germ cell tumors demonstrate focal cytokeratin immunoreactivity. GFAP positivity is not a feature of germ cell neoplasms.

GERM CELL TUMORS—PATHOLOGIC FEATURES

Gross Features

▶ Tumors are generally solid; teratomas may have a cystic component
▶ Presence of necrosis or hemorrhage usually associated with more aggressive patterns of germ cell tumor (embryonal carcinoma, yolk sac tumor, and choriocarcinoma); presence of teratomatous elements may dramatically alter the gross appearance of the lesion

Microscopic Features

▶ Histologic features are reminiscent of the germ cell tumor counterparts of these tumors arising in the ovary or testis
▶ Germinomas are composed of uniform large germ cells with vesicular nuclei, prominent nucleoli, and abundant clear cytoplasm usually associated with a prominent lymphoid infiltrate and occasional syncytiotrophoblastic-type giant cells (Fig. 10-18A)
▶ Teratomas are marked by differentiation along ectodermal, endodermal, and mesodermal cell lines; mature teratomas are composed of terminally differentiated tissues (see Fig. 10-18B); and immature teratomas are composed of incompletely differentiated tissue elements
▶ Yolk sac tumor marked by primitive-appearing epithelioid cells resembling yolk sac endoderm in a myxoid stroma with scattered eosinophilic hyaline globules (see Fig. 10-18C).
▶ Embryonal carcinoma composed of sheets and nests of large cells with prominent nucleoli, high mitotic rates, and frequent zones of necrosis (see Fig. 10-18D)
▶ Choriocarcinoma marked by proliferation of both cytotrophoblastic and syncytiotrophoblastic giant cell elements (see Fig. 10-18E).
▶ Ultrastructural features are not generally used in the routine evaluation of these neoplasms

Immunohistochemical Features

▶ Placental alkaline phosphatase positivity in germinomas
▶ Teratomas with cytokeratin and variable α-fetoprotein positivity
▶ Yolk sac tumors positive for α-fetoprotein and cytokeratins
▶ Embryonal carcinoma positive for placental alkaline phosphatase, cytokeratins and CD30
▶ Choriocarcinoma positive for HCG, human placental lactogen (HPL), and cytokeratins (syncytiotrophoblastic cells) and variably positive for placental alkaline phosphatase

Genetics

▶ Limited data regarding the cytogenetics of CNS germ cell tumors

Differential Diagnosis

▶ Differentiating one germ cell type from another
▶ Metastatic carcinoma
▶ Glioma

PROGNOSIS AND THERAPY

The prognosis and therapy are somewhat dependent on the tumor type or elements contained in a mixed germ cell neoplasm. The best prognosis is associated with pure germinomas, which are radiosensitive. Teratomas are also typically associated with a generally good outcome. Tumors containing embryonal, yolk sac, or choriocarcinoma components tend to behave in a more aggressive fashion.

PITUITARY TUMORS

CLINICAL FEATURES

The most common pituitary neoplasms are adenomas. Adenomas may arise at any age but are more common in adults and females. The signs and symptoms of

PITUITARY TUMORS—FACT SHEET

Definition

▶ Variety of tumors arising primarily in the pituitary gland region, including pituitary adenomas, granular cell tumors, and rare pituitary carcinomas

Locations

▶ Adenomas and carcinomas arise in the adenohypophyseal region
▶ Granular cell tumors arise in the neurohypophyseal region
▶ Incidence rates for pituitary adenomas range from 2% to 27% in the general population. Carcinomas are very rare lesions

Gender and Age Distribution

▶ Adenomas may develop at any age but are relatively infrequent during childhood
▶ Adenomas more common in females than in males

Clinical Features

▶ Secretory adenomas—symptoms may be related to the hormone being produced
▶ Hormonal secretion in adenomas in descending order of prevalence includes prolactin; growth hormone (GH); mixed type; adrenocorticotropic hormone (ACTH); follicle-stimulating hormone/luteinizing hormone (FSH/LH); and thyroid-stimulating hormone (TSH)
▶ Approximately 20% of adenomas are nonsecretory
▶ Other symptoms may be related to a mass effect and include visual symptoms, headaches, and hypopituitarism
▶ Approximately 3% of adenomas are associated with multiple endocrine neoplasia type I
▶ Granular cell tumors are often asymptomatic incidental findings at autopsy; rarely, they are large enough to cause visual field defects
▶ Pituitary carcinomas may be associated with excess hormonal secretion or evidence of metastatic disease

Radiologic Features

▶ Circumscribed radiologic enhancing lesions arising in the adenohypophyseal region

Prognosis and Treatment

▶ Incompletely excised tumors are likely to recur locally
▶ Invasive adenomas are defined by local infiltration of surrounding structures and are more likely to recur after incomplete excision
▶ Pituitary carcinomas are defined by noncontiguous spread of tumor and are associated with a poor prognosis
▶ Most pituitary granular cell tumors appear to be benign lesions amenable to surgical excision

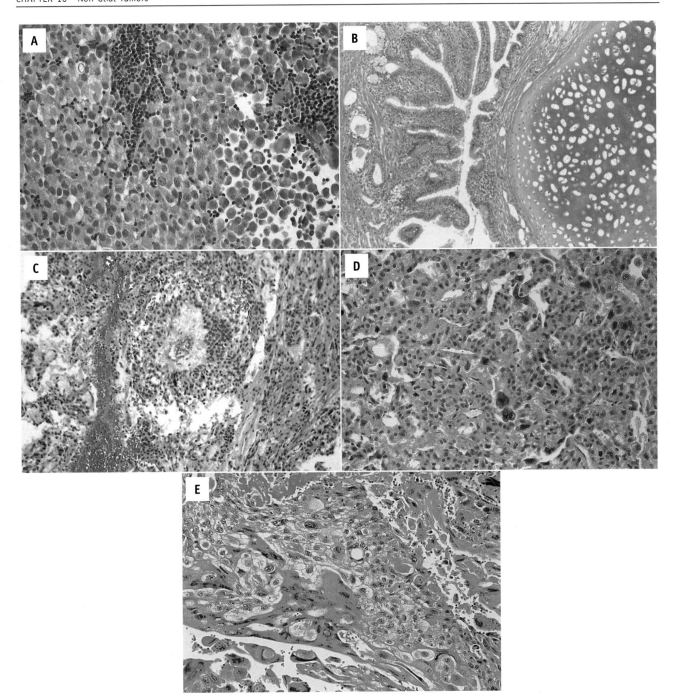

FIGURE 10-18

A, Germinoma composed of large cells with abundant cytoplasm and prominent nucleolation intermixed with benign-appearing lymphocytes. **B**, Mature teratoma with cartilaginous and respiratory airway–type tissue. **C**, Yolk sac tumor characterized by epithelioid cells and a Schiller-Duval body. **D**, Embryonal carcinoma marked by a proliferation of large atypical, prominently nucleolated cells. **E**, Admixture of syncytiotrophoblastic giant cells and cytotrophoblastic cells in choriocarcinoma.

adenoma may be related to either a mass effect (visual symptoms or headaches) or production of hormones. Approximately a fifth of adenomas are nonsecretory. There is a well-known association of pituitary adenomas with multiple endocrine neoplasia type I. Radiographically, adenomas are enhancing, circumscribed lesions arising in the adenohypophysis. Less commonly, one may encounter other tumor types, including granular cell tumors, which may be marked by a mass effect, and rarely pituitary carcinomas, which may be associated with a mass effect, evidence of excessive hormonal secretion, or occasionally metastatic disease.

PATHOLOGIC FEATURES

Grossly, most adenomas are circumscribed, unencapsulated masses. Some tumors may contain microcalcifications or evidence of amyloid deposition. Histologically, adenomas are marked by a proliferation of monomorphic-appearing cells arranged in a sheet-like configuration that results in obliteration of the normal nested architectural pattern of the neurohypophysis (Fig. 10-19A). Nuclear pleomorphism may be focally quite prominent. Cells may be architecturally arranged in a variety of alternative patterns, including acinar, ribbon-like, pseudopapillary, and rosetting (see Fig. 10-19B). Occasionally, large adenomas may undergo hemorrhagic necrosis (apoplexy). Pituitary carcinomas are defined by the presence of noncontiguous spread of the tumor. Granular cell tumors arising in the neurohypophyseal region of the gland resemble their counterparts elsewhere in soft tissue and are characterized by a proliferation of cells with abundant granular eosinophilic cytoplasm (see Fig. 10-19C). Their granularity is due to the presence of large cytoplasmic lysosomes, which can be appreciated ultrastructurally. The secretory product of the adenoma can be demonstrated by immunohistochemistry. Most adenomas also stain with a variety of cytokeratin markers and with antibody to EMA. Granular cell tumors are characteristically S-100 protein positive (see Fig. 10-19D).

DIFFERENTIAL DIAGNOSIS

Distinction of adenomas from pituitary hyperplasia and metastatic carcinoma may at times be problematic. Hyperplasia represents a proliferation of cell types and usually results in minor distortions of the normal nested architectural pattern of the adenohypophysis. These distortions can be highlighted with a reticulin stain. Carcinomas metastatic to the gland have been well documented. Typically, these tumors show features of the parent neoplasm and are frequently marked by increased mitotic activity, associated necrosis, or well-formed glandular structures. Lymphocytic hypophysitis is characterized by a prominent chronic inflammatory cell infiltrate associated with destruction of cells in the adenohypophysis and eventual fibrosis (see Fig. 10-19E). This condition is almost exclusively encountered in postpartum women and can mimic a neoplasm radiographically.

PITUITARY TUMORS—PATHOLOGIC FEATURES

Gross Findings

▶ Circumscribed, nonencapsulated mass with tan-brown coloration
▶ May contain microcalcifications or amyloid nodules
▶ Granular cell tumors are nodular, firm, tan-gray, well-demarcated but nonencapsulated masses

Microscopic Features

▶ Adenoma generally marked by proliferation of monomorphic-appearing cells arranged in a sheet-like configuration
▶ Nuclear pleomorphism or occasional binucleation may be evident in adenoma
▶ Reticulin stain in adenoma highlights absence of the normal nested architectural pattern of pituitary adenohypophysis
▶ Other architectural patterns in adenomas may be observed, including acinar, nested, ribbon-like, pseudopapillary, and rosetting
▶ Amyloid deposition and psammomatous calcifications are particularly associated with prolactinomas
▶ GH adenomas may contain cells with eosinophilic perinuclear cytokeratin filament collections called fibrous bodies
▶ Apoplexy is marked by hemorrhagic necrosis of an adenoma
▶ Carcinomas have no well-defined morphologic criteria and are marked by noncontiguous spread of tumor
▶ Granular cell tumors are characterized by cells with abundant granular eosinophilic cytoplasm

Ultrastructural Features

▶ Different subtypes contain variably sized granules ranging from 50 to 1200 nm in diameter; most granules are electron dense and round to irregular in shape
▶ Paranuclear fibrous bodies consist of aggregates of intermediate-molecular-weight filaments
▶ Granular cell tumor with prominent large cytoplasmic lysosomes
▶ Genetic abnormalities are not reliably identified in adenomas or granular cell tumors

Immunohistochemical Features

▶ Adenomas positive for cytokeratins, EMA, and a variety of pituitary hormones (ACTH, GH, prolactin, FSH, LH, and TSH), depending on the tumor type
▶ Granular cell tumors S-100 protein and vimentin positive

Differential Diagnosis

▶ Pituitary hyperplasia
▶ Lymphocytic hypophysitis
▶ Metastatic carcinoma

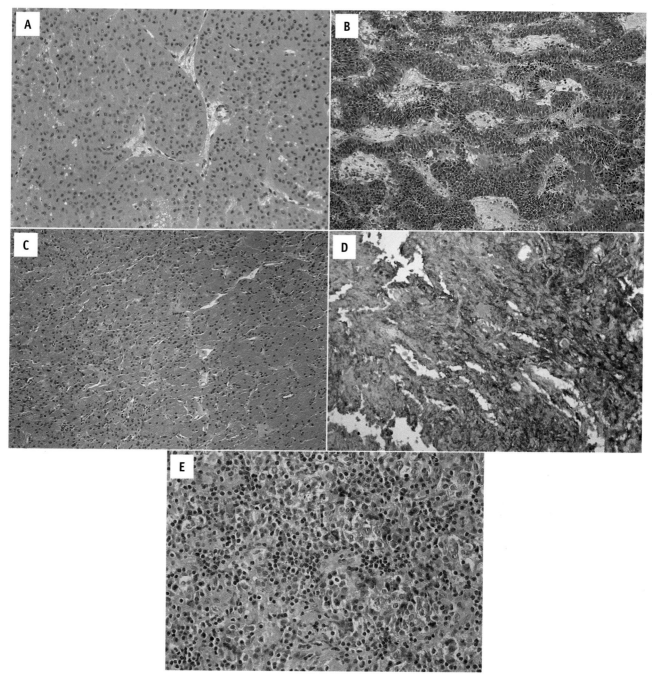

FIGURE 10-19

A, Monomorphic population of eosinophilic cells in a pituitary adenoma. **B**, Trabecular arrangement of cells in a pituitary adenoma. **C**, Granular cell tumor arising in the neurohypophysis and characterized by cells with finely granular eosinophilic cytoplasm. **D**, Diffuse S-100 immunoreactivity in a granular cell tumor. **E**, Prominent lymphocytic infiltration of the pituitary adenohypophysis in lymphocytic hypophysitis.

PINEAL TUMORS

CLINICAL FEATURES

Tumors arising as primary neoplasms of the pineal gland, besides germ cell tumors, are relatively uncom-

mon. Pineoblastomas typically develop in the first 2 decades and radiographically and morphologically resemble their counterpart embryonal tumors in the cerebellum (medulloblastoma) and cerebrum (neuroblastoma). Pineocytomas may arise at any age but have a peak incidence in adults. These tumors are generally associated with symptoms and signs related to increased intracranial pressure, neuro-ophthalmologic abnormalities, or hypothalamic dysfunction.

PINEAL TUMORS—FACT SHEET

Definition

▶ Relatively rare group of pineal parenchymal tumors, including pineoblastoma, pineocytoma, and pineal parenchymal tumor of intermediate differentiation

Incidence and Location

▶ Pineoblastomas are rare tumors that represent approximately 45% of all pineal parenchymal tumors
▶ Pineocytomas account for less than 1% of intracranial tumors and between 15% and 30% of pineal parenchymal tumors
▶ Pineal parenchymal tumor of intermediate differentiation represents approximately 10% of all pineal parenchymal tumors

Gender and Age Distribution

▶ Pineoblastomas occur in the first 2 decades of life with a slight male preponderance
▶ Pineocytomas occur at any age, but have a peak incidence in adults 25 to 35 years of age with no gender predilection
▶ Pineal parenchymal tumor of intermediate differentiation occurs at any age with a peak incidence in adulthood

Clinical Features

▶ Size and symptoms are usually related to increased intracranial pressure, neuro-ophthalmologic abnormalities, and dysfunction of the hypothalamus, brain stem, and cerebellum

Radiologic Features

▶ Pineoblastoma appears as a large, lobulated homogeneous mass that enhances with contrast
▶ Pineocytomas on computed tomographic scan are usually round demarcated masses that are hypodense and homogeneous; MRI findings include a hypointense mass on T1- and hyperintense tumor on T2-weighted images

Prognosis and Treatment

▶ Pineoblastomas have a high risk of craniospinal spread and extracranial metastasis
▶ The 3-year survival rate for pineoblastomas is 78%; the 5-year survival rate is 58%
▶ Pineoblastomas arising in the setting of retinoblastoma syndrome have a particularly poor prognosis, with survival less than 1 year
▶ Pineocytomas have a 5-year survival rate of 86%
▶ Pineal parenchymal tumor of intermediate differentiation is associated with spread within the CNS or metastasis outside the CNS

PATHOLOGIC FEATURES

Grossly, pineoblastomas are friable, soft, and poorly demarcated lesions that are frequently marked by areas of necrosis and hemorrhage. Pineocytomas tend to be better demarcated masses that are generally more homogeneous in appearance, although they may demonstrate cystic degeneration and focal necrosis. Histologically, pineoblastomas resemble embryonal tumors and may be associated with the formation of Homer Wright pseudorosettes or, less commonly, Flexner-Wintersteiner rosettes (Fig. 10-20A). Pineocytomas are characterized by a proliferation of small uniform cells resembling normal cells found in the pineal gland. These tumors may contain rosette-like structures and may rarely show evidence of neuronal, glial, or photoreceptor cell differentiation (see Fig. 10-20B). In contrast to pineocytomas, the so-called pineal parenchymal tumors of intermediate differentiation are cellular lesions devoid of rosette formations (see Fig. 10-20C). By immunohistochemistry, pineoblastomas and pineocytomas may demonstrate immunoreactivity to markers of neural differentiation, glial differentiation (GFAP), and photoreceptor differentiation (retinal S antigen).

DIFFERENTIAL DIAGNOSIS

Mostly commonly, differentiation of pineal tumors from germ cell tumors, which are more common in this location, is warranted. Gliomas are diffusely GFAP positive and generally do not stain with markers of neural differentiation. Metastatic carcinomas, which are cytokeratin positive, may enter the histologic differential.

PROGNOSIS AND THERAPY

Pineoblastomas have a propensity to spread via the cerebrospinal axis. Tumors arising in the setting of retinoblastoma syndrome have a particularly poor prognosis. The 5-year survival rate for pineocytomas is much better than that for pineoblastomas (86% versus 58%, respectively). Information regarding the behavior of pineal parenchymal tumor of intermediate differentiation is sparse, although cases of spread and extra-CNS metastasis have been documented.

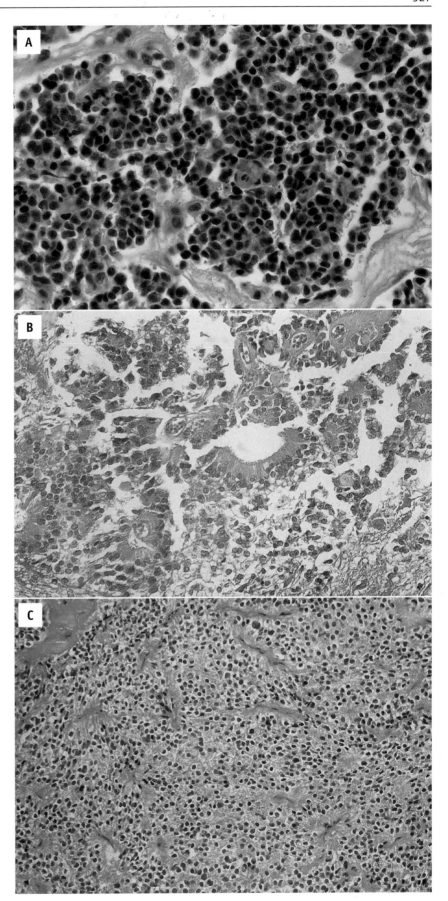

FIGURE 10-20

A, Diffuse proliferation of small embryonal cells reminiscent of medulloblastoma in a pineoblastoma. **B**, Pineocytoma marked by cells resembling normal pituicytes and focally forming rosette structures. **C**, An absence of rosette structures in a pineal parenchymal tumor of intermediate differentiation.

PINEAL TUMORS—PATHOLOGIC FEATURES

Gross Findings

▶ Pineoblastomas are friable, soft, and poorly demarcated masses that may contain areas of hemorrhage and necrosis
▶ Pineocytomas are well-demarcated, gray-tan homogeneous granular lesions that may demonstrate cystic degeneration and foci of hemorrhage

Microscopic Features

▶ Pineoblastomas resemble medulloblastomas and are marked by a proliferation of small rounded cells with a high nuclear-to-cytoplasmic ratio
▶ Pineoblastomas may be associated with Homer Wright and Flexner-Wintersteiner rosettes
▶ Pineoblastomas frequently demonstrate necrosis and prominent mitotic activity
▶ Pineocytomas are marked by a proliferation of small uniform cells resembling mature pineocytes
▶ Pineocytomas may contain rosette structures marked by nucleus-free areas with a delicate meshwork of cell processes in the center
▶ Pineocytomas generally have low mitotic rates, and necrosis is only rarely noted
▶ Rare evidence of neuronal, glial cell, or photoreceptor differentiation may be observed
▶ Pineal parenchymal tumors of intermediate differentiation are highly cellular lesions devoid of rosettes

Ultrastructural Features

▶ Pineoblastomas are marked by a lack of significant differentiation and resemble primitive neuroectodermal tumors
▶ Pineocytomas have membrane-bound electron-dense granules and clear vesicles within the cytoplasm
▶ Pineocytomas may demonstrate synaptic-type junctions in cytoplasmic processes rich in microtubules that end in club-like extensions
▶ Retinoblastic differentiation in pineocytomas may be marked by the presence of cytoplasmic annulated lamellae, cilia, synaptic ribbons, and intracellular lumen formation

Immunohistochemical Features

▶ Pineoblastomas and pineocytomas have similar immunophenotypes and may demonstrate immunoreactivity to synaptophysin, neuron-specific enolase, neurofilament protein, class III β-tubulin, chromogranin, retinal S antigen, and rarely GFAP (in tumors with glial differentiation)

Genetics

▶ Pineoblastomas are associated with deletion of chromosome 11q

Differential Diagnosis

▶ Glioma, including pineal cysts
▶ Germinoma or other germ cell tumor because of location
▶ Metastatic carcinoma

CRANIOPHARYNGIOMA

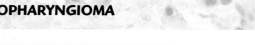

CLINICAL FEATURES

Craniopharyngiomas are epithelioid neoplasms that generally arise in the sellar region. They constitute approximately 1.2% to 4.6% of intracranial tumors and follow a bimodal distribution with a peak incidence in childhood and a second peak in middle-aged adults. Symptoms are generally related to compression of adjacent structures.

CRANIOPHARYNGIOMA—FACT SHEET

Definition

▶ Epithelial tumor arising in the sellar region from Rathke's pouch epithelium

Incidence and Location

▶ Account for 1.2% to 4.6% of intracranial tumors; 0.5 to 2.5 new cases per million population per year
▶ Account for 5% to 10% of intracranial tumors in children
▶ Most arise in the suprasellar or intrasellar region

Gender and Age Distribution

▶ Bimodal distribution with peaks in childhood and adults older than 50 years
▶ Papillary craniopharyngiomas occur almost exclusively in adults
▶ No gender predilection

Clinical Features

▶ Most common manifestations include visual disturbances, endocrine deficiencies, diabetes insipidus, cognitive impairment, and signs related to increased intracranial pressure

Radiologic Features

▶ Computed tomographic scan marked by contrast enhancement of solid tumor and calcifications
▶ T1-weighted MRI may show cystic areas, which are homogeneous and hyperintense, and solid components, which are isointense

Prognosis and Treatment

▶ Generally benign, with a 60% to 93% 10-year recurrence-free survival rate
▶ Recurrence is related to the extent of surgical resection
▶ Tumor greater than 5 cm in diameter marked by a worse prognosis
▶ Prognostic behavior of papillary tumors versus adenomatous tumors debated, with some literature suggesting a better prognosis for papillary lesions
▶ Rare documentation of malignant transformation to squamous cell carcinoma after radiotherapy

PATHOLOGIC FEATURES

Craniopharyngiomas are generally solid neoplasms that may have a variable cystic component. The cystic component is frequently filled with lipid- and cholesterol-rich, brown thick fluid. Calcifications are a frequent finding. Most tumors are marked by an adenomatous pattern characterized by proliferation of nests and cords of squamoid cells (Fig. 10-21A and B). The nests are rimmed by palisades of basaloid cells. Less commonly, the tumors may have a papillary architectural pattern with squamoid cells and pseudopapillae. Spillage of cyst fluid may elicit a xanthogranulomatous inflammatory response.

DIFFERENTIAL DIAGNOSIS

Craniopharyngiomas, especially those with a cystic component, may resemble epidermoid cysts. Epidermoid cysts, in contrast to craniopharyngiomas, are filled with keratin material and have cells that contain keratohyaline granules. Tumors marked by a prominent xanthogranulomatous response may mimic other

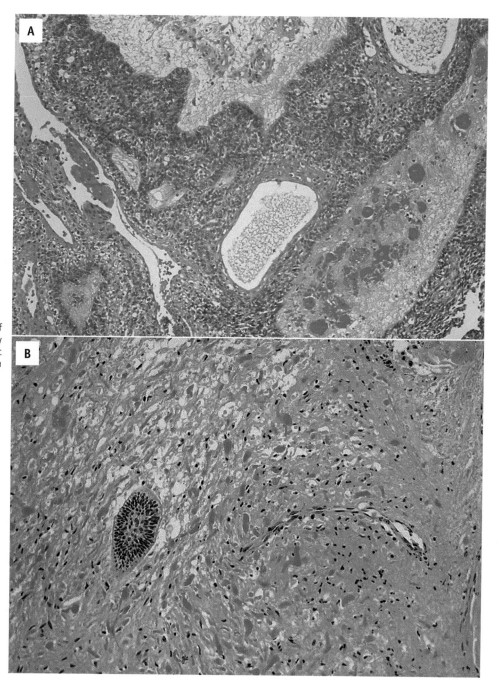

FIGURE 10-21

A, Craniopharyngioma composed of cords of squamous cells rimmed by peripheral basaloid cells. **B**, Prominent gliosis and Rosenthal fiber formation adjacent to a craniopharyngioma.

CRANIOPHARYNGIOMA—PATHOLOGIC FEATURES

Gross Findings
► Generally solid tumors with a variable cystic component
► The adamantinomatous variant is frequently calcified
► Cysts filled with lipid- and cholesterol-rich "machine oil–like" fluid

Microscopic Features
► The adamantinomatous variant consists of cords and nests of squamous epithelial cells with peripheral palisaded nuclei and central stellate reticulum
► The adamantinomatous variant is associated with compact keratin material, fibrosis, dystrophic mineralization, and lipid and cholesterol cleft formation (xanthogranulomatous inflammation)
► Papillary tumors are marked by sheets of squamous epithelium with separations forming pseudopapillae
► Calcification, keratin material, and xanthogranulomatous inflammation are less commonly seen with the papillary variant

Ultrastructural Features
► Tumor cells containing bundles of intermediate filaments and desmosomal junctions

Immunohistochemical Features
► Positive for both high- and low-molecular-weight keratins.

Genetics
► Not known

Differential Diagnosis
► Epidermoid cyst
► Xanthogranulomatous inflammation of the sella

PARAGANGLIOMA—FACT SHEET

Definition
► Endocrine tumor associated with segmental or collateral autonomic ganglia

Incidence and Location
► Paragangliomas of the CNS are uncommon; most are manifested as an intradural spinal mass in the filum terminale region

Gender and Age Distribution
► Most occur in adults with a mean age between 40 and 50 years
► Slight male preponderance
► Jugulotympanic paragangliomas have a female preponderance

Clinical Features
► Spinal tumors are characterized by lower back pain, radicular pain, and sensory motor deficits, including sphincter disturbances
► Glomus jugulare tumors extend into the cranial cavity (approximately 40%) and cause progressive hearing loss, cranial nerve palsies, and signs related to the production of catecholamines (hypertension, sweating, palpitations)

Radiologic Features
► Most tumors are isodense and homogeneously enhancing on computed tomographic scan
► MRI studies show both hypointense and isointense areas with respect to the spinal cord on T1-weighted images and a contrast-enhancing and hyperintense tumor on T2-weighted images

Prognosis and Treatment
► The majority of filum terminale tumors are slow-growing lesions curable by gross total resection
► Tumors arising in other locations are more likely to recur locally (approximately 50%) and metastasize (5%)
► Histologic features are not predictive of clinical behavior

---

inflammatory, non-neoplastic lesions that may occasionally involve the sellar region.

PROGNOSIS AND THERAPY

Craniopharyngiomas are usually amenable to surgical resection. They generally behave in a benign fashion but recur if incompletely excised. Rare case reports of malignant transformation to squamous cell carcinoma, particularly after radiotherapy, have been documented in the literature.

PARAGANGLIOMA

CLINICAL FEATURES

Paragangliomas are neuroendocrine tumors that most commonly arise in association with ganglionic seg-

ments. Only rare cases of these tumors have been described arising in the intracranial vault. The filum terminale region of the spinal cord is a fairly common location. Most paragangliomas develop in adults. In patients with spinal cord tumors, the most common manifestations include lower back pain, sensory motor deficits, and sphincter dysfunction.

PATHOLOGIC FEATURES

The appearance of paragangliomas is somewhat uniform irrespective of the site of origin. Grossly, these tumors tend to be somewhat circumscribed, red-brown soft tissue masses. Histologically, they are composed of cells arranged in nests or lobules limited by a single layer of S-100 protein–positive sustentacular cells (Fig. 10-22A and B). Their nested architectural pattern is referred to as Zellballen. Nuclear pleomorphism may be focally

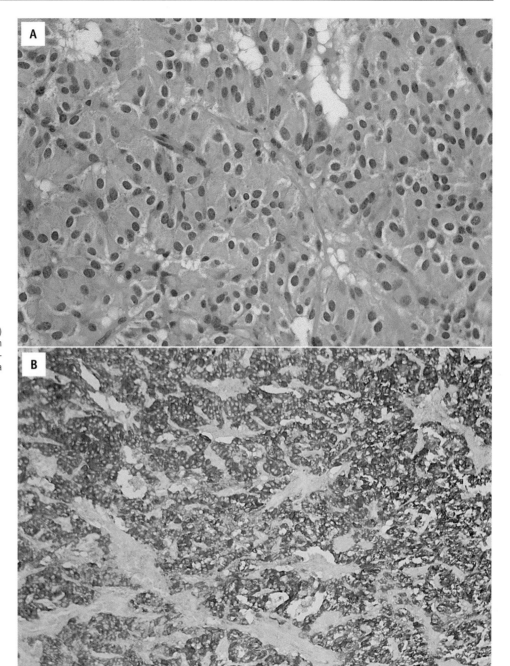

FIGURE 10-22

A, Nests of tumor cells (Zellballen) separated by small blood vessels in a paraganglioma. **B**, Diffuse chromogranin immunoreactivity in a paraganglioma.

PARAGANGLIOMA—PATHOLOGIC FEATURES

Gross Findings

▶ Cauda equina tumors are intradural and attached either to the filum terminale or less commonly to the caudal nerve roots
▶ Oval to elongated, encapsulated shape; red-brown soft tissue masses
▶ Cystic component may be present

Microscopic Features

▶ Arrangement of chief cells in nests or lobules (Zellballen)
▶ Nests of lobules are surrounded by a single layer of sustentacular cells
▶ Delicate fibrovascular network between nests and lobules
▶ Nuclear pleomorphism may be focally prominent and represents degenerative change
▶ Intermixed ganglionic cells may be present
▶ Necrosis may occasionally be noted, as can scattered mitotic figures
▶ Rarely, other architectural patterns can be observed, including pseudorosetting, adenomatous, angiomatous, spindled, oncocytic, and melanocytic variants

Ultrastructural Features

▶ Dense secretory granules (100 to 400 nm) in chief cells
▶ Chief cells may contain prominent mitochondria with typical features and perinuclear collections of intermediate filaments

Immunohistochemical Features

▶ Chief cells are generally positive for synaptophysin, neuron-specific enolase, chromogranin, and neurofilament
▶ Perinuclear keratin immunoreactivity may be present
▶ Sustentacular cells are S-100 protein positive and may stain with GFAP

Genetics

▶ Association with chromosomes 11q and 3p
▶ May be seen in association with von Hippel–Lindau disease and in multiple endocrine neoplasia types IIa and IIb

Differential Diagnosis

▶ Ependymomas, including myxopapillary ependymoma
▶ Meningioma
▶ Schwannoma

ependymomas/myxopapillary ependymomas, meningiomas, and schwannomas. In most cases, the histologic appearance of the paraganglioma is distinct enough to warrant easy differentiation. Immunohistochemistry may also be helpful. In contrast to ependymomas, GFAP immunoreactivity is confined to only the sustentacular cells of paraganglioma. Schwannomas demonstrate diffuse positive S-100 immunoreactivity, in contrast to the S-100 immunoreactivity of sustentacular cells in paragangliomas. Meningiomas do not stain for markers of neural differentiation.

PROGNOSIS AND TREATMENT

Most paragangliomas have a good prognosis and are amenable to surgical resection. Incompletely excised tumors may recur locally, and only rare cases have been known to metastasize. Unfortunately, the histologic appearance of the lesion is not predictive of its clinical behavior.

METASTASIS

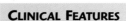

CLINICAL FEATURES

Metastases are the most common tumors of the CNS. They can occur at any age, and the clinical findings are dependent on the location and size of the lesions. Most metastases are situated either in the arterial border zones of the cerebral hemispheres or in the leptomeninges. Tumors are frequently multifocal and often involve more than one vascular distribution.

PATHOLOGIC FEATURES

Grossly, most parenchymal-based metastases are circumscribed lesions (Fig. 10-23A-C), in contrast to high-grade gliomas, which are typically infiltrative in nature. Metastatic lesions generally demonstrate the features of the parent tumor. The immunohistochemical profile is often consistent with the primary lesion.

DIFFERENTIAL DIAGNOSIS

The differential diagnosis for metastatic disease is quite extensive. One of the most common considerations is distinction of a metastasis from primary malignant glioma. Most metastatic lesions do not stain with GFAP antibody but demonstrate evidence of keratin immunoreactivity. However, care must be taken with regard to

prominent. Occasional tumors may demonstrate necrosis and sometimes mitotic figures. Ultrastructurally, the cells are marked by the presence of numerous dense secretory granules. By immunohistochemistry, the chief cells, which compose the bulk of the tumor, stain with markers of neural differentiation, including synaptophysin, neuron-specific enolase, and chromogranin.

DIFFERENTIAL DIAGNOSIS

The main differential diagnosis includes other tumors that frequently arise in the filum terminale region:

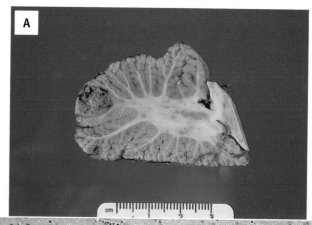

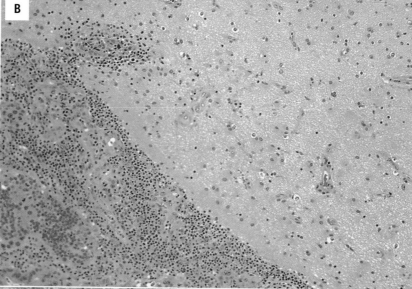

FIGURE 10-23

A, Well-circumscribed metastatic adenocarcinoma of lung origin in the cerebellum. **B**, Typical well-demarcated interface of metastatic carcinoma and the adjacent reactive brain parenchyma. **C**, Infiltrating squamous cell carcinoma involving the dura and extending directly from the nasal cavity.

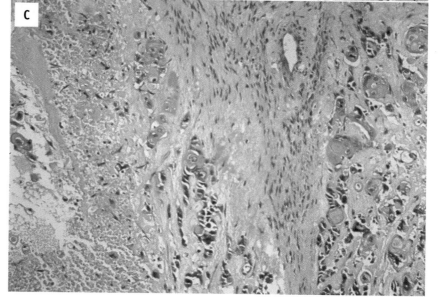

METASTASIS—FACT SHEET

Definition

▶ Tumors that spread from outside the CNS (discontinuous spread)

Incidence and Location

▶ Most common tumor of the CNS
▶ Intracranial metastasis present in approximately a fourth of individuals with systemic cancer in autopsy series
▶ Annual incidence of metastatic tumors: 4.1 to 11.1 per 100,000 population annually
▶ Approximately 80% of brain metastases are located in the arterial border zones of the cerebral hemispheres; 15% are in the cerebellum
▶ Majority of cases are multifocal and involve multiple vascular distributions
▶ Involvement may occasionally be predominantly leptomeningeal/dural based and associated with leptomeningeal carcinomatosis

Gender and Age Distribution

▶ Incidence increases with age
▶ Slight male preponderance

Clinical Features

▶ Dependent on location; most commonly consist of focal neural deficits, headaches, and mental disturbances

Radiologic Features

▶ Discrete, isodense or hypodense masses with focal enhancement and surrounding edema
▶ At least half the patients have multiple lesions
▶ On MRI studies, metastases are hypodense on T1-weighted images and hyperintense and contrast enhancing on T2-weighted images

Prognosis and Treatment

▶ Prognostic factors include age (younger better), Karnofsky score (higher better), number and location of lesions, sensitivity of lesions to therapy, and progression of the primary neoplasm
▶ Mean survival of patients with multiple brain metastases treated with radiation is 3 to 6 months
▶ Solitary metastases may be amenable to surgical excision and have a better prognosis

METASTASIS—PATHOLOGIC FEATURES

Gross Findings

▶ Discrete well-circumscribed gray-white or tan mass
▶ Hemorrhage associated with metastatic melanoma, choriocarcinoma, renal cell carcinoma, and lung carcinoma
▶ Leptomeningeal-based lesions may form nodules

Microscopic Features

▶ Lesions classically well demarcated from adjacent reactive gliotic and edematous parenchyma
▶ Vascular proliferative changes may be observed adjacent to tumors
▶ Tumors generally demonstrate features of the parent tumor

Ultrastructural Features

▶ Related to tumor type

Immunohistochemical Features

▶ Generally reflective of tumor type
▶ Caution using some keratin markers (such as AE1/AE3), since there is some cross-reactivity with glioblastoma multiforme; likewise, rare metastases may be GFAP positive
▶ Often difficult to tell primary by histologic appearance

Genetics

▶ Reflective of the parent tumor
▶ Metastatic lesions may demonstrate genetic alterations associated with metastasis and tumor type, such as c-erb-B2 in breast carcinoma and CD44R1 in colon carcinoma

Differential Diagnosis

▶ Malignant glioma
▶ Lymphoma
▶ Primary sarcoma
▶ Primary melanoma
▶ Medulloblastoma

tomas and other primitive neuroectodermal tumors from metastatic small cell carcinoma may also be difficult and is frequently dependent on the clinical history. Many small cell carcinomas also demonstrate some evidence of keratin immunoreactivity.

the choice of keratin markers for the purpose of sorting this differential diagnosis by immunohistochemistry. Certain keratin markers such as the cytokeratins AE1/AE3 demonstrate considerable immunoreactivity with gliomas and are therefore not useful in differentiating carcinoma from high-grade astrocytoma. Other differential diagnostic considerations include lymphoma. Metastatic lymphoma more commonly involves the leptomeninges, in contrast to the parenchymal-based location of most primary CNS lymphomas. Cases of primary sarcoma or melanoma may also arise in the CNS. Distinction of these tumors from metastasis may be difficult on histologic grounds and generally requires careful evaluation of the patient. Distinction of medulloblas-

SUGGESTED READINGS

Meningiomas

Carneiro SS, Scheithauer BW, Nascimento AG, et al: Solitary fibrous tumor of the meninges: A lesion distinct from fibrous meningioma: A clinicopathologic and immunohistochemical study. Am J Clin Pathol 1996;16:217-224.

Louis DN, Scheithauer BW, Budka H, et al: Meningiomas. In Kleihues P, Cavence WK (eds): Tumours of the Nervous System. Lyon, France, IARC Press, 2000, pp 175-184.

Mahmood A, Caccamo DV, Tomecek FJ, Malik GM: Atypical and malignant meningiomas: A clinicopathological review. Neurosurgery 1993;33:955-963.

Perry A, Scheithauer BW, Stafford SL, et al: "Malignancy" in meningiomas: A clinicopathologic study of 116 patients with grading implications. Cancer 1999;85:2046-2056.

Perry A, Stafford SL, Scheithauer BW, et al: Meningioma grading:
An analysis of histologic parameters. Am J Surg Pathol
1997;21:1455-1465.

Smith DA, Cahill DW: The biology of meningiomas. Neurosurg Clin
North Am 1994;5:201-215.

Mesenchymal Tumors

Chang SM, Barker FG II, Larson DA, et al: Sarcomas subsequent to
cranial irradiation. Neurosurgery 1995;36:685-690.

Mena H, Ribas JL, Pazeshkpour GH, et al: Hemangiopericytoma of
the central nervous system: A review of 94 cases. Hum Pathol
1991;22:84-91.

Perry A, Scheithauer BW, Nascimento AG: The immunophenotypic
spectrum of meningeal hemangiopericytoma: Comparison with
fibrous meningioma and solitary fibrous tumors of meninges. Am
J Surg Pathol 1997;21:1354-1360.

Winek RR, Scheithauer BW, Wick MR: Meningioma, meningeal
hemangiopericytoma (angioblastic meningioma), peripheral
hemangiopericytoma, and acoustic schwannoma: A comparative
immunohistochemical study. Am J Surg Pathol 1989;13:251-261.

Hemangioblastoma

Filling-Katz MR, Choyke PL, Oldfield E, et al: Central nervous
system involvement in von Hippel-Lindau disease. Neurology
1991;41:41-46.

Lodrini S, Lasio G, Cimino C, Pluchino F: Hemangioblastomas:
Clinical characteristics, surgical results and immunohistochemical
studies. J Neurosurg Sci 1991;35:179-185.

Mills SE, Ross GW, Perentes E, et al: Cerebellar hemangioblastoma:
Immunohistochemical distinction from metastatic renal cell
carcinoma. Surg Pathol 1990;3:121-132.

Neumann HPH, Lips CJM, Hsia YE, Zbar B: Von Hippel-Lindau
syndrome. Brain Pathol 1995;5:181-193.

Wizigmann-Voss S, Plate KH: Pathology, genetics and cell biology of
hemangioblastomas. Histol Histopathol 1996;11:1049-1061.

Melanocytic Lesions

Brat DJ, Giannini C, Scheithauer BW, Burger PC: Primary
melanocytic neoplasms of the central nervous system. Am J Surg
Pathol 1999;23:745-754.

Maken GWJ, Eden OB, Lashford LS, et al: Leptomeningeal
melanoma of childhood. Cancer 1999;86:878-886.

O'Brien TF, Moran M, Miller JH, Hensley SD: Meningeal
melanocytoma: An uncommon diagnostic pitfall in surgical
neuropathology. Arch Pathol Lab Med 1995;119:542-546.

Reyes-Muglia M, Chou P, Byrd S, et al: Nevomelanocytic
proliferations in the central nervous system of children. Cancer
1993;72:2277-2285.

Chordoma

Forsyth PA, Cascino TL, Shaw EG, et al: Intracranial chordomas: A
clinicopathological and prognostic study of 51 cases. J Neurosurg
1993;78:741-747.

Gay E, Sekhar LN, Rubinstein E, et al: Chordomas and
chondrosarcomas of the cranial base: Results and follow-up of 60
patients. Neurosurgery 1995;36:887-897.

Matsuno A, Sasaki T, Nagashima T, et al: Immunohistochemical
examination of proliferative potentials and the expression of cell
cycle–related proteins of intracranial chordomas. Hum Pathol
1997;28:714-719.

O'Connell JX, Renard LG, Liebsch NJ, et al: Base of skull chordoma:
A correlative study of histologic and clinical features of 62 cases.
Cancer 1994;74:2261-2267.

York JE, Kaczaraj A, Abi-Said D, et al: Sacral chordoma: 40-year
experience at a major cancer center. Neurosurgery 1999;44:74-80.

Choroid Plexus Tumors

Berger C, Thiesse P, Lellouch-Tubiana A, et al: Choroid plexus
carcinomas in childhood: Clinical features and prognostic factors.
Neurosurgery 1998;42:470-475.

Coffin CM, Wick MR, Braun JT, Dehner LP: Choroid plexus
neoplasms. Clinicopathologic and immunohistochemical studies.
Am J Surg Pathol 1986;10:394-404.

Newbould MJ, Kelsey AM, Arango JC, et al: The choroid plexus
carcinomas of childhood: Histopathology, immunocytochemistry
and clinicopathological correlation. Histopathology 1995;26:137-
143.

Tacconi L, Delfini R, Cantore G: Choroid plexus papillomas:
Consideration of a surgical series of 33 cases. Acta Neurochir
1996;138:802-810.

Neurocytoma

Figarella-Branger D, Pellissier JF, Daumas-Duport C, et al: Central
neurocytomas: Critical evaluation of a small-cell neuronal tumor.
Am J Surg Pathol 1992;16:97-109.

Gyure KA, Prayson RA, Estes ML: Central neurocytoma: A
clinicopathologic study with p53 and MIB1
immunohistochemistry. J Surg Pathol 1997;2:277-282.

Hassoun J, Söylemezoglu F, Gambarelli D, et al: Central
neurocytoma: A synopsis of clinical and histological features.
Brain Pathol 1993;3:297-306.

Söylemezoglu F, Scheithauer BW, Esteve J, Kleihues P: Atypical
central neurocytoma. J Neuropathol Exp Neurol 1997;56:551-556.

Yasargil M, von Ammon K, von Deimling A, et al: Central
neurocytoma: Histopathologic variants and therapeutic
approaches. J Neurosurg 1992;76:32-37.

Embryonal Tumors

Bergmann M, Pietsch T, Herms J, et al: Medulloblastoma: A
histological, immunohistochemical, ultrastructural and molecular
genetic study. Acta Neuropathol 1998;95:205-212.

Burger PC, Yu IT, Tihan T, et al: Atypical teratoid/rhabdoid tumor
of the central nervous system: A highly malignant tumor of
infancy and childhood frequently mistaken for medulloblastoma:
A Pediatric Oncology Group study. Am J Surg Pathol
1998;22:1083-1092.

Gianaspero F, Rigobello L, Badiali M, et al: Large-cell
medulloblastomas: A distinct variant with highly aggressive
behavior. Am J Surg Pathol 1992;16:687-693.

Hart MN, Earl KM: Primitive neuroectodermal tumors of the brain
in children. Cancer 1973;32:890-897.

Rorke LB, Trojanowski JQ, Lee VM-Y, et al: Primitive
neuroectodermal tumors of the central nervous system. Brain
Pathol 1997;7:765-784.

Schwannoma

Casadei GP, Komori T, Scheithauer BW, et al: Intracranial
parenchymal schwannoma. J Neurosurg 1993;79:217-222.

Casadei GP, Scheithauer BW, Hirose T, et al: Cellular schwannoma:
A clinicopathologic, DNA flow cytometric, and proliferation
marker study of 70 patients. Cancer 1995;75:1109-1119.

Celli P, Cervoni L, Tarantino R, Fortuna A: Primary spinal
malignant schwannomas: Clinical and prognostic remarks. Acta
Neurochir 1995;135:52-55.

Léger F, Vital C, Rivel J, et al: Psammomatous melanotic
schwannoma of a spinal nerve root: Relationship with the Carney
complex. Pathol Res Pract 1996;192:1142-1146.

Swanson PE, Scheithauer BW, Wick MR: Peripheral nerve sheath
neoplasms: Clinicopathologic and immunochemical observations.
Pathol Annu 1995;30(Pt 2):1-82.

Lymphoma

Camilleri-Bröet S, Davi F, Feuillard J, et al: AIDS-related primary
brain lymphomas: Histopathologic and immunohistochemical
study of 51 cases. Hum Pathol 1997;28:367-374.

Camilleri-Bröet S, Martin A, Moreau A, et al: Primary central
nervous system lymphomas in 72 immunocompetent patients.
Am J Clin Pathol 1998;110:607-612.

Freilich RJ, DeAngelis LM: Primary central nervous system
lymphoma. Neurol Clin 1995;13:901-914.

Liebowitz D: Epstein-Barr virus and cellular signaling pathway in lymphomas from immunosuppressed patients. N Engl J Med 1998;338:1413-1421.

Miller DC, Hochberg FH, Harris NL, et al: Pathology with clinical correlations of primary central nervous system non-Hodgkin's lymphoma, the Massachusetts General Hospital experience 1958-1989. Cancer 1994;74:1383-1397.

Histiocytic Tumors

Andriko J-AW, Morrison A, Colegial CH, et al: Rosai-Dorfman disease isolated to the central nervous system: A report of 11 cases. Mod Pathol 2001;14:172-178.

Babu R, Lansen T, Chadburn A, Kasoff S: Erdheim-Chester disease of the central nervous system. J Neurosurg 1997;86:888-892.

Belen D, Colak A, Ozcan O: CNS involvement of Langerhans cell histiocytosis, report of 23 surgically treated cases. Neurosurg Rev 1996;19:247-252.

Haddad E, Sulis ML, Jabado N, et al: Frequency and severity of central nervous system lesions in hemophagocytic lymphohistiocytosis. Blood 1997;89:794-800.

Cysts

Bejjani GK, Wright DC, Schessel D, Sekhar LN: Endodermal cysts of the posterior fossa: Report of 3 cases and review of the literature. J Neurosurg 1998;89;326-335.

Graziani N, Dufour M, Figarella-Branger D, et al: Do the suprasellar neurentric cyst, the Rathke cleft cyst and the colloid cyst constitute the same entity? Acta Neurochir 1995;133:174-180.

Harrison MJ, Morgello S, Post KD: Epithelial cystic lesions of the sellar and parasellar region: A continuum of ectodermal derivatives? J Neurosurg 1994;80:1018-1025.

Mathiesen T, Grane P, Lindgren L, Lindquist C: Third ventricle colloid cysts: A consecutive 12-year series. J Neurosurg 1997;86:5-12.

Germ Cell Tumors

Felix I, Becker LE: Intracranial germ cell tumors in children: An immunohistochemical and electron microscopic study. Pediatr Neurosurg 1990;16:156-162.

Jennings MT, Gelman R, Hochberg F: Intracranial germ-cell tumors: Natural history and pathogenesis. J Neurosurg 1985;63:155-167.

Kraichoke S, Cosgrove M, Chandrasoma PT: Granulomatous inflammation in pineal germinoma: A cause of diagnostic failure at stereotaxic brain biopsy. Am J Surg Pathol 1988;12:655-660.

Rueda P, Heifetz SA, Sesterhenn IA, Clark GB: Primary intracranial germ cell tumors in the first two decades of life. A clinical, light microscopic, and immunohistochemical analysis of 54 cases. Perspect Pediatr Pathol 1987;10:160-207.

Pituitary Tumors

Asa SL: Tumors of the Pituitary Gland, 3rd ed. Washington, DC, Armed Forces Institute of Pathology, 1998.

Pernicone PJ, Scheithauer BW, Sebo TJ, et al: Pituitary carcinoma: A clinicopathologic study of 15 cases. Cancer 1997;79:804-812.

Saeger W, Lüdecke DK: Pituitary hyperplasia: Definition, light and electron microscopical structures and significance in surgical specimens. Virchows Arch A 1983;399:277-287.

Schaller B, Kirsch E, Tolnay M, Mindermann T: Symptomatic granular cell tumor of the pituitary gland: Case report and review of the literature. Neurosurgery 1998;42:166-171.

Teears RJ, Silverman EM: Clinicopathologic review of 88 cases of carcinoma metastatic to the pituitary gland. Cancer 1975;36:216-220.

Pineal Tumors

Fauchon F, Jouvet A, Paquis P, et al: Parenchymal pineal tumors: A clinicopathological study of 76 cases. Int J Radiat Oncol Biol Phys 2000;46:959-968.

Mena H, Rushing EJ, Ribas JL, et al: Tumors of pineal parenchymal cells: A correlation of histological features, including nucleolar organizer regions with survival in 35 cases. Hum Pathol 1995;26:20-30.

Schild SE, Scheithauer BW, Haddock MG, et al: Histologically confirmed pineal tumors and other germ cell tumors of the brain. Cancer 1996;78:2564-2571.

Schild SE, Scheithauer BW, Schomberg PJ, et al: Pineal parenchymal tumors: Clinical, pathologic and therapeutic aspects. Cancer 1993;72:870-880.

Craniopharyngiomas

Crotty TB, Scheithauer BW, Young WF, et al: Papillary craniopharyngioma: A clinicopathological study of 48 cases. J Neurosurg 1995;83:206-214.

Paulus W, Honegger J, Keyvani K, Fahlbusch R: Xanthogranuloma of the sellar region: A clinicopathological entity different from adamantinomatous craniopharyngioma. Acta Neuropathol 1999;97:377-382.

Paulus W, Stockel C, Krauss J, et al: Odontogenic classification of craniopharyngiomas: A clinicopathological study of 54 cases. Histopathology 1997;30:172-176.

Tateyama H, Tada T, Okabe M, et al: Different keratin profiles in craniopharyngioma subtypes and ameloblastomas. Pathol Res Pract 2001;197:735-742.

Weiner HL, Wisoff JH, Rosenberg ME, et al: Craniopharyngiomas: A clinicopathological analysis of factors predictive of recurrence and functional outcome. Neurosurgery 1994;35:1001-1011.

Paraganglioma

Horoupian DS, Kerson LA, Saintz H, Valsamis M: Paraganglioma of cauda equina. Cancer 1974;33:1337-1348.

Moran CA, Rush W, Mena H: Primary spinal paragangliomas: A clinicopathological and immunohistochemical study of 35 cases. Histopathology 1997;31:167-173.

Sonneland PR, Scheithauer BW, LeChago J, et al: Paraganglioma of the cauda equina region: Clinicopathologic study of 31 cases with special reference to immunocytology and ultrastructure. Cancer 1986;58:1720-1735.

Metastasis

Bouffet E, Doumi N, Thiesse P, et al: Brain metastasis in children with tumors. Cancer 1997;79:403-410.

Hwang T-L, Close TP, Grego JM, et al: Predilection of brain metastasis in gray and white matter junction and vascular border zones. Cancer 1996;77:1551-1555.

Kleinschmidt-DeMaster BK: Dural metastases. A retrospective surgical and autopsy series. Arch Pathol Lab Med 2001;125:880-887.

Mrak RE: Origins of adenocarcinomas presenting as intracranial metastases. An ultrastructural study. Arch Pathol Lab Med 1993;117:1165-1169.

Nussbaum ES, Djalilian HR, Cho KW, Hall WA: Brain metastasis. Histology, multiplicity, surgery and survival. Cancer 1996;78:1781-1788.

11 Skeletal Muscle and Peripheral Nerve Disorders

Mark L. Cohen

INTRODUCTION TO SKELETAL MUSCLE

Skeletal muscle, which represents 40% of the weight of a reasonably fit human, has one major function: converting food into force. The unit of contraction in skeletal muscle is the *sarcomere*, a 2.5-µm-long lattice of interdigitating thick (myosin) and thin (actin) filaments, the latter anchored to Z discs. Z discs (visible by light microscopy as cross-striations) keep adjacent sarcomeres aligned and linked to the outer membrane of the muscle fiber. A *myofibril* consists of a series of sarcomeres (10,000 per inch) attached to each other beginning at a muscle's origin and ending at its insertion. Each muscle fiber that we recognize under the light microscope is a multinucleated syncytium consisting of parallel arrays of a thousand or so myofibrils (Fig. 11-1A). Grossly visible muscles are composed of (roughly) parallel arrays of thousands to millions of muscle fibers (the gastrocnemius muscle, for example, contains about a million fibers). Although the number of muscle fibers within a muscle is fairly static, the number of myofibrils within each of these muscle fibers is dynamic and is thus responsible for changes in muscle size with activity (or lack thereof) and aging.

Muscles work through adenosine triphosphate (ATP)-dependent movement of actin along myosin. Despite heavy dependence on ATP, very little is stored within muscle, so efficient metabolism of glycogen and lipids is necessary to provide this energy substrate. Two major types of muscle fibers have evolved: those capable of generating large amounts of force quickly (*fast twitch*) and those capable of generating force over a more protracted interval (*slow twitch*). Slow-twitch muscle fibers, being more dependent on a steady supply of oxygen, contain greater amounts of myoglobin and thus appear redder than fast-twitch fibers do (dark meat versus light meat in your average turkey). Slow-twitch fibers also contain more lipid and mitochondria than fast-twitch fibers do; however, the latter contain more glycogen and myofibrillary adenosine triphosphatase (ATPase). This difference has been used to histochemically separate fibers into type 1 (low myofibrillary ATPase) and type 2 (high myofibrillary ATPase) based on the stability of this enzyme to alkaline incubation. Subsequently discovered acid-stable isoenzymes of myofibrillary ATPase demonstrate the reverse, with type 1 fibers staining darkly and type 2 fibers showing a range of pallor that allows subdivision of these fibers into types 2a, 2b, and 2c. Muscles composed of single fiber types are found in some animals (a hummingbird's wings and a clam's catch muscles), but not in humans (although the relative proportions of type 1 and 2 fibers vary depending on the primary function of the muscle).

Each muscle fiber is innervated by a motor axon originating from an anterior horn neuron within the spinal cord. A single anterior horn cell innervates anywhere from several hundred to several thousand muscle fibers, depending on the precision and force needed to accomplish the required muscle functions. These *motor units* are interspersed among each other within muscle to form a mosaic pattern best visualized by ATPase staining (see Fig. 11-1B). The rate and pattern of neuronal firing determine the fiber type through induction of gene expression patterns. Innervation is also needed to maintain sarcomeric balance. In the absence of such stimulation, the 1% to 2% of muscle protein that degenerates daily is not replaced, and the motor unit atrophies (see Fig. 11-2A). If reinnervated by axonal sprouting from adjacent motor units (within about a 2-month window), denervated muscle fibers can regain normal size and shape, although their type will conform to that of the adjacent motor unit. This change is manifested electrophysiologically as large and polyphasic motor unit action potentials and pathologically as fiber-type grouping, or interruption of the normal mosaic pattern by single-type fiber groups (see Fig. 11-1C).

Although it is a truism that we are entering the molecular age of myology, patients will continue to have symptoms and signs of muscle dysfunction, clinicians will almost certainly continue to evaluate these patients with anatomic-physiologic algorithms, and pathologists will indubitably continue to receive biopsy specimens without any of this information. Nevertheless, efficient pathologic diagnosis of muscle disease is only possible with some knowledge of the clinical manifestations. Age at onset and duration of symptomatology are probably most important, followed closely by whether the dysfunction is predominantly progressive or episodic. This information can then be integrated into an anatomic-pathophysiologic approach to diagnosis, as outlined in Table 11-1.

Even though this table oversimplifies a very complex set of disorders, it provides a serviceable starting point when confronting a muscle biopsy specimen. Several diseases covered in this chapter highlight the clinical and pathophysiologic heterogeneity of skeletal muscle

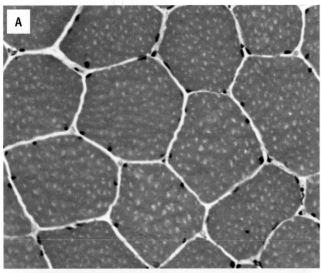

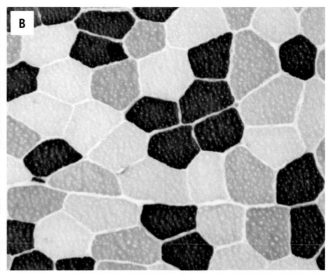

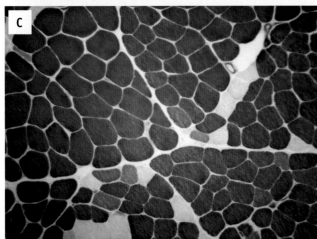

FIGURE 11-1

A, Transverse section of frozen skeletal muscle demonstrating multiple peripheral nuclei within each muscle fiber. Ice crystal ("waffle") artifact is also apparent. **B**, ATPase histochemical staining (pH 4.6) demonstrates a mosaic pattern of type 1 (dark), type 2A (light), and type 2B (intermediate) fibers within all normal human muscles. **C**, Reinnervated muscle demonstrating fiber-type grouping by ATPase histochemical staining.

TABLE 11-1

Anatomic-Physiologic Approach to Diagnosis

Site of Primary Defect	Progressive Disease	Episodic Disease
Neuron/peripheral nerve	Denervation atrophy	—
Neuromuscular junction	Autoimmune myasthenia	—
Muscle membranes	Muscular dystrophies	Channelopathies
	Channelopathies	
Sarcomeres	Congenital myopathies	—
Energy metabolism	Acid maltase deficiency	McArdle's disease
	Mitochondrial diseases	CPT II deficiency
		Mitochondrial diseases
Exogenous: toxic	—	Acute quadriplegic myopathy
Exogenous: inflammatory	Dermatomyositis	—
	Polymyositis	
Unknown (?degenerative)	Inclusion body myositis	—

CPT II, carnitine palmitoyltransferase II.

diseases. As indicated in Table 11-1, mitochondrial damage may be manifested as either progressive loss of muscle function or episodic dysfunction (exercise intolerance, cramps), although patients usually exhibit both. Both myotonic dystrophy and central core disease are characterized by progressive disease punctuated by episodic crises (myotonic crisis and malignant hyperthermia, respectively).

One cannot get far in the discussion of muscle diseases before entering the somewhat arcane world of specimen processing, histochemical staining, and electron microscopy. These techniques should be seen as important aids to diagnosis rather than as obstacles to understanding. Table 11-2 attempts to put this concept into perspective by introducing the diseases covered in this chapter in terms of the type of preparations necessary to make presumptive (P) and definitive (D) diagnoses of each. (Note that a D not preceded by a P indicates a diagnosis that is unlikely to be considered in the absence of a compelling clinical history.) In the body of this chapter, I follow the usual order of discussing histochemical features before ultrastructural abnormalities; this table lists electron microscopy first. My rationale is that ultrastructural examination can be performed on tissue received in formalin with minimal loss of information (as long as the tissue was not subjected to paraffin embedding for histologic processing). "Ancillary studies" subsumes tests not usually performed in anatomic laboratories (e.g., genetic testing, biochemical studies, immunoblot analysis).

Note that among these 16 exemplary muscle diseases, histochemical staining provides diagnostic information that is not obtainable by ultrastructural examination for only 2 (denervation atrophy and McArdle's disease). Note also that only about half these diseases can be definitively diagnosed with full histologic, histochemical, and ultrastructural evaluation. For the remaining 50%, we end up in Plato's cave with our radiologic colleagues—suggesting diagnoses and recommending further testing.

Which of the multitude of histochemical stains is worth performing as a routine battery on every muscle biopsy? I would venture that each of the authors contributing to this text would answer this question differently, although many would agree on the essentials. A recent textbook on neuropathology techniques recommends an even dozen: hematoxylin-eosin (H&E), acid phosphatase, myofibrillary ATPase (at 3 pH levels), Gomori trichrome, NADH-tetrazolium reductase (NADH-TR), succinate dehydrogenase (SDH), cytochrome oxidase (COX), oil red O, periodic acid–Schiff (PAS), and myophosphorylase. In our laboratory, we routinely perform four of these stains: H&E, ATPase (pH 4.6), Gomori trichrome, and COX. In potential metabolic disease, we stain for myophosphorylase and perform electron microscopy. All vacuolar myopathies are evaluated ultrastructurally, thereby obviating the need for PAS, oil red O, and acid phosphatase stains. NADH-TR, SDH, and COX are all oxidative enzyme stains that assess various components of the electron

TABLE 11-2
Preparations for Presumptive and Definitive Diagnoses

	Paraffin H&E	EM	Histochemistry	Ancillary Studies
Denervation	P	P	D	—
Autoimmune myasthenia	—	—	—	D
Periodic paralysis	—	P	—	D
Myotonic dystrophy	P	—	—	D
Duchenne's dystrophy	P	—	—	D
LGMD	P	—	—	D
Nemaline myopathy	P	D	D	—
Central core disease	—	D	D	—
Acid maltase deficiency	P	P	P	D
McArdle's disease	—	P	D	—
CPT II deficiency	P	P	P	D
Mitochondrial disease	—	P	P	D
Acute quadriplegic myopathy	—	D	—	—
Dermatomyositis	D	—	—	—
Polymyositis	P	—	—	D
Inclusion body myositis	P	D	—	—

CPT II, carnitine palmitoyltransferase II; D, definitive; LGMD, limb-girdle muscular dystrophy; P, presumptive.

transport chain. Of these, COX provides the greatest sensitivity. We confirm abnormalities on COX histochemistry by electron microscopy, followed by recommendations for definitive biochemical and genetic testing.

Ideally, processing of a muscle biopsy specimen consists of dividing the muscle into four portions: a small aliquot fixed in glutaraldehyde or half-strength Karnovsky's glutaraldehyde/paraformaldehyde solution and three roughly equal quantities of muscle embedded transversely in OCT embedding media (Miles Scientific) and flash-frozen in liquid nitrogen–cooled isopentane (2-methylbutane) for histochemistry; placed in a sterile container or aluminum foil, flash-frozen in liquid nitrogen, and stored at −80° C; or fixed in formalin and embedded longitudinally in paraffin for routine light microscopy. Because focal abnormalities (e.g., inflammatory infiltrates) are best visualized within paraffin-embedded specimens, these specimens are serially sectioned at approximately 100-μm intervals with sections stained with H&E or left unstained on charged slides for possible immunohistochemistry. Thus, the pathologist receives frozen transverse muscle sections stained with H&E, ATPase, Gomori trichrome, and COX, accompanied by perhaps a half dozen paraffin-embedded H&E-stained longitudinal sections. These slides may then be approached as follows:

Paraffin-embedded H&E-stained sections: Inflammation? Endomysial fibrosis? Degeneration or regeneration of muscle fibers (or both)? Cytoplasmic vacuoles?

Frozen transverse H&E-stained sections: Abnormalities in fiber size and shape? Distribution of these abnormalities? Presence and prevalence of fibers with centralized nuclei? Endomysial fibrosis? Degeneration or regeneration of muscle fibers (or both)?

ATPase histochemical stain: Abnormalities on H&E staining involving one or both fiber types? Fiber-type grouping? Target fibers?

Gomori trichrome stain (Confession: this is a tinctorial rather than a histochemical stain because it is not dependent on enzyme activity. When performed on frozen sections, muscle fibers and collagen are green, nuclei are purple, and mitochondria/T tubules/sarcoplasmic bodies are red): Endomysial fibrosis? Ragged red fibers? Nemaline rods? Rimmed vacuoles? Sarcoplasmic bodies?

Cytochrome C oxidase (complex IV) histochemical stain (type 1 fibers normally stain darker than type 2 fibers): Fibers with increased subsarcolemmal or cytoplasmic staining? Prevalence of COX-negative fibers? Central cores? Multi-minicores?

It has oft been stated that what separates the novice from the master pathologist is the latter's ability to recognize artifacts of tissue handling and processing. Muscle biopsy interpretation is frequently complicated by one or more of the following:

1. Hypercontraction of fibers caused by handling of the muscle before fixation/freezing—these fibers may be indistinguishable from hypercontracted fibers secondary to acute myofiber necrosis. In true muscle disease, regenerating muscle fibers can usually be found on careful inspection, although in rare instances, definitive resolution is not possible.

2. Ice crystal artifact as a result of poor (slow) freezing—when mild, holes left in muscle fibers may be confused with vacuolar degeneration. The latter is usually more varied in size and, on careful inspection, not optically empty (clear). When severe, freezing artifact can render the biopsy specimen uninterpretable. In such cases, thawing and refreezing the muscle may ameliorate the problem. In particularly refractory instances, one can process some of the muscle for electron microscopic analysis. Although not amenable to histochemical analysis, the semi-thin sections often show enough morphologic preservation to render a diagnosis.

3. A single focus of atrophic or degenerated fibers in an otherwise normal-appearing biopsy specimen—the former is usually due to proximity of the muscle sample to a tendinous insertion; the latter may be due to muscle trauma before biopsy, occasionally iatrogenic (biopsy of muscle used for electrophysiologic testing).

We now turn to a survey of skeletal muscle pathology.

DENERVATION ATROPHY

CLINICAL FEATURES

Although denervation atrophy is not a disease unto itself, it is among the most common diagnoses rendered on muscle biopsy specimens. Thus, its elimination from consideration represents the first step in the analysis of muscle biopsy specimens. Elderly patients with neuropathies often have clinical and laboratory features suggestive of muscle disease—weakness that is not obviously distal, elevated creatine kinase, and unreliable physical findings.

DENERVATION ATROPHY—FACT SHEET

Definition
▶ Anatomic separation of skeletal muscle fibers from their motor nerves

Incidence and Location
▶ Common; specific incidence dependent on cause
▶ Distal weakness usually predominates

Gender and Age Distribution
▶ Dependent on cause; peaks include infancy (spinal muscular atrophy) and advancing age (peripheral neuropathies, radiculopathies, motor neuron disease)

Clinical Features
▶ Distal-predominant muscle weakness (except in spinal muscular atrophy)
▶ Gross atrophy of muscle in severe cases
▶ Decreased tendon reflexes
▶ Accompanying sensory loss (in most neuropathies and radiculopathies)

Prognosis and Treatment
▶ Dependent on cause

PATHOLOGIC FEATURES

The cardinal histopathologic feature of denervation atrophy is "small group atrophy"—clusters of a few to several angulated muscle fibers in proximity (but not adjacent) to each other. These fibers appear smaller than the intervening normal (or occasionally hypertrophic) muscle fibers, and all of the fibers within a group appear to have shrunk by approximately the same amount (Fig. 11-2A). Occasional degenerating and regenerating muscle fibers may accompany these changes without invoking dual pathology. In long-standing denervation, such as accompanies some hereditary neuropathies, histopathologic features indistinguishable from those of myopathy may be encountered ("pseudomyopathic changes of chronic denervation") (see Fig. 11-2B). Severely atrophic fibers, having lost all of their sarcomeres, remain as bundles of nuclei that may resemble lymphocyte aggregates on superficial inspection. In infants with spinal muscular atrophy, denervated fibers are usually rounded rather than angulated and may be so atrophic that they resemble macrophages (see Fig. 11-2C).

ANCILLARY STUDIES

Histochemistry

ATPase histochemistry demonstrates that atrophic fibers within small groups are all of the same fiber type and that small groups of both fiber types are present within the biopsy specimen (although type 2 fiber groups usually predominate because their greater reliance on phasic neural input results in more rapid atrophy after denervation). On reinnervation of atrophied muscle fibers, sarcomeric reconstitution is initially accompanied by target fiber formation (see Fig. 11-2D). After complete reconstitution, the reinnervated fibers switch type based on that of the parent neuron, thereby resulting in large groups of similarly typed fibers (see Fig. 11-1C).

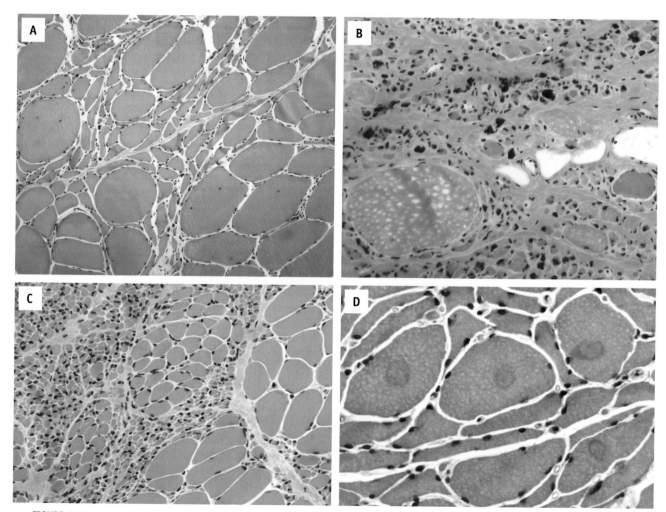

FIGURE 11-2

A, Denervated muscle demonstrating groups of angular atrophic muscle fibers. **B**, "Pseudomyopathic" changes in a patient with chronic denervation atrophy secondary to hereditary neuropathy. Bundles of muscle nuclei within markedly atrophic fibers should not be mistaken for lymphocytic infiltrates. **C**, Muscle biopsy from an infant with spinal muscular atrophy demonstrating rounded atrophic fibers resembling macrophages. **D**, Sarcomeric reorganization after reinnervation manifested as "target fiber" formation.

vation and are discussed in the second part of this chapter.

DENERVATION ATROPHY—PATHOLOGIC FEATURES

Microscopic Findings
- ▶ Decrease in diameter of muscle fibers
- ▶ Bimodal fiber size distribution
- ▶ Groups of small angulated (adults) or rounded (infants) fibers
- ▶ Fiber-type grouping in long-standing cases

Histochemical Findings
- ▶ Esterase: denervated fibers are dark
- ▶ Target fibers in ≈25% of cases
- ▶ Trichrome: smudgy appearance in center of fiber
- ▶ ATPase: central clearing
- ▶ Oxidative: central clearing with peripheral condensation

Ultrastructural Features
- ▶ Redundant basal lamina

Genetics
- ▶ Dependent on cause. Most infantile and childhood cases are autosomal recessive (Werdnig-Hoffmann disease); most adult cases are sporadic or acquired

Pathologic Differential Diagnosis
- ▶ Type 2 fiber atrophy secondary to disuse
- ▶ Type 1 fiber atrophy in some metabolic myopathies

AUTOIMMUNE MYASTHENIA ("MYASTHENIA GRAVIS")

CLINICAL FEATURES

Myasthenia gravis is a disease of young women and older men that is generally manifested as ptosis that worsens as the day wears on. A history of slowly progressive "weakness" can usually be elicited, which on further investigation generally represents fatigability rather than fixed weakness. Oculobulbar symptomatology predominates early in patients with true autoimmune myasthenia, whereas patients with the Lambert-Eaton myasthenic syndrome usually experience more fatigue in the proximal leg muscles along with decreased deep tendon reflexes and autonomic dysfunction. The majority of patients with generalized autoimmune myasthenia have antibodies against acetylcholine receptors, and about two thirds have thymic hyperplasia. Thymoma is discovered in approximately 15% of patients. Small cell carcinoma of the lung is found in about 50% of patients with the Lambert-Eaton myasthenic syndrome. Patients with cancer-associated

Ultrastructural Features

Loss of sarcomeric protein with preservation of sarcolemmal membranes results in cells with folded, redundant basal lamina.

DIFFERENTIAL DIAGNOSIS

It is important to distinguish denervation atrophy from the type-specific atrophy encountered commonly in disuse (type 2 fiber atrophy) or uncommonly in specific muscle diseases (e.g., type 1 fiber atrophy in myotonic dystrophy, central core disease). Although ATPase histochemistry is required for a definitive differential diagnosis, type-specific atrophy virtually never occurs as small group atrophy, but is usually distributed evenly within the muscle.

Much has been written concerning distinguishing targets from cores in muscle fibers. It is likely that absolute distinctions are neither possible nor necessary because the contexts in which the two are encountered provide more distinguishing information than histochemical and ultrastructural analysis does.

PROGNOSIS AND THERAPY

The prognosis and treatment depend on the underlying disease responsible for the loss of muscle inner-

---

AUTOIMMUNE MYASTHENIA ("MYASTHENIA GRAVIS")—FACT SHEET

Definition
- ▶ Acquired autoimmune disease of the (postsynaptic) neuromuscular junction

Prevalence and Location
- ▶ ≈200 cases per million
- ▶ Oculobulbar symptoms usually predominate

Gender and Age Distribution
- ▶ Female preponderance in children and young adults
- ▶ Male preponderance in patients older than 50 years

Clinical Features
- ▶ Insidious onset of weakness and fatigability beginning in the oculobulbar muscles in more than 50% of patients
- ▶ Acetylcholine receptor antibodies in 50% (ocular) to ≈85% (generalized)
- ▶ Thymic hyperplasia in 65%
- ▶ Thymoma in ≈15%

Prognosis and Treatment
- ▶ Cholinesterase inhibitors for symptom control
- ▶ Immunosuppressive therapy
- ▶ Plasma exchange, intravenous immune globulin (useful for myasthenic crises, but effects are short lived)
- ▶ Thymectomy (in cases of thymoma)

myasthenia usually have serum antibodies that bind to voltage-gated calcium channels.

PATHOLOGIC FEATURES

Muscle histology is usually normal in autoimmune myasthenia and Lambert-Eaton myasthenic syndrome. Large collections of lymphocytes (lymphorrhages) within muscle have been reported, but they are so rare that they render histologic analysis of muscle virtually useless.

ANCILLARY STUDIES

Ultrastructural Features/Immunohistochemistry

Immunoelectron microscopic analysis of neuromuscular junctions may demonstrate inaccessibility of acetylcholine receptors.

PROGNOSIS AND THERAPY

In patients with myasthenic syndromes in the absence of cancer, the prognosis is favorable. Cholinesterase inhibitors (e.g., pyridostigmine) are used for symptom relief. Thymectomy may lead to improvement in patients with thymoma. The mainstay of therapy is immunosuppression,

with plasma exchange and intravenous immune globulin used in the treatment of myasthenic crises.

PERIODIC PARALYSIS

CLINICAL FEATURES

The periodic paralyses are the first-described and best-understood group of diseases resulting from inherited ion channel mutations and are thus often referred to as "channelopathies." The periodic paralyses have historically been classified on the basis of serum potassium levels during attacks, although ongoing genetic studies may eventually result in reclassification based on which ion channels (sodium, potassium, calcium) are primarily affected. Among the periodic paralyses, the most common is hypokalemic periodic paralysis. This autosomal dominant disease usually starts in childhood, with attacks of weakness typically lasting hours to days and often triggered by carbohydrate ingestion. In hyperkalemic periodic paralysis, attacks typically occur after (not during) exercise and do not last as long (minutes to hours). The ocular and respiratory muscles are usually spared. Although the frequency of attacks in both types of periodic paralysis tends to decrease with age, a fixed vacuolar myopathy may develop.

AUTOIMMUNE MYASTHENIA ("MYASTHENIA GRAVIS")— PATHOLOGIC FEATURES

Microscopic Findings
▶ Usually normal
▶ Lymphorrhages (very rare)

Histochemical Findings
▶ Occasionally type 2 atrophy

Ultrastructural Features
▶ Routine electron microscopy normal

Genetics
▶ Sporadic

Immunohistochemical Features
▶ Immunoelectron microscopy of neuromuscular junctions may demonstrate reduced density of acetylcholine receptors

Pathologic Differential Diagnosis
▶ N/A
▶ The clinicopathologic differential diagnosis includes Lambert-Eaton myasthenic syndrome and botulism

---

PERIODIC PARALYSIS—FACT SHEET

Definition
▶ Episodic muscle weakness caused by intermittent inexcitability of muscle fibers secondary to ion channel dysfunction

Incidence and Location
▶ ≈1 case/million/year
▶ Generalized limb weakness/paralysis

Gender and Age Distribution
▶ No gender predilection
▶ Generally develops in childhood or adolescence

Clinical Features
▶ Hyperkalemic:
  ▶ Weakness lasting minutes to hours
  ▶ Often precipitated by rest after exercise
  ▶ Cold-induced myotonia may occur
  ▶ Frequency of attacks diminishes with age
▶ Hypokalemic:
  ▶ Weakness lasting 12 to 24 hours
  ▶ Often precipitated by carbohydrate ingestion

Prognosis and Treatment
▶ The hypokalemic variant more frequently eventuates in degenerative myopathic changes with permanent residual weakness
▶ Treatment is aimed at preventing fluxes in serum potassium concentration

PATHOLOGIC FEATURES

Except for patients in whom fixed weakness with vacuolar changes has developed, muscle biopsy specimens appear normal by H&E staining.

ANCILLARY STUDIES

Histochemistry

Trichrome staining may disclose subsarcolemmal aggregates of red-staining granular material (Fig. 11-3A). Although these aggregates may superficially resemble the "ragged red" fibers seen in mitochondrial disorders, the two processes can be distinguished by oxidative enzyme staining, which highlights mitochondrial proliferations but not tubular aggregates.

Ultrastructural Features

Tubular aggregates appear as densely packed tubules arising from the sarcoplasmic reticulum, usually in a subsarcolemmal location (see Fig. 11-3B).

Other

Specific sodium, potassium, and calcium channel mutations are associated with the periodic paralyses. The potassium level at initial evaluation, as well as the presence or absence of associated clinical findings or a family history thereof, provides a useful guide to which mutations are likely to be responsible. The presence of a channel protein mutation confirms the diagnosis.

DIFFERENTIAL DIAGNOSIS

Neither vacuolar degeneration nor tubular aggregates are pathognomonic for periodic paralysis, although they help substantiate the diagnosis in clinically suspicious cases. Tubular aggregates may be seen in association with other channelopathies, including myotonic disorders such as myotonia congenita and paramyotonia congenita, and in malignant hyperthermia. They have also been reported in alcoholic myopathy and congenital myasthenic syndromes and constitute the diagnostic hallmark of familial "tubular aggregate myopathy." Autophagic vacuolar degeneration may also occur as a nonspecific finding in a variety of myopathies and is commonly seen as a manifestation of lysosomal toxicity associated with drugs such as colchicine, chloroquine, and amiodarone (see Fig. 11-3C). T-tubule–associated

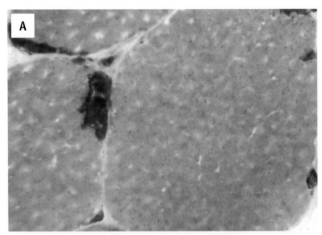

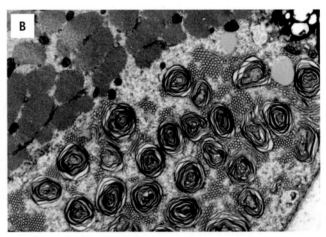

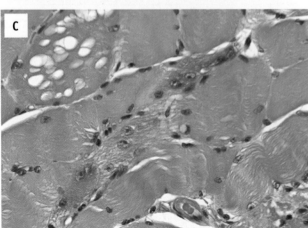

FIGURE 11-3

A, Trichrome histochemical staining demonstrates subsarcolemmal tubular aggregates in a patient with periodic paralysis. **B**, Densely packed subsarcolemmal arrays of tubular aggregates arising from the sarcoplasmic reticulum in a patient with periodic paralysis. **C**, Vacuolar myopathy may be seen in a variety of toxic and metabolic conditions, but it must be distinguished from the more common ice crystal artifact.

PERIODIC PARALYSIS—PATHOLOGIC FEATURES

Microscopic Findings

▶ H&E may be normal or may show vacuolar changes within muscle cells

Histochemical Findings

▶ Tubular aggregates appear as collections of red subsarcolemmal granules on trichrome stain

Ultrastructural Features

▶ Proliferation and dilatation of the sarcoplasmic reticulum and T-tubular system
▶ Tubular aggregates may be seen in otherwise unaffected fibers

Genetics

▶ Autosomal recessive
  ▶ Hyperkalemic: *SCN4A* (17q23) sodium channel
  ▶ Hypokalemic: *CACNA1S* (1q32) calcium channel, *SCN4A* (17q23) sodium channel, *KCNE3* (11q13-14) potassium channel

Pathologic Differential Diagnosis

▶ Tubular aggregates:
  ▶ Other channelopathies, including myotonia and paramyotonia congenita, and malignant hyperthermia
  ▶ Alcoholic myopathy
  ▶ Congenital myasthenic syndromes
  ▶ Familial "tubular aggregate myopathy"
▶ Vacuolar degeneration:
  ▶ Nonspecific autophagic (lysosomal) vacuoles
  ▶ Drug-induced vacuolar degeneration
  ▶ Lysosomal storage disorders

MYOTONIC DYSTROPHY (TYPE 1)—FACT SHEET

Definition

▶ Multisystem disease characterized by myotonia, progressive muscle wasting, and a range of potential systemic manifestations

Incidence and Location

▶ 5 to 6 cases/100,000 population/year
▶ Facial and distal muscle weakness predominates

Gender and Age Distribution

▶ No gender predominance
▶ Typically develops in the third or fourth decade; 10% present with neonatal hypotonia

Clinical Features

▶ Weakness and wasting of facial muscles with ptosis
▶ Extremity weakness and atrophy begin distally
▶ Clinical myotonia with myotonic discharges on electromyography
▶ Heart block, cardiomyopathy, cataracts, hypersomnia, diminished intellect, gonadal atrophy, frontal balding, dysphagia, constipation, and diabetes mellitus may develop

Prognosis and Treatment

▶ Diaphragmatic weakness may lead to respiratory failure
▶ Cardiac arrhythmias may lead to sudden death
▶ Early pacemaker insertion is critical; respiratory therapy is supportive

---

vacuoles identical to those of periodic paralysis may be seen in drug-related hypokalemia, such as may occur with diuretics, laxatives, and amphotericin B.

PROGNOSIS AND THERAPY

Progression to permanent fixed weakness with myopathic changes occurs in a minority of patients but is more common with the hypokalemic variant. Treatment of acute attacks depends on the serum potassium level. Patients with hyperkalemic paralysis may respond to a single dose of acetazolamide, whereas oral potassium is the treatment of choice for hypokalemic attacks. Acetazolamide may be useful in preventing attacks of either kind, although multicenter trials on management of the periodic paralyses are in early stages.

MYOTONIC DYSTROPHY (TYPE 1)

CLINICAL FEATURES

Myotonic dystrophy is unusual among the primary muscle diseases in that patients generally present with

distal rather than proximal extremity weakness and wasting. Facial muscle wasting with ptosis leads to a distinctive "hatchet face" appearance that is virtually diagnostic. Myotonic discharges on the electromyograph cinch the diagnosis, which can be confirmed by genetic testing. Although patients classically come to medical attention in early adulthood, the age at diagnosis and the severity of the disease correlate with the size of an unstable trinucleotide repeat expansion. Infants with large (>1000 repeat) expansions present with neonatal hypotonia. These severe congenital cases nearly always arise from trinucleotide expansion during oogenesis within an affected mother, although rare cases of large spermatogenic expansion have been reported.

Additional clinical features of type 1 myotonic dystrophy include heart block, cardiomyopathy, cataracts, hypersomnia, low IQ, gonadal atrophy, diabetes, frontal balding (in both males and females), swallowing difficulties, and constipation.

PATHOLOGIC FEATURES

Routine light microscopy reveals striking central nuclear migration within most (but not all) muscle fibers (Fig. 11-4). Longitudinal sections may show distinctive chains of nuclei within the central region of myofibers. Angular atrophic fibers are present throughout the muscle but are disposed randomly rather than

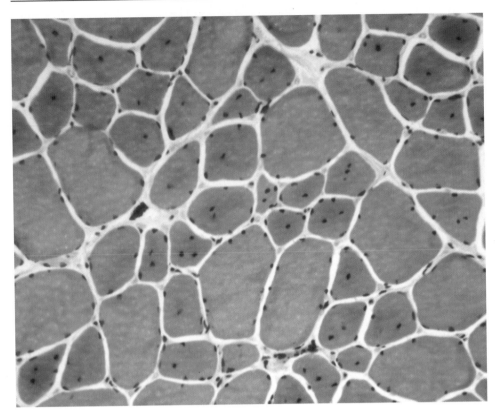

FIGURE 11-4

Muscle biopsy specimens from patients with myotonic dystrophy (type 1 or type 2) demonstrate striking central nuclear migration within the majority of muscle fibers.

MYOTONIC DYSTROPHY (TYPE 1)—PATHOLOGIC FEATURES

Microscopic Findings
► Central nuclear migration in a majority of fibers
► Widespread fiber atrophy without grouping

Histochemical Findings
► Selective type 1 fiber atrophy

Ultrastructural Features
► Nonspecific

Genetics
► CTG repeat expansion involving the *DMPK* gene (chromosome 19) in nearly all cases

Pathologic Differential Diagnosis
► When present in full, the histologic features are virtually pathognomonic
► In neonatal cases, the histology may be nonspecific
► In advanced cases, dystrophic features supervene

---

in groups. Dystrophic features supervene in advanced cases.

In infants with neonatal hypotonia, the histopathologic features are nonspecific. Before the molecular genetic era, neonatal diagnosis was accomplished by biopsy of the baby's mother, in whom diagnostic features are usually present even in the absence of symptomatology.

ANCILLARY STUDIES

Histochemistry

ATPase staining shows that the atrophic fibers are type 1.

Other

Genetic analysis is the preferred diagnostic modality and demonstrates CTG expansion within the *DMPK* gene on chromosome 19.

DIFFERENTIAL DIAGNOSIS

Although both central nuclear migration and muscle fiber atrophy may be seen in a wide variety of muscle diseases, the severity of the nuclear changes combined with the type 1 selectivity of the fiber atrophy is distinctive.

Myotonic dystrophy type 2, also known as proximal myotonic myopathy, is a more recently described genetic disease that has many clinical similarities to myotonic dystrophy type 1, but different gene expansion (untranslated CCTG on chromosome 3). These patients are more likely to come to biopsy, which shows many of the features seen in type 1 myotonic dystrophy.

PROGNOSIS AND THERAPY

The severity of the disease correlates directly with the size of the trinucleotide repeat expansion. The most common cause of death is respiratory failure secondary to pneumonia, diaphragmatic weakness, or both. Cardiac arrhythmias, usually secondary to atrioventricular block, are the second leading cause of death. Although the indications for pacemaker placement are not clearly defined, abnormal PR intervals or documented dysrhythmias (or both) should prompt referral to a cardiologist.

DUCHENNE'S MUSCULAR DYSTROPHY

CLINICAL FEATURES

Duchenne's muscular dystrophy becomes clinically apparent in early childhood. Initially, these young boys are clumsy and have trouble running; later, they have difficulty climbing stairs. Hip and knee extensor weakness is manifested as the Gower sign, whereby the child climbs up his thighs to arise from a lying or sitting position. Although calf hypertrophy is considered to be one of the hallmarks of Duchenne's muscular dystrophy, it is not specific. Progressive, mainly proximal, muscle weakness leads to wheelchair dependence in most boys by the age of 12 years.

PATHOLOGIC FEATURES

Muscle biopsies performed early in the disease may show only scattered hypereosinophilic and regeneration fibers with fiber splitting, although endomysial fibrosis is usually apparent (Fig. 11-5A). As the disease progresses, there is a disproportionate increase in the amount of endomysial fibrosis and fat within the muscle. Focal lymphocytic infiltrates may be seen, particularly in the early stages, and should not be taken as evidence of an inflammatory myopathy.

ANCILLARY STUDIES

Histochemistry

Trichrome staining highlights hypercontracted fibers and endomysial fibrous tissue.

Ultrastructural Features

Disruption of myofibrillary architecture can be seen, although this finding is nonspecific.

Immunohistochemistry

In Duchenne's muscular dystrophy, there is complete absence of immunoreactivity for dystrophin, with the exception of rare clusters of "revertant fibers" (see Fig. 11-5B). In Becker's muscular dystrophy (the milder

---

DUCHENNE'S MUSCULAR DYSTROPHY—FACT SHEET

Definition
▶ X-linked dystrophy of muscle caused by mutations resulting in the absence of dystrophin

Incidence and Location
▶ 1 case per 3500 live male births
▶ Shoulder, pelvic, and extremity muscles

Gender and Age Distribution
▶ Nearly exclusively males
▶ Peak age of onset between 2 and 5 years

Clinical Features
▶ Clumsiness progressing to weakness with calf hypertrophy
▶ Joint contractures, kyphoscoliosis, and diminished pulmonary function
▶ Wheelchair bound by age 12
▶ Cardiomyopathy with conduction defects and congestive failure (late)
▶ 20% have IQ less than 70

Prognosis and Treatment
▶ Usually fatal by the late teens/early 20s as a result of pneumonia compounded by cardiac involvement
▶ Therapy is currently supportive, although molecular therapies are evolving

---

DUCHENNE'S MUSCULAR DYSTROPHY—PATHOLOGIC FEATURES

Microscopic Findings
▶ Early—hyaline fibers with densely opaque cytoplasm, fiber splitting
▶ Later—degeneration and regeneration of muscle fibers with disproportionate endomysial fibrosis
▶ Focal lymphocytic inflammation may be present

Histochemical Findings
▶ Hyaline fibers best visualized on H&E and trichrome stains, where they appear smudged and homogeneous

Ultrastructural Features
▶ Disruption of myofibrillary architecture

Genetics
▶ Intragenic dystrophin deletions (Xp21) in 65% with a frameshift
▶ Duplications in ≈10%, presumed frame-shifting point mutations in 25%
▶ About a third of cases arise from new (somatic) mutations

Immunohistochemical Features
▶ Complete absence of dystrophin immunoreactivity, with the exception of rare clusters of "revertant fibers"

Pathologic Differential Diagnosis
▶ Becker's muscular dystrophy
▶ "Limb-girdle" muscular dystrophies

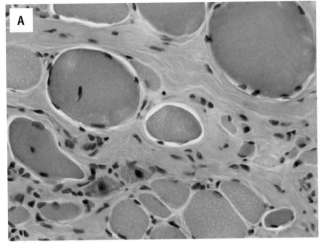

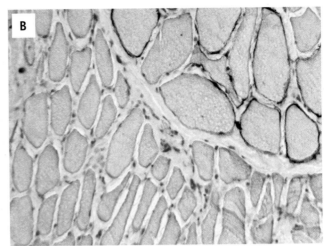

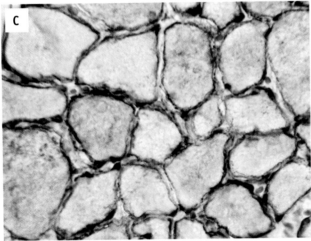

FIGURE 11-5

A, Muscle biopsy specimen from a young boy with Duchenne's muscular dystrophy demonstrating endomysial fibrosis. **B**, Dystrophic immunohisto-chemical staining demonstrates complete absence of reactivity within the majority of muscle fiber in Duchenne's muscular dystrophy. Groups of positively staining "revertant fibers" may be present and do not alter the diagnosis. **C**, Boys with Becker's muscular dystrophy may demonstrate weak or apparently normal dystrophin immunoreactivity.

variant of dystrophinopathy), immunostaining may be reduced or normal (see Fig. 11-5C).

Other

Immunoblot analysis of skeletal muscle confirms the complete absence of dystrophin in Duchenne's muscular dystrophy and the abnormally short dystrophin in Becker's muscular dystrophy. Genetic analysis of the X chromosome can be used to diagnose dystrophinopathy in the majority of boys. Frame-shifting dystrophin mutations resulting in a premature stop codon cause Duchenne's muscular dystrophy, whereas non–frame-shifting deletions result in the milder (Becker) phenotype.

DIFFERENTIAL DIAGNOSIS

The histopathologic features of the muscular dystro-phies are relatively nonspecific. Absence of immuno-reactivity for dystrophin is virtually diagnostic of Duchenne's muscular dystrophy, although confirmatory immunoblotting is recommended. Apparently decreased or normal immunoreactivity may be seen in a large number of autosomally inherited dystrophies, as well as Becker's muscular dystrophy. The clinical course of Duchenne's

muscular dystrophy is fairly uniform and parallels the degree of damage seen within the biopsy specimen. There-fore, immunostaining for dystrophin in an ambulatory patient older than 12 years is rarely, if ever indicated.

PROGNOSIS AND THERAPY

Duchenne's muscular dystrophy is relentlessly pro-gressive. Death occurs as a result of a combination of cardiomyopathy with conduction defects, respiratory weakness, and pneumonia. Although these patients rarely used to live beyond the age of 20 years, supportive therapies have increased their life expectancy approxi-mately 10 years. Specific therapies are not yet available, but molecular approaches are encouraging.

LIMB-GIRDLE MUSCULAR DYSTROPHIES

CLINICAL FEATURES

Similar to the dystrophinopathies, patients with limb-girdle muscular dystrophies present with progressive

LIMB-GIRDLE MUSCULAR DYSTROPHIES—FACT SHEET

Definition

▶ Heterogeneous group of autosomally determined, face-sparing, proximally predominant, progressive muscular dystrophies

Incidence and Location

▶ ≈8 cases/million population/year
▶ Pelvic or shoulder girdle weakness predominates
▶ Most common types are calpainopathy (LGMD2A), dysferlinopathy (LGMD2B), and sarcoglycanopathies (LGMD2C-F)

Gender and Age Distribution

▶ No gender predominance
▶ Age at onset varies greatly (usually first to third decade)

Clinical Features

▶ Normal intelligence
▶ Calf hypertrophy (except dysferlinopathy)
▶ Elevated creatine kinase
▶ Variable rate of progression, some with cardiac (LGMD2C) and respiratory (LGMD2I) involvement

Prognosis and Treatment

▶ Prognosis is variable
▶ Treatment is supportive at present; molecular studies are ongoing

proximal weakness, usually with onset during childhood. Unlike Duchenne's and Becker's muscular dystrophy, limb-girdle muscular dystrophies are transmitted as autosomal disorders, usually recessive. Because the general term "limb-girdle muscular dystrophy" is used to describe any noncongenital dystrophic myopathy not caused by a primary dystrophin abnormality, there is considerable variation in clinical features among the specific genetic diseases, although the pathologic features show more similarities than differ-

ences. The most common limb-girdle muscular dystrophies are the sarcoglycanopathies (themselves a group of at least four subtypes), dysferlinopathy (one mutation, several clinical forms), and calpainopathy.

PATHOLOGIC FEATURES

By and large, all these diseases have dystrophic features (degeneration and regeneration of muscle fibers with endomysial fibrosis) virtually indistinguishable from those seen in the dystrophinopathies, thus necessitating immunoblot or genetic analysis (or both) for diagnosis. Pathologic clues to the diagnosis include lobulated type 1 fibers in calpainopathy (Fig. 11-6A) and (sometimes) inflammatory infiltrates in dysferlinopathy (see Fig. 11-6B).

ANCILLARY STUDIES

Histochemistry

ATPase histochemical staining is useful to confirm that the lobulated fibers seen in calpainopathy are type 1. Rimmed vacuoles and rod-like structures have been described in trichrome-stained sections from some patients with rare subtypes of limb-girdle muscular dystrophy (telethoninopathy and myotilinopathy, respectively).

Immunohistochemistry

Cryostat- or paraffin-reactive antibodies (or both) to a variety of these proteins are becoming available. Currently, diagnosis of these unusual diseases generally requires that frozen muscle be sent to specialized laboratories where either immunoblot or genetic analysis or both can be performed.

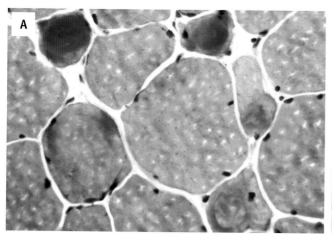 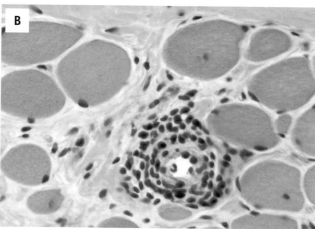

FIGURE 11-6

A, Lobulated muscle fibers in a patient with calpainopathy (limb-girdle muscular dystrophy type 2A). **B,** Perivascular lymphocytic inflammation in an adult patient with dysferlinopathy (limb-girdle muscular dystrophy type 2B). Scattered inflammatory infiltrates may be seen in a variety of muscular dystrophies and should not prompt a diagnosis of primary inflammatory muscle disease.

LIMB-GIRDLE MUSCULAR DYSTROPHIES—PATHOLOGIC FEATURES

Microscopic Findings

▶ Degeneration and regeneration of muscle fibers with endomysial fibrosis
▶ Inflammation may be present in dysferlinopathy
▶ Lobulated type 1 fibers reported in calpainopathy

Histochemical Findings

▶ Nonspecific

Ultrastructural Features

▶ Nonspecific

Genetics

▶ 90% autosomal recessive (10 subtypes, LGMD2A-J)
▶ 10% autosomal dominant (5 subtypes, LGMD1A-E)

Immunohistochemical Features

▶ Loss of immunoreactivity with antibodies to corresponding normal muscle proteins
▶ Secondary reduction in dystrophin immunostaining (sarcoglycanopathies)
▶ Defective proteins coded by mutant genes may be detectible by immunoblot analysis

Pathologic Differential Diagnosis

▶ X-linked muscular dystrophies
▶ Inflammatory myopathies

DIFFERENTIAL DIAGNOSIS

In boys, the primary differential diagnostic consideration is dystrophinopathy, particularly Becker's muscular dystrophy (once immunostaining for dystrophin excludes Duchenne's muscular dystrophy). In dysferlinopathy, an erroneous diagnosis of inflammatory myopathy should be avoided through attention to the dystrophic features accompanying the inflammatory changes, particularly in patients who come to medical attention later in life.

PROGNOSIS AND THERAPY

Despite marked variability in the prognosis of individual diseases within this group, the general rule of earlier onset equals worse prognosis tends to hold. Sarcoglycanopathies are usually manifested in early childhood with a Duchenne-like phenotype ("severe childhood autosomal recessive muscular dystrophy"), calpainopathy usually occurs in late childhood, and dysferlinopathy often does not develop until adulthood. However, adult onset may be seen in virtually any of the limb-girdle muscular dystrophies. Certain sarcoglycanopathies (β, δ) appear to confer a higher risk of cardiomyopathy. At present, no specific therapies are available for any of the limb-girdle muscular dystrophies.

NEMALINE MYOPATHY

CLINICAL FEATURES

Nemaline myopathy was one of the first congenital/structural myopathies described and is a well-known cause of infantile hypotonia (the "floppy infant"). In these babies, facial and respiratory weakness helps distinguish nemaline myopathy from the many other causes of floppiness in babies. Currently, six different clinical forms of nemaline myopathy consisting of at least five distinct genetic diseases are recognized. These variants range from severe neonatal forms with the fetal akinesia sequence to adult-onset cases with isolated neck extensor weakness (the "dropped-head" sign). Thus, the pathologist must always peruse the muscle biopsy specimen for these sometimes subtle, but distinctive cytoplasmic structures.

PATHOLOGIC FEATURES

Light microscopic changes usually consist of muscle fiber atrophy without grouping. Careful examination of the atrophic fibers may reveal focal subsarcolemmal regions of increased refractivity (Fig. 11-7A).

NEMALINE MYOPATHY—FACT SHEET

Definition

▶ Myopathy with rod-shaped structures within muscle fibers (Greek *nema* = thread)

Incidence and Location

▶ ≈1 case/500,000/year
▶ Proximal weakness predominates

Gender and Age Distribution

▶ No gender predominance noted
▶ Onset from birth through adulthood; most become clinically apparent in the neonatal period or during childhood

Clinical Features

▶ Classic: floppy infant with facial and respiratory weakness
▶ Range: severe congenital forms with fetal akinesia and neonatal respiratory insufficiency to adult-onset forms with isolated head-drop

Prognosis and Treatment

▶ Earlier-onset cases are usually more severe
▶ Overall mortality is ≈20%, with death caused by respiratory insufficiency during the first year of life
▶ Aggressive supportive therapy may result in clinical stabilization with age

---

NEMALINE MYOPATHY—PATHOLOGIC FEATURES

Microscopic Findings
▶ Atrophic fibers without grouping; may contain small subsarcolemmal areas of increased refractivity

Histochemical Findings
▶ Trichrome: reddish purple thread-like inclusions within the sarcoplasm, often within atrophic fibers
▶ ATPase: type 1 fiber predominance and atrophy/hypotrophy

Ultrastructural Features
▶ Intracytoplasmic (and rarely intranuclear) rod-shaped structures composed of Z-band–like material, often accompanied by sarcoplasmic disruption

Genetics
▶ At least five different genetic diseases, including autosomal dominant and autosomal recessive forms

Immunohistochemical Features
▶ Sarcoplasmic rods react with antibodies to α-actinin

Pathologic Differential Diagnosis
▶ Nemaline bodies may form in fibers that have lost thick filaments for a variety of reasons. Specifically, they have been reported in association with central core disease and inflammatory myopathies

---

ANCILLARY STUDIES

Histochemistry

Although nemaline myopathy was first described on formalin-fixed, paraffin-embedded sections, the thread-like inclusions are much more easily seen on trichrome histochemical staining of frozen sections, where they show up as reddish purple against the light blue-green color of the muscle cytoplasm (see Fig. 11-7B). The proportion of muscle fibers containing these structures varies greatly from case to case but is often more than 50% of the fibers.

Ultrastructural Features

Electron microscopy frequently reveals striking osmiophilic rod-shaped inclusions that tend to be both subsarcolemmal and perinuclear (see Fig. 11-7C). Rarely, intranuclear inclusions are identified and signify a worse prognosis. Sarcomeric disruption is also usually seen in patients with severe weakness.

Immunohistochemistry

Immunohistochemical analysis has demonstrated a wide variety of skeletal muscle proteins within nemaline rods, although the most constantly stained protein is α-actinin type 2.

DIFFERENTIAL DIAGNOSIS

Nemaline rods may form in response to the loss of thick filaments within muscle fibers and may therefore be encountered in myopathies resulting from other causes. Specifically, nemaline rods have been reported in patients with inflammatory muscle diseases and in association with muscle cores in central core disease.

PROGNOSIS AND THERAPY

The classic neonatal form of the disease carries a 20% mortality rate, usually secondary to respiratory failure during the first year of life. The other 80% of these infants show clinical stabilization or even improvement, thus underscoring the value of aggressive supportive therapy. Later-onset cases tend to be less severe. Light microscopic findings do not correlate with clinical disease severity or genotypic analysis.

CENTRAL CORE DISEASE

CLINICAL FEATURES

The clinical spectrum of central core disease ranges from apparent normalcy to severe weakness resulting

---

CENTRAL CORE DISEASE—FACT SHEET

Definition
▶ Congenital myopathy with extensive areas in muscle fibers devoid of oxidative activity

Incidence and Location
▶ Reported to be one of the most frequent forms of congenital myopathy; true incidence not known because of wide phenotypic variability
▶ Facial, neck, and proximal limb weakness with generalized hypotonia

Gender and Age Distribution
▶ No gender predilection reported
▶ Usually becomes clinically apparent in infancy or early childhood

Clinical Features
▶ Slowly progressive or nonprogressive weakness with hypotonia
▶ Often develops in association with skeletal abnormalities (hip dislocation, scoliosis)
▶ Children more severely affected than their parents
▶ Respiratory insufficiency and cardiomyopathy are rare
▶ Highly associated with malignant hyperthermia

Prognosis and Treatment
▶ Functional improvement is common, even in severe cases
▶ Treatment is supportive and preventive (avoidance of stress, including medications, which might trigger episodes of malignant hyperthermia)

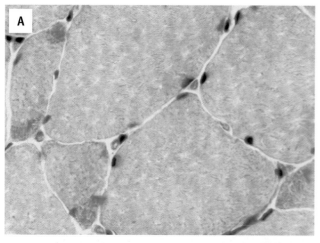

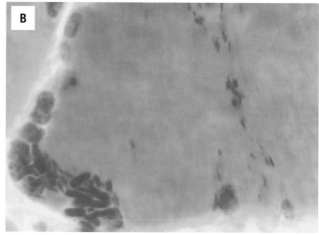

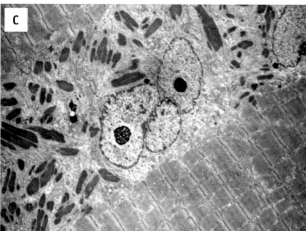

FIGURE 11-7

A, Nemaline rods may be appreciable on routine hematoxylin-eosin staining as focal areas of increased subsarcolemmal refractivity. **B**, On Gomori trichrome–stained sections, nemaline rods appear purplish red. **C**, By ultrastructural examination, nemaline rods appear as striking osmiophilic structures resembling Z-disk material.

in the need for ambulatory assistance. At initial evaluation, children tend to be more severely affected than their parents, thus suggesting the possibility of a trinucleotide repeat disease with genetic "anticipation." The proximal limb muscles, facial muscles, and neck flexors are most prominently involved. Initially, the weakness tends to be slowly progressive or static, but it often improves with time (which may be responsible for the appearance of anticipation). Orthopedic abnormalities are common, particularly scoliosis and congenital hip dislocation. Respiratory weakness and cardiomyopathy are rarely encountered. Malignant hyperthermia is highly associated with central core disease (but not multiminicore disease) independent of the degree of muscle weakness.

PATHOLOGIC FEATURES

Central core disease is the prototypical histochemically defined myopathy. Routinely stained muscle can appear entirely normal, although more severe cases may demonstrate nonspecific myopathic features.

ANCILLARY STUDIES

Histochemistry

Central core disease is named for the central regions of absent oxidative enzyme activity (NADH-TR, SDH, COX) within muscle fibers (Fig. 11-8). A second common, but nonspecific, finding is marked predominance (or even uniformity) of type 1 muscle fibers (usually demonstrated with ATPase histochemical stains). The closely related "multi-minicore disease" demonstrates multiple smaller regions of absent oxidative activity within muscle fibers.

Ultrastructural Features

As suggested by their histochemical features, central cores are regions devoid of mitochondria. When the myofibrillary architecture is preserved in these areas, the cores are referred to as "structured." When mitochondrial absence is accompanied by myofibrillary dissolution, the core is referred to as "unstructured." The significance of such core subtypes has not been elaborated. Central cores extend the full length of the muscle fiber; multi-minicores do not.

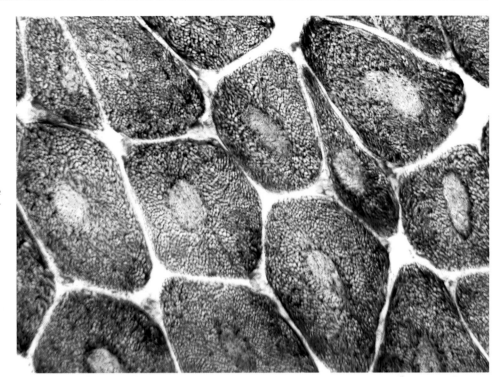

FIGURE 11-8

Loss of oxidative activity within the center of muscle fibers is the hallmark of central core disease.

CENTRAL CORE DISEASE—PATHOLOGIC FEATURES

Microscopic Findings

▶ Usually normal, but may demonstrate myopathic features in more severe cases

Histochemical Findings

▶ ATPase: type 1 fiber predominance (or even uniformity)
▶ Oxidative enzyme stains: central or peripheral cores, multiple minicores, or no cores with uniform staining

Ultrastructural Features

▶ Areas devoid of mitochondria, either with preservation (structured core) or disruption (unstructured core) of sarcomeres

Genetics

▶ Autosomal dominant
▶ Linked to ryanodine receptor gene mutations (*RYR1*, chromosome 19q13), with 50% of cases demonstrating a mutation in exons 93 to 104.

Immunohistochemical Features

▶ Cores contain a wide variety of proteins, including desmin and γ-filamin

Pathologic Differential Diagnosis

▶ Cores have been reported in hypothyroid myopathy
▶ Cores may closely resemble targets seen in neurogenic processes

Other

Dominantly inherited mutations in the ryanodine receptor gene (*RYR1*) are encountered in more than 50% of patients with central core disease. Such mutations are rare in multi-minicore disease, which has been associated with mutations in a gene associated with rigid spine syndrome (*SEPN1*).

DIFFERENTIAL DIAGNOSIS

Both central cores and multi-minicores must be distinguished from target fibers accompanying denervation atrophy. Such distinction is more easily said than done (targets are supposed to show peripheral increases in ATPase and oxidative enzyme staining). A diagnosis of core disease should be considered with trepidation in a patient showing other evidence of denervation atrophy.

PROGNOSIS AND THERAPY

Functional improvement is common even in severe cases, thus arguing for aggressive supportive therapy and avoidance of stresses that might trigger episodes of hyperthermia. This improvement may account for the observed generational differences in clinical severity at the time of diagnosis.

POMPE'S DISEASE (INFANTILE ACID MALTASE DEFICIENCY)

CLINICAL FEATURES

Acid maltase deficiency is the archetypic glycogenosis with fixed, rather than episodic muscle weakness. Although acid maltase deficiency may occur as isolated skeletal muscle weakness in children and young adults, the most common form is Pompe's disease, which is systemic and invariably fatal within the first 2 years of life. The combination of generalized hypotonia ("floppiness") and massive cardiomegaly is nearly diagnostic, but pathologic or biochemical confirmation (or both) is required.

PATHOLOGIC FEATURES

Muscle biopsy specimens show severe vacuolar degeneration of muscle fibers (Fig. 11-9A).

POMPE'S DISEASE (INFANTILE ACID MALTASE DEFICIENCY)—FACT SHEET

Definition
▶ Infantile form of acid α-glucosidase (lysosomal acid maltase) deficiency

Incidence and Location
▶ 1 to 2 cases per 100,000 live births
▶ Generalized weakness (floppiness) with massive cardiomegaly

Gender and Age Distribution
▶ No gender predominance
▶ Develops in infancy (nonclassic forms of acid maltase deficiency may occur later in life)

Clinical Features
▶ Infantile hypotonia and weakness with firm muscles, respiratory and feeding difficulties, cardiomegaly, hepatomegaly, and macroglossia

Prognosis and Treatment
▶ Invariably fatal before age 2; median survival is 6 to 8 months
▶ Treatment is supportive, although intravenous enzyme replacement trials are ongoing

---

POMPE'S DISEASE (INFANTILE ACID MALTASE DEFICIENCY)—PATHOLOGIC FEATURES

Microscopic Findings
▶ Replacement of the sarcoplasm by variably sized vacuoles containing blue-brown granular material

Histochemical Findings
▶ Vacuoles react with PAS and acid phosphatase, indicative of lysosomal glycogen storage

Ultrastructural Features
▶ Membrane-bound collections of glycogen

Genetics
▶ Autosomal recessive (chromosome 17q21-23)

Immunohistochemical Features
▶ N/A. Biochemical measurement of acid maltase in muscle establishes the diagnosis

Pathologic Differential Diagnosis
▶ X-linked vacuolar cardiomyopathy and myopathy (Danon's disease) are caused by a deficiency of LAMP-2

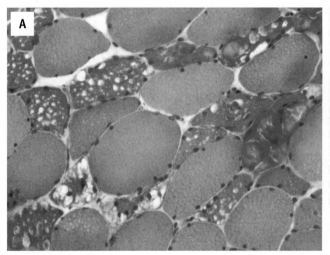
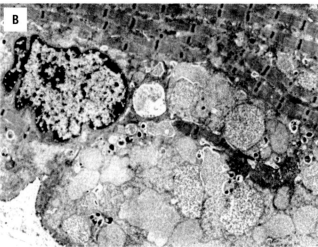

FIGURE 11-9

A, Severe vacuolar muscle fiber degeneration in an infant with acid maltase deficiency. **B,** Ultrastructural examination demonstrates massive lysosomal and nonlysosomal glycogen storage within muscle fibers.

ANCILLARY STUDIES

Histochemistry

Histochemical stains for both acid phosphatase and glycogen label the vacuoles and thus indicate accumulation of glycogen within lysosomes.

Ultrastructural Features

Electron microscopy confirms the presence of lysosomes distended with glycogen granules (see Fig. 11-9B). Muscle fibers also contain increased amounts of free glycogen.

Other

Biochemical assay of muscle α-glucosidase activity establishes the diagnosis.

DIFFERENTIAL DIAGNOSIS

The most important differential diagnostic consideration is a rare disease caused by mutation of the lysosome-associated membrane protein-2 (LAMP-2) gene on the X chromosome. These infants present with cardiomegaly, mental retardation, and vacuolar myopathy. Ultrastructurally, vacuoles contain membranous debris in addition to glycogen. α-Glucosidase levels are normal.

PROGNOSIS AND THERAPY

The median survival is 6 to 8 months. Although no specific therapy exists as of this writing, enzyme replacement trials are yielding encouraging preliminary results.

McARDLE'S DISEASE

CLINICAL FEATURES

Among the rare nonlysosomal glycogenoses, McArdle's disease (glycogenosis type V) is the most prevalent. Although an astute physician may suspect the diagnosis before biopsy, the need for specific histochemical staining for pathologic diagnosis requires that the pathologist be familiar with the clinical manifestations of this disease. It also underscores the importance of good communication between the clinician and pathologist in evaluation of the patient.

A disease of energy metabolism, McArdle's disease is characterized by pain, stiffness, and cramps after exercise. Myoglobinuria accompanies these symptoms in about 50% of patients. Patients with myophosphorylase deficiency usually come to medical attention during childhood, but the disease may go unrecognized for many years, especially in patients who do not manifest myoglobinuria. The "second-wind phenomenon," in which exer-

---

cise tolerance improves after about 10 minutes of activity, is characteristic of the nonlysosomal glycogenoses.

PATHOLOGIC FEATURES

The light microscopic features of McArdle's disease are usually quite subtle and consist of subsarcolemmal vacuoles easily ascribed to artifact. If the biopsy specimen is obtained during a myoglobinuric episode, myofiber necrosis may also be present.

ANCILLARY STUDIES

Histochemistry

The subsarcolemmal vacuoles stain with PAS, but not with acid phosphatase. Myophosphorylase is deficient in all but regenerating muscle fibers.

Ultrastructural Features

Subsarcolemmal vacuoles are composed of nonlysosomal (free) glycogen granules. Because the amount of free glycogen may vary widely among children with and without muscle disease, this finding is not specific.

DIFFERENTIAL DIAGNOSIS

The pathologic features of McArdle's disease are subtle, so awareness of this entity coupled with a low

McARDLE'S DISEASE—PATHOLOGIC FEATURES

Microscopic Findings

▶ Linear or crescent-shaped subsarcolemmal vacuoles

Histochemical Findings

▶ Vacuoles are strongly PAS positive but do not contain acid phosphatase
▶ Necrotic and regenerating fibers may be seen during myoglobinuric episodes
▶ Myophosphorylase absent from (non-regenerating) muscle fibers

Ultrastructural Features

▶ Subsarcolemmal accumulations of non–membrane-bound glycogen

Genetics

▶ Autosomal recessive (11q13), more than 33 distinct mutations— *R49X* nonsense mutation in exon 1 most common in North America

Immunohistochemical Features

▶ N/A. Biochemical analysis of muscle is definitive

Pathologic Differential Diagnosis

▶ Although several other nonlysosomal glyocogenoses involve muscle, myophosphorylase deficiency defines McArdle's disease
▶ Failure to detect myophosphorylase may occur after prolonged specimen storage at room temperature or after death

CARNITINE PALMITOYLTRANSFERASE II DEFICIENCY—FACT SHEET

Definition

▶ Impairment of organ function secondary to a deficiency of carnitine palmitoyltransferase II

Incidence and Location

▶ Incidence unknown—one of the most common inherited disorders of lipid metabolism
▶ Generalized weakness with myoglobinuria

Gender and Age Distribution

▶ Male preponderance (≈5:1) in the young adult form
▶ The young adult form is most common, the infantile/early childhood form is unusual, and the perinatal form is rare

Clinical Features (Young Adult Form)

▶ Recurrent myoglobinuria is usually precipitated by heavy exercise. It may also be precipitated by cold, infections, emotional stress, and fasting. The frequency of attacks may vary greatly; patients are usually asymptomatic between attacks. Creatine kinase is normal between attacks and is markedly elevated during attacks in ≈90% of patients

Prognosis and Treatment

▶ The prognosis in adult forms is generally excellent, as long as renal failure is avoided
▶ Intravenous glucose infusions are beneficial in improving exercise tolerance, although oral glucose is not. A carbohydrate-rich diet has been recommended

threshold for myophosphorylase histochemical staining is required to make the diagnosis. However, the pathologist must also avoid making an erroneous diagnosis of McArdle's disease based on loss of myophosphorylase activity after prolonged specimen storage at room temperature or after death. In acid maltase deficiency, much of the glycogen within muscle fibers is bound within lysosomal membranes.

PROGNOSIS AND THERAPY

Patients with McArdle's disease generally do well as long as myoglobinuric renal failure is avoided. Mild, fixed proximal muscle weakness develops in about a third of patients. Oral ingestion of sucrose before exertional activity improves exercise tolerance, as does a program of moderately low-intensity aerobic conditioning.

CARNITINE PALMITOYLTRANSFERASE II DEFICIENCY

CLINICAL FEATURES

Thus far, three distinct forms of carnitine palmitoyltransferase II (CPT II) deficiency have been delineated.

The most common ("adult form") is manifested in young adults as recurrent myoglobinuria, usually precipitated by heavy exercise. Much less common is the "infantile form," which (despite the name) is manifested in early childhood as fasting-induced hypoglycemia, hepatic failure, cardiomyopathy, and peripheral neuropathy. The least common (perinatal) form occurs similarly soon after birth and is rapidly fatal.

PATHOLOGIC FEATURES

During myoglobinuric attacks, acutely necrotic muscle fibers are readily identified, as are fibers containing intracytoplasmic vacuoles. Between attacks, however, the muscle nearly always appears normal.

ANCILLARY STUDIES

Histochemistry

Intracytoplasmic vacuoles stain bright red with oil red O.

CARNITINE PALMITOYLTRANSFERASE II DEFICIENCY—PATHOLOGIC FEATURES

Microscopic Findings

▶ Vacuolar myopathy with acutely necrotic fibers during attacks; usually normal between attacks

Histochemical Findings

▶ Oil red O: vacuoles bright red
▶ Toluidine blue: vacuoles pale green

Ultrastructural Features

▶ Increased skeletal muscle lipid (most cases)

Genetics

▶ Autosomal recessive (1p32); more than 25 mutations, *S113L* being most common

Pathologic Differential Diagnosis

▶ Primary and secondary carnitine deficiency
▶ Very long chain acyl-CoA dehydrogenase deficiency
▶ Other very rare defects in fatty acid oxidation

Ultrastructural Features

Intracytoplasmic vacuoles appear pale green in semithin sections; ultrastructural examination demonstrates large cytoplasmic lipid droplets.

Other

CPT II activity can be measured with approximately 100 mg of frozen skeletal muscle. Tandem mass spectrometry, performed on peripheral blood, may show elevated long-chain acylcarnitines.

DIFFERENTIAL DIAGNOSIS

Primary and secondary carnitine deficiency states demonstrate abundant lipid accumulations within muscle fibers. Clinically, however, these diseases are characterized by fixed, progressive weakness rather than episodic weakness. Very long chain acyl-CoA dehydrogenase deficiency may appear identical to CPT II deficiency and therefore requires bioassay for exclusion, as do other very rare defects in fatty acid β-oxidation.

PROGNOSIS AND THERAPY

As long as renal failure secondary to rhabdomyolysis can be avoided, the long-term prognosis in the common adult form of CPT II deficiency is generally excellent. Intravenous glucose helps improve exercise tolerance, although oral glucose does not.

MITOCHONDRIAL ENCEPHALOMYOPATHIES

CLINICAL FEATURES

Although mitochondrial proteins may be encoded by either nuclear or mitochondrial DNA, disorders involving defects in the latter account for the majority of diseases currently recognized as mitochondrial encephalomyopathies. Because nearly all mitochondria within our cells trace their ancestry back to the ovum, contain their own DNA, and are not subject to segregation rules during cell division, the clinical manifestations of mitochondrial defects are protean and may vary widely even among family members carrying identical mitochondrial mutations.

As we all learned in grade school, mitochondria are the powerhouses of the cell. It follows that tissues composed of cells with high energy requirements (brain and muscle) are most susceptible to power outages. The greater accessibility of the latter renders muscle biopsy the procedure of choice for a tissue diagnosis of mitochondrial disease.

As with other metabolic muscle diseases, good communication and a high index of suspicion are critical to diagnosis. Mitochondrial disease should be considered in any patient with a maternal pattern of inherited disease, multiorgan symptomatology, lactic acidosis, or any combination of these factors. Routine oxidative enzyme staining is recommended for pediatric muscle biopsy samples.

MITOCHONDRIAL ENCEPHALOMYOPATHIES—FACT SHEET

Definition

▶ Multisystem disorders caused by respiratory chain defects

Prevalence and Location

▶ 10 to 15 cases per 100,000 persons
▶ Weakness is usually generalized; progressive external ophthalmoplegia is common

Gender and Age Distribution

▶ No gender predilection
▶ Onset from infancy to adulthood

Clinical Features

▶ Symptoms involve multiple organ systems
▶ Progressive course with episodes of exacerbation
▶ Maternal inheritance pattern (most cases)
▶ Lactic acidosis common

Prognosis and Treatment

▶ Although the prognosis can vary widely with the clinical features, median survival for infantile-onset cases is 12 years; many die within 1 to 2 years of onset
▶ No effective therapy, although nutritional-based treatments are used

PATHOLOGIC FEATURES

Paralleling the clinical challenge, routine staining of muscle biopsy specimens may demonstrate a range of abnormalities, often quite subtle, including angular atrophic fibers or scattered granular-appearing fibers (Fig. 11-10A).

ANCILLARY STUDIES

Histochemistry

In an ironic twist of historical fate, this group of disorders is often referred to as the "ragged red" fiber myopathies. In fact, ragged red fibers (seen on trichrome staining) are encountered in a very small minority (<5%) of patients with mitochondrial myopathy (see Fig. 11-10B). COX histochemical staining is somewhat more sensitive and may show either a "ragged" appearance of muscle fibers in which mitochondria are present in increased numbers or absence of activity in fibers containing mitochondrial mutations involving complex IV of the electron transport chain (see Fig. 11-10C).

Ultrastructural Features

Ultrastructural examination of muscle biopsy specimens may demonstrate increased numbers of mitochondria in subsarcolemmal or intermyofibrillary locations or mitochondrial pleomorphism with or without mitochondrial inclusions (or both) (see Fig. 11-10D).

Other

Biochemical or genetic analysis, or both, is required to confirm and specify the mitochondrial defect.

DIFFERENTIAL DIAGNOSIS

Muscle mitochondrial dysfunction may occur as a secondary phenomenon in a wide variety of muscle dis-

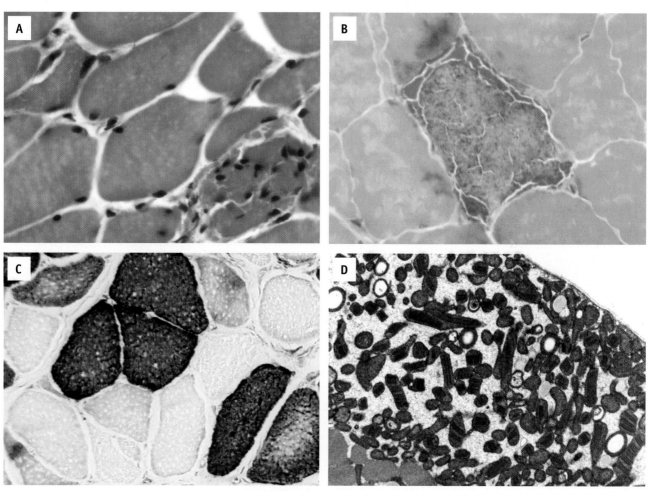

FIGURE 11-10

A, Light microscopic findings may be subtle in patients with mitochondrial myopathy and consist of scattered atrophic or granular-appearing muscle fibers (or both). **B,** Gomori trichrome staining demonstrating the elusive "ragged red" fiber signifying subsarcolemmal mitochondrial proliferation. **C,** The prevalence of muscle fibers lacking cytochrome oxidase activity may be increased in patients with mitochondrial disease. **D,** Subsarcolemmal proliferations of abnormal-appearing mitochondria may be seen within scattered muscle fibers in patients with mitochondrial myopathy. Occasionally, paracrystalline ("parking lot") mitochondrial inclusions are present.

MITOCHONDRIAL ENCEPHALOMYOPATHIES—PATHOLOGIC FEATURES

Microscopic Findings

▶ Atrophic fibers; scattered necrotic, granular, or regenerating fibers

Histochemical Findings

▶ Trichrome: ragged red fibers (rare)
▶ Cytochrome oxidase–deficient fibers

Ultrastructural Features

▶ Increased numbers of mitochondria, especially subsarcolemmal
▶ Mitochondrial pleomorphism with or without inclusions

Genetics

▶ Sporadic, autosomally (nuclear DNA–encoded proteins), or maternally (mitochondrial DNA–encoded proteins) inherited deletions, duplications, or point mutations affecting respiratory chain proteins, tRNA, or rRNA

Pathologic Differential Diagnosis

▶ Other inflammatory, metabolic, and congenital/structural myopathies or systemic diseases/therapies with secondary mitochondrial changes (zidovudine, aging)

ACUTE QUADRIPLEGIC MYOPATHY—FACT SHEET

Definition

▶ Acute weakness developing in the intensive care setting

Incidence and Location

▶ ≈25% of critically ill patients undergoing mechanical ventilation for longer than 1 week
▶ More likely to occur with sepsis, corticosteroid therapy, or both
▶ Proximal weakness predominates and may be asymmetric

Gender and Age Distribution

▶ Female preponderance
▶ Mean age ≈65, with a wide distribution

Clinical Features

▶ Rapid onset of diffuse, sometimes asymmetric weakness and muscle wasting that may lead to difficulty in ventilatory weaning

Prognosis and Treatment

▶ Neuromuscular dysfunction resolves within 3 weeks in approximately half of patients; in the majority of the remainder it resolves within a year
▶ Aggressive rehabilitation therapy may facilitate recovery. Prevention is recommended through restriction of corticosteroid therapy in critically ill patients to disorders in which they have been clearly demonstrated to significantly improve patient outcome

---

eases (especially the inflammatory myopathies) and as a consequence of pharmacotherapy with certain agents (e.g., zidovudine). Because mitochondrial defects accumulate with time, morphologic manifestations of these defects are seen with increased frequency during aging. Indeed, many researchers believe that we are only as old as our mitochondria!

PROGNOSIS AND THERAPY

The protean manifestations of this group of diseases are reflected in similarly protean prognostic implications. The median survival for patients with infantile-onset encephalomyopathy is 12 years, although many die within 1 to 2 years.

ACUTE QUADRIPLEGIC MYOPATHY

CLINICAL FEATURES

To date, acute quadriplegic myopathy has been reported exclusively in the critical care setting, which explains the alternative appellation—critical illness myopathy. This myopathy is usually recognized when a critically ill patient cannot be weaned off the ventilator because of diffuse flaccid paralysis, including paralysis of the diaphragmatic and intercostal muscles. Two of the three following conditions are usually required to produce this disorder: corticosteroid therapy, neuromuscular blockade, and severe systemic illness such as sepsis.

PATHOLOGIC FEATURES

Routinely stained sections may show features of rhabdomyolysis, but they often demonstrate muscle fiber atrophy without necrosis (Fig. 11-11A).

ANCILLARY STUDIES

Histochemistry

ATPase staining reveals that the atrophic muscle fibers are nearly entirely type 2. Muscle fibers may show central pallor on all histochemical stains.

Ultrastructural Features

A striking selective loss of thick filaments is seen within atrophic fibers (see Fig. 11-11B).

Immunohistochemistry

Decreased myosin heavy-chain immunostaining may be detectable within affected fibers.

DIFFERENTIAL DIAGNOSIS

Light microscopic findings are nonspecific, but the ultrastructural features are virtually pathognomonic.

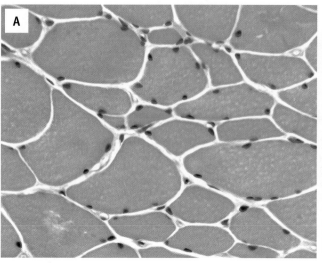
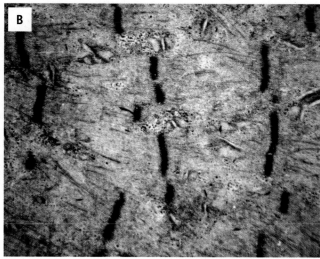

FIGURE 11-11

A, Light microscopic findings in patients with acute quadriplegic myopathy may be subtle and resemble those of denervation atrophy. **B**, Ultrastructural examination of muscles from patients with acute quadriplegic myopathy demonstrates selective loss of thick (myosin) filaments within atrophic fibers.

ACUTE QUADRIPLEGIC MYOPATHY—PATHOLOGIC FEATURES

Microscopic Findings

▶ Prominent atrophy of muscle fibers (often >50% of fibers)
▶ Necrotic fibers may be present

Histochemical Findings

▶ ATPase: type 2 fibers may be more affected. May demonstrate central pallor
▶ Trichrome: fibers appear more purple than green
▶ Oxidative: may show central pallor

Ultrastructural Features

▶ Selective loss of thick filaments (A-band loss)

Immunohistochemical Features

▶ Myosin heavy chains deficient within pale zones

Pathologic Differential Diagnosis

▶ Light microscopic changes are nonspecific; electron microscopic features are virtually pathognomonic in the right clinical setting
▶ Selective myosin loss may be seen in infantile myotubular myopathy, in infantile cytochrome oxidase deficiency, and occasionally in chronically denervated fibers

---

Depletion of myosin heavy chains may occasionally be encountered in chronic denervation and has been reported in infantile myotubular myopathy and infantile cytochrome oxidase deficiency.

PROGNOSIS AND THERAPY

On cessation of corticosteroid therapy or neuromuscular blockade (or both), recovery of muscle strength occurs within 3 weeks in approximately 50% of patients; the majority of the remainder regain normal strength within a year. Treatment is supportive. Prevention is recommended through restriction of corticosteroid use in critically ill patients to disorders in which they have clearly been demonstrated to significantly improve patient outcome.

DERMATOMYOSITIS

CLINICAL FEATURES

Patients present with proximal muscle weakness that has developed over a period of weeks to months. A characteristic rash precedes or accompanies the weakness. Although mild to moderate weakness is the rule, rare patients may progress to quadriparesis. Sensation is preserved, but reflexes may be difficult to elicit in patients with advanced weakness. Children may present with "misery," defined as irritability, flushing, fatigue, and withdrawal. Gait problems secondary to flexion contracture of the ankles may also develop in children.

PATHOLOGIC FEATURES

Dermatomyositis is a bit of a misnomer because the inflammation in both skin and muscle consists predominantly of inflammation of small vessels with secondary ischemic damage to the myofibers. The vascular damage is complement mediated and thus results in a mixed inflammatory infiltrate in which lymphocytes are accompanied by plasma cells and eosinophils (Fig. 11-12A). Ischemic damage to muscle is reflected by necrosis and phagocytosis of muscle fibers, which may occur in groups (microinfarcts). Sublethal ischemic stress is manifested as fiber atrophy at the interface of the muscle fascicle and the perimysium ("perifascicular atrophy") because these

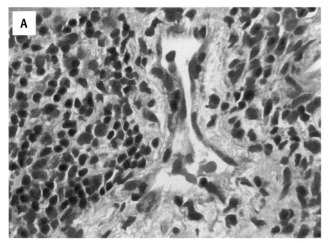

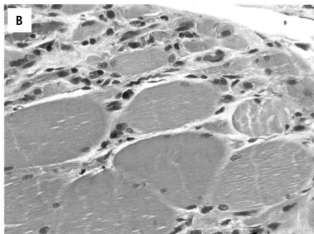

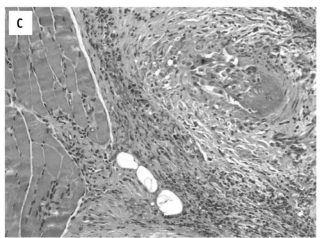

FIGURE 11-12

A, Muscle biopsy specimen from a patient with dermatomyositis demonstrating a mixed inflammatory infiltrate consisting of lymphocytes, plasma cells, and scattered eosinophils. **B**, Ischemic stress in dermatomyositis causes preferential atrophy and degeneration in muscle fibers located at the periphery of muscle fascicles. **C**, Skeletal muscle vasculitis in a patient with polyarteritis nodosa. Note that the caliber of arteries affected in patients with systemic vasculitis is considerably larger than the small perimysial vessels targeted in dermatomyositis.

DERMATOMYOSITIS—FACT SHEET

Definition
▶ Humorally mediated microangiopathy with ischemic necrosis of muscle fibers

Incidence and Location
▶ ≈5 to 10 cases/million/year
▶ Proximal weakness predominates

Gender and Age Distribution
▶ Most common inflammatory myopathy of childhood, but may be seen at all ages
▶ Female-to-male ratio of ≈3:2

Clinical Features
▶ Characteristic rash precedes or accompanies weakness in more than 90%
▶ "Misery" common in childhood cases
▶ Ankle contractures may be seen in children

Prognosis and Treatment
▶ Frequency of cancer is increased for 3 years after onset (adult cases)
▶ "Overlap syndrome": dermatomyositis plus either scleroderma or mixed connective tissue disease
▶ Weakness responds to immunosuppressive therapy in most patients

---

DERMATOMYOSITIS—PATHOLOGIC FEATURES

Microscopic Findings
▶ Inflammation of perimysial blood vessels and interfascicular septa
▶ Plasma cells and eosinophils may accompany lymphocytes
▶ Necrosis and phagocytosis of muscle fibers, commonly in groups (microinfarcts)
▶ Perifascicular atrophy (diagnostic even without inflammation)

Histochemical Findings
▶ Nonspecific

Ultrastructural Features
▶ Endothelial swelling, fibrin thrombi, tubuloreticular inclusions in endothelial cells

Immunohistochemical Features
▶ Admixture of T and B cells
▶ Complement activation on capillaries

Pathologic Differential Diagnosis
▶ Myositis accompanying collagen vascular disorders
▶ Systemic vasculitic syndromes

fibers are at the distal end of the blood supply (see Fig. 11-12B). Perifascicular atrophy is so characteristic of dermatomyositis that many experts consider its presence diagnostic, even in the absence of inflammation.

ANCILLARY STUDIES

Ultrastructural Features

Ultrastructural examination demonstrates pathologic changes in the microvasculature of the muscle, including endothelial swelling, tubuloreticular inclusions in endothelial cells, and luminal fibrin thrombi.

Immunohistochemistry

Immunohistochemical stains show an admixture of both B and T cells around blood vessels. Complement activation and deposition on capillaries can be demonstrated by immunofluorescence.

DIFFERENTIAL DIAGNOSIS

The myositis accompanying a variety of collagen vascular diseases may demonstrate histopathologic and immunocytochemical features identical to those of dermatomyositis and must therefore always be considered in the clinical differential diagnosis. It is important to distinguish dermatomyositis from systemic vasculitis involving skeletal muscle because treatment of the latter is usually performed on an emergency basis and is more aggressive. Although clinical correlation is required, systemic vasculitic involvement of skeletal muscle nearly always affects larger epimysial arteries and arterioles (see Fig. 11-12C).

PROGNOSIS AND THERAPY

In most patients, the weakness and rash respond to immunosuppressive therapy. In adults, an increased risk of cancer persists for 3 years after onset. "Overlap syndrome," defined as dermatomyositis accompanied by either scleroderma or mixed connective tissue disease, develops in some patients.

POLYMYOSITIS

CLINICAL FEATURES

It is safe to say that no more controversial disease presently exists in the world of muscle pathology than polymyositis. Depending on whom one reads, polymyositis is regarded either as the most common muscle disease in adults or as virtually nonexistent. As molecular genetic analysis continues to broaden the

POLYMYOSITIS—FACT SHEET
Definition
▶ HLA-restricted, antigen-specific, cell-mediated immune response against muscle fibers
Incidence and Location
▶ ≈1 to 5 cases/million/year
▶ Proximal muscle weakness predominates
Gender and Age Distribution
▶ Average age at onset of 37 years
▶ Rare under age 18
▶ More prevalent (2:1) in women between 20 and 40 years of age
Clinical Features
▶ Muscle weakness developing over a period of weeks to months, with proximal weakness predominating
▶ Oculobulbar muscles rarely affected
▶ Sensation and reflexes normal
▶ Elevation of plasma creatine kinase
Prognosis and Treatment
▶ May be associated with other autoimmune/collagen vascular diseases, rarely with cancer
▶ Treated with immunosuppressive therapies; about a third are left with varying degrees of disability

spectrum of dystrophic myopathies, many of which may contain inflammatory infiltrates, and as inclusion body myositis is recognized with increased frequency, it is likely that polymyositis will become, if not a nonexistent entity, at least a diagnosis of exclusion.

Currently, polymyositis is usually diagnosed clinically in adults in whom proximal muscle weakness develops over a period of weeks to months, accompanied by elevations in serum creatine kinase.

PATHOLOGIC FEATURES

The classic histopathologic hallmark in polymyositis is lymphocytic inflammation surrounding and invading otherwise healthy-appearing muscle fibers (Fig. 11-13). Both rimmed vacuoles (as seen in inclusion body myositis) and other types of inflammatory cells (as seen in dermatomyositis) should be absent. Endomysial fibrosis is said to be a feature of chronic polymyositis, but this raises the probability of a dystrophic myopathy with epiphenomenal inflammation.

ANCILLARY STUDIES

Histochemistry

There are no specific histochemical features of polymyositis. Rimmed vacuoles on trichrome staining are

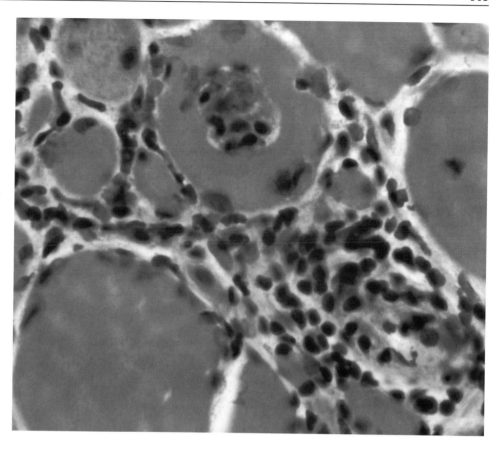

FIGURE 11-13

The histopathologic hallmark of polymyositis is lymphocytic inflammation surrounding and invading otherwise healthy-appearing muscle fibers. Note the absence of plasma cells and eosinophils within the inflammatory infiltrate.

POLYMYOSITIS—PATHOLOGIC FEATURES

Microscopic Findings

► Focal lymphocytic infiltrates surround and invade healthy muscle fibers
► Eosinophils, neutrophils, plasma cells rarely seen
► Endomysial connective tissue increased in chronic cases
► Rimmed vacuoles absent

Histochemical Findings

► Nonspecific

Immunohistochemical Features

► Association of CD8+ T cells with MHC class I–positive muscle fibers

Pathologic Differential Diagnosis

► Endomysial inflammation may be seen in several muscular dystrophies (fascioscapulohumeral, Duchenne's, dysferlinopathy, congenital), as well as in association with certain drugs (D-penicillamine, zidovudine)
► Other inflammatory diseases of muscle include infectious myositis, eosinophilic myositis, granulomatous myositis, and macrophagic myofasciitis

---

incompatible with the diagnosis, and increased numbers of COX-negative fibers (>3%) should raise serious doubts.

Immunohistochemistry

Those who favor stringent criteria for the diagnosis of polymyositis require demonstration of the CD8/ MHC-I (class I molecules of the major histocompatibility complex) relationship, which is the intimate association of CD8+ T cells with muscle fibers demonstrating upregulation of MHC-I.

DIFFERENTIAL DIAGNOSIS

In addition to inclusion body myositis, dermatomyositis, and dystrophic myopathies with endomysial infiltrates, polymyositis needs to be distinguished from other inflammatory diseases of muscle, including infectious myositis (in which polymorphonuclear leukocytes predominate), eosinophilic myositis, granulomatous myositis, and macrophagic myofasciitis. Rare drug reactions may include inflammatory infiltrates within skeletal muscle.

PROGNOSIS AND THERAPY

It is likely that the prognostic data regarding polymyositis are colored by the differing definitions of the disease used in the various studies. It has been estimated that approximately a third of patients will be left with some degree of disability. First-line treatment consists of corticosteroids. A poor response to corticosteroids is a good indication that another disorder may be responsible for the patient's problems.

INCLUSION BODY MYOSITIS

CLINICAL FEATURES

Inclusion body myositis is the most common muscle disease in patients older than 50 years. In younger patients, inclusion body myopathy is usually encountered only in rare, familial forms. When compared with the other inflammatory muscle diseases, the rate of symptom progression in inclusion body myositis is considerably slower. Patients often do not come to medical attention for several years. Early involvement of the quadriceps and ankle dorsiflexors resulting in frequent falls is common, as is early involvement of the wrist and finger flexor muscles leading to difficulty holding onto objects. Approximately half the patients have swallowing difficulties, and muscle atrophy may be prominent and lead to a clinical diagnosis of motor neuron disease.

INCLUSION BODY MYOSITIS—FACT SHEET

Definition
▶ Progressive age-related muscle disease with degenerative and inflammatory features

Incidence and Location
▶ 1 to 5 cases/million/year
▶ Early involvement of quadriceps and wrist/finger flexors

Gender and Age Distribution
▶ The most common muscle disease in patients older than 50 years
▶ Unusual familial variants encountered in younger patients
▶ More common in males (3:1)

Clinical Features
▶ Indolent onset (years) of weakness
▶ Distal and asymmetric weakness may be seen
▶ Swallowing difficulties in 40% to 60%
▶ Facial weakness in about a third of patients
▶ Muscle atrophy may be prominent

Prognosis and Treatment
▶ Poorly responsive to immunosuppressive therapies
▶ 50% wheelchair bound after 10 years

PATHOLOGIC FEATURES

Both inflammatory cell invasion of muscle fibers and groups of atrophic fibers are seen on routine sections. Endomysial fibrous tissue may be increased, with marked fibrofatty replacement seen in advanced cases. Inclusion bodies consist of intracytoplasmic vacuoles within muscle fibers surrounded by basophilic granules ("rimmed vacuoles") (Fig. 11-14A). The granules are dissolved during paraffin embedding, so they can be appreciated only in cryostat sections.

ANCILLARY STUDIES

Histochemistry

On trichrome staining the perivacuolar granules are red; ragged red fibers indicative of mitochondrial proliferation may also be seen. Oxidative enzyme stains confirm the presence of mitochondrial proliferation and dysfunction (increased COX-negative fibers). Congo red staining may reveal deposits around vacuoles, but epifluorescent signal amplification is required.

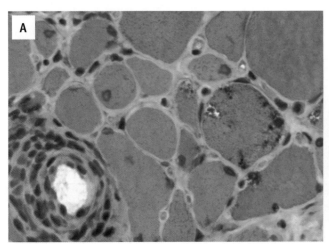
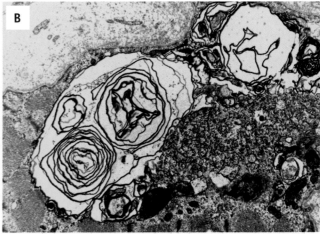

FIGURE 11-14

A, Muscle biopsy specimen from a patient with inclusion body myositis demonstrating perivascular lymphocytic inflammation and intramuscular vacuoles surrounded by granular basophilic material. **B,** On ultrastructural examination, the perivacuolar granular material is composed of (diagnostic) tubulofilamentous aggregates.

INCLUSION BODY MYOSITIS—PATHOLOGIC FEATURES

Microscopic Findings

▶ Endomysial inflammation invading non-necrotic fibers
▶ Groups of atrophic fibers
▶ Intracytoplasmic vacuoles rimmed with granular material

Histochemical Findings

▶ H&E: basophilic granules only visualized on frozen sections
▶ Trichrome: granular material stains red; ragged red fibers may be present
▶ Oxidative: increased numbers of cytochrome oxidase–negative fibers
▶ Congo red with epifluorescence reveals deposits around vacuoles

Ultrastructural Features

▶ 15- to 18-nm tubulofilamentous inclusions in cytoplasm, nuclei, or both

Genetics

▶ Unusual familial myopathies may show rimmed vacuoles without inflammation

Immunohistochemical Features

▶ Intracytoplasmic inclusions react with a variety of antibodies usually associated with neurodegenerative diseases, including β-amyloid, tau, and ubiquitin

Pathologic Differential Diagnosis

▶ Polymyositis (if inclusions not recognized)
▶ Rimmed vacuoles may also be seen in oculopharyngeal muscular dystrophy, familial distal myopathies (hereditary inclusion body myositis), and chronic denervation

---

Ultrastructural Features

The diagnostic ultrastructural feature of inclusion body myositis is the presence of 15- to 18-nm tubulofilamentous inclusions within muscle cytoplasm, nuclei, or both (see Fig. 11-14B). Amyloid filaments may also be appreciated by electron microscopy.

Immunohistochemistry

The inclusions of inclusion body myositis react with antibodies to proteins usually associated with neurodegenerative diseases, including β-amyloid, hyperphosphorylated tau protein, and ubiquitin.

DIFFERENTIAL DIAGNOSIS

If the inclusions are not recognized, an erroneous diagnosis of polymyositis may be made. On rebiopsy after failed immunosuppressive therapy, the number of muscle fibers containing inclusion bodies is often increased, although the amount of inflammation may be less. Conversely, it is important to establish that intramuscular vacuoles are associated with either amyloid (by epifluorescent Congo red staining) or tubulofila-

mentous inclusions (by ultrastructural examination) before making the diagnosis.

Rimmed vacuoles identical to those seen in inclusion body myositis may occur in patients with oculopharyngeal muscular dystrophy, familial distal inclusion body myopathy, or chronic denervation.

PROGNOSIS AND THERAPY

Inclusion body myositis is poorly responsive to immunosuppressive therapies, with half of patients becoming wheelchair dependent after 10 years.

INTRODUCTION TO PERIPHERAL NERVES

Like skeletal muscle, the peripheral nerve is a monofunctional system that conducts electrical signals from neurons to end-organs (muscle, skin, viscera, etc.) and vice versa. Structurally, the wiring system analogy also applies inasmuch as axons neither begin nor end in the peripheral nerve itself, but consist of very long, thin extensions of neuronal cytoplasm. Natural selection has bequeathed us three populations of axons: those measuring approximately 10 to 12 μm in diameter, 4 to 6 μm in diameter, and 0.5 to 1.5 μm in diameter (Fig. 11-15C). The two larger populations are insulated by specialized cytoplasmic extensions of Schwann cells that form myelin sheaths. As in the CNS, this insulating layer markedly increases conduction velocity along the axons and provides some protection from perturbations in the extracellular environment. The smallest axons remain unmyelinated, although they are surrounded by cytoplasmic extensions of nonmyelinating Schwann cells ("Remak cells").

Peripheral nervous system myelin is similar but not identical to that of CNS myelin. The dominant membrane proteins differ, thus accounting for distinct autoimmune demyelinating diseases of the peripheral and central nervous systems. In addition, in a normal peripheral nerve, one Schwann cell contributes to the myelination of a single axon (in contrast to the promiscuity of normal oligodendroglial cells). Myelination of more than one axon by a single Schwann cell is evidence of axonal sprouting and implies previous axonal degeneration.

Myelinated fibers are used to transmit motor signals and "large fiber" sensory modalities (primarily vibration and proprioception). These populations are routinely examined during electrophysiologic testing. Most unmyelinated fibers transmit pain and temperature signals to the CNS. A subpopulation of unmyelinated axons are responsible for executing autonomic functions, although autonomic and sensory fibers cannot be distinguished morphologically or by routine immunohistochemical techniques.

Normal proportions of these axonal populations vary from nerve to nerve, from the uniform large myelinated axons in motor nerve roots to the predominantly

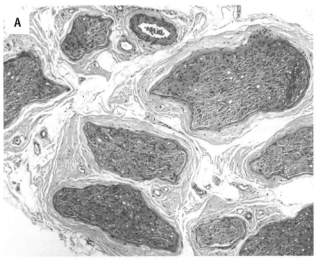

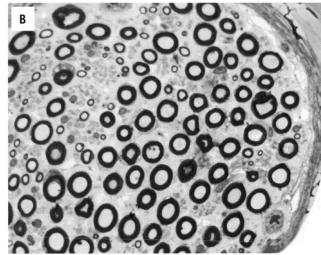

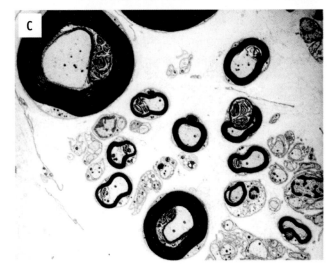

FIGURE 11-15

A, The sural nerve is composed of several nerve fascicles, each delineated from the epineurium by a dense collar of modified Schwann cells ("the perineurium"). **B**, On toluidine blue–stained, plastic-embedded sections, myelin sheaths are darkly stained but axons are not. **C**, Three axonal populations compose the sural nerve: large myelinated fibers, small myelinated fibers, and unmyelinated fibers.

unmyelinated fibers in distal sensory nerves such as the sural nerve. Morphometric analysis has demonstrated alterations in the relative proportions of these axonal populations with age. Only a few nerves have been studied in enough detail to allow meaningful conclusions to be drawn regarding morphometric alterations, so extreme caution is advised when examining nerves for which such information is not available.

By far the most commonly biopsied nerve is the sural nerve, which is composed entirely of sensory fibers (supplying the lateral aspect of the foot). These axons join others to form the tibial nerve, which contributes to the medial portion of the sciatic nerve. They then ramify through the lumbosacral plexus before finding their parent neurons in lower lumbar and upper sacral dorsal root ganglia (the majority of sural nerve axons originate from S1 neurons). The sural nerve consists of 8 to 10 fascicles, each composed of several hundred myelinated fibers and several thousand unmyelinated fibers held together by 5 to 10 layers of modified Schwann cells and fibroblasts making up the perineurium. The perineurium serves two important physiologic functions: it forms the nonvascular component of the blood-nerve barrier (similar to the choroid plexus in the CNS), and it holds the endoneurial contents

together by maintaining pressure higher than that in surrounding tissue. This last physiologic phenomenon is well demonstrated by traumatic neuromas, in which the endoneurial contents literally spew out into the surrounding connective tissue. Histologically, the perineurium separates endoneurium from epineurium (all the connective tissue elements that lie between fascicles) (see Fig. 11-15A). Of greatest interest in the epineurium are the 50- to 200-μm arterioles that supply the perineurium and endoneurium. Although not apparent on routine histologic sections, the endoneurium is supplied by a complicated plexus of arterioles; occlusion of any one vessel rarely leads to infarction. Instead, the effects of vascular compromise are indirect and often quite subtle.

As with skeletal muscle, the pathologist should approach peripheral nerve disease systematically: Is the primary damage to the Schwann cell/myelin component or to the neuron/axonal component of the peripheral nerve? If the latter predominates, does the process primarily affect small myelinated and unmyelinated fibers, or are all axonal populations affected?

Diseases predominantly affecting Schwann cells/myelin:

Acute inflammatory demyelinating polyradiculoneuropathy

Chronic inflammatory demyelinating polyradiculoneuropathy

Paraproteinemic neuropathy

Charcot-Marie-Tooth disease, type 1

Diseases predominantly affecting small myelinated and unmyelinated axons:

Amyloid neuropathy

Diabetic polyneuropathy

HIV-associated polyneuropathy

Diseases affecting all axonal populations:

Vasculitic neuropathy

Lumbosacral plexopathy

Charcot-Marie-Tooth disease, type 2

Although the number of stains used in the interpretation of peripheral nerve biopsy specimens pales in comparison with skeletal muscle, nerve biopsies seem to generate even greater anxiety, probably because of the requirement for special preparations to adequately assess the endoneurial compartment, coupled with the need to make inferences about structures not directly visualized at the light microscopic level (the axons). One-micron plastic-embedded sections are generally stained with a metachromatic dye such as methylene or toluidine blue, which leaves the axons unstained (see Fig. 11-15B). Thus, myelinated axons appear as donut holes and unmyelinated axons do not appear at all (without resorting to oil immersion, neurofilament immunostaining, or electron microscopy). As in the CNS, axons can exist devoid of myelin, but the reverse is not true. We are left using patterns of myelin loss and associated pathologic changes to make inferences concerning the axonal population. To turn inferences into facts requires electron microscopy, nerve-teasing studies (whereby individual axons are separated in glycerin and stained with osmium tetroxide and their patterns of myelin loss are assessed and tallied), the generation of frequency histograms, and sometimes all three!

The good news is that in the modern era of electrophysiology, nerve biopsies are rarely performed to assess the endoneurial compartment (although a general familiarity with this compartment occasionally provides useful information). Nerve biopsies are instead performed in an attempt to find a treatable cause for the clinical/electrophysiologic abnormalities. Of the nine exemplary peripheral nerve diseases covered in this section, diagnostic nerve biopsies are typically carried out for two: vasculitic and amyloid neuropathy. Either of these diagnoses can easily be made on routinely embedded, sectioned, and stained sections of peripheral nerve (although a good Congo red stain helps considerably in the latter).

With this in mind, let us begin our examination of peripheral nerve pathology.

ACUTE INFLAMMATORY DEMYELINATING POLYRADICULONEUROPATHY

CLINICAL FEATURES

Acute inflammatory demyelinating polyneuropathy is so often manifested as Guillain-Barré syndrome that many use the two terms interchangeably. Guillain-Barré syndrome consists of rapidly evolving symmetric weakness with areflexia, variable autonomic dysfunction, and mild sensory signs.

PATHOLOGIC FEATURES

Light microscopic findings classically include endoneurial lymphocytic inflammation and macrophage infiltration (Fig. 11-16A). The pathologic changes are usually

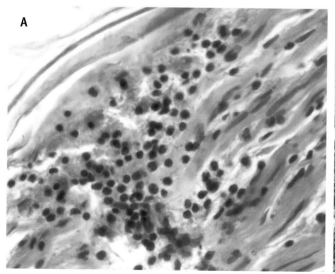
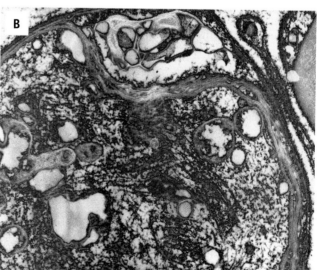

FIGURE 11-16

A, Although scattered lymphocytes are commonly encountered within the epineurium, endoneurial lymphocytic inflammation is always abnormal and usually signifies the presence of autoimmune/inflammatory neuropathy. **B,** Macrophage-mediated lysis with stripping of myelin sheaths from otherwise normal-appearing axons is the diagnostic hallmark of acute inflammatory demyelinating polyradiculoneuropathy.

ACUTE INFLAMMATORY DEMYELINATING POLYRADICULONEUROPATHY—FACT SHEET

Definition
▶ Rapidly progressive ascending polyradiculoneuropathy

Incidence and Location
▶ ≈2 cases/100,000 population/year
▶ Proximal and distal weakness with frequent cranial nerve involvement

Gender and Age Distribution
▶ Male preponderance, ≈1.5:1
▶ Incidence increases with age, with a peak in the 60s

Clinical Features
▶ Progressive weakness of more than two limbs, areflexia, and progression for no more than 4 weeks
▶ Mild sensory signs, raised CSF protein without pleocytosis ("albuminocytologic dissociation")
▶ Dysautonomia may occur
▶ Respiratory failure in ≈25% of cases
▶ Antecedent infection in ≈75% of cases

Prognosis and Treatment
▶ 80% ambulatory at 6 months and have good recovery at 2 years
▶ Early mortality is ≈5%
▶ Poor prognostic signs include severity at nadir, amplitude of compound motor action potentials on nerve conduction studies, early need for intubation, and age older than 50 years
▶ General treatment includes respiratory care, early treatment of autonomic dysfunction, prevention of deep venous thrombosis, and good nursing care
▶ Intravenous immunoglobulin and plasmapheresis are the mainstays of immunomodulatory treatment at present; corticosteroid therapy is not indicated

---

ACUTE INFLAMMATORY DEMYELINATING POLYRADICULONEUROPATHY—PATHOLOGIC FEATURES

Microscopic Findings
▶ Endoneurial mononuclear infiltrate, with macrophages predominating
▶ Schwann cell proliferation 1 to 2 weeks after onset
▶ Endoneurial lymphocytes are usually rare

Ultrastructural Features
▶ Macrophage-mediated demyelination with vesicular myelin degeneration surrounding normal-appearing axons

Genetics
▶ Sporadic

Immunohistochemical Features
▶ Immunostaining for lymphocytes and macrophages may reveal subtle endoneurial infiltrates

Pathologic Differential Diagnosis
▶ Macrophage-mediated demyelination is seen only in acute and chronic inflammatory demyelinating polyradiculoneuropathy; onion bulb formations support the latter
▶ Epineurial lymphocytes are nonspecific

---

most severe in the nerve roots, with rather subtle alterations in peripheral nerve biopsy specimens.

ANCILLARY STUDIES

Ultrastructural Features

Macrophage-mediated demyelination is the sine qua non of acute inflammatory demyelinating polyradiculoneuropathy (see Fig. 11-16B).

DIFFERENTIAL DIAGNOSIS

When endoneurial lymphocytes are present in the context of acute macrophage-mediated demyelination, the diagnosis can be made with certainty. Epineurial lymphocytes are not sufficient because they may be seen in normal nerves and a variety of other neuropathic conditions.

PROGNOSIS AND THERAPY

Most patients (≈80%) regain the ability to walk unaided after 6 months. Approximately 5% die in the acute phase of the disease secondary to respiratory failure. Meticulous supportive care is critical. Specific therapies include plasma exchange and intravenous immune globulin.

CHRONIC INFLAMMATORY DEMYELINATING POLYRADICULONEUROPATHY

CLINICAL FEATURES

Approximately 50% of patients with chronic inflammatory demyelinating polyradiculoneuropathy are found to initially have the classic triad of symmetric proximal and distal weakness progressing over a period of more than 2 months, preferential impairment of large fiber sensory modalities, and decreased deep tendon reflexes. The other 50% usually have various components of the triad or asymmetric motor or sensory impairment (or both).

PATHOLOGIC FEATURES

Paraffin-embedded sections demonstrate lymphocytic endoneurial inflammation in about 50% of cases.

CHRONIC INFLAMMATORY DEMYELINATING POLYRADICULONEUROPATHY—FACT SHEET

Definition

▶ Proximal and distal weakness with sensory abnormalities and hyporeflexia evolving over a period of at least 2 months

Incidence and Location

▶ ≈1 case/100,000 population/year
▶ Both proximal and distal weakness

Gender and Age Distribution

▶ Male preponderance, ≈1.5:1
▶ Broad age distribution (≈50 ± 20 years)

Clinical Features

▶ Usually symmetric proximal and distal weakness; sensory deficits can be prominent
▶ Cranial nerve palsies (especially VII) in about a third
▶ 90% have elevated CSF protein with a normal cell count
▶ Hyporeflexia or areflexia
▶ May be progressive or relapsing and remitting

Prognosis and Treatment

▶ Improvement with corticosteroids in 40% to 95%; spontaneous improvement may also occur. Intravenous immune globulin and plasma exchange may result in improvement within days to weeks, although chronic immunosuppression may be needed in refractory or relapsing cases

CHRONIC INFLAMMATORY DEMYELINATING POLYRADICULONEUROPATHY—PATHOLOGIC FEATURES

Microscopic Findings

▶ Lymphocytic infiltration of the endoneurium (≈50% of cases), thinly myelinated axons, lipid-laden macrophages, and onion bulb formations (≈25% of cases)

Ultrastructural Features

▶ Macrophage-mediated demyelination with onion bulb formations

Genetics

▶ Sporadic

Immunohistochemical Features

▶ Leukocyte common antigen demonstrates endoneurial lymphocytes in greater than normal numbers (three to four per fascicle cross section)

Pathologic Differential Diagnosis

▶ Normal epineurial lymphocytes
▶ May be superimposed on diabetic, paraproteinemic, or HIV infection
▶ Hereditary sensory and motor neuropathy (demyelinating types)

Epineurial lymphocytic inflammation may be seen in up to 75% of nerve biopsy samples but is not specific.

ANCILLARY STUDIES

Semi-thin Sections

Decreased myelinated fiber density accompanied by demyelinated or thinly myelinated axons suggests the presence of demyelination. "Onion bulb" formations indicative of repeated demyelination and remyelination are seen in approximately 25% of cases (Fig. 11-17).

Ultrastructural Features

Redundant Schwann cell processes around normal, thinly myelinated or unmyelinated axons constitute the "onion bulbs" seen in a minority of nerve biopsy specimens. Macrophage-mediated demyelination is also seen in a minority of nerve biopsy samples. High cerebrospinal fluid (CSF) protein levels and autopsy studies indicate that demyelination is most prominent in the proximal nerve roots, which are rarely sampled clinically.

Immunohistochemistry

Immunohistochemical stains with antibodies against pan-lymphocyte antigens highlight endoneurial lymphocytes within paraffin-embedded sections. Scattered lymphocytes may be encountered in healthy patients, so care is recommended in the interpretation of immunohistochemical studies.

DIFFERENTIAL DIAGNOSIS

The major differential diagnostic consideration is Charcot-Marie-Tooth disease (hereditary sensory and motor neuropathy). Because both may contain scattered lymphocytes, the major difference between the two disease pathologies is the uniform involvement of nerve fascicles in Charcot-Marie-Tooth disease in contrast to the usually uneven fascicular damage encountered in acquired inflammatory neuropathy. Chronic inflammatory demyelinating polyradiculoneuropathy may sometimes be superimposed on preexisting axonal neuropathies (e.g., diabetic, paraproteinemic, and human immunodeficiency virus/acquired immunodeficiency syndrome [HIV/AIDS]-associated neuropathies).

PROGNOSIS AND THERAPY

The clinical course in chronic inflammatory demyelinating polyradiculoneuropathy may be monophasic, relapsing/remitting, or progressive. Corticosteroid

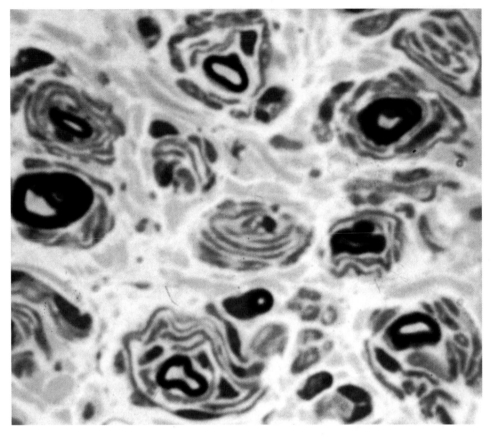

FIGURE 11-17
Redundant Schwann cell proliferations ("onion bulb formations") signify the repeated episodes of demyelination in the myelination experienced by patients with chronic inflammatory demyelinating polyradiculoneuropathy.

therapy has been associated with improvement in many patients. Intravenous immune globulin and plasmapheresis often induce significant clinical responses within a few days to several weeks. Spontaneous improvement may also occur.

PARAPROTEINEMIC NEUROPATHY

CLINICAL FEATURES

Antibody-producing plasma cells, on which we depend so heavily for protection against microbial assaults, are not themselves immune to the dysfunctions of growth and regulation that accompany the aging process. When these dysfunctions include populations of cells still capable of secreting functional antibodies, patients are subject to a plethora of possible adverse consequences. Problems associated with increased circulating immunoglobulins (variably referred to as paraproteinemias, dysproteinemias, and gammopathies) result either from the physical consequences of increased immunoglobulin levels within the body (e.g., amyloidosis) or from specific autoimmune properties of these antibodies. The (nonamyloidotic) neuropathies account for a significant proportion of this latter category, although antibody specificities have been elucidated in only a minority. The best-characterized paraproteinemic neuropathy occurs in patients with monoclonal IgM

PARAPROTEINEMIC NEUROPATHY—FACT SHEET
Definition
▶ Neuropathy associated with a monoclonal gammopathy
Prevalence and Location
▶ Prevalence may be as high as 1 in 1000 patients older than 50 years
▶ Distal, symmetric sensorimotor polyneuropathy
Gender and Age Distribution
▶ Male preponderance
▶ Increases with age; related to the incidence of monoclonal gammopathies
Clinical Features
▶ Usually mild, slowly progressive symmetric distal weakness
▶ ≈20% are painful with severe sensory loss and paresthesias
Prognosis and Treatment
▶ The prognosis and therapy are largely dependent on the underlying disease process. Cytotoxic immunomodulation may be effective in relieving symptoms

antibodies possessing anti-MAG (myelin-associated glycoprotein) activity.

The prevalence of paraproteinemic neuropathy increases with age and may be as high as 1 in 1000 for people older than 50 years. In a biopsy series of elderly patients

(65 years and older) with peripheral neuropathy, paraproteinemias were the second most common cause (vasculitis was the most common). Because the clinical manifestations of paraproteinemic neuropathies are generally nonspecific (distal symmetric sensorimotor polyneuropathy), a search for paraproteins should be part of the clinical evaluation of adult-onset polyneuropathies.

PATHOLOGIC FEATURES

Light microscopic abnormalities are nonspecific and usually include both myelin and axonal loss, without inflammation. Vasculitis may be associated with neuropathies secondary to cryoglobulinemia.

ANCILLARY STUDIES

Ultrastructural Features

The paraproteinemic neuropathies are the electron microscopist's dream (or nightmare) inasmuch as a variety of distinctive ultrastructural alterations have been associated with some of these diseases. Widening of the outer myelin lamellae is typically seen in patients with IgM-associated polyneuropathy, whereas loss of myelin compaction is reported in the POEMS syndrome (polyneuropathy, organomegaly, endocrinopathy, M protein, and skin changes), although uncompacted

---

PARAPROTEINEMIC NEUROPATHY—PATHOLOGIC FEATURES

Microscopic Findings
▶ Usually noninflammatory (except in cryoglobulinemia)
▶ Myelin or axonal loss (or both)

Ultrastructural Features
▶ Widened myelin lamellae (IgM)
▶ Uncompacted myelin lamellae (POEMS)
▶ Capillary deposits (cryoglobulinemia)

Immunohistochemical Features
▶ Direct immunofluorescence may show immunoglobulin deposition

Pathologic Differential Diagnosis
▶ Widened myelin lamellae may rarely be seen in acute and chronic inflammatory demyelinating polyradiculoneuropathy

---

myelin lamellae are not specific to this syndrome. Endoneurial cryoglobulin deposits may be seen in patients with cryoglobulinemic neuropathy.

Immunohistochemistry

Direct immunofluorescence with antibodies directed against circulating immunoglobulin may show deposits within the nerve biopsy specimen, especially in cases with IgM anti-MAG activity (Fig. 11-18).

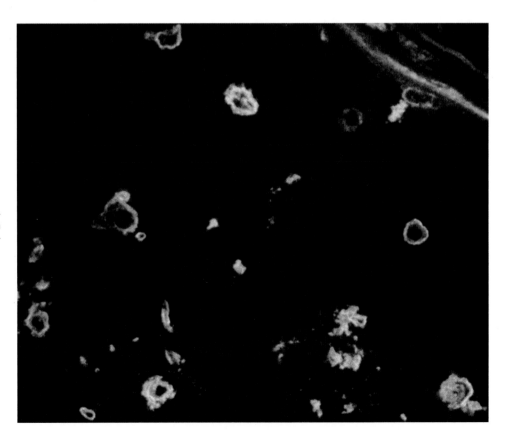

FIGURE 11-18
Direct immunofluorescence demonstrating IgM binding to myelin sheaths in a patient with paraproteinemic neuropathy.

DIFFERENTIAL DIAGNOSIS

The light microscopic abnormalities are nonspecific. Evaluation for cryoglobulinemia should be part of the clinical laboratory evaluation of peripheral nerve vasculitis. Ultrastructural abnormalities of myelin compaction are strongly suggestive of paraproteinemic neuropathies, but they may be encountered in other neuropathic disorders as well, particularly immunerelated demyelinating neuropathies. Well-executed immunofluorescent studies are diagnostic in the small subset of these disorders in which class-specific immunoglobulin deposits can be definitively identified within the myelin sheaths.

PROGNOSIS AND THERAPY

The overall prognosis depends predominantly on the disease process responsible for the paraproteinemia. Disease progression may be modified by immunomodulatory therapies, although some forms (e.g., anti-MAG–associated neuropathy) seem to be resistant to therapy.

AMYLOID NEUROPATHY

CLINICAL FEATURES

Amyloid neuropathies, both hereditary and acquired, are classically manifested as "small fiber" neuropathies;

that is, the clinical syndrome is dominated by selective abnormalities in pain and temperature sensation along with autonomic dysfunction. Painful dysesthesias are common. Autonomic symptoms include bowel and bladder dysfunction, impotence, and orthostasis. Symptoms related to dysfunction of other organs may be prominent, especially cardiac (cardiomyopathy, arrhythmia) and renal (nephritic syndrome, renal failure).

PATHOLOGIC FEATURES

Endoneurial and vascular amyloid deposits may be striking (Fig. 11-19). Relative preservation of large myelinated fibers may be appreciable.

ANCILLARY STUDIES

Histochemistry

Congo red staining demonstrates metachromasia with birefringence. Abdominal fat pad biopsy can be performed to confirm the nerve biopsy findings.

Ultrastructural Features

Long, unbranched fibrils measure 7 to 10 nm in width.

Immunohistochemistry

Although immunotyping of the amyloid deposits might occasionally be useful, there tends to be a lack of specificity in immunohistochemical assays.

AMYLOID NEUROPATHY—FACT SHEET

Definition
- ▶ Peripheral neurologic dysfunction related to endoneurial amyloid deposits

Incidence and Location
- ▶ Neuropathy occurs in ≈25% of patients with acquired AL amyloidosis (rare) and defines patients with familial amyloidotic polyneuropathy (also rare)
- ▶ Distal sensorimotor polyneuropathy with autonomic dysfunction

Gender and Age Distribution
- ▶ No gender predilection
- ▶ Onset in third (familial) or sixth to seventh (sporadic) decades

Clinical Features
- ▶ Dissociated sensory loss (which may be painful) followed by distal weakness (which may be asymmetric)
- ▶ Autonomic disturbances are frequent and early (diarrhea, constipation, orthostatic hypotension)
- ▶ Cardiac and renal involvement is common

Prognosis and Treatment
- ▶ Median survival is 2 years (sporadic) to 10 years (familial)
- ▶ Symptomatic treatment, including cardiac pacing and hemodialysis, is important. Eradication of bone marrow plasma cells has improved survival in sporadic AL amyloidosis, whereas early liver transplantation in familial cases has yielded encouraging results

---

AMYLOID NEUROPATHY—PATHOLOGIC FEATURES

Microscopic Findings
- ▶ Axonal neuropathy with preferential loss of small-caliber fibers accompanied by endoneurial amyloid deposits that vary in size and number

Histochemical Findings
- ▶ Congo red staining demonstrates metachromasia with birefringence

Ultrastructural Features
- ▶ Unbranched 7- to 10-nm fibrils of indeterminate length

Genetics
- ▶ Familial cases are most commonly seen in Portugal, Sweden, Japan, and France, where they demonstrate autosomal dominant inheritance, with most being secondary to transthyretin mutations (chromosome 18). The Val30Met mutation is by far the most common

Immunohistochemical Features
- ▶ Theoretically important, but incompletely specific

Pathologic Differential Diagnosis
- ▶ None; findings may be confirmed with abdominal fat pad biopsy

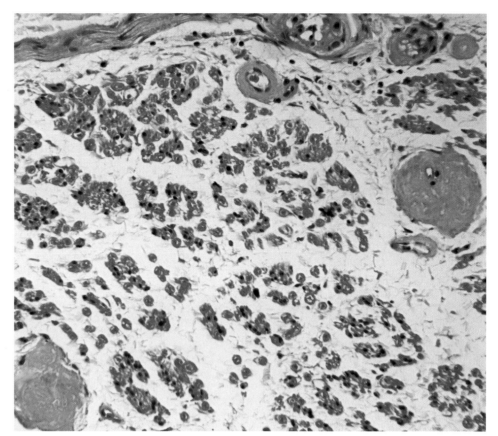

FIGURE 11-19
Endoneurial and vascular deposits of amorphous eosinophilic proteinaceous material ("amyloid") in a patient with multiple myeloma.

Other

Most familial amyloid polyneuropathies result from transthyretin mutations. Because the Val30Met substitution accounts for the majority of these mutations, it can be assayed when this is a consideration.

DIFFERENTIAL DIAGNOSIS

Renaut bodies, or fibroelastotic subperineurial thickenings, may resemble amyloid deposits. However, they do not stain metachromatically with Congo red and consist of concentrically arranged fibroblasts rather than straight filaments by electron microscopy.

PROGNOSIS AND THERAPY

The median survival after diagnosis is 10 years in familial amyloidotic polyneuropathy but only 2 years in acquired cases. Early liver transplantation has shown encouraging results in familial transthyretin amyloidoses, whereas eradication of marrow plasma cells has extended survival in sporadic amyloid neuropathy. Cardiac pacing and hemodialysis are required in most patients.

DIABETIC POLYNEUROPATHY

CLINICAL FEATURES

Patients with diabetes may suffer from a variety of peripheral nerve abnormalities. The most common is length-dependent axonal sensorimotor polyneuropathy, which is usually manifested as pain and paresthesias in the lower extremities. Physical examination discloses some degree of motor deficit in about a third of patients. Gait abnormalities may be seen in about 15% of patients at initial evaluation. Autonomic abnormalities are common; when they are the initial manifestations (postural hypotension, bowel or bladder dysfunction, erectile dysfunction), the syndrome is often referred to as "diabetic autonomic neuropathy."

PATHOLOGIC FEATURES

Diabetic polyneuropathy is often considered the prototype of axonal neuropathy because it demonstrates loss of large, small, and unmyelinated fibers. At the same time, these pathologic features are entirely nonspecific. Although many reports mention thickening and hyalinization of the perineurium and endoneurial blood vessels, such features are also common in nerve biopsy specimens from nondiabetic patients.

DIABETIC POLYNEUROPATHY—FACT SHEET

Definition

▶ Length-dependent symmetric sensorimotor polyneuropathy associated with diabetes/impaired glucose tolerance

Incidence and Location

▶ Affects less than 10% of diabetics at diagnosis, but nearly 50% of diabetics after 25 years (or 4 of 100 adults in the United States)
▶ Sensory dysfunction and weakness predominant in the distal end of the lower extremity

Gender and Age Distribution

▶ Slight male preponderance (≈1.5:1)
▶ Mean age at onset in the sixth decade; range from the third to the ninth decade

Clinical Features

▶ Usually manifested as pain and paresthesias in the lower extremities. Motor deficits can be elicited in about a third of patients. Gait disturbances are seen in ≈15%. A subset has erectile dysfunction, postural hypotension, urinary disturbances, or any combination of these findings ("diabetic autonomic neuropathy")

Prognosis and Treatment

▶ Diabetes is the leading cause of nontraumatic lower extremity amputations in the United States; foot complications develop in 25% of patients at some point
▶ The best treatment is prevention through strict glycemic control. A variety of medications have been used for pain control (e.g., amitriptyline, gabapentin). Fastidious foot care is essential to prevent complications

---

DIABETIC POLYNEUROPATHY—PATHOLOGIC FEATURES

Microscopic Findings

▶ Axonal degeneration with hyalinization of endoneurial vessels, although both are nonspecific

Ultrastructural Features

▶ Thickening and reduplication of vascular basement membranes

Pathologic Differential Diagnosis

▶ The pathologic features are nonspecific. Biopsies are only used if another form of neuropathy is suspected

---

ANCILLARY STUDIES

Ultrastructural Features

Thickening and reduplication of basement membranes may be seen, but this finding is relatively nonspecific.

DIFFERENTIAL DIAGNOSIS

Because the histopathologic features are nonspecific, biopsy is used only to exclude a superimposed treatable neuropathy such as chronic inflammatory demyelinating polyradiculoneuropathy.

PROGNOSIS AND THERAPY

No specific therapies for diabetic polyneuropathy currently exist, although many are under development. Strict glycemic control in diabetics has been shown to delay the onset of neuropathy and slow its progression. Severe sensory impairment with loss of trophic function leads to foot ulcers, which often progress to gangrene necessitating amputation.

HIV-ASSOCIATED DISTAL SENSORY POLYNEUROPATHY

CLINICAL FEATURES

HIV-infected individuals may suffer a variety of peripheral nervous system complications, although

---

HIV-ASSOCIATED DISTAL SENSORY POLYNEUROPATHY—FACT SHEET

Definition

▶ Symmetric, predominantly sensory, neuropathy associated with HIV infection

Incidence and Location

▶ Clinical neuropathy occurs in 10% of HIV-infected patients and up to 35% of those with AIDS; as many as half of HIV-infected patients have electrophysiologic evidence of peripheral nerve dysfunction
▶ Distal lower extremity pain predominates

Gender and Age Distribution

▶ Male preponderance (≈4:1)
▶ Age at onset is 40 ± 7 years

Clinical Features

▶ Gradual onset of painful feet with tingling and numbness in the toes
▶ May progress proximally over a period of several months to involve the ankles or knees
▶ Severe dysesthetic pain often develops
▶ Reflexes may be depressed or increased, the latter indicating concomitant myelopathy
▶ Distal weakness may occur in advanced cases

Prognosis and Treatment

▶ Median survival in the pre-HAART (highly active antiretroviral therapy) era was 6 months
▶ Patients now survive longer, but there is no specific treatment of the neuropathy
▶ Some patients progress into a numb, but pain-free, state over time

distal sensory polyneuropathy occurring in advanced HIV/AIDS is the most common. As with diabetic polyneuropathy, patients generally have pain and paresthesias in the distal end of the lower extremities. Progression tends to be rapid, with severe dysesthetic lower extremity pain often developing within months. Deep tendon reflexes may be depressed or increased; the latter indicates concomitant myelopathy. Although sensory symptoms dominate the clinical picture, distal weakness may occur in advanced cases.

PATHOLOGIC FEATURES

Peripheral nerve biopsy specimens show nonspecific axonal degeneration. Although both epineurial and endoneurial lymphocytic infiltrates may be identified, neither correlates with clinical severity.

ANCILLARY STUDIES

Ultrastructural Features

Tubuloreticular inclusions have been described in endothelial cells, perineurial cells, and macrophages, but they are nonspecific.

DIFFERENTIAL DIAGNOSIS

Toxic axonal degeneration secondary to antiretroviral therapy is pathologically identical to AIDS-associated distal sensory neuropathy and must be excluded clinically. Acute inflammatory demyelinating polyradiculoneuropathy usually occurs at seroconversion. Chronic inflammatory polyradiculoneuropathy is typically encountered with moderately advanced HIV disease. Both show macrophage-mediated myelin stripping on ultrastructural examination.

HIV-ASSOCIATED DISTAL SENSORY POLYNEUROPATHY— PATHOLOGIC FEATURES

Microscopic Findings
▶ Epineurial or endoneurial perivascular lymphocytic infiltrates, which do not correlate with the severity of the neuropathy
▶ Acute and chronic axonal degeneration

Ultrastructural Features
▶ Tubuloreticular inclusions in endothelial cells, macrophages, and perineurial cells

Pathologic Differential Diagnosis
▶ Antiretroviral toxic neuropathy
▶ Inflammatory demyelinating polyradiculoneuropathy

PROGNOSIS AND THERAPY

No specific treatment currently exists. Some patients progress to a numb, but pain-free, state.

VASCULITIC NEUROPATHY

CLINICAL FEATURES

Advances in noninvasive investigation of peripheral nerve disease have led to marked changes in the indications for (and demographics of) nerve biopsy specimens in clinical practice. Peripheral nerve biopsies are used predominantly to determine the cause of peripheral nerve dysfunction. In adults, particularly elderly adults, the answer is usually found in the epineurium and most often entails vasculitic damage to the epineurial arterioles. It is not unreasonable to assume, until proved otherwise, that a nerve biopsy in an adult patient is being performed to "rule out" vasculitis, either systemic or restricted to the peripheral nervous system ("nonsystemic vasculitic neuropathy").

The "classic" manifestation of vasculitic neuropathy is "mononeuritis multiplex," in which patients experience peripheral nerve dysfunction affecting different regions of the body over time. In fact, mononeuritis multiplex is seen at initial evaluation in less than 50% of patients with systemic vasculitis affecting the peripheral nervous system and in fewer than 1 in 5 patients with nonsystemic vasculitic neuropathy. Nevertheless, careful

---

VASCULITIC NEUROPATHY—FACT SHEET

Definition
▶ Ischemic peripheral nerve damage secondary to vascular inflammation

Incidence and Location
▶ Overall incidence unknown; found in 25% of biopsies performed for disabling neuropathies in patients older than 65 years
▶ Distal accentuation of weakness, but proximal weakness present

Gender and Age Distribution
▶ Female preponderance: ≈1.5:1
▶ Broad age distribution: ≈60 ± 15 years

Clinical Features
▶ Nearly all patients present with a painful neuropathy, and weakness often follows the onset of pain by hours or days
▶ Asymmetry in 75% (systemic) to 98% (nonsystemic)
▶ Mononeuritis multiplex in 15% (nonsystemic) to ≈50% (systemic)

Prognosis and Treatment
▶ In systemic vasculitic neuropathy, depends on underlying disease
▶ For nonsystemic vasculitic neuropathy, ≈90% 5-year survival rate with relapses and moderate disability in about 50% of cases
▶ Treatment is with corticosteroids, cyclophosphamide, or both

clinical examination of patients with sensorimotor polyneuropathy usually discloses some degree of asymmetry in the degree of peripheral nerve dysfunction. An additional clue to the diagnosis is the presence of pain in affected regions. Although pain eventually develops in many sensory and sensorimotor neuropathies, its presence at initial evaluation suggests vasculitic neuropathy.

PATHOLOGIC FEATURES

Epineurial arterioles vary from about 50 μm to about 400 μm in diameter. Although the diagnosis of systemic versus nonsystemic vasculitic neuropathy requires careful clinical investigation, there is a tendency to see the larger epineurial arterioles involved in the former (Fig. 11-20A) and the smaller epineurial arterioles involved in the latter. Because skeletal muscle arterioles may also be affected in either condition, concurrent muscle biopsy increases the likelihood of being able to make a diagnosis, as does the use of serial sectioning.

A "soft" sign of vasculitic neuropathy is fascicular and subfascicular variability of peripheral nerve damage (see Fig. 11-20B) or (very rarely) infarction of a nerve fascicle. This variability implies a vascular, rather than metabolic or inherited cause of the peripheral nerve damage. In the proper clinical context, such a vascular pattern of nerve injury would support a clinical diagnosis of vasculitis.

ANCILLARY STUDIES

Ultrastructural Features

Although rarely used for the diagnosis of vasculitic neuropathy, ultrastructural examination may reveal

---

VASCULITIC NEUROPATHY—PATHOLOGIC FEATURES

Microscopic Findings
- Lymphoplasmacytic inflammation of epineurial arterioles, with medial and intimal necrosis
- May be focal, segmental, or both
- Fascicular and subfascicular variability in axonal loss secondary to nonuniform peripheral nerve ischemia
- Perineurial or endoneurial neovascularization (or both) may occur

Ultrastructural Features
- May reveal endothelial cell necrosis in biopsy samples in which light microscopy shows inflammation without necrosis

Genetics
- Sporadic

Immunohistochemical Features
- T cells predominate

Pathologic Differential Diagnosis
- Epineurial perivascular inflammation is common and nonspecific
- Chronic inflammatory demyelinating polyradiculoneuropathy demonstrates both epineurial and endoneurial infiltrates, without vascular necrosis
- Infectious causes should be excluded clinically, pathologically, or both
- Lymphoma should be excluded

---

endothelial cell necrosis not apparent on light microscopy.

Immunohistochemistry

T cells predominate within the inflammatory infiltrate. Despite publications asserting that immunofluo-

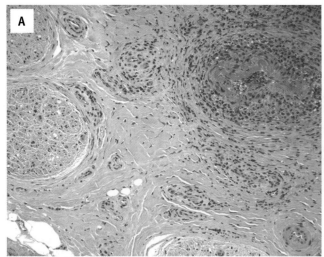
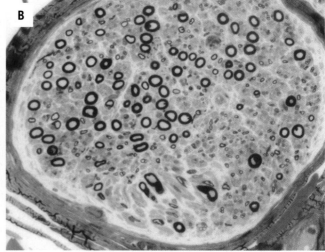

FIGURE 11-20

A, Fibrinoid necrosis of epineurial arteries in a patient with rheumatoid vasculitis. **B**, Subfascicular axonal loss suggests proximal ischemic peripheral nerve damage, typically seen in patients with peripheral nervous system vasculitis.

rescent studies for complement components increases diagnostic sensitivity, problems with specificity limit the utility of this approach.

DIFFERENTIAL DIAGNOSIS

As in other regions of the body, it is important to establish that the vessel wall is the target of the immune attack and not just an innocent bystander encountered by immune cells on their way to the actual target. Vascular necrosis or reactive endothelial changes, or both, should be identified because perivascular inflammation is common and nonspecific. Once the vasculitic nature of the inflammatory process has been established, it is important to be sure that the immune cells appear cytologically benign and polyclonal or to follow up any concerns with a battery of immunostains to exclude lymphomatous peripheral nerve involvement (or both). Lymphomatous peripheral neuropathy may occur in the absence of systemic lymphoma, either as a single (mass) lesion or as part of a diffuse process (neurolymphomatosis).

PROGNOSIS AND THERAPY

Patients with nonsystemic vasculitic neuropathy are treated with corticosteroids, cyclophosphamide, or both. Relapses resulting in moderate disability occur in about half. The 5-year survival rate is approximately 90%. In systemic vasculitic neuropathy, the prognosis and therapy depend on the underlying disease process.

LUMBOSACRAL RADICULOPLEXOPATHY

CLINICAL FEATURES

Although classically associated with type 2 diabetes mellitus, where it is also referred to as "diabetic amyotrophy," lumbosacral radiculoplexopathies are also encountered in nondiabetic patients. In both groups the disease is associated with weight loss, followed by severe pain and weakness in the hip and thigh that may remain unilateral or spread to involve the other lower extremity. Although motor symptoms predominate, the autonomic and sensory systems are also involved, with 50% of patients manifesting autonomic dysfunction.

PATHOLOGIC FEATURES

Peripheral nerves show vasculitis involving endoneurial and small epineurial blood vessels.

LUMBOSACRAL RADICULOPLEXOPATHY—FACT SHEET

Definition
▶ Asymmetric sensorimotor deficit involving the lower limbs both proximally and distally

Incidence and Location
▶ Occurs in ≈15% of diabetic patients; the incidence in nondiabetic patients has not been established
▶ Lower extremity, usually proximal predominant

Gender and Age Distribution
▶ Male preponderance among diabetic patients (≈1.5:1); no gender predominance in nondiabetic patients
▶ Median onset in the seventh decade; range from the third to the ninth decades

Clinical Features
▶ Severe pain and weakness develop abruptly and focally in the hip and thigh, but quickly spread to involve both the proximal and distal portions of the lower extremities. Autonomic symptoms (orthostatic hypotension, erectile dysfunction, and bowel and bladder problems) develop in about half
▶ CSF protein is elevated

Prognosis and Treatment
▶ Although improvement occurs in almost all, recovery is usually incomplete, with persistent pain and weakness
▶ Treatment is symptomatic because no proven therapy currently exists

---

LUMBOSACRAL RADICULOPLEXOPATHY—PATHOLOGIC FEATURES

Microscopic Findings
▶ Multifocal axonal degeneration with focal perineurial thickening and focal microvasculitis

Immunohistochemical Features
▶ Leukocyte markers confirm vascular inflammation

Pathologic Differential Diagnosis
▶ Chronic inflammatory demyelinating polyradiculoneuropathy
▶ Systemic vasculitis involving peripheral nerves

ANCILLARY STUDIES

Semi-thin Sections

One-micron sections demonstrate multifocal (as opposed to diffuse) fiber loss, consistent with ischemic necrosis.

Immunohistochemistry

Immunostaining with antibodies to lymphocyte markers highlights vasculitic inflammation.

DIFFERENTIAL DIAGNOSIS

Differential diagnostic considerations include chronic inflammatory demyelinating polyradiculoneuropathy (which may be superimposed on diabetic polyneuropathy) and systemic vasculitis involving the peripheral nervous system. In the former, the inflammation is perivascular, not vasculitic, and in the latter, the vasculitic process involves larger epineurial arterioles.

PROGNOSIS AND THERAPY

In both diabetic and nondiabetic patients, the illness is monophasic, with improvement occurring in almost all. The improvement, however, is incomplete, with persistent pain and weakness in most and wheelchair dependence in many. Current treatment is entirely symptomatic, although trials with immunomodulatory therapies are ongoing.

CHARCOT-MARIE-TOOTH DISEASE

CLINICAL FEATURES

The typical story elicited from a patient with Charcot-Marie-Tooth disease (also known as hereditary sensory and motor neuropathy) is one of slowly progressive distal weakness, usually beginning in childhood. Both muscle atrophy and sensory impairment develop over time, but dominance of distal lower extremity symptoms and signs persists. Hammertoes and pes cavus are common in all forms of the disease; palpable nerve enlargement and tremor are usually confined to the most common form, CMT1.

PATHOLOGIC FEATURES

The most common forms of the disease (CMT1 and CMTX) are characterized by a reduction in the number of both large and small myelinated fibers, with "onion bulb" formations involving most of the remaining fibers. These collars of redundant Schwann cells are not seen in young children, but develop over time and lead to an increase in caliber of the affected nerve fascicles. The less common axonal form (CMT2) demonstrates axonal degeneration with frequent regenerative axonal clusters, but rare or absent onion bulb formations.

CHARCOT-MARIE-TOOTH DISEASE—FACT SHEET

Definition

▶ A pathologically and genetically heterogeneous group of sensory and motor neuropathies characterized by distal limb weakness and wasting
▶ Subdivided into demyelinating (autosomal dominant = CMT1, X-linked dominant = CMTX) and axonal (CMT2)

Prevalence and Location

▶ ≈20 cases/100,000 persons; CMT1 predominates (≈3:1:1)
▶ Distal lower extremity weakness and wasting

Gender and Age Distribution

▶ Males more severely affected in CMTX, otherwise no gender predilection
▶ Onset in the first or second decade; may not come to medical attention until later

Clinical Features

▶ Distal muscle weakness and atrophy with decreased reflexes and minimal sensory symptoms. Pes cavus and hammertoes are common. Palpable nerve enlargement in 50% and essential tremor in ≈30% of CMT1 patients

Prognosis and Treatment

▶ Early age of onset and the degree of axonal damage predict a more severe course, but most patients experience very slow progression with normal longevity, a minority becoming wheelchair dependent. No specific therapies are currently available, although ascorbic acid has shown promising results in animal studies

---

CHARCOT-MARIE-TOOTH DISEASE—PATHOLOGIC FEATURES

Microscopic Findings

▶ CMT1, CMTX: increased size of nerve fascicles with a reduction in the number of both large and small myelinated fibers and onion bulb formations involving most of the remaining myelinated fibers (except in young children)
▶ CMT2: axonal degeneration with frequent regenerating clusters

Ultrastructural Features

▶ CMT1, CMTX: onion bulb formations
▶ CMT2: onion bulbs absent or rare

Genetics

▶ CMT1 (autosomal dominant):
  ▶ Duplication of 17p11.2 (*PMP22* gene, CMT1A, 70%)
  ▶ Point mutations in the myelin protein 0 gene (1q22-33, CMT1B, 20%)
  ▶ Point mutations in the *LITAF* gene (16p12-13, CMT1C, <10%)
  ▶ Point mutations in the *EGR2* gene (10q21-22, CMT1D, rare)
▶ CMTX (X-linked dominant): more than 200 mutations in the connexin 32 gene
▶ CMT2 (autosomal dominant): A (1p36), B (3q13), C (?), D (7p14)

Pathologic Differential Diagnosis

▶ CMT1, CMTX: chronic inflammatory demyelinating polyradiculoneuropathy, Dejerine-Sottas syndrome (in infantile cases)
▶ CMT2: Pathologic features are nonspecific

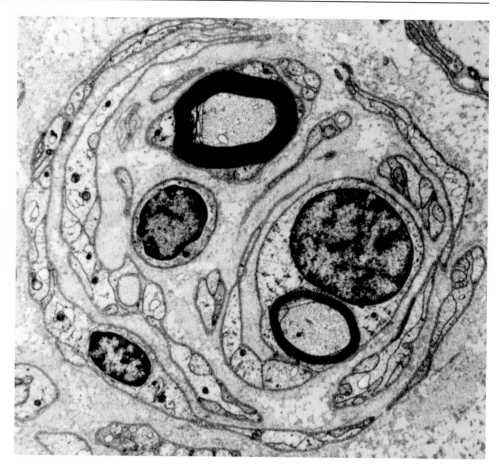

FIGURE 11-21

Typical "onion bulb formations" consisting of multiple redundant Schwann cell layers around thinly myelinated and demyelinated axons in a patient with Charcot-Marie-Tooth disease.

ANCILLARY STUDIES

Ultrastructural Features

Semi-thin and thin sections confirm the presence of onion bulb formations in CMT1 and CMTX (Fig. 11-21).

Other

Genetic analysis has shown mutations in a variety of myelin-related and unrelated proteins (see the pathologic features box). Mutation analysis eliminates the need for biopsy in all but the most atypical cases and has even enabled prenatal diagnosis in some instances.

DIFFERENTIAL DIAGNOSIS

The pathologic features of CMT2 are nonspecific, although some have suggested that the abundance of regenerative axonal clusters in young patients is distinctive. CMT1 and CMTX may appear identical to severe early-onset hereditary sensory and motor neuropathy (Dejerine-Sottas syndrome). In older patients, the critical differential diagnosis is with acquired, treatable, chronic inflammatory demyelinating poly-

radiculoneuropathy. Although the name implies that inflammation would be useful, many cases of chronic polyradiculoneuropathy demonstrate little or no inflammation at biopsy, whereas some cases of CMT containing small numbers of lymphocytes have been reported. The major pathologic difference between these two diseases is variability in the severity of damage among nerve fascicles in chronic inflammatory demyelinating polyradiculoneuropathy and absence of such variability in CMT.

PROGNOSIS AND THERAPY

Most CMT patients experience very slow disease progression and normal longevity. Earlier age at onset predicts a more severe course, with a minority of such patients becoming wheelchair dependent. Specific therapies are not currently available.

SUGGESTED READINGS

General Muscle/Denervation Atrophy

Dawson TP, Neal JW, Llewellyn L, Thomas C: Neuropathology Techniques. London, Arnold, 2003, pp 197-220.
Karpati G: Structural and Molecular Basis of Skeletal Muscle Diseases. Basel, ISN Neuropath Press, 2002.

Karpati G, Hilton-Jones D, Griggs RC: Disorders of Voluntary Muscle, 7th ed. Cambridge, Cambridge University Press, 2001.

Autoimmune Myasthenia

Keesey JC: Clinical evaluation and management of myasthenia gravis. Muscle Nerve 2004;29:484-505.

Riggs AJ, Riggs JE: "Guessing it right," John A. Simpson, and myasthenia gravis: The role of analogy in science. Neurology 2004;62:465-467.

Wirtz PW, Nijnuis MG, Sotodeh M, et al: The epidemiology of myasthenia gravis, Lambert-Eaton myasthenic syndrome and their associated tumours in the northern part of the province of South Holland. J Neurol 2003;250:698-701.

Periodic Paralysis

Davies NP, Hanna MG: The skeletal muscle channelopathies: Distinct entities and overlapping syndromes. Curr Opin Neurol 2003;16:559-568.

Kullmann DM, Hanna MG: Neurological disorders caused by inherited ion-channel mutations. Lancet Neurol 2002;1:157-166.

Pandey HK, Riggs JE: Channelopathies in pediatric neurology. Neurol Clin 2003;21:765-777.

Myotonic Dystrophy

Erginel-Unaltuna N, Akbas F: Improved method for molecular diagnosis of myotonic dystrophy type 1 (DM1). J Clin Lab Anal 2004;18:50-54.

Meola G: Clinical and genetic heterogeneity in myotonic dystrophies. Muscle Nerve 2000;23:1789-1799.

Schoser BG, Schneider-Gold C, Kress W, et al: Muscle pathology in 57 patients with myotonic dystrophy type 2. Muscle Nerve 2004;29:275-281.

Duchenne's Muscular Dystrophy

Emery AE: The muscular dystrophies. Lancet 2002;359:687-695.

Mathews KD: Muscular dystrophy overview: Genetics and diagnosis. Neurol Clin 2003;21:795-816.

Muntoni F, Torelli S, Ferlini A: Dystrophin and mutations: One gene, several proteins, multiple phenotypes. Lancet Neurol 2003;2:731-740.

Limb-Girdle Muscular Dystrophies

Brown SC, Torelli S, Brockington M, et al: Abnormalities in alpha-dystroglycan expression in MDC1C and LGMD2I muscular dystrophies. Am J Pathol 2004;164:727-737.

Kirschner J, Bonnemann CG: The congenital and limb-girdle muscular dystrophies: Sharpening the focus, blurring the boundaries. Arch Neurol 2004;61:189-199.

Zatz M, de Paula F, Starling A, et al: The 10 autosomal recessive limb-girdle muscular dystrophies. Neuromuscul Disord 2003;13:532-544.

Nemaline Myopathy

Goebel HH: Congenital myopathies at their molecular dawning. Muscle Nerve 2003;27:527-548.

Ryan MM, Ilkovski B, Strickland CD, et al: Clinical course correlates poorly with muscle pathology in nemaline myopathy. Neurology 2003;60:665-673.

Sanoudou D, Frieden LA, Haslett JN, et al: Molecular classification of nemaline myopathies: "Nontyping" specimens exhibit unique patterns of gene expression. Neurobiol Dis 2004;15:590-600.

Central Core Disease

Giampetro DM, Prayson RA, Friedman NR, et al: Pathologic quiz case: A slow and awkward child. Arch Pathol Lab Med 2004;128:481-482.

Mathews KD, Moore SA: Multiminicore myopathy, central core disease, malignant hyperthermia susceptibility, and RYR1 mutations: One disease with many faces? Arch Neurol 2004;61:27-29.

Quinlivan RM, Muller CR, Davis M, et al: Central core disease: Clinical, pathological, and genetic features. Arch Dis Child 2003;88:1051-1055.

Acid Maltase Deficiency

DiMauro S, Lamperti C: Muscle glycogenoses. Muscle Nerve 2001;24:984-999.

Hermans MM, van Leenen D, Kroos MA, et al: Twenty-two novel mutations in the lysosomal alpha-glucosidase gene (GAA) underscore the genotype-phenotype correlation in glycogen storage disease type II. Hum Mutat 2004;23:47-56.

van den Hout HM, Hop W, van Diggelen OP, et al: The natural course of infantile Pompe's disease: 20 original cases compared with 133 cases from the literature. Pediatrics 2003;112:332-340.

Winkel LP, Kamphoven JH, van den Hout HJ, et al: Morphological changes in muscle tissue of patients with infantile Pompe's disease receiving enzyme replacement therapy. Muscle Nerve 2003;27:743-751.

McArdle's Disease

Amato AA: Sweet success—a treatment for McArdle's disease. N Engl J Med 2003;349:2481-2482.

Gordon N: Glycogenosis type V or McArdle's disease. Dev Med Child Neurol 2003;45:640-644.

Haller RG, Vissing J: No spontaneous second wind in muscle phosphofructokinase deficiency. Neurology 2004;62:82-86.

Carnitine Palmitoyltransferase Deficiency

Sigauke E, Rakheja D, Kitson K, et al: Carnitine palmitoyltransferase II deficiency: A clinical, biochemical, and molecular review. Lab Invest 2003;83:1543-1554.

Vockley J, Whiteman DA: Defects of mitochondrial beta-oxidation: A growing group of disorders. Neuromuscul Disord 2002;12:235-246.

Wieser T, Deschauer M, Olek K, et al: Carnitine palmitoyltransferase II deficiency: Molecular and biochemical analysis of 32 patients. Neurology 2003;60:1351-1353.

Mitochondrial Encephalomyopathies

DiMauro S, Schon EA: Mitochondrial respiratory-chain diseases. N Engl J Med 2003;348:2656-2668.

Oldfors A, Tulinius M: Mitochondrial encephalomyopathies. J Neuropathol Exp Neurol 2003;62:217-227.

Rollins S, Prayson RA, McMahon JT, et al: Diagnostic yield of muscle biopsy in patients with clinical evidence of mitochondrial cytopathy. Am J Clin Pathol 2001;116:326-330.

Taylor RW, Schaefer AM, Barron MJ, et al: The diagnosis of mitochondrial muscle disease. Neuromuscul Disord 2004;14:237-245.

Acute Quadriplegic Myopathy

Ruff RL: Why muscle atrophy in acute quadriplegic myopathy is rapid and severe. Ann Neurol 2004;55:161-163.

Sander HW, Golden M, Danon MJ: Quadriplegic areflexic ICU illness: Selective thick filament loss and normal nerve histology. Muscle Nerve 2002;26:499-505.

Sieb JP, Gillessen T: Iatrogenic and toxic myopathies. Muscle Nerve 2003;27:142-156.

Dermatomyositis

Dalakas MC, Hohlfeld R: Polymyositis and dermatomyositis. Lancet 2003;362:971-982.

Grogan PM, Katz JS: Inflammatory myopathies. Curr Treat Options Neurol 2004;6:155-161.

Mastaglia FL, Garlepp MJ, Phillips BA, et al: Inflammatory myopathies: Clinical, diagnostic and therapeutic aspects. Muscle Nerve 2003;27:407-425.

Polymyositis

Bronner IM, Linssen WH, van der Meulen MF, et al: Polymyositis: An ongoing discussion about a disease entity. Arch Neurol 2004;61:132-135.

Kissel JT: Misunderstandings, misperceptions, and mistakes in the management of the inflammatory myopathies. Semin Neurol 2002;22:41-51.

Inclusion Body Myositis

Amato AA, Gronseth GS, Jackson CE, et al: Inclusion body myositis: Clinical and pathological boundaries. Ann Neurol 1996;40:581-586.

Askanas V, Engel WK: Proposed pathogenetic cascade of inclusion-body myositis: Importance of amyloid-beta, misfolded proteins, predisposing genes, and aging. Curr Opin Rheumatol 2003;15:737-744.

Vattemi G, Engel WK, McFerrin J, et al: Endoplasmic reticulum stress and unfolded protein response in inclusion body myositis muscle. Am J Pathol 2004;164:1-7.

Peripheral Nerve—General

Dawson TP, Neal JW, Llewellyn L, Thomas C: Neuropathology Techniques. London, Arnold, 2003, pp 221-237.

Mendell JR, Kissel JT, Cornblath DR: Diagnosis and Management of Peripheral Nerve Disorders. New York, Oxford University Press, 2001.

Midroni G, Bilbao JM: Biopsy Diagnosis of Peripheral Neuropathy. Boston, Butterworth-Heinemann, 1995.

Acute Inflammatory Demyelinating Polyradiculoneuropathy

Chio A, Cocito D, Leone M, et al: Guillain-Barré syndrome: A prospective, population-based incidence and outcome survey. Neurology 2003;60:1146-1150.

Dalakas MC: Intravenous immunoglobulin in autoimmune neuromuscular diseases. JAMA 2004;291:2367-2375.

Winer JB: Guillain-Barré syndrome. Mol Pathol 2001;54:381-385.

Chronic Inflammatory Demyelinating Polyradiculoneuropathy

Sander HW, Latov N: Research criteria for defining patients with CIDP. Neurology 2003;60:S8-S15.

Vallat JM, Tabaraud F, Magy L, et al: Diagnostic value of nerve biopsy for atypical chronic inflammatory demyelinating polyneuropathy: Evaluation of eight cases. Muscle Nerve 2003;27:478-485.

Paraproteinemic Neuropathies

Kissel JT, Mendell JR: Neuropathies associated with monoclonal gammopathies. Neuromuscul Disord 1996;6:3-18.

Vital A: Paraproteinemic neuropathies. Brain Pathol 2001;11:399-407.

Amyloid Neuropathies

Adams D: Hereditary and acquired amyloid neuropathies. J Neurol 2001;248:647-657.

Vucic S, Chong PS, Cros D: Atypical presentations of primary amyloid neuropathy. Muscle Nerve 2003;28:696-702.

Diabetic Polyneuropathy

Lozeron P, Nahum L, Lacroix C, et al: Symptomatic diabetic and non-diabetic neuropathies in a series of 100 diabetic patients. J Neurol 2002;249:569-575.

Polydefkis M, Griffin JW, McArthur J: New insights into diabetic polyneuropathy. JAMA 2003;290:1371-1376.

Toth C, Brussee V, Cheng C, et al: Diabetes mellitus and the sensory neuron. J Neuropathol Exp Neurol 2004;63:561-573.

HIV-Associated Neuropathies

Brew BJ: The peripheral nerve complications of human immunodeficiency virus (HIV) infection. Muscle Nerve 2003;28:542-552.

Morgello S, Estanislao L, Simpson D, et al: HIV-associated distal sensory polyneuropathy in the era of highly active antiretroviral therapy: The Manhattan HIV Brain Bank. Arch Neurol 2004;61:546-551.

Vasculitic Neuropathies

Chia L, Fernandez A, Lacroix C, et al: Contribution of nerve biopsy findings to the diagnosis of disabling neuropathy in the elderly: A retrospective review of 100 consecutive patients. Brain 1996;119:1091-1098.

Collins MP, Periquet MI, Mendell JR, et al: Nonsystemic vasculitic neuropathy: Insights from a clinical cohort. Neurology 2003;61:623-630.

Griffin JW: Vasculitic neuropathies. Rheum Dis Clin North Am 2001;27:751-760, vi.

Lumbosacral Radiculoplexopathies

Dyck PJ, Windebank AJ: Diabetic and nondiabetic lumbosacral radiculoplexus neuropathies: New insights into pathophysiology and treatment. Muscle Nerve 2002;25:477-491.

Said G, Lacroix C, Lozeron P, et al: Inflammatory vasculopathy in multifocal diabetic neuropathy. Brain 2003;126:376-385.

Charcot-Marie-Tooth Disease

Hattori N, Yamamoto M, Yoshihara T, et al: Demyelinating and axonal features of Charcot-Marie-Tooth disease with mutations of myelin-related proteins (PMP22, MPZ and Cx32): A clinicopathological study of 205 Japanese patients. Brain 2003;126:134-151.

Pareyson D: Diagnosis of hereditary neuropathies in adult patients. J Neurol 2003;250:148-160.

Passage E, Norreel JC, Noack-Fraissignes P, et al: Ascorbic acid treatment corrects the phenotype of a mouse model of Charcot-Marie-Tooth disease. Nat Med 2004;10:396-401.

Vallat JM: Dominantly inherited peripheral neuropathies. J Neuropathol Exp Neurol 2003;62:699-714.

Index

Note: Page numbers followed by f indicate figures;
those followed by t indicate tables.

A

Abducens nerve (CN VI), 5f, 9
Abrasions, scalp, 73
Abscess
  brain, 289-290, 289f, 290f
    actinomycotic, 297-298
    nocardial, 298-299
  epidural, 299-301
  spinal
    epidural, 299-301
    in tuberculosis, 222
  subdural, 299-301
Absidia, 305
Acanthamoeba infections, 329
Accessory nerve (CN XI), 5f, 9
Acetazolamide, for periodic paralysis, 545
Acetyl Co-A, mitochondrial production of, 386
Acetylcholine, neurons producing, 12, 12f
Acetylcholinesterase, amniotic fluid, in neural tube defect screening, 97
N-Acetylglucosamine deficiency, 339, 340
Acid lipase deficiency, 371-372
Acid maltase deficiency, 348. *See also* Lysosomal storage disorders.
  in Pompe's disease, 369-371, 554-555
  infantile, 554-555
Acid phosphatase, in liposomal storage disorders, 342, 346f
Acidemia, hyperpipecolic, 376
Acidophils, pituitary, 22, 24f
Acoustic schwannomas (neuromas), 512-514
  in type II neurofibromatosis, 162, 163f, 165, 512
Acquired immunodeficiency syndrome. *See* Human immunodeficiency virus infection.
Actin, 537
Actinomycosis, 297-298
Acute disseminated encephalomyelitis, 216-217, 217f
  fulminant, 217-218, 219f
  vs. acute (Marburg-type) multiple sclerosis, 212
Acute hemorrhagic leukoencephalitis, 217-218, 219f
Acute inflammatory demyelinating polyradiculoneuropathy, 567-568, 567f

Acute multiple sclerosis, 207-208, 210-213
Acute neuronal cell change, 39, 39f, 40f
Acute quadriplegic myopathy, 559-560, 560f
Addison's disease, adrenoleukodystrophy and, 182, 185, 185f, 186f
Adenohypophysis, anatomy of, 5, 22, 24f
Adenoma, pituitary, 522-524, 525f
Adenoma sebaceum, in tuberous sclerosis, 165
Adenosine triphosphate. *See* ATP.
Adenoviruses, 327
Adrenal insufficiency, adrenoleukodystrophy and, 182, 185, 185f, 186f
Adrenoleukodystrophy, 181-185, 182f-186f
  neonatal, 374t, 375t, 376, 380-383, 383f
  vs. Schilder's disease, 214
  X-linked, 374-375, 374t
Adrenomyeloneuropathy, 182-185
Adult neuronal ceroid lipofuscinosis, 365-368, 366t
Adult Refsum's disease, 374t, 375t, 384-385. *See also* Peroxisomal disorders.
African trypanosomiasis, 334-335
Age-related changes, nonpathologic, 32, 32t, 33f-35f
Aicardi's syndrome, 122, 122f, 124, 128
AIDS dementia complex, 324-326, 325f. *See also* Human immunodeficiency virus infection.
Alanine metabolism, peroxisomes in, 374
Alcohol abuse, 418-419
  alcoholic dementia and, 418
  amblyopia and, 394, 414
  central pontine myelinosis and, 408-411
  fetal alcohol syndrome and, 124, 418-419
  holoprosencephaly and, 108, 109
  midline cerebellar degeneration and, 413, 413f
  Wernicke-Korsakoff syndrome and, 411-413, 412f, 418
ALDP mutations, in X-linked adrenoleukodystrophy, 375
Alexander's disease, 181, 193-194, 194f-198f
Alglucerase, for Gaucher's disease, 354
Alobar holoprosencephaly, 110-111, 111f, 113, 113f. *See also* Holoprosencephaly.

Alpha motor neurons, 12
α–Fetoprotein, in neural tube defect screening, 97
Alphaviruses, 322-323
Aluminum intoxication, 416t
Alveus, 20, 21f
Alzheimer type II astrocytes, 13-15, 14f
  in hepatic encephalopathy, 406, 407
  in hypoxic-ischemic encephalopathy, 407
  in urea cycle disorders, 400, 400f
Alzheimer's disease, 223-232
  age at presentation of, 223
  amyloid deposition in, 224-230, 226f, 227f, 229f-232f
  ancillary studies in, 230-231
  apolipoprotein ε4 allele in, 224, 231
  CERAD scores in, 225
  cerebral angiopathy and, 60
  clinical features of, 223-224
  corticobasal degeneration and, 256
  course of, 232
  diagnostic criteria for, 225
  differential diagnosis of, 231-232
  epidemiology of, 223
  familial, 223
  genetic factors in, 223-224
  genetic testing for, 231
  granulovacuolar degeneration in, 225, 230f
  Hirano bodies in, 225, 230f
  imaging studies in, 230-231
  in Down syndrome, 157, 158, 159
  inheritance of, 223
  laboratory tests for, 230-231
  Lewy body variant of, 237-239, 239f
  neurofibrillary tangles in, 224, 225, 228f, 229f
  overview of, 223, 224
  pathologic features of, 32, 224-230, 224f-232f
    gross, 224, 224f, 225f
    microscopic, 224-230, 226f-232f
  prognosis of, 223, 232
  radiologic features of, 223
  senile plaques in, 32, 224-225, 226f-229f. *See also* Senile plaques.
  staging of, 225
  treatment of, 223, 232
  vascular dementia and, 44-45
Amebiasis, 328-329
American trypanosomiasis, 334-335

I